phy·si·cian

Books by Richard Leviton

Anthroposophic Medicine Today
Seven Steps to Better Vision
The Imagination of Pentecost
Brain Builders
Weddings by Design
Looking for Arthur

phy·si·cian

Medicine and the Unsuspected Battle for Human Freedom

Richard Leviton

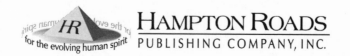

HAMPTON ROADS
PUBLISHING COMPANY, INC.

Cover design by Marjoram Productions
Cover art by Matthew Friedman

For information write
Hampton Roads Publishing Company, Inc.
1125 Stoney Ridge Road
Charlottesville, VA 22902

Or call: 804-296-2772
FAX: 804-296-5096
e-mail: hrpc@hrpub.com
Web site: www.hrpub.com

If you are unable to order this book from your local
bookseller, you may order directly from the publisher.
Quantity discounts for organizations are available.

Library of Congress Catalog Card Number: 99-95409

ISBN 1-57174-168-2

10 9 8 7 6 5 4 3 2 1

Printed on acid-free paper in the United States

Dedication

Judith A. Lewis, R.N., N.D.
Ira M. Golchehreh, L.Ac., O.M.D.
Rev. Leon S. LeGant
—*three superb masters of the* physis

Table of Contents

PART II

The *Physis*cal Truth: Self *and* Environment

CHAPTER 3

CHAPTER 4

The Holographic Human:
Probable Locations of the Body / 227

A Matrix of Connection for Complex Energy Systems • Personality and Biography Written in a Palm Print • The Holographic Paradigm: Distributing Information • Maybe the World Is a Splendidly Detailed Illusion • The Mind at the End of the Palm • Energy Meridians Flowing through the Hands • The Zones of the Sole: Reflexing the Body Map on the Feet • The Little Human in the Ear • The Geography of the Eye: Another Body Map in the Iris • Micro-acupuncture Holograms in the Body • Stems and Branches into the Cosmos • Palpating the Big Open Mind on the Stomach • The Energy Fields of Life and Their Celestial Antennae • The Psychoenergetic Terrain: Mind and Body Meet in the Meridians • The Meridian Is the Hyphen in the Word "Psycho-Somatic" • Searching for the Master Template • The Palm at the End of the Mind • The Human Is a Mirror Image of the Spiritual World • The Human Is a Living Picture of the Universe • The Cosmic Composition of the Human Being • The Geomythics of Environment: Aboriginal Dreamtime and World Making • Song Lines for the Eternal Ones of the Dream • The Ancestors Dreamed the World into Being • Spirituality and Landscape Breathe Together • Opossum Dreaming Is but Another Aspect of Yourself • Standing Up for Gaia: The Deep Ecological World without Boundary • Lovelock's Geophysiology and the Planetary Physician • The Essential Theoretical Basis for Practicing Planetary Medicine • An Act of Ecological "Self-Realization" • "I am part of the rain forest protecting myself"

CHAPTER 5

Mysteries of the Body: Remaking Our
Inner Environment / 295

Participating in the Life of the Body • Making Pleasure-Inducing Drugs in Your Head • Biology Is Dramatically Mutable through Acts of Consciousness • Placebo Response—The Therapy of Expectant Belief • Reinterpreting the "Mere" Placebo Effect • Placebo—The Benign Lie That Heals • Laughter and the Chemistry of Healing • A Non-drug with Specific Intent • PNI—Awakening the Self-Healing Competency • "Your unconscious mind may be smarter than you" • Yogic Vigilance in the Face of a Body That Listens • The Exceptional Patient— Key to the Miracle of Healing • The Quantum Blueprint for Healing • Multiple Identities Bloom in the Human Psyche • Mysteries of the Coma: Time-Out with the Dreambody • Doorway into an Awareness of Life beyond the Body • A Father's Love—Life inside His Son's Coma • The Conscious Imagination of a Healthy Environment

PART III

*Physis*cian Healings: Self *as* Environment

The Physician and the Struggle for Control of the Environment

In a remarkable, unsuspected, and dramatic sense, today's physician is the key player in millennial struggle for definition and ownership of the human soul. A profound philosophical, even metaphysical, battle over human consciousness and spiritual freedom is being played out in the seemingly unlikely field of American health care.

Physician is about the politics and philosophy of medicine as exemplified in the struggle between two approaches to practicing it—conventional, or allopathic, medicine and alternative, or empiric, medicine. The book explores the consequences to the human body, mind, and spirit of medical treatment under one or the other medical approach. It proposes that a medical system can either support or obstruct the spiritual unfolding of a person.

Specifically, the book argues that conventional medicine operates in a way contrary to spiritual unfolding and at this point in Western history is a prime obstacle to healthy human soul life. By this, I don't mean individual doctors practicing conventional medicine, but rather the sum total and effect on an individual of conventional medicine as a system or thought form. Conventional medicine typically denies human awareness, consciousness, and/or the soul any legitimate role in biology, other than as an ineffectual bystander.

Physician also looks at the ramifications for our environmental policy as a result of the prevailing medical paradigm, proposing that the world-view (of the inner world, the body and its functions) implicit in a medical system *necessarily* dictates a corresponding way of viewing the outer world. Both the body and the world are seen as primarily mechanistic, devoid of consciousness or soul, or, if they are accorded any consciousness, they have no primacy in the affairs of the body or environment.

Environment has two faces, that of the body and its immunological domain, and that of the outer world, and its ecological domain. This book argues that a medical practice (and its paradigm) has ramifications in both expressions of the environment, and that what a physician does can determine the destiny of either or both expressions.

The link between the two realms—human health, or immunology, and outer health, or ecology—is consciousness. Does a medical paradigm permit or prohibit consciousness in finding a place to reside in the environment, be it the body or the physical world? Physicians and their practices, whether allopathic or alternative, have a great deal to do with the outcome.

The Prevailing Model of Separateness

The book is divided into three parts.

- Part I, "The Physicians' Conspiracy: Self *versus* Environment," is about the attitude of *separateness* promoted by conventional medicine in which consciousness is cut off from its habitat (body and world) and given no fundamental role in organic life.

This part looks at ways in which allopathic medicine achieves a political agenda against alternative practices under the misleading banner of therapeutic efficacy. The status of alternative medicine is presented, supported by statistical studies of usage and popularity. Ways in which mainstream media bias consumers in favor of conventional medicine and against alternative are analyzed. Indications of some degree of organized, perhaps conspiratorial, activity on the part of conventional medical interests seeking to control the medical marketplace are presented.

Further, the *inner* orientation of conventional medicine is examined—seeing its practices and attitudes as a unity—and here the book calls upon metaphysical and occult sources to establish its viewpoint. The suggestion is made, following indications of Austrian spiritual philosopher Rudolf Steiner (1861-1925), that medicine can either support or hinder the presence and influence of the human soul in the body, which is to say, it can either help or hurt the spiritual unfoldment of the human individual. The argument is presented that allopathy seeks to drive the soul (and with it, consciousness) out of the body, leaving the human a kind of spiritually bereft organic automaton. This same attitude is then transferred to how modern industrialized societies treat their physical outer environments.

The historical roots of this struggle between two medical views is traced back to classical Greece and followed through periods of American history up to the present, indicating that it is a profound, deeply entrenched dialectical issue. The prevalence of conventional medicine has ramifications for how we relate to our environment, both bodily and the physical world; it encourages us to think that human self, or consciousness, is set against and separate from the world (and body).

How Natural Medicine Fosters an Attitude of Relatedness

- Part II, "The *Physis*ical Truth: Self *and* Environment," is about the concept of *relatedness* (human body, consciousness, and world) fostered by alternative medicine.

This part examines the principles and practices of alternative medicine in depth, identifying its key philosophical positions with respect to both inner (immunological) and outer (ecological) environments. The term *physis* is a word from classical Greek medical thinking, originally used to designate the life force running the body, what acupuncturists call *Qi*.

The doctor or physician was the one trained in the management of this life force for the benefit of the patient—the *physis* manager, if you like. To manage the *physis*, you must understand it; you must see it as a living, dynamic, interactive energy, not as something you drug, suppress, kill, or transplant. Almost by definition, the classical *physis* manager is more like what today we think of as an alternative medicine physician. The alternative or natural medicine physician aspires to this same degree of understanding of life force as a healing energy in the practice of medicine.

The struggle between medical paradigms is in essence a struggle for the control of the *physis,* which, the book argues, is the biological foundation for consciousness. Which approach will prevail, that of the *physis* manager or *physis* killer? Today's physician—*physis*cian—is pivotal in the outcome.

Chapters in this section document the various energy connections between the human body and the outer world, making its case through discussion of disciplines such as biometeorology (the effect of weather on health), geopathology (the effect of earth energies on health), and electromagnetism (the effects, both good and bad, of electromagnetic energy, both natural and human-made, on health).

This section also goes into the concept of the "holographic human." This is the idea that not only is the human body affected by subtle environmental energies, but the places where these effects are registered in the body are multiple and holographic. Examples pertinent here include "body maps" from acupuncture, iridology, reflexology, and palmistry, in which information about the whole system is available in miniaturized maps of this system (the eye, soles of feet and palms, the ear, tongue, solar plexus).

Chinese medicine explains how these holographic body maps are connected to outer environmental energies and form a kind of continuous feedback loop. Evidence is presented suggesting that the physical world, like the human body, has subtle energy systems and centers, and that these, too, are responsive to consciousness.

The model of esoteric physiology proposed by Rudolf Steiner takes this idea even further with the suggestion that the human organization (physical body and subtle energy system) is in fact a miniature world, a little cosmos, in which organs and organ processes are interconnected with larger environmental energies and processes, even events in the solar system, and beyond, including the spiritual worlds.

This part then documents how consciousness can be creatively used to remake the human physical environment, drawing upon examples of psycho-neuro-immunology, the placebo effect, multiple personality syndrome, coma studies, and other examples of the formative effect of consciousness upon matter.

- Part III, *"Physis*cian Healings—Self *as* Environment," shows how medicine, appropriately used, can reunite the inner and outer environments, restoring the essential *unity* between immunology and ecology and restoring consciousness to its rightful place of efficacy.

Modalities such as homeopathy, music therapy, and anthroposophic medicine are explored to support a model of the human subtle energy body, sometimes called the etheric body, and to show how both the human and the physical world share this feature, both participating in a larger interactive energy matrix.

Why Pandora's Covenant Must Be Renewed

One of the principal metaphors developed in the book is that of Pandora's covenant, based on the well-known Greek myth of Pandora and her box. Most people know the story of Pandora: against better advice, she opened a box and released all the world's miseries, sins, and illnesses. Put simply, I have adapted (or interpreted) this myth for the purposes of illustrating a spiritual issue pertaining to medicine.

I propose we view Pandora as a representation of the human soul; the "miseries, sins, and illnesses" she released from her box as the planetary microbial kingdom; and the covenant as an agreement between the soul and the world's microbes to produce health or illness, as desired, for spiritual purposes. Modern conventional medical practices have broken this covenant between the soul and the microbial kingdom, producing potentially disastrous consequences, including an abrogation of human freedom.

Using the Greek myth of Pandora's Box, this part probes the meaning and spiritual dimensions of illness and the underlying question of *why* there is illness in the first place. If illness has a spiritual origin and/or purpose, how is this purpose conveyed to the physical body? The book suggests that subtle aspects of the human organization (the etheric and astral body) make arrangements with the microbial kingdom to execute a spiritual agenda through illness. Support for this concept is presented by way of discussing the pleomorphic theory of microbiology, which proposes that microbiological organisms shift their nature and form from benign to pathogenic within the human body according to changes in biochemical conditions, which in turn reflect changes in the emotional and mental tenor of the person.

The expression of a soul or spiritual agenda through an illness process is regarded as a profound act of human freedom, the freedom to resolve soul intentions, or karma, through biology and incarnation. A medical paradigm can either support or block this activity, thereby aiding or hindering human spiritual unfoldment. The book argues that allopathy seeks to block this process by interfering inappropriately with the disease process through its toxic medicines and invasive procedures.

The book further proposes that the larger purpose of this karma/disease process is to prepare the human soul for the incarnation of Christ Consciousness—fully awake, synoptic cognition, as exemplified by the Christ—in the flesh. The book argues that this was the purpose of the Mystery of Golgotha, the public initiation process, including crucifixion, transfiguration, and ascension, of the Christ. In this context, Christ is viewed as a cosmic being, what Rudolf Steiner called a cosmic fact, rather than as the ideological possession of a single religion or dogmatic belief system.

Conventional medicine, at its deepest level, seeks to block the entry of the Christ Consciousness into the world (both inner and outer) through the human soul and into the human body. The irony is that on the surface conventional medicine has no awareness of this intention, yet, still, its medical practices seek to achieve this intention. There is a reason why the intense dialectic between medical approaches is played out on North American soil, as opposed to European. Certain esoteric factors of the North American landscape and its ancient past explain why this struggle for control of the prevailing medical paradigm is being played out specifically *here* in the U.S.

Conventional medicine itself represents only the topmost layer of a proposed multilevel conspiratorial hierarchy, seeking to block the incarnation of the Christ in the body. The book dissects the conspiracy theory at four levels of expression, from the outer political and financial to the inner occult machinations of forces, both planetary and extraterrestrial.

In short, there is a political issue blocking the threshold to a spiritual issue. The political issue is the control of the American medical marketplace, an annual one trillion dollar-plus honeypot, and the suppression of true freedom of choice by the consumer. *Physician* explains how Americans do not yet have access to a free, open, and unencumbered medical marketplace in which all medical modalities compete openly and on the basis of their innate therapeutic merits. Instead, the U.S. has a de facto state-endorsed single medical modality—conventional allopathy—instituting a kind of backdoor socialized medicine.

Medical licensing laws, insurance reimbursements, and FDA regulation of medical information about alternative medicine and its medicines all act in favor of allopathy and contrary to the interests of any alternative approach. Triple-bypass surgery does not compete openly and fairly with chelation therapy (a slow infusion of amino acids to bind up and remove calcium plaque deposits in the blood vessels) as an approach to correcting heart disease.

You can get chelation in some states, but in most cases you'll be paying for it yourself, even though its demonstrated efficacy is higher than that of bypass for producing long-term resolution of heart disease. Of course, some may prefer bypass to chelation, and this is fine. The issue is not, finally, which is more medically efficacious, but that medical consumers should be allowed to *choose* which modality to use to improve their health.

Both should be allowed to flourish, or fail, without governmental obstruction in the medical marketplace. Allopathic and alternative practices (provided either have demonstrated efficacy) should be allowed to operate *freely* in the marketplace. Consumers, not the government, will choose which modalities to employ. Consumers should have more, not less, information about alternative therapeutics and substances with which to make informed choices. At present, we do *not* have that free and open choice.

Consumer choice is the fundamental issue in the struggle for the control of the environment because it is the threshold of the spiritual and occult issues that really drive the struggle. Block consumer choice and you can ensure the predominance of allopathic medical procedures, which *Physician* demonstrates are inimical to human spiritual unfolding. Control the medical marketplace and you thereby control the human soul, and the planet.

Physician proposes that a major occult battle for control of the human soul (consciousness) and its future is being waged in America today through a struggle between two approaches to medicine. *Physician* exposes the dynamics and high stakes of this struggle—the spiritual freedom of the human soul within biology—thereby empowering the reader to make a conscious, informed choice in favor of medical rights and freedom, thereby enabling each individual to contribute to the renewing of Pandora's covenant.

CHAPTER 1

Militarized Medicine:
The Political Agenda
of Conventional Medicine

Defining the Alternative:
Natural Healing and Holistic Medicine

What most people know as natural, holistic medicine is called "alternative" mainly for the purposes of maintaining a political and therapeutic distinction with respect to what is now regarded as "conventional" medicine. Historically, alternative medicine has always been the mainstream, primary form of medical care and what we know as conventional medicine is a recent development and intrusion into a therapeutic continuity encompassing thousands of years of practice.

More specifically, alternative medicine (or "natural," "traditional," "holistic," "complementary," "integrated," "essential" medicine) includes at least forty modalities such as acupuncture, Ayurveda, herbalism, naturopathy, homeopathy, dietary/nutritional, chiropractic, osteopathy, color and music therapy, hydrotherapy, reflexology, and many others. Acupuncture, which is part of traditional Chinese medicine, has a traceable history of about 5,000 years; homeopathy has a 200-year documented history; reflexology and color and music therapy were practiced in classical Greece, and even Egypt.

Naturopathy, as an umbrella category for a variety of disciplines, derives from the mid-nineteenth-century hydrotherapy spas and herbal sanitariums—the nature cure or *Naturheilkunde*—of Central Europe run by the *Naturartz,* the nature doctor, such as the Swiss priest/healer Sebastian Kneipp (1824-1897). The nature doctor worked with natural, gentle healing agents, such as pure air, water, sunshine, food (usually vegetarian), and herbs (including homeopathic remedies) to stimulate the body's innate ability to purge itself of poisons and heal itself. The nature doctor honored the *vis medicatrix naturae,* the inborn healing power of nature, working through the body, and used therapeutic approaches that did not mask, suppress, obscure, or hinder this power, but rather that supported and stimulated it.

Alternative medicine, writes medical philosopher and historian Richard Grossinger in *Planet Medicine,* "describes the general and continuous emergence of systems of treatment in opposition to a universal technological medicine." As such, this domain includes both ancient and folk medicines "that reassert themselves from era to era, as well as idiosyncratic medicines that may derive, at least in part, from aspects of the scientific model." Alternative medicine, Grossinger says, is at once art, science, philosophy, and craft.

Conventional medicine, which refers to the "heroic" use of strong doses of metals, chemicals, and synthetic substances, antibiotics, high-tech surgery, radiation, transplantation, and other severe measures that are almost always toxic when overused, has only been with us for about one century. More rightfully, we should say that conventional medicine has emerged as an alternative (usurper, some might say) to traditional, natural, holistic medicine.

The emphasis of conventional medicine is upon war (against pathogens) and not repair (of the body). Disease, for conventional medicine, is regarded as an invasion of the body by an enemy; thus treatment is retaliation via magic biochemical bullets, such as drugs or vaccines, to eliminate or kill the "enemy" as in the *war on cancer.* Medicine increasingly has become one-sided in its focus, having lost sight of the whole person; instead, it strives to address only the body's individual components.

Keeping the *whole* person in sight is the key to alternative medicine, or natural healing. In this approach to therapeutics, a person has a discomfort or illness, not, as conventional medicine sees it, a disease has a body. Alternative medicine—shall we call it natural healing, for this discussion—places the individual foremost in the diagnosis and treatment of any illness. The overall organization of the human being—body, mind, emotions, soul, and spirit—makes up this individual, yet the total is still more than the sum of its parts, for consciousness is what animates the organism, and self-consciousness is what comprises the individual. Natural healing never construes health or illness in terms of parts or components; it is always a matter of assessing in what ways an individual has shifted into a state of systemic imbalance and by what means the natural balance of the person may be restored.

This individual has a reservoir of basic life energy, called *physis* in the classical Greek medical tradition, from which came the term *physician,* meaning the one who manages the *physis.* The *physis* is the human organism's innate ability to keep itself in dynamic balance (or homeostasis), to heal when it's sick, to restore when it's depleted, and to thrive when it's given the proper nourishment. You might consider the *physis* to be the human organism's inborn intelligence of health and vitality, its homeostatic regulator. Natural therapeutics *support* the *physis,* the human organism's physical ability to heal itself; these approaches do not seek to kill a disease (as does conventional medicine), but to strengthen the body's ability to transmute its ill-health-producing effect and restore itself to health. In effect, what the ancients knew as *physis,* we call immune system vitality today. This subject is discussed in more detail later in this chapter.

There is yet another, distinctly political, reason for using the term "alternative" with respect to traditional, natural healing. Medicines that rightfully belong under this rubric are most often less expensive and more effective, and produce little or no side effects while supporting the immunological vitality of the individual than the approaches of conventional medicine. In fact, the therapeutic track record for much of conventional medicine, with the exception of emergency room care for trauma, accidents, and broken bones, is quite poor, while the "iatrogenic" (doctor- or hospital-generated ill health effects) results are distressingly high.

Cultural analyst Ivan Illich once called this iatrogenic effect our *medical nemesis:* modern industrial/technological medicine had become so estranged from the *physical* reality of the human individual that it was now accomplishing "the expropriation of health," Illich contended. Illich was remarkably prescient: his critique of industrialized medicine, first published in 1976, is 100% apt today, more than twenty years later. The medical establishment is now a major threat to health: it has become pathogenic medicine that is undermining of and counterproductive to health, said Illich. Modern medicine is now a "sick-making" institution. Medicine, Illich adds, as if anticipating our time, could become "a prime target for political action that aims at an inversion of industrial society."

"During the last generations the medical monopoly over health care has expanded without checks and has encroached on our liberty with regard to our own bodies." Along the same lines, that which was once noble about the medical profession, "the ability to provide comfort and compassion," physician/epidemiologist Leonard A. Sagan, M.D., notes in *The Health of Nations,* "is rapidly being eroded in favor of increasingly sophisticated, mechanical, and dehumanized treatment of unproven benefit."

The Rapid Rebirth
of Alternative Medicine in America

In the field of medicine, if for nothing else, the 1990s will be remembered as the decade for alternative medicine's rapid return to validation and widespread public usage in North America. But it was also a time for mounting opposition by establishment medicine, for multiple reasons to be explored throughout this book. In many respects, it is a paradox: alternative medicine is entering the mainstream *and* conventional medicine is fighting to stop this by marginalizing every modality. Alternative medicine is growing and being inhibited in an intense dialectic with the patient's health—physical, emotional, moral, spiritual—at stake.

Since 1990, the evidence has been mounting that alternative medicine is growing rapidly in popularity and usage in the United States. The trend favoring alternative medicine really began in the late 1960s, coincident with the interest in natural foods, meditation, alternative fuels technology, and agrarian lifestyles. Despite the fervent reluctance of the mainstream media and conventional medicine moguls to admit it, it is statistically provable that alternative medicine (otherwise known as "natural," "holistic," or "complementary" medicine) is now no longer a "folk" tradition practicing on the therapeutic fringes, but a legitimate and financially significant component of the overall American (and global) medical scene.

When the *New England Journal of Medicine* published the results of a groundbreaking study of the health care preferences of Americans, the results alarmed doctors of conventional medicine but delighted holistic physicians. According to the results of a 1991 telephone survey of 1,539 American adults, 34% admitted they had used at least one "unconventional," (i.e., not common in the practice of most M.D.s) medical therapy in the previous year. Most typically they had consulted holistic doctors for relief of chronic rather than emergency conditions, such as anxiety, obesity, back problems, depression, or chronic pain.

The highest use of unconventional medicine was among white persons aged 25 to 49 with college educations and high incomes. Of this sample group, 72% said they did not inform their conventional M.D. of their consultations with "alternative" practitioners and that they had paid for most of these services out of their own pockets. In a country where third-party reimbursements for medical costs is the unquestioned norm, this is a remarkable initiative by health care consumers.

Extrapolated to the U.S. population, the study estimated that in 1990, Americans made an estimated 425 million office visits to nontraditional, holistic physicians, spending $13.7 billion in fees and paying for $10.3 billion of this themselves. Given a 1992 American population of 256 million, the study results suggest that some 87 million men and women broke stride with health care orthodoxy and sought out the alternative. "The frequency of use of unconventional therapy in the United States is far higher than previously reported," wrote David M. Eisenberg, M.D., the lead researcher. The *Journal*, never an ally of natural medicine, reluctantly concluded that "unconventional medicine has an enormous presence in the U.S. health care system."

These facts alarmed the allopathic doctors because for decades they have been institutionally and professionally aligned against such "deviations" from therapeutic norms. They had vigorously promoted the public view that holistic, complementary, empiric, and natural medicines were just inches short of "unscientific quackery." Now a statistical study published in their own peer review journal was telling them their patients thought differently and were willing to pay for their rebellious thoughts, too. Erik L. Goldman, journalist for *Internal Medicine News and Cardiology News,* a publication for the medical specialist, comments: "A growing number of Americans, dissatisfied with the care they receive from established medical sources, are seeking treatment—unbeknownst to their physicians—from a wide range of 'alternative' providers."

The evidence of widespread acceptance of alternative medicine is borne out in a series of subsequent supportive studies throughout the decade, a representative sampling of which follows.

- *SELF* magazine polled its readers, mostly upmarket, well-educated, professional, fortysomething women, about their opinions and practices regarding alternative medicine. When *SELF* asked its readers if they had ever consulted an alternative practitioner, 84% said yes. When asked what they thought of alternative medicine in general, 53% said sometimes it works, sometimes not, but 36% admitted they have more faith in it than in conventional medicine; 8% worried about possible dangers in its use; and only 2% were openly skeptical. So much for the "unproven quackery" issue that opponents of alternative medicine so often insist on.

Among the most popular alternative therapies consulted are chiropractic (60%), massage (58%), herbalism (42%), relaxation techniques (40%), acupuncture (30%), and reflexology (24%). But among those disciplines *SELF* readers haven't yet tried but would like to, acupuncture ranked highest.

Regarding cures with alternative therapies, 75% said they knew someone (including themselves) who had been cured, while only 25% said they had been disappointed by the results. Then came the clincher: When asked on a scale of 1 to 5, with 5 being the highest, how much confidence do you place in conventional medicine, only 11% gave it the highest marks. But when asked the same question about alternative medicine, 30% ranked it in category 5. In other words, these health care consumers have *three times more confidence* in alternative medicine than in conventional.

- Of people living in the San Francisco Bay Area of California, 41% tried alternative medicine at least once in 1994, according to a poll of 600 adults conducted in April 1995. This is far above the national average of 34%, which surprised many when first cited in 1993 (based on 1990 figures). Most popular among the disciplines consulted are herbs and vitamins, relaxation techniques, massage, chiropractic, and macrobiotics. Interest in acupuncture is soaring in California, with 4,500 licensed practitioners, or one-half of the nation's total, at work in this state.

Of those who tried alternative medicine, 54% said they were "very satisfied" and 80% said they would do it again; 51% said they were "likely to try" alternative treatments soon. More women (46%) than men (37%) made those office visits, yet 51% of both sexes said they were favorably considering making an appointment. Why is alternative medicine's popularity growing so rapidly? Because it works, is affordable, and doesn't fill your life with side effects.

- According to U.S. government data, between 1987 and 1992, the second fastest growing field in U.S. health care was alternative medicine. Listed as "Offices and Clinics of Health Practitioners—Not Listed Elsewhere," this category includes acupuncturists, dietitians, midwives, naturopaths, nutritionists, nurses, Christian Science practitioners, and twelve other specialties. This category, representing 22,260 offices, grew by 163.1% (from 12,044 offices) compared to the number of new offices of conventional doctors, which grew by only 56.3%; dentists, which grew by 47.9%; and osteopaths, which grew by 71.7%. The number of chiropractic offices expanded by 80.7%, from 20,065 to 27,329. The category with the greatest growth was in home health care, which grew by 244%; this category, incidentally, is often provided by nurses, who tend to be more open to alternative medicine approaches.

- Mass market sales of medicinal herbs in U.S. drugstores and supermarkets grew by 35% in 1994, worth $106.7 million in sales. Topping the list were garlic, whose drugstore sales grew by 40% to $12.9 million, and ginseng, whose sales climbed by 28% to $31.1 million. Their sales in food stores were even higher: garlic sales in retail food outlets grew by 40% to $12.9 million and ginseng leaped by 63% to $11.8 million. Even more impressive was acidophilus (taken as a "probiotic" bacteria, beneficial to the intestines) whose drugstore sales soared by 140% and whose food store sales expanded by 57%. The U.S. vitamin and dietary supplement market was estimated in 1995 to be $4 billion a year, and was growing at the rate of 15% each year.

- Worldwide, sales of herbal medicines (called phytomedicines outside the U.S.) are equally booming, estimated at $12.4 billion for Europe, Japan, Asia, and North America. In Europe, sales of herbal medicines are allocated according to these categories: cardiovascular, 27.2%; digestive, 14.4%; respiratory, 15.3%, tonics, 14.4%; sedative, 9.3%; and others. In Germany, for example, one-third of all nonprescription drugs are herbal and *Ginkgo biloba* (as a circulatory agent) leads the pack with annual sales of $280 million, followed by horse chestnut (for the blood) with $103 million. Herbal sales worldwide are expected to continue growing by 8% to 15% during the next five years, depending on the region.

- A survey released in March 1998 (conducted by Celestial Seasonings, a leading herbal tea manufacturer), announced that based on polling of 500 people, aged 35 to 54, 37% use herbal supplements. This was a tenfold increase in usage since 1990, Celestial Seasonings reported.

- According to *Natural Foods Merchandiser,* an industry trade publication, 1997 natural products sales totaled $14.8 billion, of which $2.6 billion were for nutritional supplements—a 19.5% increase over 1996.

- The demand for alternative medicine is 39% higher than the supply. In July 1995, the Seattle-King County Department of Health in Washington State surveyed 759 patients to assess their use of alternative medicine. Of those polled, 77% were women, 26% were Asian, 67% were aged 20 to 49, and 35% had no health insurance. The study showed that 19% had used some form of alternative medicine in the past year and 58% would use such treatments if they were "affordable and convenient."

Of those polled, 13% said they had consulted at some time an acupuncturist, 33% a chiropractor, 24% a massage therapist, 18% a naturopath, while 44% said they had used any form of alternative medicine at least once. The difference between the number of one-time users (19%) and future possible usage (58%, if "affordable and convenient") indicates a "potential unmet demand" of 39% of patients for alternative medicine.

- Estimated U.S. retail sales of homeopathic medicines for 1994 was $165 million, a 25% increase over 1993. The number of

U.S. homeopathic practitioners has grown from 200 in 1970 to about 2,000 in 1995. And a 1991 analysis of 107 controlled clinical trials of homeopathy, published in the *British Medical Journal,* showed that in 77% of cases, the use of homeopathy for numerous common health problems produced positive results.

- A 1998 nationwide telephone survey of 1,000 Americans by the Stanford Center for Research in Disease Prevention at Stanford University showed that 69% of those polled had used some form of alternative medicine at least once in the past year. The poll further reported that 56% thought their insurance provider should cover any of the nineteen alternative treatments listed in the questionnaire, while 55% of those who said they used alternative medicine said this usage had enabled them to reduce their use of conventional medicine.

- Another poll conducted by the Stanford Center for Research in Disease Prevention, this time involving 1,035 Americans, found that 40% had used some form of alternative medicine in the previous year. The focus of this poll was to ascertain *why* Americans were using alternative medicine. Chief among the answers were the following: higher educational levels among the users, poorer health status, a holistic attitude about health, and some form of "transformational" experience that had predisposed them to alternative medicine's more encompassing standpoint, or a specific health problem for which alternative medicine was known to be competent.

- Yet another study (a 1998 survey of 1,500 Americans conducted by Landmark Healthcare, Inc.) edged the number of adults using alternative medicine up to 42%. The study announced that 47% of those polled were willing to pay increased insurance premiums to get coverage for alternative modalities, and, even more impressive, that 67% believed that the availability of such care is a key factor in how they select a provider.

- Growth in usage in Canada has consistently exceeded that of the U.S. An August 1997 telephone survey of 1,200 adult Canadians (conducted by the Angus Reid Group of Toronto) showed an 81% growth in the usage of alternative medicine by

Canadians since 1992. The group stated that the increase was 76% for adults aged 35 to 54 years, but 146% for those aged 18 to 34. Further, the group stated that 42% of Canadians, as of 1997, use alternative medicine, while 66% advocate the Canadian government should support alternative medicine as a cost-savings measure.

• Another Canadian study released in late 1997 by *Maclean's* magazine and *CBC News* reported that 57% of those polled had used alternative medicine at least once, that 47% had become more receptive to this medical approach since 1992, and that 25% would trust an herbal remedy over a conventional prescription drug.

The Cost-Savings Edge: Efficacy Plus Affordability

With American health care costs exceeding $1 trillion a year, alternative medicine's stunning cost-savings advantage is beginning to attract notice. In fact, it is not an exaggeration to state that alternative medicine could save Americans literally billions a year in health care costs. If, as a taxpayer, you're wondering if there isn't some way to reduce the $1 trillion-plus annual price tag for American health care, here are some startling figures on how cost-effective alternative medicine could be if we gave it a free run in the medical marketplace.

For asthma, the cost of medications, doctors' visits, and hospitalizations is about $10 billion a year, but with alternative medicine, using allergy-elimination diets plus nutritional supplements, the savings would be about $3 billion. Consider atherosclerosis: Conventional medicine gives various kinds of surgery and drugs, costing $30 billion annually. Alternative approaches, including nutrition and chelation, would save taxpayers about $9 billion. Regarding chronic ear infections, the combined cost of office visits, antibiotics, and ear tubes for about 100,000 children is $650 million. Using allergy-elimination diets, estimated savings would be $487.5 million, with a 75% reduction in the recurrence of ear infections.

How about heart attacks? Conventional treatment includes clot-dispersing drugs that cost between $500 million to $1 billion a year, or about $2,600 a dose. The recommended alternative therapy involves a $5 dose of intravenous magnesium, producing cost savings of close to $1 billion. The annual cost for nonsteroidal anti-inflammatory drugs for osteoarthritis is between $2 billion and $4 billion.

Alternative therapies, involving nutrition and dietary modification, would shave about $1 billion from this. Conventional treatments for peptic ulcer cost $2 billion a year, while alternative therapies produce healing at one-third the cost, saving $1.33 billion. Finally, there can be cost savings on prostate enlargement treatments. Conventional therapy, involving surgery ($5,000/operation) and Proscar ($540/year) cost $2 billion a year to treat two million men. Alternative therapy costs about $150 a person, saving $2.78 billion annually.

The Mainstream Is Deserting Conventional Doctors

While a new medical paradigm is being birthed (or born again) in America through the acceptance of alternative medicine, the inevitable deconstruction of the *ancien régime* of allopathy is increasingly apparent.

- A survey of 70,000 readers of *Consumer Reports,* probably the largest survey conducted to date on the doctor-patient relationship, reveals that many patients feel their conventional M.D.s are not open to their questions or views and don't give them enough (or any) advice on how to have a healthy lifestyle. The survey shows that too many conventional doctors don't know how to talk with their patients or how to work with them cooperatively in the healing process. These are "potentially serious problems," the study concluded. The greatest patient grumbling is in the area of chronic ailments for which no standard treatment is available. In the past year, 23% of patients were dissatisfied with their conventional doctor over poor results for chronic headache, 28% for lower back pain, 15% for depression, 14% for arthritis and intestinal problems, 12% for allergies, and 11% for cancer and respiratory problems.

- Patients of mainstream M.D.s are also complaining about problems in the examining room. Many doctors, they feel, do not put the patient first. Among the patient gripes with their regular doctors, 29% said the M.D. didn't seek their opinion or explain lifestyle changes that might improve the problem; 26% complained their doctors didn't go over the possible side effects of the drugs; 22% said their doctors never took a complete medical history; 20% discouraged patient questions; and 15% didn't seem to care about the patient's emotional well-being. The writing is definitely on the waiting-room walls.

- A survey of 600 people dramatically shows that patients are asking questions, demanding information, and keeping their alternatives open. In this group, 65% asked their doctors to explain unfamiliar terms; 62% asked about side effects and alternatives to the drugs prescribed; 50% wanted to know about risks in surgery; 48% did their own independent research on their condition. The survey also showed that 44% asked about alternatives to the standard tests or surgery; 44% wanted to know about other treatments available; 43% queried their M.D.'s experience in similar cases; 36% wrote their questions down in advance; 26% took notes on their office visit; 25% complained that what their doctor recommended wasn't working; 19% asked to see their medical records. Clearly the days of the passive, compliant patient are history.

- Conventional doctors aren't listening to their patients, concluded another poll of 750 American adults conducted by Roper Starch Worldwide in August 1995. This study indicated that an increasing number of patients believe their mainstream physicians are not listening to them. The chief problem in doctor-patient communication is that physicians do not explain matters clearly, said 34%; and that they do not listen, said 12%. The prime behavioral fault of conventional doctors is that they're too rushed (30%), too hard to reach (19%), and they speak too technically (11%). Nearly one-third (30%) of the women polled said doctors took women's health complaints less seriously than men's. When asked for their response to a doctor's suggestion, only 51% said they would follow it, while 34% said they would seek a second opinion and do their own research first.

- It is seemingly contradictory, but other statistics show that conventional doctors are beginning to make referrals to the competition. When the American Board of Family Practice and the

American Board of Medical Specialties recently polled 572 family practice physicians and internists as to whether they would ever refer patients to practitioners of alternative medicine, more than half said they would.

Of the doctors polled, 80% were males and 42% were in their forties (of whom 72% were highly open to referrals), and 94% said they would refer patients for at least one unconventional therapy; 77% were willing to recommend up to four therapies; 36% actually practiced one unconventional therapy; and 19% practiced two. High on the list of referral specialties were relaxation techniques, biofeedback, therapeutic massage, hypnosis, and acupuncture. Of the therapies practiced by polled physicians, the two most popular categories were relaxation techniques and lifestyle/diet.

• Sometimes, patients have to take medical research into their own hands and buck the intransigence of conventional medicine. An inspiring example of medical care consumers taking research and treatment into their own hands was brought dramatically, and cinematically, to the American attention in 1992 with the popular film *Lorenzo's Oil*. Based on a true story, the film presented the struggles and successes of Augusto and Michaela Odone, parents of a son, named Lorenzo, who was diagnosed with a rare, incurable nerve-degeneration disease called adrenoleukodystrophy, or ALD.

Against the pessimism, indifference, intractability, and vested research interests of the medical establishment, the Odones researched and discovered a cure (based on two natural oils, high in erucic and oleic acids) for halting and partially reversing the slow, painful death by nerve demyelinization that ALD precipitates in boys aged five to ten. The Odones were clearly intelligent but not medical practitioners, scientists, or Ph.D. researchers, but no matter, their son's life—and that of hundreds of others—was at stake and that was sufficient motivation to rally all their intellectual resources.

"We respectfully claimed the right to have an independent mind and to study everything available in the literature, formulate hypotheses, and test them," Michaela Odone told *The New York Times*. Her message to parents is straightforward and politically daunting: "Realize that your interests and the doctors' interests are not parallel." Naturally, scientists, M.D.s, and other supporters of the AMA-dominated medical status quo have sought to discredit, qualify, question, and generally undermine the Odones' message, claiming that the movie version outruns science, conveying a false, damaging, and "scary" message to average parents.

Probably not, as many groups of parents, with children suffering from various obscure, under-researched, and generally rare diseases have since taken heart from the Odones' politically catalytic act and started underwriting research on their own. The Gelblum family launched the Canavan Disease Foundation out of their Manhattan home and raised $111,000 for research on behalf of their son. Canavan Disease is an apparently genetically driven brain deterioration that afflicts young children. "You can't just sit back and hope for a discovery," states Orren Alperstein Gelblum. "You have to make it happen." Or as another mother with an afflicted child—Cheryl Volk, director of the Association for Neurometabolic Disorders—puts it: "I almost consider it to be an underground movement. There are so many families desperate to do something, who feel they have to do it all themselves."

- There is criticism, even dissension, from within the ranks of conventional medicine, specifically, from the cancer doctors (called oncologists), usually the most conservative of the allopathic rank and file.

According to a study released by the Competitive Enterprise Institute (CEI), the FDA may be the cancer patient's worst enemy. The CEI polled 160 oncologists and found that 76% declare the FDA should not restrict information about unconventional, or "off-label," uses of approved drugs and devices.

Yet in its current "reign of censorship," the FDA has strenuously suppressed the free flow of information about new cancer treatments, about 70% of which involve off-label uses. The CEI poll also showed that 47% agreed that the FDA's five-year lag time in drug approval costs lives; 66% said that FDA policy has directly obstructed their ability to provide top care to at least one cancer patient. Oncologists believe that cancer patients will die because doctors cannot learn of new, effective treatments, because of the FDA's heavy-handedness about the spread of information. The study further revealed that 76% believe that the FDA should not restrict information about new uses for drugs and devices, 61% favored the FDA allowing physicians to use unapproved drugs and devices, and 21% had a totally unfavorable opinion of the FDA.

According to the *New England Journal of Medicine,* television's portrayal of emergency allopathic medicine may glamorize the treatments at the sacrifice of accuracy. The researchers analyzed ninety-seven episodes of *E.R., Chicago Hope,* and *Rescue 911,* three highly popular television shows that constantly portray heroic chest thumping and last-minute cardiac resuscitations of dying patients by skilled doctors and nurses; *E.R.* alone has an estimated 35 million viewers. However, the researchers found that at least sixty of these episodes, which presented "seemingly authentic detail," actually quite misrepresented the emergency room realities.

On TV, only 17% of those receiving CPR are elderly, yet in "real life," the majority of cases are old people; on TV, about 75% of cases requiring CPR derived from accidents, in real life 75% to 95% are caused by underlying heart disease; and while 66% of CPR patients on TV survive, the reality is more like 7% to 15%. The "real life" version of CPR is gruesome, violent, undignified, and may entail broken bones, the researchers noted; television's glamorized version of amazing medical successes succeeds only in fabricating an illusory picture of allopathic competence. On the other hand, it may be illusory and medically meretricious, but as imagistic propaganda it's a fabulous boon to allopathy.

Medical Licensing: The Key to *Un*freedom of Choice in Health Care

There may be steady gains in the acceptance and legitimation of alternative medicine in the U.S., but it still lags noticeably behind Europe, where it is full speed ahead for *all* effective medical approaches. European nations, lacking the obstructive interference of antipatient organizations such as the FDA, National Institutes of Health, and National Cancer Institute, are allowing alternative medicine to find its rightful place in the medical marketplace. U.S. health care would benefit enormously from following the European example.

About 49% of French and 46% of German patients use some form of alternative medicine. Homeopathy use in France grew from 16% of the population in 1982 to 36% in 1992. The British market for homeopathic medicine is growing by 20% annually, and in Greece and Portugal, by 30%. In Belgium, 84% of homeopathic and 74% of acupuncture treatments are provided by conventional doctors, while in Holland, 47% of M.D.s use alternative medicine and in Germany, 77% of pain clinics use acupuncture. In Denmark, reflexology is the most popular modality, while in Belgium, France, and Holland, it is homeopathy. In Germany, more than 70% of practitioners prescribe herbal medicines, drawing from 67,000 different commercially registered products. In most cases, herbal prescriptions (worth about $1.7 billion annually at retail prices) are paid for by public health insurance.

A prime means by which the conventional medicine establishment is keeping the U.S. lagging far behind Europe regarding the mainstreaming of alternative medicine is the *political* use of medical licensing. The licensing of individuals to practice medicine in any specialty is done at the state, not federal, level. Naturopaths, for example, may legally practice in Connecticut, but not Massachusetts; in New Hampshire, but not Vermont; in Nevada, but not California. The real politics of medicine is not about who is going to pay the $1 trillion annual health care bill, but why there isn't a cheaper, more effective alternative. Alternative medicine, as many now know, is that more effective alternative, yet the key issues nobody is talking about are these: why is it not more widely available in *every* state and why are the insurance companies not paying for it when it would save them money?

The reason is a little-known political fact that took shape in the 1920s and has never been changed since, called the medical practices acts. These were similar laws passed by all the states to ensure that only M.D.s could be licensed and thus legitimately practice medicine. The idea was to deliberately set up a medical monopoly that favored conventional doctors. The idea was also to keep homeopaths, naturopaths, herbalists, and chiropractors out of the marketplace by regulating the licensing of physicians.

The practical result is that there is no free and open competition in the American medical marketplace. You have the right to choose your physician, provided it is an allopathic M.D., but you cannot, in most cases, choose between an M.D. and a naturopath and expect to get insurance reimbursement. In fact, there are barely a dozen states where you can even legally choose a naturopath and only about thirty-five where you can get acupuncture from a licensed practitioner.

Freedom of choice is available in most areas of American life except medicine. There it is tightly held by the conventional medical establishment and the strong economic and political interests supporting it. Repeal of the medical practices acts, at the state level, would throw the medical marketplace open to free competition among all the medical specialties—for the first time in 100 years. The alternative would quickly become the new mainstream, just as it did in 1830s America when the M.D.s had a similar "death grip" on medicine and were faced with honest competition from a new wave of homeopaths and herbalists. What happened 160 years ago ought to happen again: "The public, disgusted with the maltreatment it was receiving, stripped the licensed profession of its legal protection and threw the practice of medicine open to all comers," says medical historian Harris Coulter in *Divided Legacy: Twentieth Century Medicine—The Bacteriological Era.*

There are positive signs of change, though they come only after considerable struggle, even oppression. There are now nine states (Alaska, Washington, North Carolina, South Dakota, New York, and Oklahoma were among the first) in which the medical practice acts have been amended (since 1990) to accommodate the demand for alternative medicine. In at least two of these states (New York and North Carolina), this change in the legal status of alternative medicine came only after great travail, cost, suppression, licensure revocation, and enormous grass-roots politicking by concerned citizens.

New York's law is fairly representative of the others. It guarantees that the medical practice act shall not be construed to effect or prevent "the physician's use of whatever medical care, conventional or nonconventional, which effectively treats human diseases, pain, injury, deformity, or physical condition." It also stipulates that at least two of the eighteen physician members of the State Board for Professional Medical Conduct must be those for whom alternative medicine represents a "significant portion" of their practice. Legislative initiatives in at least another six states are at various stages of success or failure, but the remaining 75% to 80% of the states are still legally beholden to the conventional medicine status quo.

Medical licensing laws and federal reimbursement programs severely limit open competition among medical modalities and keep the cost of American health care exorbitant, states medical analyst Sue Blevins in a policy analysis from the Cato Institute of Washington, D.C.

Since their introduction in the 1870s, licensing laws have limited the supply of health care providers, thereby limiting competition and increasing doctors' incomes, Blevins explains. Government policies, which strongly favor (and reward) conventional medicine, are largely responsible for the escalation of health care costs and the lack of a wide range of choices in medical services. In addition, there is "little actual evidence that medical licensing improves quality [of care] or protects the public," says Blevins. The result is a "government-imposed medical monopoly," supported by the tax dollars of all Americans, including the 33% who consult alternative practitioners.

Consider how licensing regulations restrict the public's access to nonphysician health care providers, such as midwives. There are 10,000 midwives in the U.S., but thirty-six states either restrict or prohibit their activities. "Americans' low usage of midwifery does not correlate with high-quality birth outcomes," Blevins says, because the U.S. has the world's second highest rate of Caesarean sections and has the fifth highest infant mortality rate among industrialized nations. Midwife-assisted births could save Americans $2.4 billion annually if only 20% of women used them.

Nurse practitioners are another case in point. These are registered nurses (R.N.s) with advanced training. Research indicates that almost 80% of adult primary care and about 90% of child care services could be safely provided by nurse practitioners. A 1993 Gallup poll reported that 86% of consumers would willingly use nurse practitioners for all their basic medical services. Further, we could be saving $6.4-$8.75 billion a year if nurse practitioners were more widely used. But they're not because "many states impose scope-of-practice regulations that prevent nurses from practicing independently as primary care providers," says Blevins. This action suppresses the full potential demand for them because they are not legally free to compete.

Whether you like it or not, tax dollars directly subsidize conventional medical schools, but not alternative schools such as chiropractic or naturopathic colleges, says Blevins. Today only 5% of medical school income comes from tuition and fees; the rest comes from state and federal government subsidies. Of the $23 billion that U.S. medical schools received in 1992, $2.7 billion came from state and local governments, and $10.3 billion came from the federal government.

Tax dollars support the medical monopoly through other means, too, such as research, training, and teaching grants from agencies such as the National Institutes of Health, and Medicare and Medicaid reimbursements, which cover only conventional medicine. The time for reform is at hand, urges Blevins. Even if you do not particularly favor alternative medicine, she argues, the medical monopoly goes against the capitalist grain of free, unrestricted, non-monopolistic competition in the marketplace. When it comes to medicine in this country, we haven't seen that for over 125 years. "Breaking the anti-competitive barriers of licensing laws and federal reimbursement regulations will provide meaningful health reform, increase consumer choice, and reduce health care costs," states Blevins.

The True Market Value of a Federal Imprimatur

Licensing reform through amending medical practices acts at the state level is a slow, expensive, and charged political process. Some states take up the initiative and fail, which is to say, the efforts are successfully blocked by the allopathic establishment. It would seem that conventional allopathy is fighting a rearguard action, the last defense of grumpy old men defending their economic turf, using the media to spew forth pejoratives against the rising stars of alternative medicine. There is a kind of schizoid approach to news coverage regarding this dialectic, even in a supposedly (or formerly) left-liberal newspaper as the *New York Times*.

On the same day, this newspaper had an article reporting on the nation's first government-supported naturopathic clinic in Washington State. The coverage was mostly objective, fair, and factual. The King County Council had unanimously voted to request $1-$2 million in federal funding to subsidize the clinic's annual operation. Natural medicine, including dietary supplements, herbs, enzymes, acupuncture, and other alternative treatments, which may once have been considered on the "fringe" of health care, is now "reaching the mainstream," reported *The New York Times*. Yet on the Op-Ed page of that same issue, a physicist and biologist railed against this project (which, incidentally, would put alternative treatments within reach of low-income people), claiming it was tantamount to "buying snake oil with tax dollars." It was an allopathic propaganda set piece with all the red-flagged pejoratives and slanders so typical of this kind of opinion-making.

The usual words and insinuations were bandied about: magic, shaman, faith healer, miracle cures, placebo effect, magical notions, charlatans. The authors suggest that alternative medicine is "superstition masquerading as science" and that the "sensational accounts of amazing health benefits" attributed to alternative medicine "were once the stuff of tabloids." Alternative medicine is not science, but a snake oil machination and therapeutic sleight of hand that ignores natural law and achieves its small successes thanks to the power of patient belief. Then the writers deliver their editorial *coup de grace:* "Giving a federal imprimatur to such techniques invites deception."

The authors were referring to minuscule federal funding (about $14 million annually) now allocated for research and evaluation of alternative medicine. This use of the term *imprimatur* has a beautiful propagandistic irony, for there is a far stronger case to be made (as Sue Blevins and Harris Coulter have already done, above) that if the U.S. government is giving its seal of approval and imprimatur to a form of medicine, it is to conventional allopathy. In this case, it is a gesture of support worth about $1 trillion a year.

The Ideology of Illness: Analyzing Mainstream Medical Attitudes

In the uncritical American mainstream, it's clear that the allopathic medical paradigm still prevails. So deeply entrenched is this dominant mode of perception, that it's become nearly invisible, hidden powerfully within the language and images by which the mainstream media reports medical events. One needs to school oneself in the mechanics of propaganda, and for this, we can take useful counsel from the recent history of chiropractic in the U.S.

One of the landmark days in the recent history of alternative medicine in the U.S. was August 27, 1987. On that day, District Judge Susan Getzendanner found the American Medical Association (AMA) and fourteen associated parties guilty of waging a conspiracy against chiropractors to contain and eliminate them entirely, in violation of the Sherman Antitrust law. According to chiropractor Chester Wilk, D.C., who spearheaded the antitrust lawsuit, the fourteen litigators probably cost AMA at least $15 million. But even better, it exposed some of their propaganda methods for a later day. The AMA may have failed to quash chiropractic, but there's always chelation and oxygen therapy, biological dentistry, and alternative cancer therapies.

The AMA's conspiracy against chiropractic began in 1963 with the secret formation of their Committee on Quackery, says Dr. Wilk. During the 1960s, disparaging press came in all directions against chiropractic, and it became obvious to Dr. Wilk, when he studied the phrases, cliches, and cases cited that they were the rotten fruit of an increasingly predictable negative propaganda campaign. What he learned then about the AMA's techniques is just as valuable today. Next time you read something highly critical of alternative medicine, keep this in mind.

All of the "information" against chiropractic fell into seven categories: innuendoes that implied wrongdoings but couldn't be proved; material taken out of context to create an unfavorable image; half-truths manipulated to support false conclusions; obsolete material no longer representative of how chiropractors think or practice; obscure sources, off-the-cuff comments by practitioners never claiming to represent the field; incidental exceptions to the rule presented as if they are standard examples; and outright lies, because, as the Nazi propagandists knew so well, "the more outrageous the falsehood, the more believable it becomes," says Dr. Wilk.

Mass-market journalism, typified by publications like *Time, Newsweek, Discover,* and *U.S. News & World Report,* in addition to television and newspaper medical reporting, habitually reinforces allopathic conceptions of disease, causation, and therapeutic efficacy, shaping thoughts and attitudes (like political propaganda) most typically below the threshold of the public's analytical awareness.

While allopathy unarguably has as many therapeutic and procedural marvels as it has excesses, the crucial point here is that the *enforced* marketplace monopoly of both allopathic practice and thinking has serious consequences for how we regard health, illness, the physician-drug-medicine interface between them, and the nature and prospects of healing itself. Unless we are vigilant, this monopoly also blinds us to critical, analytical, and creative thinking about alternatives beyond the intellectual range of its medical world-view—which is only one of at least two. And when we forego our consideration of legitimate medical alternatives, typified by empiric, holistic medicine, we shortchange our environment, both inner and outer, our body and our world. In other words, a medical paradigm has in all senses an environmental impact.

You need to appreciate the fact that a paradigm is an intellectual environment. Harris Coulter's rigorous analysis of the hidden economic factors in Western and American medical history schools us in the necessarily *political* nature of medical therapeutics. Now that we understand that there is an underlying political dimension to therapeutic issues, the next step is to appreciate how that political struggle is played out before us (and within our thinking) in mainstream attitudes about medicine as reflected in the popular media. After all, what keeps the allopathic domination largely in play is our *uncritical* acceptance of many of its attitudes.

We may think we are alert to bias in journalism, but I am continually surprised at how subtle and pervasive—and frankly skillful—the allopathic bias in mainstream medical journalism has become. Even when you catch the loaded word or prejudiced phrase, deeper insinuations still lurk within. Our efforts at critical reading reap a high reward. When we free ourselves from the conceptual trance state into which allopathy has inducted us, we are well on the way to changing the balance of power and influence between the allopathic, or rationalist, and the empiric, or holistic, views of medicine; we enter a position in which we can allow both to find their *natural,* unmanipulated level in the medical care marketplace. As Coulter documents, in this struggle between the allopathic and holistic medical views, we are dealing with two paradigms of therapeutics—broad, all-encompassing patterns of thinking and acting.

By definition, a paradigm is so big, so inclusive, that normally we can't see it; rather, it's an ideological environment in which we unquestioningly live. Because the biases of allopathy are buried so deeply—and cleverly—in the quotidian language of journalism and daily speech, invariably we miss its concept-shaping power. Allopathic ideology lives in our language, most acutely in the attitudes and phrases in mainstream and popular science journalism. If we're not assiduously critical in our reading, we may become susceptible to the hidden ideology of illness implicit in the language of medical journalism. And if we unknowingly become intellectually colonized by allopathic ideology, we may gravely shortchange our own prospects for full health, self-care, self-responsibility, medical rights, and health-care consumer freedom of choice. We may miss our rightful chance to participate in the politics of medicine.

A great deal is at stake depending on which paradigm we live within. A paradigm represents a consensual view of the world, a culturally pervasive way of framing the world into some standardized form of coherence. But a paradigm's ubiquity basically guarantees its invisibility; without our noting it, the paradigm's assumptions become equated with "common sense." It's difficult, then, for us to perceive it critically because our words, concepts, attitudes, and habits of thinking are so deeply colored by its pervasive filtering of data.

The parameters of a paradigm—allopathy, in this case—encompass everything, from how we think about ourselves, our health, how we understand causality, agency, and the nature of action, to how we position and act upon our environment. A paradigm is an intellectual environment. The parameters of a paradigm exist in our minds like an invisible electrified fence; they are there to keep our thoughts bounded within one heavily grazed pasture, to prevent them from wandering off into another paradigmatic pasture. The fence is invisible because it's subconscious, subliminally erected in words and sentences, in our thinking processes and expectations.

Only vigilance will save us from falling asleep to other critical views and healing opportunities. So we must be like the feminists and affirmative-action advocates in the 1970s who rigorously analyzed school textbooks for gender and racial biases. We need to analyze mass-market journalism for its allopathic biases. When we momentarily step outside the charged words and metaphors of a medical ideology, when we distance ourselves from the seductive allopathic icons and learn to survey with a critical eye typical, representative articles in magazines like *Time, Newsweek, U.S. News & World Report,* and *Discover,* we'll appreciate the astonishing, even alarming, degree to which allopathy dominates our public discussion of medical issues.

Were the American Medical Association itself to edit the medical articles in these mass market publications, it couldn't arrive at a better endorsement—an advertisement for the paradigm, in effect—of their own values and assumptions of practice than we can find in a handful of randomly selected articles.

In this chapter we will browse these magazines critically like textual anthropologists examining their journalistic biases as a way of teasing out the hidden values, core attitudes, and implicit positions of the allopathic model of health and illness embedded in the language itself. Then we'll examine a few of the consequences—patients suing their doctors and diagnostic dead ends in the face of new baffling diseases—of working under this enforced view. This is both an eye-opening introduction to the subtlety of the allopathic ideology and an urgent task of conceptual liberation, without which we would be unable to reposition our environment in more positive, creative, and empiric terms.

The Military Occupation of Your Body

The phenomenon of disease is usually couched in adversarial, military language. A *Time* cover story on the immune system ("The Battle inside Your Body") reminds us that the immune system is an efficient guard dog that "fights off disease" because we must "stop that germ." Immunology is battle, conflict, aggression, and, one hopes, victory. *Time*'s cover art, viewed by millions worldwide, shows a man looking inside his chest at a boxing match in which the "white-cell wonder" (the lymphocytes of the immune system) slugs the "vicious virus" with biochemical gusto.

This immunological confrontation between good white cells and bad invader germs happens independently inside the man's body while he watches like a neglectful landlord wondering what the tenants are squabbling about. He is passive, aloof, alienated, and not immediately relevant to the battle, even though it's all on his behalf. He is disenfranchised from his biological being.

The article's description of the immune system is studded with words evocative of warfare: enemies, jungle, lethal, target, prey, predators, constant siege, invade, assault, destroying, alien, biological warfare, battle-manager, move in for the kill, carnage. The "vicious viruses" are framed apocalyptically as a terrorist's amalgam all in one entity. We may be oblivious to the fact, but our immunological Marines are staging a ferocious counterattack within us on our behalf, implies *Time*.

So laden is *Time*'s snappy prose with the military metaphor that in the article's first five paragraphs alone adjectival variations on the adversarial theme are repeated twenty-eight times. In the midst of the verbal crossfire is a central photograph of a two-month-old infant receiving an inoculation from a headless white-frocked physician. Surely this is one of allopathy's most cherished, potent icons: the absolutely vulnerable newborn being biochemically protected against bacterial invasion by the beneficent doctor, who generically (as the doctor's individual head isn't shown) represents the entire medical establishment. Newborn human life is saved, nurtured, and protected by modern (mostly male) medicine. This icon, in conjunction with the cover image, reinforces the belief in the staunch efficacy of Western medicine against disease, its insatiable, monolithic "enemy."

In a similar story from *Newsweek* ("Young Survivors in a Deadly War") we learn this (italics added): "More and more *young* people are *beating* cancer but many find that *getting well* is only half the *battle.*" The tacit message? Our only rational response to cancer is pugilistic: we fight to win, we beat it, and young people have the necessary spunk to do it; health, even remission, must be acquired, as if purchased like another consumer good: we "get" wellness by going to the doctor and paying for it. Wellness is a market commodity and allopathic medicine is its stock exchange. The wartime pall is reiterated in more than a dozen *battle*-laden words in this two-page article with words like fought, racked, afflicted, veterans, outcast, and combat.

"The flu virus looks like the head of a Roman mace"

Implicit in the proliferation of military rhetoric is the concept that disease—a product of nature's fulsome cornucopia of pathogens—is inimical to human life and well-being. Pathogens and disease agents are the shadow side of nature, the predatory "man-eating" faces of a hostile environment, and must be kept at bay, if not decisively eradicated. As allopathy portrays it, microbial pathogens are our "tiny foes," grim, bizarre, bullying mechanistic creatures who are "mankind's deadliest enemy," destructive agents that evince "Machiavellian tactics" in subverting our organic domestic harmony, as *Time* phrases it. It's as if the microbial world were teleologically obsessed with the ruination of humanity.

Disease's malefic agent is a faceless bureaucrat representing an inexorable biological destiny written in genetics. Consider *Time* on colon cancer, after lung cancer the "second most deadly form of the disease." *Time* opens with a tabloid headline worthy of an Agatha Christie detective story: "New *Clues* to Detecting a *Killer*— Researchers *zero in* on the *genetic causes* of colon cancer." Medicine is a question of mysteries and sleuthing; the M.D. is Hercule Poirot working magisterially on our case; he will detect the clues leading to the identification of the culprit. The cancer in question is vicious, a cold-blooded killer; our heroic interventionists are focusing their high-powered rifle sights (the nuance of "zero in") on the assailant. But don't worry, it's a robotic mechanical killer—it's genetic, meaning, beyond our control.

Since colon cancer is genetically caused, its etiology is out of our hands; it's our forebears' fault and not our responsibility; or as *Time* puts it, it's caused by a "faulty gene" or "genetic defect" that "triggers" the infection. Our genome is factory-damaged, imperfect, flawed during production even before we received the goods (i.e., were born), preprogrammed in earlier generations to destroy us today; the regrettable defect then impassively, automatically *triggers* the condition. When it's genetic we're off the hook: victims of course, but not to blame, not responsible. It's all impersonal and mechanistic: no body, no soul is involved, no human, conscious agent, just an anonymous, shadowy force pulling the cancer trigger with double-stranded fingers.

Thus the human body and its interdependent organic systems are more like an inert, insentient machine assembled from pieces, according to this view. As such, the body breaks down like a defective product. The immune system goes "awry, makes errors, gets confused, often entirely on its own," says *Time*. It can "overrespond, fail to respond, or turn against the body, usually for genetic reasons." Whose immune system is it, anyway? Surely not ours if it operates with a mind of its own. In other words, like *Time*'s cover man with his chest open, we have this ambivalent, frequently incompetent, and always inscrutable mechanism ratcheting noisily within us, its origin and purpose veiled in that mysterious past that allopathy metaphorically calls "genetics." When allergies make their "airborne assault" it's the result of "aberrant functioning" of the immune system, says *Time*. Millions of Americans sneeze and suffer, "victimized by errant genes."

The victim mentality is so pervasive it reaches down into the molecular level of the human genome: the human as patient is betrayed at the foundations of biology by aberrant, inimical nucleotides. But allergy victims will strike back. *Time*'s full-page illustration depicts a face with a clenched fist instead of a nose, as if to say, "In your face, pollen grains, mold spores, and dust-mite dung!"

With Huntington's disease, says *Discover,* "Things start to go *awry* in the brain,*" a circumstance that requires teams to research "when the brain function first turns *abnormal,*" to identify that portentous moment when "this gene kicks in." The image we take away is that neurological illnesses are caused by nanotechnology failures that deconstruct the integrity of the human mechanism. Genetic clock-work is by definition beyond our reach, control, or intervention; it acts, often aberrantly, and we passively receive its results, and often suffer. We must be precise: genetic "defects" may be beyond the patient's reach, but not the physician's, aided with the innovations of gene therapy. *Discover* waxes bleak when it likens Huntington's to "the ticking of a time bomb in the genes," portraying this concept in a full-page illustration of a dynamite bomb strapped to a nucleotide within a double-helix strand of DNA. The message is clear: Nature is treacherous, dangerous, nasty, subversive, malevolent, and *antihuman.*

This attitude fosters a distrust of nature and our internal biological environment. It's a distrust that approaches the old Gnostic revulsion for the human body as the jailer of the human spirit, for the infernal processes of nature, and by logical extension, the whole of the natural world. Environment itself, both interior and exterior, is unfriendly to human life, and must be aggressively controlled, if not fought. Our bodies are polluted, defective, inimical to the human spirit, and we live unilaterally "at risk," *Discover* insists, repeating its grim view excessively, using "at risk" twenty-five times and "risk" fourteen times in the same story. Philosophically, *Discover* tells us that incarnation (literally, life in the flesh) is at best a conditional risk.

When we take our cues from this kind of reporting, no wonder our latent fear of embodiment can escalate into the kind of uncontrollable panic we might experience were we to discover ourselves airborne passengers in a terribly defective jumbo jet. It's the perennial dialectic of human rationality against nature's irrationality, of physician against pathogen. Viruses, says *Time,* are our "ancient enemies," the "agents of all these infections." The language of opprobrium is heaped high on these invisible microbial miscreants: they are "scourges, tiny attackers," full of "malevolence and mischief" evincing a "much greater capacity for evil" than good.

"The flu virus looks like the head of a Roman mace," says *Time.* Not only is there a first cause that precipitates our organic discomforts—genetic defects—but microbial scourges are malevolent and evil. The ancient struggle between good and evil, light and darkness is waged in our bodies in an organic morality play in which our physicians become our priests and redeemers.

Nature may be purposefully plotting against us, the allopathic logic implies. The defect might be intentional, part of a cursed teleology from our phylogenetic beginnings. "Exorcising a Damnable Disease"—here the infernal hostility of nature is raised to a near religious ardency in another *Discover* story about Tourette's syndrome, a neurological dysfunction characterized by spasms, noises, and outbursts of obscenities. Nature has such apparent negativity and demoniac intentions that only an exorcism can save us from biological damnation. In *Discover's* eschatology, disease *is* damnation, organic retribution for original sin. "Indeed, those who have Tourette's in its full-blown form do seem possessed, if not by a demon, then by *something* altogether alien—and something that speaks," notes *Discover.*

Disease is not only debilitating, it can even be dehumanizing, according to allopathic perception. That's the nuance of *Discover's* "alien." In *Discover's* "The Ticking of a Time Bomb in the Genes," we learn that Huntington's disease is, according to patients, "terrible, dreadful, incurable, the most horrible thing I can think of" and "one of the worst diseases of mankind." Nobody with compassion will deny that the *experience* of a condition like Huntington's is dreadful, but to categorically state that the condition itself is devoid of personal meaning or relevance may be closing the door to insight at the crucial moment we need to keep it open. Is *Mother* Nature that heartlessly horrible? And is the organic world itself, the context for Huntington's, so devoid of mercy and good will? These are vital questions—or perhaps, foregone conclusions—implicit in the statements of the Huntington's patients.

For allopathy, disease is a biological anomaly with malicious antihuman intent, a pathogenic invader from outside, from outside reason—the predator, terrorist, and madman in the environment— that "wreaks such havoc" in our lives when it bursts the cellular gates. We find this assumption again in *Discover's* treatment of Alzheimer's disease. "Alzheimer's *victims fail* in a pattern that's a *deadly reversal* of childhood development." The tone is quite negative and pessimistic. Not only are people with Alzheimer's victims, but they are failed victims, their productive lives terminated without a clue. By this logic, an Alzheimer's diagnosis means not only an immedicable and certain death by senility, but, as the phrase "deadly reversal of childhood development" implies, an evolutionary regression, a psychobiological atavism to a time before even childhood—a reversal into death.

The Doctors' Screenplay: In Search of the Good Patient

Since we can't trust nature or the organic processes in our body, we can't trust ourselves to know how to heal. The role of the patient is clearly delineated in this primal icon: we are the suffering, afflicted *victim,* the passive supplicant awaiting medical palliatives and allopathic salvation. An ideology of aggression, militarism, and combat necessarily victimizes; there is a combative agent who wins and a subdued recipient who loses. We may think it's pathogenic nature that loses, but it's us. The irony is that allopathy makes all patients into victims; it's the only role permitted us.

Here's how *Newsweek* subtitled a major story on depression: "It is *hitting* young adults *harder* than ever before, but researchers are gaining new understanding of the emotional *disorder* that *afflicts* millions" (italics added). Let's work out the nuances in this powerful single sentence. The illness is violent and assaultive, like a brickbat that hits hard; it's chaotic, soulless, and deranged, victimizing the public as indiscriminately as an exploding bomb. It hits, afflicts, and disorders—this is its core energy: it's entropic.

Allopathy cultivates the victim mentality in the petri dish of the hospital. The descriptive language for the patient's role is emotionally loaded to evoke immediate sympathy and condolence. The patient is biologically decimated, forlorn, passive, paralyzed, incapable of self-rescue: victimized. One man is "leaning on crutches, racked by bone cancer," while another "in the throes of disease, he didn't dare look beyond tomorrow." "I know there's this big fight going on in there," said a young woman patient. She was pictured lying forlornly in a hospital bed pointing to her stomach; she was waiting for medicine to rescue her life. Victims racked by pain haven't the spunk to dare a better outcome; their perspective is foreshortened, their future foreclosed.

Meanwhile, experts "help survivors navigate a wilderness of dilemmas." The "expert," presumably a physician, becomes the psychopomp, conducting the patient's soul through the underworld of illness. Our victimization is senseless, irrational, and merciless, another baffling act in an apparently godless world.

The agon of biology versus humanity is keenly pitched into pathos by the *Time* tragedians in their cover story on viruses. Several family members were simultaneously diagnosed with cancer. The family was "stunned, stricken," reeling under the "macabre coincidence" and this "unbelievable misfortune"; now "the afflicted family is living on the edge." Cancer is the ultimate robbery, the quintessential housebreak. In the face of this affront, our only option is to seek redress through the authorities.

The passivity before the medical pharaohs that is required of the good (and miserable) patient comes across in this charged phrase like something out of Bertold Brecht: "Confronting their doctors, the victims asked . . . " In this scheme, disease is meaningless; it has no inherent or existential relationship to its recipient; it's more like a bad draw in a lottery. There is no cognitive palliative for its victims, either, no rational explanation, no spiritual teleology that accounts for why them, why this way, and why now. Allopathy doesn't offer that kind of salvation; it only promises magic bullets.

As a patient, there's nothing positive I can do—other than to get used to living on the edge. As patients, we must turn for "hope" to the medical authorities. Angrily, we may confront them, these bureaucrats of our biological destiny. One patient perfectly summarized the paradigmatic expectations when she said: "If they can find out what triggered me." The fourfold passivity and alienation in this declaration is awesome. The woman is dependent on outside authorities (they) to determine what electrochemical glitch in her wiring involuntarily produced (triggered) this condition; that the whole enterprise is fraught with uncertainty and conditionality she perfectly expressed in her dependent preposition, *if*. The patient is insignificant, a minuscule statistic in a data compilation, appended to the end of the description as an afterthought: *me*. If any eight words concisely express the lament of the allopathic patient, this woman's statement does.

The patient is isolated, in both knowledge and identity, from the disease. She doesn't know much about it, nor does she identify with it. She's intellectually disenfranchised by the medical vocabulary and she's alienated from her medical condition, not to mention her body and the healing process. If relief happens, it's attributable to the ubiquitous, salvific *they* of the medical establishment. Allopathy doesn't speak about healing, anyway. Instead, there are victories, decisive wins, triumphs, and good, even "stunning" results, but that's all part of "disease-management" that delivers the magic bullets to their intended targets. But we don't hear about healing; rarely is there a plan for a postdisease restoration of the body or lifestyle.

The only legitimate activity permitted the good patient is to make consumer selections at the medical smorgasbord of drugs, technological interventions, and experimental surgeries. "A patient opted for the expensive therapies," said *Time,* referring to an $80,000 one-time procedure. The virtues of consumerism are translated into the perquisites of the sickroom. Victims all, nature has hijacked us, holding us hostage in the hospital as we fervently await our antibiotically armed rescuers. And don't worry about the bill for that $80,000 procedure; the insurance company will pay for it; and if something goes wrong, you can always sue the doctor, the hospital, or the drug company. When the patient is cast as a passive, disenfranchised, minimally conscious victim who participates neither in the process of healing nor in payment for services, the powers that be, namely the physicians, hospitals, drug and insurance companies, take care of the rest—and quite profitably.

"My Doctor, His Drugs, My Heroes," Keens the Chorus of Patients

In all fairness, it must be said that the medical establishment does want to rescue us, reimbursable patients as we might be, but strictly on its terms. The mainstream press mythologizes the male M.D., creating a heroic icon. Virologists are "prominent," their experimental strategies are "working fantastically," their new vaccines are "quite effective" and "advanced," and top surgeons have "even attempted the daunting feat" of some new surgical intervention. A Genentech scientist is "not discouraged" because biogenetics research is "explosive" and "promising."

The Nobel Prize vindicates this rash of medical heroism: every new Nobel awarded further validates the paradigm. If Gerald Edelman, who says the mind (and consciousness) emerges from the physiological brain as a by-product, gets a Nobel in physiology/medicine for this view, he must be right. Only highly credentialed authorities from government, industry, or the academic world are reliable, quotable sources for "explanations," only AMA-commissioned M.D.s can "unravel the mysteries," only accredited "researchers" get quoted in *Time*.

The allopathic doctor and medical researcher are our staunch allies in the battle against nature. The M.D. will outwit and manipulate nature on our behalf, taking all the requisite "steps toward a brave new world," as *Time* informs us. "The rush is on to treat neural disorders with brain implants," states *Time's* lead for a piece on transplanting adrenal gland tissue into the brain to palliate Parkinson's and other neurological dysfunctions. The rush is on, the headline tells us, meaning it's urgent, moving fast, and must be supported now and without question but with open arms, journalistic praise, and funding dollars.

Consider this congeries of upbeat commendation in only five paragraphs of *Time's* coverage: even more remarkable developments; promising research; predicted; rapid surgical advances; there is no question; first used successfully; there is no danger; they are accepted; heartening Parkinson's results; sees a braver new world ahead; fetal brain grafts offer a better bet. All of this is abetted by the victimized patient's own grateful testimony: "I have hope where there was no hope before."

The message is that modern medicine can do practically anything; it's invincible. Surgeons perform "a dazzling daylong operation" severing Siamese twins; they "gamble against uncertain odds" and "in a bold bid to save a leg, transplant a knee." Surgeons outwit our immune systems, too, according to *Discover:* "By changing a body's sense of itself, Suzanne Ildstad is able to *trick it* into accepting transplanted organs." In its heroic quest to fix dysfunctional bodies, allopathy can reconfigure human identity at the molecular level.

Let's study this icon carefully. Most often, the M.D. is male, the patient is female. What's particularly evident is a simultaneous mythopoeic exaltation of the white male M.D. and the "victimization" of the suffering female patient. This produces an environment that allopathic critic Robert Mendelsohn, M.D., characterized as "mal(e)practice" and radical feminists are wont to call "malev(i)olence." In *Newsweek's* feature on headaches, three of the four opening-page photographs show women "afflicted" with headaches, strapped into high-tech medical equipment. The patriar-

chal icon is reinforced as we see two white-clad male physicians leaning over a woman in a hospital bed. This woman is completely passive, her eyes closed; she's surrounded by a shopping cart of drugs
and a roomful of sophisticated instruments, as she receives her "first
step" in migraine treatment, which is an injection of an antiheadache
drug. Another photo shows a smug male M.D., amid several female
patients, who is credited with "controlling (their) cluster attacks."

The mythology is unmistakable here. The *victim* (medical
patient) is *female,* the presumed "weaker," *passive* sex, who is *ravaged* (attacked) by the invasive headaches that the skillful male
doctor *controls* by an injection made available by the wonders of
modern pharmaceutical research. More women in medicine may
be the best way to counteract the "insufferable paternalism" of
male medicine, comments Natalie Angier in *The New York Times,*
particularly in allopathy's most body-invasive territory, gynecology,
where many male M.D.s tend to be sexist, insensitive, and take an
assembly-line approach. "As Americans become shrewder and
more skeptical about the health care business, and as they lose
patience with the gruff imperiousness displayed by many practicing physicians, some are beginning to suspect that the best guarantee against insufferable paternalism in a doctor is to make sure
the doctor is a woman." This would be a good step, but more
women doctors per se doesn't resolve the problem of allopathically indoctrinated physicians—who can be female—because a medical paradigm transcends gender differences.

With male M.D.s smiling beneficently from their hero's perch,
their magic silver bullets (drugs and technology) are exalted as well.
Their biochemical pharmacopoeia is apotheosized in typical *Time,
Newsweek,* and *Discover* stories. "New drugs and advancing research
offer hope for 45 million chronic victims," states *Newsweek.* This
attitude swells into almost religious tones through the use of a word
like "hope" in the context of victims and drugs. Nature brings
damnation by pathology but allopathic drugs offer *hope.*
Cyclosporine, a drug used to confuse the immune system so it won't
reject transplanted organs, is canonized as a "miracle" with "dramatic results." Interleukin 2 shows "promising results" and "spectacular successes." Vaccines are "the most powerful preventive
measures in medicine . . . well-known medical triumphs," writes
Newsweek's Terence Monmaney. "Of all the approaches drugs have
been the AIDS patient's greatest objects of hope," says *Time.*

We are urged to remember this simple catechism: the best news is always the latest, experimental, miracle drug. As one elated medical researcher declared in *Time,* the key to successful treatment "will probably be discovering at what point in the life cycle of the virus a drug will be effective." Medical palliation *a priori* means a drug or surgery; thus, medical progress means new, more, faster, more efficient drugs. A new anticholesterol drug called lovastatin is fanfared as "a potent new ally" for millions of Americans "in their battle against heart disease, the nation's No. 1 killer," *Time* announces. Says one happy recipient, a 54-year-old woman: "I really believe that it's saving my life." Not only is the drug powerful, even, in an abstracted sense, sexually virile ("potent"), but its name itself—*lova*statin—testifies to its *heart*-warming goodness.

Uncritical boosterism about a new drug can sometimes produce a grim scenario. Consider the case of Halcion, the most widely prescribed sleeping pill in the world. *Time,* in a piece called "Sweet Dreams or Nightmare?" showed us the darker side of what happens when a passive female medical victim momentarily wakes up from her drugged trance and takes action. Halcion is a high-profile miracle drug, sold in ninety countries, with annual sales of $250 million, and used regularly by about 7 million Americans who can't sleep.

A middle-aged woman was arrested for murdering her mother, but was later acquitted because she was deemed "involuntarily intoxicated" and therefore not responsible for her actions. She'd been taking Halcion to sleep better for over a year under her doctor's prescription; she may have slept better but Halcion also made her paranoid, agitated, and sporadically amnesiac. When she got out of custody and off the drug, the woman sued Upjohn, Halcion's maker, for $21 million for promoting "a defective drug" and failing to warn the public of its "severe and sometimes fatal adverse reactions."

The passive female victim, dependent on drugs to regulate a fundamental biological function (sleep), gets victimized yet again by a *defective* drug. Not only is she dependent on drugs to enhance what should be normal biological function, but the drug itself is defective and further aberrates her already skewed system. Note that it isn't the defectiveness of the drug *ideology* that she indicts, only that one specific drug is flawed. Meanwhile, her dependency, passivity, and victim status remain untouched because now she needs the lawyers to handle her tort against Halcion.

"We can dissect and demystify it. Then we can defeat it."

The patient is alienated and abstracted from the organic life that has suddenly "gone awry" inside the body. As nature is combative, aggressive, and ruthless, so shall allopathy be unrelentingly fierce in its retaliation. Where is safety in this battle zone? For that matter, where exactly is the patient within this Armageddon of malevolent biology and salvific physicians? Presumably somewhere in the mind, hidden snugly inside the brain; that's the patient's place of safety, the mind, where s/he sits fearful and shriveled in an attic corner of the body estate.

The patient's tactical retreat to the brain reinforces the classic Cartesian mind-body dualism that has exacerbated Western thinking for several centuries. Of course, allopathy is founded and rationalized on this separation of mind and body. The body acts, the mind observes, the person suffers, while doctors with drugs manipulate the interface. We await the outcome of this battle from the schizoid safety of our sundered organic unity—up in our head somewhere. Allopathy vigorously separates mind and body, regarding them as twin mechanistic entities in the human organism; psychiatrists correct the mind, physicians fix the body. Yet paradoxically, allopathy discounts the survival of the mind, or consciousness, beyond the confines and duration of the body; nor is it particularly willing to grant human consciousness a discrete single location in the brain.

Descartes may have claimed the pineal gland is the seat of the human soul, but neuroanatomists have distributed (and fractionated) consciousness by function throughout the cortex. Human consciousness is a fleeting, provisional epiphenomenon of the organic brain, neuroscientists assert, an end product entirely dependent on its host environment for existence. When the brain dies, our consciousness dissipates. Highly commended popular science books like *Consciousness Explained* by Tufts University's Daniel C. Dennett and *Bright Air, Brilliant Fire* by Nobel Prize winner Gerald Edelman, further entrench this reductionist view.

But there is a knotty problem in all this epistemological bravado. If mind-body unity is disallowed and consciousness is dependent on the brain, which is a perishable, vulnerable organism, then where, exactly, are we permitted to be within the human organism? Presumably, the diminutive *me* of the equation, the repository of self-consciousness, huddles somewhere in the gray convolutions of the cortex as the much assailed, ineffectual, passive holder of awareness. But why should consciousness huddle even in the brain? This three-pound universe is no less organic, mutable, and perishable than the rest of the human organism. Why should consciousness be permitted here and nowhere else in the body? There is something arbitrary and thus contradictory with this special privilege.

The ontology of allopathy essentially disallows *human* consciousness (which is self-aware, reflexive, responsive, individualized consciousness) tenancy rights anywhere. It will permit mechanical, reactive, generic computerlike intelligence, mainly because it's easily reprogrammed. Ultimately, allopathy seems to construe the human as a robotic, preprogrammed homunculus. For allopathy, consciousness is, adapting Arthur Koestler's famous term, "the ghost in the machine."

Allopathy has strong opinions about the origin, location, and efficacy of consciousness. Allopathy implies that human consciousness is isolated in the brain, arising secondarily and dependently from matter, from processes of the brain. With the termination of organic matter, consciousness instantly dissolves and the self vanishes, this view argues. The self is an illusory creation of bodily location and agency; consciousness is its (enfeebled) tool. Because consciousness is matter-dependent, it has no efficacy or sovereignty, no power over bodily matter; that means it cannot be wielded by its possessor, the human tenant.

The tenant, or self, can be proprioceptively aware of its organic suffering but powerless to respond on its own, through itself; response is permissible only through *extra*bodily, external, extracarnational agencies, whether these are medicines or procedures. Allopathy schools us in believing that humans are not capable of using consciousness in self-directed, *intra*bodily activities, such as healing from within. Spontaneous remissions and miraculous cures are anomalous quirks of an otherwise mechanistic nature. The bodily environment is a given: pre-created, preformed, predetermined; it can be polluted but not re-created, lived in but not regenerated.

Even this colony of consciousness lodged in the brain is subject to mechanical breakdown. If this island of consciousness produces, for example, schizophrenia, there are corrective pills. "We can do for schizophrenia what we've done for so many major illnesses," commented Dr. Samuel Keith, chief of the National Institute of

Mental Health's National Schizophrenic Plan, quoted in *Time*. "We can dissect and demystify it. Then we can defeat it."

The redemptive virtues of allopathy are displayed vividly in a recent *Time* cover story on mental illness. First, *Time* paints as bleak, desperate, and vile a picture of schizophrenia as possible. Schizophrenia is "this most devilish of mental illnesses," "terrifying," "devastating," "insidious," a "shadowy land of waking nightmares, fiendish voices" in which patients are "tormented by demons and at times lost to reality," "wrestling with inner demons," and "hounded by a frightening spirit." According to the article, the condition has remained tragically immedicable, excepting the former miracle drug, Thorazine, which doesn't work so well anymore and produces nasty side effects. Doctors and drugmakers have made "impressive strides" while researchers are "working furiously" to perfect the drug-based treatment approach.

Into this picture of suffering patients and heroic researchers comes the "remarkable drug" clozapine, a true pharmaceutical *deus ex machina*. Patients using clozapine experience an "awakening to reality after many years of being lost in the darkness." The implication here is that clozapine is the chemical tool for waking up, gaining more consciousness, becoming cognitively competent, and of course for "regained hope." Our conscious relations with "reality" will be mediated successfully and expertly by this new drug. Clozapine "brings patients back to life," says *Time*, implying that life, hope, and awakening to reality are equivalent events that can best be mediated by this mind-altering drug. The *Time* journalist described postschizophrenia clozapine patients at a dance, then imaginatively extrapolated their regeneration along these lines: "The revelers were, in a sense, the laughing, dancing embodiments of a new wave of drug therapy that is revolutionizing the way doctors are dealing with this most devilish of illnesses."

Clozapine is the neurotransmitter-suppressing face of redemption and joy everlasting that will stamp out the evil in this world—and in our heads—in an agape celebrated by doctors, patients, and drug companies. Sandoz, the Swiss pharmaceutical giant who engineered the drug, couldn't have written a better public relations sentence to capture the redemptive miracle of clozapine than this (my italics added): "For doctors, patients, and *anguished* families who have *coped* for years with schizophrenia, the *arrival* of a new drug that can *dramatically help* even a portion of the *victims* is cause for *elation*."

Here's how I read *Time*'s script for what is virtually an allopathic passion play: The entire medical community—caregivers and victims—has suffered miserably but stoically awaiting the messianic appearance of the miracle drug; its competence is shocking and bold, the victims' response should be celebratory and joyous. If this isn't enough, *Time* adds: "One patient in ten responds to the drug so dramatically that the effect is like being *reborn.*" In the domain of allopathy, even consciousness can be fixed.

Creating a Nation of Medical Victims

A medical paradigm is a philosophy of matter that has consequences in all aspects of our lives—especially so when it is enforced by law. Allopathy inevitably fosters passivity, dependency, and therapeutic impotence among its patients. Individuals become patients, forgetting that healing, ultimately, is self-generated. Allopathy discourages our active engagement in the processes of health, illness, and healing, and it disallows consciousness any effective role in the bodily environment, putting the *physis* in thrall to antibiotics.

When a medical regime denies the efficacy of consciousness in what is by nature a fundamentally human environment (in this case, the body), it relegates the human identity to outlaw status; when the self loses its psychobiological imprimatur, human immunology starts to erode into a form of allopathy-induced automatic dependency. As far as human free will, immunological vitality, spiritual development, and life-purpose fulfillment, it's a dead end from here on in. The physician commandeers the human *physis,* leaving the patient with but the husk of life.

This enforced passivity requires a surrendering of our active responsibility for causality and outcome—but this is a metaphysically perilous position to assume. Restitution from disease (which isn't necessarily the same as health and well-being) results from the skillful application of magic bullets and technological interventions by omniscient physicians. The trouble is, if we are so vulnerable that we must be perpetually rescued by our doctors, we are also liable to victimization by this capricious, ambivalent class of heroes—but we've learned to accommodate this diminution, discovering that victim status has its peculiar advantages.

We are becoming a nation of victims wallowing in a "great mass of annoyance, grievance, and blame" in which mastery of victim chic can be highly remunerative, contends social critic Charles Sykes. "Portraying oneself as a victim has become an attractive pastime . . . this squalling howl of grievance has become a national chorus." Examining America in the politically correct early 1990s, in which the victim ethos is fueled by "a hypersensitivity so delicately calibrated that it can detect racism in the inflection of a voice," Sykes reports: "I hear America whining." When misbehavior can be redefined as disease, growing numbers of the newly diseased have flocked to myriad new support groups.

The mantra of participants in this burgeoning politics of victimization is *I am not responsible; it's not my fault,* says Sykes, highlighting a core value of allopathic therapeutics. "The ethos of victimization has an endless capacity not only for exculpating one's self from blame, washing away responsibility in a torrent of explanation—racism, sexism, rotten parents, addiction, and illness—but also for projecting guilt onto others. The new culture reflects a readiness not merely to feel sorry for oneself, but to wield one's resentments as weapons of social advantage and to regard deficiencies as entitlements to society's deference." Wounds are an asset, dysfunction is a growth industry, victimization is a ticket to entitlement, and illness is a serviceable excuse for all manner of public misconduct in this epidemic of disability, argues Sykes. But the "unmovable unwillingness to accept responsibility" and the simultaneous propensity to blame (and sue) others may be indicative of the decay of the American character, signs that we are generating a "society of resentful, competing, and self-interested individuals who have dressed their private annoyances in the garb of victimism."

A nation of litigious, politically correct victims as the product of allopathic environmentalism is not a healthy polity by any means. Morally, it's an opportunistic infection of human character. It generates a metaphysically degenerate and intellectually disempowered state of mind, qualities entirely inappropriate for the demands of true democracy.

An Environment of No Responsibility: A Prescription for Malpractice

One of the major consequences of this enforced domination of the medical marketplace by allopathy is a consumer revolt called malpractice and the extensive litigation it entails. In recent years medical injury, malpractice litigation, and huge court-awarded financial settlements have become the norm in American medicine. America may have the world's most sophisticated medical machine, but that high-tech machine is cranking out damages and costing a fortune. And patients have found a way to feed back their views into the system, through suing their doctors.

Still, it's not an ideal outlet for consumer dissatisfaction, for it keeps in place the patient's attitude of no responsibility for the outcome or difficulties of the medical case. The constantly escalating costs of malpractice (insurance premiums; court-awarded settlements; defensive medicine and a proliferation of sophisticated, expensive tests; and higher patient fees) is a significant factor driving up the annual cost of American medical care.

While finger pointing and blame casting predominates—patients blame the doctors, doctors blame the lawyers, lawyers blame the insurers, insurers criticize the patients—this complex situation is the inevitable result of enforcing an unresponsive medical paradigm on health-care consumers. Allopathy, the paradigm of contraries and dialectics, itself generates all this opposition expressed through an epidemic of malpractice. The allopathic rationalists may have temporarily won the juridical day in America, but their clientele is beginning to protest at the grass-roots level.

When allopathy encourages patient passivity, dependency, and a victim identity in the context of an armamentarium of drugs, procedures, and instrumentation, malpractice litigation becomes the only option for allopathic victims to exact retribution for their mishandling and the failure of medical interventions. Filing malpractice torts becomes the only safety valve, the only feedback option for a nation of litigious victims whereby patients, forced to take their health care within this tightly insulated, politically mandated situation, can register their dissatisfaction.

The litigation reflex is an innate component of the adversarial dialectic of allopathy: physician against infection, patient against doctor—and doctor against patient, at least defensively. This is the insurrection of the patients against the passive relationship they're put into by their physician: they can either consent or fail to consent to what the doctor says, then sue them later if things go wrong. Modern allopathy transforms the patient from a living, dynamically mysterious organic individuality into a mechanistic pathology, a reduction that's utterly disempowering, even alienating, severing us from our true human beingness.

The malpractice "epidemic" is, at heart, an insistence by patients that this imbalance in the therapeutic exchange must be redressed and the patient must be allowed and encouraged to participate in the creation of one's health. Yet the responsibility cuts both ways. If patients feel clinically disempowered, they must acknowledge, too, their own complicity in creating this medical disenfranchisement.

So the litigation reflex breeds defensive medicine, high-tech predictive, preemptive diagnostic methods in ever increasing amounts. Doctors, fearing patient suits for malpractice or misdiagnosis, order more tests, invariably very expensive, to cover all therapeutic contingencies; this in part is what's driving the upwardly spiraling costs of medical care. Are the doctors responsible for driving up costs or are the patients culpable for refusing to take responsibility for the etiology and treatment of their conditions, or are the insurance companies to blame for gouging both doctors and patients with high premiums?

The trouble is this self-contained malpractice loop doesn't resolve the core issue that's really fueling it: namely, the fact that all the players are exempted from taking true responsibility for their actions and for bearing the financial consequences of their medical decisions. It's a revolving door of cost deferments: doctors order expensive operations and tests, hospitals bill insurance companies for patient services, physicians bill insurers for their malpractice claims, and insurers raise premiums for patients and doctors alike. It's always somebody else's fault; it's always someone else who will pay the bill. The high incidence of malpractice claims is more a symptom than the problem itself; it's a symptom of the core attitude in allopathic medicine whereby the recipient of care is exempted from true responsibility for the activities and consequences of healing.

In some areas the allopathic malpractice dilemma is putting additional financial strain and pressure on empiric, holistic practitioners, making it harder to secure adequate coverage and putting them on the defensive. In this respect, allopathic malpractice may be hindering accessibility (and certainly third-party reimbursement for) alternative therapies. But there's a bright side to allopathic malpractice, too. The growing volume of claims and torts, coupled with the escalating costs of malpractice insurance premiums for conventional practitioners, is driving a financial and therapeutic wedge into the heart of the allopathic monopoly; when it cracks open, space will be created for the burgeoning empirical, holistic disciplines for whom the incidence of malpractice, in fact or allegation, is minimal.

One wedge that is helping to crack open the edifice is the $4 billion silicone breast implant settlement owed to about 400,000 women plaintiffs by Dow Corning and its insurance companies. Although the FDA recognized silicone leakage from the implants as early as 1982, it took them a decade to order the implants off the market, during which time, thousands of women came down with what is now being called Silicone Implant Disease. The silicone implant disaster is only one of many big dollar fiascoes that beset the medical devices industry in the 1990s.

Suing America's High-Tech Medical Machine

During the 1980s, increasing attention was focused on the incidence of malpractice in America, in terms of claims, litigation, and awards. The conclusion was that something was desperately wrong in the heart of conventional medicine that so much patient distrust and dissatisfaction would be vented in this emotionally fraught, financially exhaustive manner.

The atmosphere of malpractice and the habit of litigation in American medicine have emerged at an accelerating rate since the 1950s. An estimate by the American Medical Association put the total cost of professional liability in 1984 at $13.7 billion—about 15% of the costs of physicians' services. The medical system is entangling doctors, patients, lawyers, and insurance companies in a tightly drawn knot of high-expense, high-risk, high-defense practice, lucrative suits, and an increasingly displeased, litigious clientele. Patients aren't satisfied with their health care and they're telling doctors about it in court. The malpractice crisis has serious implications for the viability of allopathic medicine in America. If the incidence of malpractice claims is any barometer, conventional medicine has grown almost uncontrollably injurious—and combative. Its politically enforced medical mandate is backfiring; its therapeutic edifice is crumbling under its own weight.

What's fueling this confrontational attitude of patients and doctors? New medical technologies breed more patient injuries; these produce more legal suits, higher insurance premiums, and higher physicians' fees, as the atmosphere of health care becomes permeated by alienation and distrust. This estrangement will only deepen if the marketing plans of Courtscan are successful. Beginning in late 1993, Philadelphia M.D.s were offered a computerized database service (for $80 a month) to screen the legal history of their patients; Courtscan could search through all 802,000 lawsuits and judgments filed in Philadelphia in the past decade and inform the M.D. in sixty seconds if a given patient had a record of instigating malpractice litigation and was therefore malpractice prone.

While the malpractice crisis continues to mount its damaging statistical critique of conventional medicine, the overall impact on holistic, empiric medicine in the long term may be favorable. Malpractice claims against holistic practitioners—in osteopathy, chiropractic, homeopathy, naturopathy, midwifery, acupuncture—are minimal. Their fees are much lower than allopaths, their cost-effectiveness considerably higher, and holism's modality itself—no drug, no surgery, no high-tech invasive procedures, cordial communication and patient rapport—tends to insulate practitioners from legal action.

While many homeopaths and naturopaths view malpractice insurance as superfluous, acupuncturists either pay exorbitant rates or can't get insurance at all. Chiropractors have no problem because they run their own insurance company, while osteopaths are recognized by mainstream insurers as an acceptable risk. Home-birth midwifes, however, are walking an insurance tightrope. Regardless of their short-term problems, alternative-complementary care practitioners agree that the malpractice crisis may be the golden opportunity that finally puts empiric holism on the medical map of America.

Of the socioeconomic factors driving the increase in doctors' fees, two-thirds of the pressure came from liability costs. In 1992 the American Medical Association estimated that American physicians were spending $5.6 billion a year in malpractice premiums, representing 1% of that year's estimated $817 billion national health care expenditures. Concomitantly, physicians were ordering an additional $15 billion per year of tests and procedures specifically as defensive tactics to avoid future litigation from patients.

What's driving this torturous climate of malpractice? "The big issue is that the physician-patient relationship has broken down by virtue of modern technology and our increasing medical special-ization," explains Laurence Tancredi, Ph.D., professor of medicine and law at the University of Texas at Houston, and co-author of *Dangerous Diagnostics.* Physicians resort to diagnostic-predictive testing (worth about $15.5 billion a year) as a form of defensive medicine as more patients file huge malpractice-liability suits and insurance companies raise their rates.

The proliferation of high-tech, high-risk, high-expense diagnostic tests is driving a huge wedge into this already fractured relationship. The escalating costs of malpractice premiums influences the way physicians make decisions about patients, says Tancredi. The result is "defensive medicine," a self-protective practice that favors an overuse of diagnostic tests and that now costs consumers about $15.5 billion annually. The climate is such that a physician who doesn't use all the available tests is likely to be sued if anything goes wrong. "The threat of litigation drives the practice of testing in the health care system," Tancredi says. "Physicians are inclined to offer tests as soon as they are available, for litigation has established the physician's obligation to warn patients of potential problems if it is possible to gather such information through diagnostic technologies."

Physicians increasingly order more diagnostic tests, says Tancre-di, simply to establish a defensive precourt legal record of having performed appropriate medical protocol. "The tendency is to do these tests more and more, even in situations where there are only minimal indications. Some of these tests, like catheterization, are invasive, and expose the patient to more possibilities of injury. This in turn can generate more malpractice suits. So this high-technolo-gy diagnostic milieu further alienates patients."

The Allopathic Propaganda Machine Disparages the Unconventional

Medical licensing laws effectively keep the alternative practi-tioners out of the mainstream and malpractice claims keep many doctors (or drug companies) in court. But despite the proven pub-lic interest in the services of alternative practitioners, the main-stream media quite successfully keeps the public from learning the true therapeutic merits of its specialties.

Reasonable questions come to mind: Is the medical world in fact flat? Is our only alternative to fall off the edge of the world if biochemical allopathy cannot fix our problem? If allopathic journalism is all we read or watch on television, we'll certainly believe that if mainstream medicine can't save us, nothing will. It's not that the alternatives are unsatisfactory; they do not exist—at least that's what the M.D.s want us to think. Holism is a chimera, a hoax, an icon gilded in quackery.

Options from the fields of alternative, eclectic, complementary, holistic, and natural health are unilaterally ignored or derided by *The New York Times*, the *Wall Street Journal*, *Time*, *Newsweek*, *Discover*, and their media allies. As far as allopathy is concerned, such modalities—homeopathy, acupuncture, herbalism, naturopathy, massage, chiropractic—either officially don't exist or their efficacy is so unreliable, their scientific validation so potholed, their practitioners so suspect, that it's just too inconsequential to mention in print. When *Time* or *Newsweek* acknowledge holistic protocols, most often it's couched in sarcasm and scorn.

"Preying on AIDS patients," headlined *Newsweek*, showing us how "quacks peddle false hopes to sufferers of the deadly disease." *Newsweek*'s language is derisive as it lambastes the field in a generic denunciation. Its word list for holistic practices fulminates with barbs and darts: *worthless, worms, scams, mischief, blatant hucksterism, disinformation, nostrums, fraud, bogus, most absurd, vague, troublesome, kooky, purported panaceas, untested, bizarre, dubious, unproven*. AIDS patients are warned against being "ready prey for hundreds of quack doctors peddling half-truths and false hopes," while AIDS activists are exhorted to "step up the war on the fools and rascals waiting to exploit them." When at last *Newsweek* abandons fustian for details, it excoriates a "self-appointed therapist-herbalist" for charging an $80 fee; it chastises a nonagenarian healer because he once had his medical license revoked for two months; it provisionally exempts vitamin supplements, acupuncture, and macrobiotics from the Grand Inquisitor's pyre only because they are "basically harmless."

Editors of *Time* and *Newsweek* surely must assume a remarkable degree of intellectual complacency among their allopathically colonized readers, because in an accompanying article we learn how the FDA is cutting troublesome regulatory and licensing "red tape" to speed up the release of experimental drugs. In other words, if the experimental drugs and procedures are allopathic, that's okay; if they're from the empiric world, they're suspect. Testing procedures are "unnecessarily slow" and the tangle of "laborious regulation" has kept "promising medications" from severely ill patients.

"A new FDA rule offers hope to needy patients," says *Newsweek*.

This pithy sentence, which encapsulates the allopathic assumption, must be handled with caution. The truth behind the FDA's decision to release new drugs faster, one surmises, is inverted. Drug companies wishing to cut down on the formidable research, testing, labeling regulations, and multimillion-dollar investment required for new drugs, somehow persuaded the FDA to allow AIDS patients to become human guinea pigs for presumably inadequately tested new drugs. AIDS patients are the newest "afflicteds" after all "who are desperately ill and have no alternative therapy." In a strange way *Newsweek* spoke sagely when it advised AIDS activists to be vigilant against "the fools and rascals waiting to exploit them." It merely omitted to tell them that these same fools and rascals have the FDA's sanction.

Consider the way two major national publications recently handled the status of late-twentieth-century natural medicine in their cover stories barely two months apart. When we read these reports critically, the allopathic biases, both in word choice and assumption, become clear. *U.S. News & World Report* discussed "unconventional medicine" (acupuncture, hypnosis, and biofeedback), meaning practices "long dismissed by mainstream doctors" but which now seem to offer "wonder cures from the fringe." Qualified support from the scientific community is trickling in: M.D.s are tolerating acupuncture, though with suspicion; some of the approaches might work, but notwithstanding, mainstream doctors are yielding to patients' demands for options. Meanwhile, Western scientists can't explain the operation of these practices, and anyway the "proof isn't there" so it's probably all placebo effect and "a sugar pill for the mind."

Time followed with its "New Age of Alternative Medicine," telling readers why biofeedback and other "offbeat" treatments from "the believable to the bizarre" (and worth $27 billion a year in consumer spending) are "catching on." *Time*'s coverage of the options was comprehensive and its patronizing, cynical, and dismissive attitude was equally wide-ranging. Like *U.S. News & World Report*, the *Time* article reads as if the patriarchs of allopathy and the magnates of the pharmaceutical industry were reading—editing?—the text carefully, breathing over the shoulders of a magazine staff assiduously careful not to offend allopathic proprieties. Reflexology is incomprehensible and its mumbo-jumbo stretches credence to the breaking point, says *Time*. Clinical hypnosis is a semi-respectable update of the old magician's hocus pocus; biofeedback embodies "the mystical in gadget form." Even chiropractic isn't spared the scorn. Most M.D.s still "wince" at the mention of "back-crackers," and aside from some salutary benefit to the lower back, "there is no proof—aside from reams of anecdotal testimony—that the method works."

Of course *Time* failed to mention how in 1987 the AMA lost a landmark eleven-year antitrust violation suit filed by the unscientific back-crackers against the AMA's unfair monopolistic practices. The chief danger of the "cult" (alternatively: wild thicket; lush, enchanted forest; health care *a la carte*) of alternative medicine "aside from wasting money, is that the patients get so carried away with unconventional cures that they dismiss regular medicine entirely," concludes *Time*. That's a political, economic consideration, not a therapeutic one.

The allopathic propaganda machine rolls on, infiltrating national newspapers such as *The New York Times* and taking advantage of its reputation for high editorial standards and "objective" reporting. In mid June 1996, *The New York Times* ran a lengthy two-part, front-page review of alternative medicine; it dished out the usual pejoratives and disparagements. But you could discern the cracks in the dike of suppression; you could feel the writer's ideological discomfort just beyond the pejorative facade. They hate to admit it, but alternative medicine is now "a big business and a powerful force in modern medicine" supported from the ground up by an estimated 33% to 40% of Americans.

The *Times* deployed the customary terms of dismissal: *fringes, untested, unregulated, therapies based on whims or discredited science, once obscure treatments, folk remedies, a reliance on anecdotes, snake oil, quackery,* and said that the term *alternative medicine* is a species of "Orwellian newspeak, implying it is a viable option." Frankly, the article, coming at this time in the decade, makes you fume and laugh, in cycles. They can't deny the social and economic significance of the medical alternatives and they know its potential financial threat to their $1 trillion annual honeypot. The propagandistic skein is nearly transparent; you can almost count the days remaining in which they can count on gullible readers.

One prominent "quack buster," Stephen Barrett, M.D., a board member of the National Council against Health Fraud and who always seems on hand for the requisite pejorative, commented:

"Quackery isn't necessarily about selling products and services—it's about *selling misbeliefs*. For a quack to thrive, he has to *promote unwarranted distrust* [italics added]." There is not a better description of what "quack busters" and allopathic propagandists do than these two sentences. It seems to be perennially so, that the one who complains loudest about fraud or immorality is in fact the most fraudulent or immoral.

It is allopathy's hired journalistic guns and their obliging "experts" who promote unwarranted distrust and who sell misbeliefs; in accordance with the Machiavellian nature of politics and propaganda, they simply invert the process and criticize their opponents for precisely what they are guilty of doing. Their only ploy is to throw pejoratives at it and hope that there are still enough sufficiently stupid readers to be taken in by their juvenile propagandistic dismissal. They have already lost the war, and while they know it, they will never admit it; as the ship of allopathy sinks and the sharks of truth circle, their bluster and bravado is an empty, feckless pose.

Time, Newsweek, and *The New York Times* may be the first to warn us of holistic quackery and alternative health care fraudulence, but they are monolithically reticent to discuss the possibility that the quack busters themselves may be practicing a dangerous form of "medical McCarthyism," even purveying deception themselves. That's the critical position taken by Sharon Bloyd-Peshkin where she discusses in *Vegetarian Times* America's "health fraud cops" and "health care vigilantes." Bloyd-Peshkin examines the rhetoric, sponsorship, activities, and vested interests of numerous mainstream U.S. medical "quack buster" organizations—National Council against Health Fraud, American Council on Science and Health, Consumer Health Information Research Institute, Committee for the Scientific Investigation of Claims of the Paranormal—and finds them a lot less scientifically objective than they claim. In some cases they're nothing more than strong-armed public relations officers for establishment medicine posing as independent public watchdogs and "consumer advocates," but basically helping to suppress controversial information.

"The quack busters' role in this suppression is to convince the public, often with the aid of a gullible press, that medicine other than the status quo is fraudulent," writes Bloyd-Peshkin. "Never mind that they don't have their facts straight when they're actually forced to provide facts. Most of the time, quack busters get away with forcefully stating their views as though they were facts. The quack busters, who purport to save us from deception, are themselves purveyors of deception."

Conspiracy Theories:
When Paranoia Becomes Sociology?

All of this makes one reasonably wonder: if alternative medicine was this popular by the mid-1990s, why is it constantly slandered, belittled, and marginalized in the mainstream press? The answer may be shocking to some.

There are forces arrayed to block the full incorporation of alternative medicine into the mainstream. It is as intensely protected and secretive as the Pentagon's war machinations in the early days of Vietnam before *The New York Times* blew the Pentagon's cover by publishing the "Pentagon Papers" in the late 1960s. Now one might say the machinations have moved across the Potomac to the FDA and National Institutes of Health, which are to alternative medicine what the Pentagon was to the anti-Vietnam protesters. Why do the media keep belittling the subject and marginalizing its merits? Are these "forces" organized? Evidence exists to suggest that they are organized and may represent a kind of medical conspiracy.

The proposition of conspiracy theories underlying government actions, UFO cover-ups, and other scenarios in which powerful interests collude against the public, was both gaining attention in the 1990s and being marginalized to the far right of the militia groups. The "paranoid style" has always flourished in American culture, notes journalist Michael Kelly in a *New Yorker* article on the subject. The argument is that "sinister, antidemocratic forces have wormed their way into the inner workings of government" where they have subverted the legitimate interests of the public in favor of their own arcane agendas of power, financial gain, and severe secrecy. Both the John Birchers of the 1960s and the Idaho militias of the 1990s contend that a cabal of wealthy, superpowerful planners work behind the scenes to launch the inimical "New World Order" upon an oblivious population.

There is a new variation on our American style of perennial paranoia: "pure fusion paranoia," says Kelly, where the conspiracists on the political left and right "meet in paranoia." Left and right dissolve, leaving only "unanimity of belief in the boundless, cabalistic evil of the government and its allies." This theme is emphasized frequently in the highly popular television drama, *The X-Files,* in which two FBI agents are chartered to investigate the paranormal. More often than not, their research comes up against a brick wall of silence, suppression, and secrecy regarding an ultrahidden government agency interfacing with ETs, UFO technology, and unlawful biological experiments. In other words, a fair measure of the paranormal activities emanate from other branches of the government itself.

For the most part, political conspiracy theories tend to have a blind spot with regard to possible or alleged government machinations in the field of medicine. As an exception, a recent poll of 1,000 black Americans in five cities revealed that about one-third believed (another 33% wasn't sure, and only 33% disputed the theory) that HIV was developed in a government laboratory and distributed through minority populations (including theirs) both in the U.S. and Africa as a form of deliberate germ-warfare genocide.

For the most part, among the public that accords any validity to organized conspiracies of silence and suppression, very little of this paranoid state of mind is at present usefully focused on what the allopathic medical interests may be up to. However, it may one day turn out that when it comes to medicine, paranoia is sociology. Proving a conspiracy exists is tantamount to unveiling and disempowering it; at this point, the best we can responsibly say is that evidence strongly supports the proposition that there is an organized, systematic collusion among the allopathic powers to keep the medical market in their hands. In that work, the media is, as criminologist Elaine Feuer aptly points out, "an instrument for government propaganda."

If you wish to pursue the medical conspiracy idea, talk to investigative journalist Joseph Lisa. Lisa has spent the last twenty-five years probing the veiled machinations behind what he describes as the systematic harassment of practitioners of alternative medicine. In his book, *The Assault on Medical Freedom,* Lisa draws on numerous formerly secret medical industry documents to expose the "dirty politics and dirty tricks" behind this organized assault. The FDA, the large pharmaceutical drug companies, the allopathic physicians' trade groups, and the insurance industry all seem to be cooperating in "a massive propaganda campaign" to discredit alternative medicine and to persecute its drugless alternatives to toxic conventional drugs, claims Lisa. *Medlock* is what Lisa calls this weblike collusion of financial interests among the state and federal governments, pharmaceutical and insurance industries, and organized allopathy.

In fact, according to Lisa's research, the allopathic "propaganda machine" has been working behind the scenes since 1963, when the American Medical Association (AMA) established its Committee on Quackery. Another, related, initiative followed this in 1964, known as the Coordinating Conference on Health Information, a network of governmental officials and allopathic medical industry representatives. The implicit goal in either case was to position all *economic competitors* to conventional medicine—chiropractic, acupuncture, homeopathy, naturopathy, vitamin therapy, cell therapy—as "quacks." The priority targets, Lisa explains, do not use standard pharmaceutical drugs in their practice, which makes them *direct economic competition* to conventional medicine, which prefers to dominate the market.

In the years since 1963, the "quack busting" groups would change names, shift their cover slightly, and reemerge as new deceptively consumer-friendly watchdog groups such as the National Council against Health Fraud (1984). In 1983, according to Lisa's documents, the FDA and the Pharmaceutical Advertising Council (representing at least twenty-six drug companies) initiated a joint effort, called the Public Service Anti-Quackery Campaign, to universally discredit alternative medicine. It was conceived to be a clearinghouse on medical quackery, which, of course, in the view of its allopathic founders only encompassed the suspect realm of alternative medicine. Its board consisted of well-known "quack busters," M.D.s who made their living as attack dogs for conventional medicine. In reality, this was an anticompetitive alliance (and thus in violation of antitrust laws) designed to use the FDA as an instrument to go after targets identified by the drug industry as financially injurious to their trade.

Then in 1986 came the infamous October Plan, says Lisa. In October 1986, yet another new "quack buster" group was organized, this time called Public Issues in Health Care Choices; it later changed its name to Emprise, Inc. In effect, this group drew up a comprehensive shopping hit list of those practices, products, remedies, substances, and individuals in the alternative medicine world—known to them as the realm of "health fraud" requiring "strategic enforcement"—that they deemed worthy of "investigation and evaluation" and FDA harassments, interdictions, propaganda, disinformation, and armed raids. The list was virtually an inventory of everything alternative medicine had to offer: acupuncture ("unproven"), megavitamin therapy ("a nutritional scam"), chelation therapy ("dangerous . . . one of the Top Ten Health Frauds"), as well as at least twelve diagnostic tests and many dozens of biological substances, remedies, and therapeutic programs.

Agencies as diverse as the IRS, Customs, the U.S. Attorney's Office, state departments of justice and bureaus of narcotics and enforcement, among others, subsequently executed raids in seven states against what they described as "dangerously mislabeled prescription drugs." According to Lisa, these dangerous substances included, in part, coenzyme Q10, germanium, essiac, Hoxsey herbs, hydrogen peroxide, laetrile, and selenium.

Based on his research, Lisa contends that "I not only found that there was a major campaign against every single aspect of alternative medicine, I was also able to analyze the data for a common denominator that would explain why organized medicine felt compelled to attack these entities." That common denominator is any form of drugless healing arts, that is, medicine not beholden to patented drugs. It's about money, not therapies, in other words.

"The vested interests want the whole pie and thus more of the profits available in the health-care marketplace," says Lisa. Financial greed and the desire to protect market share is driving the "illegal propaganda campaign" against all the medical alternatives not beholden to the 3,000 toxic drugs catalogued in the *Physicians' Desk Reference*. The result, says Lisa, not holding back any punches, "is nothing less than an enforced totalitarian medical-pharmaceutical police state."

America's Medical Gulag—Attacking Alternative Doctors for Healing Patients

Lisa's provocative thesis was buttressed by the investigative work of criminologist Elaine Feuer, who published her damaging findings in *Innocent Casualties: The FDA's War Against Humanity*. Here Feuer shows how the FDA systematically suppresses truthful information about vitamins, minerals, and other nutritional substances and actively suppresses new companies who seek to market these, especially if they encroach upon the big-dollar diseases such as cancer or AIDS. "The entire orthodox medical establishment," says Feuer, "is threatened by alternative medicine."

The conflict has little to do with science and "everything to do with economics." After all, clinical studies continue to build the case that dietary supplements and botanicals could be successfully used to manage if not reverse most diseases without the cost, toxicity, or side effects of conventional drugs, says Feuer. One well-known physician, upon converting to alternative methods, reduced his prescriptions for pharmaceutical drugs by 90%, Feuer notes. The economic writing is very plainly on the wall as to what would happen if this trend began to multiply.

The implications are obvious: alternative medicine could bankrupt the pharmaceutical industry and deconstruct the medical ideology of allopathy as well. Like Lisa, Feuer is incisive, if not blunt: the FDA is as dangerous as the worst disease and represents an "undercover dictatorship," she asserts. Feuer quotes a former FDA commissioner named Herbert Ley, M.D., who cynically explains the FDA's modus operandi: "The thing that bugs me is that the people think the FDA is protecting them. It isn't. What the FDA is doing and what the public thinks it's doing are as different as night and day." What the FDA is doing, says Feuer, is protecting the economic interests of big medicine at the expense of the health freedoms of 260 million Americans.

Despite the growing favor in which alternative medicine is held by between 34% and 41% of the American public, it is the subject of an all-out war by the conventional medical establishment. In its better moments, this establishment seeks to marginalize, trivialize, and dismiss alternative medicine as feckless folk remedies, without scientific basis. In its grimmer moments, using the FDA as its attack dog, the allopathic establishment stages SWAT-team raids on alternative medicine clinics, breaking down doors and seizing records at gunpoint.

This was the grim experience of licensed doctor Jonathan Wright, M.D., of Tacoma, Washington, in May 1992. He was dispensing nutritional supplements and injecting B vitamins for better absorption at his clinic. Twelve FDA agents in flak vests and ten county policemen knocked down his office doors and burst into his clinic in a commando raid, pointing guns at staff and patients. They followed this with a fourteen-hour search of the premises, after which they seized over

$100,00 in medicines, supplies, records, equipment, even the computer's hard drive. It has been known since as the notorious "B Vitamin Bust." Within 24 hours of this day of infamy in Tacoma, the White House received 2,000 faxes protesting the outrageous raid; eventually, that number swelled to 20,000.

In late 1995, Dr. Wright was exonerated of all charges, his inventory returned by the FDA, and he remains in business. Other well-regarded physicians in New York, North Carolina, Texas, and elsewhere have similarly been harassed, attacked, invaded, subpoenaed, or even indicted for practicing alternative medicine. Most have survived but at great expense; in some cases, the exoneration has taken a decade of legal effort.

So we must ask: why such a disparity between public attitude and governmental policy?

During the Communist era, political dissidents were routinely arrested, subjected to mock trials, imprisoned, and often murdered in the remote Gulags of the Soviet Union, a political travesty exposed by Alexandr Solhenitzsyn in *The Gulag Archipelago.* Thanks to the FDA, conventional medicine trade groups, state medical boards, and the big drug companies, America has its own Gulag for doctors who deviate from the enforced norms and who practice alternative medicine. What the Soviet Union accomplished through state-imposed tyranny, American medicine accomplishes through licensing, regulations, and the FDA: the suppression of your freedom of choice in medical care.

Our American Gulag ruins alternative doctors through suppression, harassment, indictments, licensure revocation, and bankruptcy. To be a hero in this climate of medical terrorism and political intimidation, you need a lot of money, fortitude, and courage. The allopathic Gulag quite effectively blocks the entry of many helpful medical devices and substances into the marketplace, as mounting evidence now clearly shows. The ranks of the American medical Gulag grow every day.

The AMA—Adept at Looking after Medicine's Special Interests

The American Medical Association (AMA), the nation's largest physician's trade group, representing about 41% of American M.D.s, is a prime player in the medlock conspiracy and the American Gulag. You can count on the AMA to look after medicine's special interests. You may not realize it, but the AMA has its hands in every aspect of your everyday life. Founded in 1847, forty-three years after American homeopaths first organized their association, the AMA now looms as a monolithic communicator of medical information—and biases.

Each week its public relations staff sends out news releases to 4,000 medical journalists; they send video news releases to 800 TV outlets; and taped medical reports to 5,000 radio stations. There is probably no other organization on Earth that distributes more words about conventional medicine to doctors and the public than the AMA. Ever wonder why commercial television and most main-stream magazines are so sarcastic and skeptical about alternative medicine?

Just follow the paper trail out of the editor's office back to the AMA. The AMA also works hard to keep certain other words from reaching the public, such as denying public access to the National Practitioner Data Bank, run by the U.S. government, that lists all M.D.s who have committed malpractice, crimes, or ethical viola-tions. For you, the citizen, this information is off limits. To the AMA also goes a fair amount of credit for blocking health care reform in 1994.

Fortunately, the American public is waking up to the AMA's monopolistic control over information and medical practice. M.D.s are no longer the "Marcus Welby" heroes they once were. Polls show that the AMA's public approval rating fell from 59% in 1986 to 43% in 1993. The number of Americans who thought the AMA was a reliable source of information on health declined from a low of 31% in 1989 to a trough of only 23% in 1993. That year polls also showed that 70% of Americans are beginning to lose their faith in conventional doctors. It's highly unlikely they'll do it, given their his-tory, but perhaps the polls are saying it's time the AMA started look-ing after the *patients'* interests for a change.

Then there is the drug industry, America's nonstop profit center. In case you're wondering what is driving U.S. annual health care costs over the unbelievable $1 trillion mark, take a look at recent drug industry statistics to see a major contributing factor. Accord-ing to information reported in 1993, drug prices outside the U.S. were 10% to 70% lower than those charged in America; prescrip-tion drug prices rose about three times higher than inflation between 1980 and 1990 as drug makers boasted annual profits three times higher than the national average for Fortune 500 companies. Further, drug companies spend about $13,000 per U.S. physician in marketing, about 22% of their total sales (about $75.2 billion worldwide) on promotion, and $231 million to develop and patent a single drug.

It's not as if the exceptionally high drug profits are making life any easier for the sick. Patients pay exorbitantly for these "modern medical miracles." For example: a diabetic woman's monthly drug cost is $150; a heart transplant patient shells out $50 a day for anti-rejection pills; a Gaucher's disease patient needs $270,000 a year to pay for his drugs. Herbs are mostly unpatentable and thus unprofitable, so it's easier for drug companies to suppress rather than support them.

That's what keeps "The Club," or the organized conventional medicine establishment, highly profitable, says medical researcher and activist Michael L. Culbert, D.Sc., in his *Medical Armageddon: Behind the Healthcare Calamity of the Western World and How to Fix It,* "While the American expression of the Drug Trust is the focus . . . the international nature of the pharmaceutical octopus cannot be overlooked," writes Culbert, "for it has played a role, both openly and behind the scenes, not only in endlessly producing toxic synthetic compounds for human consumption, but in helping bar the development, use and, distribution of natural therapies at every turn."

A Perennial Ideological Conflict between Allopathy and Empiricism

Are there perhaps reasons beyond the venality of market control and economic share that prompt the allopathic establishment to so strenuously hit on the alternatives? The obvious political machinations of the medical-industrial complex aren't the full story.

The AMA and FDA are recent players in this dialectic. In fact their maneuverings represent only the most recent eruption of a perennial ideological conflict that has divided the medical world and characterized its history ever since Hippocrates first formulated the principles of Western medicine around 450 B.C. in Greece. "The great medical thinkers have all sought a rule or rules permitting correct interpretation of the primary data of experience. History shows that the search for interpretative rules can be conducted along two alternative lines."

Western medical history is marked by the continual struggle, antagonism, and interaction between two fundamentally different views of health, human physiology, and therapeutics—the empirical and the rationalist—explains medical historian Harris Coulter, Ph.D., who brilliantly chronicles their dialectic and the 2,500-year struggle of concept and therapeutics in Western medicine in *Divided Legacy.*

The empirical tradition took its early inspiration from the Skeptics, a Greek philosophical school of the third century B.C., that said knowledge derives from practice and hypotheses originate from experience. The empirics championed the natural *physis* of the human, by which they meant the autonomous, spontaneous, purposeful nature, the organismic vitality and living force within human biology: in short, human *life.* Symptoms, which can be innumerable, are unique to the individual; they represent positive, dynamic signs that the *physis* is already striving to heal itself. The symptom signifies the patient's innate strength, one's ability to constantly, flexibly, creatively counteract the morbific influence. The *physis* in constant, variable reactivity—that's health, that's immune response.

The empirics directly observe the patient, paying meticulous attention to her variegated symptomatology and physiological eccentricity. Each disease is a unique pattern of symptoms requiring an equally specific, individualized therapeutic response; nothing is generic in this symptomatic democracy. The therapeutic response is based on the idea of "similars," medicines that intensify the symptom pattern through energetic similarity with the symptoms (the basis of Samuel Hahnemann's nineteenth-century homeopathy, which means "like suffering, similar pathology"). Similars strengthen and promote the patient's inherent symptomatic reaction like a microdose of *arsenicum* for poisoning.

For the empirics, individualization is paramount, in symptom pattern and remedy. Health and disease are a continuum, an endless process of the *physis;* immune response is organismic and unilateral, not the function merely of one segment of the human system; the patient's physiological reality and needs are foremost; and all healing is self-healing in which the physician merely strengthens the innate *physis.* In its most formal sense, the empirics contended that the *physis* itself is the true physician and medical authority, not the doctor. Here we see how medicine is tacitly political.

If the *physis* is the healer, the patient, not the physician, is foremost, and the relationship justifies consumer medical rights and freedom of choice. The empiric view is upheld today by the homeopaths, naturopaths, herbalists, Ayurvedics—by an eclectic field of what we understand to be holistic, complementary, alternative, or natural medicine.

The assumptions of today's allopaths, in contrast, derive from the rationalist school, which began under the aegis of rigorous, if abstract, Aristotelian logic. The rationalist approach was later formulated by the Greek physician Galen (circa 129 A.D.), "one of the most influential intellectuals the world has ever produced," admits Coulter. The rationalists couldn't countenance the biological carte blanche of the empirics' *physis;* they wanted things tightly categorized, precisely defined, more regulated, more limited. They sought medical certainty in the rules of formal logic, abstract conceptions, and analytical doctrine—a priori theory, in other words. Data derived from experience—living patients—is useful only if it confirms existing ideas.

For the rationalists, the human organism is a predetermined mechanical clockwork whose vitality (or *physis*) derives from its material structure. The body passively suffers morbific assaults from the outside environment; these assaults produce symptoms, which are viewed as wounds, cuts, or pathologies, but not benign processes. Diseases are caused by external, material agents that invade the body, changing a normal physiology into a pathological one.

It's a linear, reductionistic, causal model. Diseases and their agents are finite and can be enumerated; thus only a limited number of remedies are required. Individual symptom patterns are irrelevant (and that includes the patient's past, present lifestyle, or future behavior) because the rationalist seeks the statistical mean, the commonality of symptoms among hundreds of patients. In fact, the individual patient is technically irrelevant, too; of much greater interest for the rationalist is the *Pneumocystis carinii,* or whatever specific, isolated pathology the patient's organism presents.

Rationalist therapeutics, which impose medical theory upon the given physiology, are founded on the doctrine of "contraries" which means medicines ought to oppose (combat) existing pathologies (hence, allopathy, or other/against pathology). Allopathic "contraries" in contemporary jargon are the famed magic bullets, the biomolecularly precise weapon—*anti*biotics, for example—that annihilate the microbial cause. "Contraries" suppress symptoms, beating them into biochemical submission, removing the "wound" of the symptom; the same "contrary" against *Pneumocystis carinii,* for example, is supposed to work for everybody suffering with this opportunistic pneumonia.

In this view, immunity, or the inherent physiological vitality, is most effectively imposed from outside the body by drugs; it is generic, a state-administered "communist" immunology in which everyone gets one shot of penicillin. Since healing is produced by external means, the physician is credited with the cure, in much the way the commanding general of an army takes the kudos of victory. If the physician cures the *physis,* then the physician commands medical authority and AMA political hegemony is philosophically rationalized.

Coulter's exhaustive analysis of the perennial ideological conflict between the empirics and rationalists is especially useful for his insistence on the *political* nature of the struggle. Politics isn't necessarily about truth or medical efficacy; it's about power, authority, and control. "The search for a scientific therapeutics is inhibited by the social and economic forces affecting medical practice and the medical profession. Hence it must be renewed in each generation."

Consider the universally repeated refrain of allopathy—representing today's "majority medicine"—that empirical medicine is unproven, unsubstantiated, and unscientific. Allopaths wield these three words like magic wands, making anything contrary go away. *Unproven* and *unscientific* are probably allopathy's two most potent pejoratives, casting as damaging, dismissive, and unchallenged a stigma upon offenders as the Catholic Church's fifteenth-century A.D. indictment, *witch.* And they might be as unwarranted, too, claims Coulter—politically, but not epistemologically, valid.

Is Modern Medicine "Scientific" and Are Its Claims "Proven"?

Is allopathy really *scientific*? Are the claims of modern medicine that unequivocally *proven*? Or have we been cowed—politically browbeaten—by the strident, authoritative rhetoric? Do they have the last word on what is proven?

These are the kinds of outrageous questions few people seem nervy enough to ask these days—excepting Harris Coulter. He asks them every day; his answers are bound to infuriate most doctors. "Rationalism is alien, both in spirit and structure, to the scientific method of investigation. It meets the social, economic, and organizational needs of the physicians by holding up a false ideal as 'scientific.' The majority of the profession always *imposes* an unscientific therapeutics on society."

The rationalist approach is conceptually unstable, explains Coulter. It reshapes its logical edifice according to the changing fashions of thought and medical "breakthroughs." The rationalist medical model is really very eclectic. The rationalist theory is "continually being pulled in one direction or another by developments in one or the other of its component sciences. In each case the sudden spurt of knowledge in mechanics, chemistry, or mathematics in the nineteenth century seemed to offer the physician a shortcut to therapeutic success, and knowledge from these disciplines was incorporated wholesale into medicine. The absence of a methodical test of the reliability of this knowledge meant that decades passed before physicians realized it was valueless for therapeutics.

"In the meantime the patients had to suffer." Take thalidomide, diethylstilbestrol, or DPT vaccine damages, for example. More recently, in 1991 the *Journal of the American Medical Association (JAMA)* published an article (delayed four years owing to internal AMA controversy) that announced one of the standard antimicrobial therapies for childhood ear infection (secretory otitis media) didn't work. This meant that pediatricians who had been telling parents for years that amoxicillin with decongestant antihistamine, the standard medical treatment for persistent asymptomatic middle ear infusions in infants and children, had been mistaken. According to Erdem I. Cantekin, Ph.D., writing in JAMA, this approach "is not effective."

In contrast the organon of homeopathy, Hahnemann's "science of experience," which relies on symptomatic description, has proven remarkably stable for nearly 200 years. Here what is once proven, stays proven. The empirics constantly seek new information derived from direct observation. The therapeutic hypothesis originates in experience, then it's continually tested through the physician's daily practice. Hahnemann developed homeopathy's extensive repertory through carefully monitored "provings," on healthy patients; these "provings" revealed invariable physiological realities, and the remedies work as remarkably well in 1993 as they did in 1810, when he published his *Organon.*

The observation and experience of symptomatology is para-mount for the empiric, but for the rationalist, it's the abstraction that takes precedence. Physiological facts must fit the medical the-ory and assumed pathological process or they are dismissed as irrelevant. The rationalists strive to impose a preexisting body of inferred knowledge—dogma accepted on faith, in other words—upon the human condition. Further, the allopathic diagnosis never points unambiguously to a single medicine, as does homeopathy; at best, it's approximate, dependent on the physician's judgment because "there is no necessary or immediate relationship between the diagnosis and the remedy." That's hardly scientific; it's more like guesswork.

"Nor can it be tested in practice, since all practice, observation, and experience have been reinterpreted in terms of this very hypoth-esis," continues Coulter. "They're carried along by the force of abstract ideas and very quickly move away from the actual, living patient. They're not really open to ideas from outside allopathy. They don't walk around to see what is happening; they don't practice what the empirics call 'shoe-leather epidemiology.'" The rationalist model is inherently imprecise, approximate, and unstable—it's a dogma of authority, not science. It puts the professional needs of the physician first, whereas for the empirics, the patient is always paramount. The empirical attitude, because it values every idiosyncratic symptom in determining the diagnosis, is actually more rational than the ratio-nalists, says Coulter.

"Empiricism is the ideology which best meets the needs of the physician oriented toward the scientific practice of medicine," con-cludes Coulter. "Once exposed to empiricism, the layman feels instinctively at home with it—for its reliance on sensory data, its sympathy with the lay contribution to medicine, and, not least of all, for its therapeutic efficacy."

But as Coulter makes so clear, therapeutic efficacy too often is subject to politics, and in the conflict between the empirics and rationalists, allopathic politics have wielded the upper, iron-gloved hand for the last 100 years. Consider the seventeen-year controver-sy over the comparative therapeutic efficacy of megadoses of vitamin C for cancer, proposed in the early 1970s by Nobel laureate Linus Pauling and Ewan Cameron, a Scottish surgeon, and interferon, the synthetic anticancer drug (made from recombinant DNA) forward-ed by the allopathic-pharmaceutical interests. The episode starkly reveals "the necessarily social character of medical knowledge" and "the vested interests and social objectives which it embodies," comments Evelleen Richards, senior lecturer in the Department of Science and Technology Studies at the University of Wollongong, Australia, in a brilliant analysis of the allopathic politics of medical epistemology.

Allopathy has secured for its medical knowledge a "privileged epistemological status," a "cognitive authority," contends Richards, with the effect that "the idea of neutral appraisal is a myth." Allopathy may assert its knowledge is pure science, but at best it's applied knowledge, argues Richards. Medicine is not neutral, its claims of value-neutrality and objectivity are fallacious, and its professional knowledge is "value-laden—dogmatic, biased, distorted—and its efficacy and reliability are suspect." The medical profession's "control over what is to count as knowledge, its cognitive authority, is thus clearly political in nature."

Pauling and Cameron, who were lambasted by the allopaths in a process of "professional marginalization and exclusion," were up against a stacked deck: they had to prove their therapeutic claims against a "powerful adjudicating medical community" who were also their professional opponents. They were up against "medicine's self-interested hegemony over the determination and evaluation of medical knowledge." Vitamin C is inexpensive, nonpatentable, and patient empowering, because a physician isn't required to administer it—none of which allopathy likes because it's accustomed to "medicine as an institution of social control," says Richards.

Allopathic clinical trials to adjudicate the possible efficacy of vitamin C, a holistic-empiric remedy, are inherently at odds, a function of "socioeconomic and political structuring of professional judgments." As a result, "we must expect, as recent sociology of scientific knowledge suggests, that clinical trials, no matter how rigorous their methodology, will inevitably embody the values or commitments of the assessors, and that they will not provide definitive answers."

The history of the vitamin C and cancer controversy, says Richards, "is best understood as a political struggle concerning control over the determination and evaluation of cancer treatment . . . We may infer further that the very notion of efficacy is politically defined and defended, and the practical success of a therapy is asserted and sustained by the power of the interests that sponsor and maintain it . . . . These conflicts must be treated as essentially political issues where there are *no* impartial experts."

In a climate in which medical knowledge is a political, not epistemological, struggle, the vaccination controversy is perhaps the most recent expression of this age-old dialectic. But what's really at play is a political struggle for control of the human immune system. It's about how the human *physis* shall be allowed to respond to disease, whether through empiric promotion or rationalist suppression. Shall we have empiric individuality or rationalist conformity? There's a simple equation here: *physis* equals immune response. That's why immunology is a political issue and why immunological freedom ought to be the cause célèbre for our lifetime.

"The allopathic paradigm in medicine is duplicated by the allopathic socioeconomic structure for delivering medical services," says Coulter. "The medical school curriculum is organized around disease concepts, as are hospitals, insurance company reimbursement provisions, and pharmaceutical research. We're not just talking now about an M.D. who could go one way or the other. The way that's been established for practicing allopathy for the last 150 years now has an enormous superstructure dependent upon it to make its living from a given way of perceiving the phenomena of disease."

A Salutary Awakening
from the Propaganda Trance

My intention is to point out some of the ways in which that deep-set assumption is linguistically set within our public discussion of medical issues and to suggest critical tools we might wield to disentangle ourselves from its pessimistic, disempowering attitudes. Let's review and summarize our findings about the allopathic view of the world.

The allopathic model is palliative, emphasizing the removal of symptoms and quick results. It's authoritarian, stressing management, control, and the preemptive wisdom of doctor's orders. This approach relies on mechanistic modeling, technological intervention, and organic substitution (transplantation, synthetic drugs, immunizations) using assembly-line methods typical of profit-hungry capitalism. Costs and patient-dependency escalate as disease and disability are seen "in terms of victimization and melodrama," as Walene James notes in *Immunization: The Reality Behind the Myth.*

Allopathy, as Harris Coulter outlined above, is an implicitly fragmenting system, treating mind and body separately; disease is an invasive, adversarial process, separate from the patient, whose causality is external, environmental. The whole approach focuses on labeling, controlling, and removing disease organisms such that health is the absence of disease and the result of allopathy's high-tech interventionist triumph. The attitude is "monolithic and coercive," the military rhetoric predominant, and the system turns on fear, distrust of the natural world, and "disease-scare."

It should be obvious by now that before we can put our life back in our own hands, we must penetrate the veil of allopathic propaganda embedded in our language and constantly reiterated in our mainstream media. We must "awaken from the propaganda trance and deprogram ourselves from the tyranny of what everyone knows," says James. We have to cease being "enthralled" by the mentality of attack and victimization. "We need a new paradigm of connectedness, cooperation, holism, stewardship, and self-empowerment. Our information system will have to open up to the idea of the validity of different models of reality."

Clearly one hopes that eventually the old allopathic paradigm, that politicized therapeutic ideology so expertly maintained by AMA-faithful editors, will dissolve and release its "victims" from their "afflictions." In the spirit of holistic self-empowerment, we can begin that process of disentanglement today by extricating our words, images, and thinking from the pervasive colonization of a waning ideology.

The Environment's Two Faces

Environment, the theme of this book, has two faces: our body, our world; two processes: immunology and ecology; and two domains: human and planet. Both faces are experiencing major problems, systemic dysfunction, even potential collapse, yet they needn't. Both, I contend, need reconsideration in light of our health care system—or perhaps I should say, the health care debate ought to focus its discussion around a reconsideration of the meaning and dynamics of our twofold environment of body and planet.

Medicine has effects and ramifications not only for our bodies, our physiological environment, but also for the landscape, our planetary environment. I hope this book may help shift the focus of public discussion in this underacknowledged direction. I pro-pose that the fate of both human and planetary environments is significantly contingent on our style of medical practice.

Our attitudes about and approach to our environment, both the inner, immunological terrain of the body and the outer, ecological terrain of the planet, derive from a tacit philosophy. I suggest that this implicit philosophy is largely informed and nourished by our prevailing model of medicine; or, we can best see it exemplified in the practices of Western medicine. A medical view can be appreci-ated as a philosophy of matter, as an environmental policy; a med-ical view instructs us in how to interact with matter to get desired results; it hands us the keys to apparent efficacy in our manipula-tion of matter.

In the broadest sense, there are basically two medical views in the world today. These are the *allopathic,* which is an exclusionary, mechanistic, fragmenting view that says consciousness is a passive by-product of matter, which operates by automatic, predictable laws; and the *empiric,* which is an inclusionary, organic, holistic view that says material environments are shaped and inhabited by active consciousness. At the present time in American cultural his-tory, the allopathic model predominates while the empiric flourish-es on the sociomedical fringes.

The present appalling condition of our inner and outer environ-ments is traceable in part to our allegiance to the allopathic phi-losophy of matter. Few will dispute the observation that our ecological environment is imperiled and our immunological envi-ronment is increasingly dysfunctional. In this book I propose that a primary consequence of our favoring and entrenching the allo-pathic model of environment is that a crucial life element has been omitted—in fact, denied—from the inner and outer environment. That element is human consciousness, the potency and efficacy of the mind.

The empiric model accords consciousness, or mind, full legiti-macy in its model of illness and healing, while the allopathic rele-gates it to a secondary, derivative role. I will propose in this book that to rectify the ravages of our inner and outer environment we must reinstate consciousness as a prime player in the life of matter. To help make this clear, I will describe certain aspects of empiric, holistic medicine in action as they exemplify this consciousness-affirming principle.

Much of this book will explore the contents and consequences of these two diametrically opposed medical/philosophical views as they play out their polarity in our bodies and the landscape. I say philosophical because although on the surface the topics we'll consider apparently pertain to current medical issues, at heart, basic philosophies, even epistemologies—a complete structure of reality as we conceive it—underlie and enliven this polarity. A great deal more than who will pay our monthly insurance premium is at stake in America's discussion about health care reform.

Our choice of medical practice—allopathic or empiric—is the direct result of our philosophical conclusions regarding humanity, our environment, and the dynamics of this interaction. As we choose our medical practices, so we choose how we build our minds, bodies, and souls—our inner environment of self—and how, from this context, we relate to the outer environment, our natural world. In fairness, I am not arguing for the sole ascendancy of empiric medicine and the decline of allopathic.

Far more rational and balanced would be a therapeutic blend of both, each in its appropriate therapeutic category, *freely* chosen by the informed health care consumer and *freely* sanctioned by a truly competitive and open medical services marketplace. This is not presently the case in America. Empiric medicine does not have free reign in the marketplace.

Contemplating this charged philosophical dialectic waged in the guise of medical practices, we find that consciousness is in search of an environment. But what do I mean by consciousness? Indeed, this is one of the prime questions of philosophy, both Eastern and Western; its elucidation has challenged and vexed the best and sub- tlest minds in the worlds. I don't claim to have a brilliant and orig- inal resolution to this archetypal question, but I will try to indicate some of the aspects of this big concept that I find relevant to this topic. In the strictest sense, I construe consciousness as the unique distinction of humankind.

By *consciousness,* I don't mean mere sentience, environmental or proprioceptive awareness, because animals possess that. Nor do I mean simply *mind,* as we commonly understand the term, as the ability to manipulate mental constructs; and to equate mind with consciousness is to travel in a circle, cycling round and round none the wiser. Nor do I mean consciousness as being simply our sense of self-identity, the notion of a continuity of identity, a consistent

I-ness, or a congruent personality as narrated and affirmed by the inner monologue.

To describe consciousness as "self-aware awareness" is more useful; this means "I am aware of myself being aware." It's a reflexive, self-referential kind of awareness, an awareness turned in on itself like a mirror contemplating a mirror or an inward spiral of attention. Eastern philosophies suggest that consciousness, or awareness, exists in a hierarchy of layers like the strata of an onion, each revealing a more exalted domain of cognition and being. Ultimately, the whole created universe is a field of consciousness, say the Eastern sages; matter is densified consciousness; the whole world is the manifold myriad play of consciousness; the ultimate particle is consciousness.

At this rarified spiritual level, qualities begin to blur for us: consciousness, being, light, God—they seem to be interchangeable conditions. They are aspects of what Deepak Chopra, M.D., a leading explicator of holistic medical philosophy, calls "the unified field, the self, pure Being, which is the source of all abundance and affluence in the universe . . . the mind of God, the field of all possibilities . . . a field of infinite, unbounded intelligence." However we model it, in this view consciousness is the primary, irreducible first and last principle of existence, whether its mode of expression is a human being or a planet. This is the implicit assumption underlying empiric medicine.

Of course, outside of religious and perhaps metaphysical circles, this is not how we think about humans and planet in the West. For most of us, our educational experience has consisted of a steady indoctrination in the view that matter is inert, automatic, accidental, and capable of machinelike manipulation. Consciousness may be *applied to* matter from the outside, but it does not inhabit, shape, or create matter, says allopathic thinking. Human beings *have* consciousness, of course, just as we have legs and arms, but consciousness is not what we are; it is only a possession. It is produced by the physical brain (in the same way the lungs "produce" carbon dioxide for exhalation) and it disappears when the brain (and the rest of the body) dies or is seriously incapacitated (such as in coma).

As such, says allopathy, consciousness has no legitimate role in scientific investigations; scientists consistently try to rule out its presence or effects in experiments or theories, regarding the consciousness factor as the ultimate intrusion of subjectivity and thus the contamination of all research.

As consciousness has no legitimate place in science, so has it no dwelling place or primacy in our environment, whether it's the body or planet. Our standard Western model has stripped consciousness of primacy in the world; science and allopathic medicine have exiled consciousness from the human and planetary environment. We have awareness, but that's because of prodigious efforts of our physical brain and its complex perceptual processes. We are aware that we transiently occupy complex physical organisms, but that awareness, or consciousness, is a special privilege easily revoked by illness, accident, or death.

Similarly, we are aware of the outer environment; we exert effects on it through our hands, tools, and technologies, which are the products of our mind; but this is not to say we can effect the environment directly without mediation and solely with our mind. That's magic, animism, primitive belief, superstition—and impossible, say the scientists.

These assumptions are familiar to all of us and they are implicit in the allopathic attitude toward environment, both human and planetary. They are at the heart of allopathic thinking and practice; but do they accord with our experience, intuitions, and expectations? Do we really want such an inert, mechanistic environment? I think not, as I think many men and women will once they realize what is at stake and how their views have been shaped by a particular philosophy of matter. Already a significant population is aware of the philosophical politics of medicine and is supporting empiric medicine; but an even larger population is still reluctantly in thrall to the intellectual power structure of allopathy. The health care debate and the revelation of its economic and power structure and increasingly ineffectual high-tech interventions may change many minds.

Some courage is required because empiric medicine, as it accords consciousness a primary role, asks much of the person under its care. Empiric medicine requires that we actively take responsibility for our environments; consciousness is a cocreative power that each of us is entitled, in fact expected, to wield on behalf of our environments. In this book, I will propose that prevailing allopathic attitudes be superceded by a more "magical" position that affirms that consciousness inhabits, sustains, rejuvenates, transforms, even creates environment without the mediation of external technologies or devices, but solely out of the potency of its own awareness. Under allopathy, consciousness is in search of an environment; under empiric medicine, consciousness *is* the environment.

A Medical Paradigm
Is a Political Issue

So it is important to be meticulously aware of the dynamics of the paradigm that informs our environmental policies. Allopathy, the name for conventional Western medicine, is the science of parts and fragments that divides, measures, and quantifies an inert, mechanical world; for the allopathic paradigm, matter is primary, manipulable only by mechanical or biochemical interventions.

Empiricism, the older name for what's now understood as holistic medicine, is the perception of the human and world as whole, reciprocal, mutually interdependent organisms, as complementary domains infused with intelligence and awareness. For the empiric paradigm, energy is primary, which implies that matter is manipulable by multiple means, including complementary energy configurations and directed consciousness, both of which are tools of holistic therapies. Between the two models spans a chasm across which our rights of passage are legislated by the politics of medicine.

The matter of paradigm is a profoundly *political* issue; we are dealing here intimately and profoundly with the body politic. Currently this dialectic—and our rights of passage—is being played out intensely in the politics of medical practice and licensure, the reform of which is awaiting our recognition to make it *the* political issue of the times.

Our democratic rights are compromised in areas we're not normally aware of and wouldn't think to examine for infringements. A medical view is not only philosophical, but also political and spiritual—awesomely so. Our choice (or, through passivity, nonchoice) of paradigm makes all the difference in how we experience and manage the world and how we bodily fulfill our lives. A paradigm is implicitly political—the foundation in fact of all political views, policies, and programs. The freedom of medical view (which implies the right to practice) is the *core* democratic right, because it effects us at the molecular, immunological foundations of our being. As I'll argue in this book, that fundamental democratic freedom is at present indefensibly abrogated by an *enforced*, exclusive, monopolistic allopathic medical system.

As we're painfully learning, the agricultural practice of mono-culture—single crop domination—ruins farmland, depleting its immunological vitality. Similarly, we're on the verge of learning that the medical practice of monotherapy—single therapeutic view, dominated by allopathy—ruins human health, depleting our immunological competency. Either way, whether the context is agriculture or immunology, it's a vitiation of our precious envi-ronment through practices founded on faulty premises. It all fol-lows, inevitably, from how we *position* things—our body, our ecosystem—in what conceptual framework we embed them.

The verb *position* describes an active, creative process of con-sciousness, far more dynamic an event than the verbs *perceive* or *conceive* convey, and more comprehensive, too, than the related verb *construct*. *Position* includes the functions of perception, con-ception, and construction, but takes the process further. But it's all done on the sly: we position environment, then officially deny it, pleading this is how reality really is, that it's not the relative result of our positioning. From here it's not such a great progression to victim status, in which we become victims of our own positioning; America, as we know, is increasingly (if oxymoronically) the land of the activist victim—"a nation of victims," as one commentator observes, or "a culture of complaint," in the view of another.

The pivotal issue in positioning environment, and one that sharply divides the allopathic and empiric paradigms, is conscious-ness. Consciousness—unilateral, synoptic awareness that is self-reflexive, aware of itself being aware, aware of its primal potency—is the core and foundation of being human. Is it present or is it absent? Is it competent or ineffectual, primary or secondary, active or passive? Is it commissioned or paralyzed?

The allopathic view asserts that consciousness is the secondary by-product of physical, material processes, a transient, biologically dependent bodily resident; but the empirical model argues the for-mative primacy of consciousness, that consciousness is biologically interdependent, the immortal mother of material processes. The debate comes down to a crucial metaphysical question: does matter produce and form consciousness or does consciousness effect, shape, even form, matter? Health—our inner immunological and the outer ecological—hangs in the balance. What position shall we take?

This in itself is a democratic right, however strange and disastrous when it's executed—to conceive of environment wrongly. If we decide affirmatively that human consciousness is a primogenitive, formative, residential force, legitimately occupying our environment, from T cells to mountains, then the issue of environment suddenly reconfigures and we see immunology and ecology in their correct context, as equivalent, coincident environmental concerns malleable through directed human consciousness. AIDS is an ecological concern; ozone depletion is an immunological concern; both are distortions of environment. In light of this reconfiguration, the enforced domination of one paradigm—in this case, the allopathic in our acutely medicalized America—is philosophically mistaken, sociologically criminal, and environmentally antidemocratic.

Allopathy is more than a therapeutic style. It is a philosophy, a politics, and an ideology that positions the human self (whose core is consciousness) in *opposition* to the environment, both inner and outer. Disease invades the human, creating illness; medicine overpowers the infectious agents, restoring health. That's how allopathy positions the disease-health process; it's the classic nineteenth-century germ theory as put forth by Louis Pasteur.

But for empirics—practitioners of holistic, complementary, energy medicines such as homeopathy, naturopathy, acupuncture, herbalism, and chiropractic—disease is precipitated by internal susceptibility and managed by microbial agents as a consequence of aberrations of self; healing is generated when the innate life force is encouraged to restore homeostasis and the self regains coherency. In the allopathic model, the self is disenfranchised, a passive consumer of medical care; in the empiric view, the self (or consciousness) is the prime player on whose behalf the biological drama of illness is undertaken.

The underacknowledged political dialectic of our time is being waged in medicine by physicians. Medicine is a philosophy, a paradigm of the human, and thereby tacitly political. Our health, immune function, intellect, emotionality, spirituality, and evolution, both personal and phylogenetic, hang in the balance. What is most crucially at stake is the freedom of the *physis,* the vital human life force—the autonomous, spontaneous, purposeful nature, the organismic vitality and living force within biology. Chinese medicine calls it *chi;* the Western metaphysical tradition calls it the *etheric body;* homeopathy calls it the *dynamis.* The *physis* is that aspect of the human totality that responds to the environment on behalf of the life process when presented with an infection, disease, or illness. *Physis* is the vital life spark in the physical. But whatever we call it, the *physis* is in jeopardy today.

The *physis* is in jeopardy today because modern scientific allopathy, the prevailing mechanistic, materialist model underlying Western medicine, has commandeered it. Allopathy has hijacked the human *physis* inwardly through enforced vaccinations, antibiotics, and invasive, militaristic therapeutics, and outwardly through the medical practices acts which guarantee M.D.s a virtual medical monopoly in this country and prohibit or restrict through licensure the free practice of natural *physis*-friendly therapeutics (most significantly, homeopathy, naturopathy, and acupuncture).

Allopathy has commandeered us intellectually by coloring with its biases the way we think about, understand, position, and describe illness. In practical terms, this means as individuals we do not have the choice in most instances to allow our organism—the *physis*—to respond to an illness process in any way other than the allopathic interventionist approach. This is a violation of our medical freedom and an infringement of the basic democratic right of individuality.

Following Cartesian dualistic thinking—mind versus body, matter versus spirit, environment versus self, biology versus medicine—allopathy has institutionalized—socially, therapeutically, and politically—a philosophical attitude that says the human body is an inert, unintelligent machine with a lot of plumbing manipulable only by outside biochemical, surgical, or genetic interventions. Consciousness, says allopathy, is an epiphenomenal side effect of an efficient, smoothly running system.

Since the body is a bionic machine, it can be added to (organ transplants) or subtracted from (surgical excision) according to the technical competence of the physician. Allopathy officially—and legally—keeps us fragmented and unintegrated as humans, alienated from our biological context, the body, and disempowered and disenfranchised with respect to the formative, regenerative, and biology-shaping possibilities of human consciousness.

It requires only a slight surrealistic twist to appreciate the hidden meaning in this recent newspaper headline: "Shift Is Historic: Federal Decision Allows Doctors to Prescribe Drugs to End Life." Technically, the headline referred to a federal appeals court decision in New York State allowing physician-assisted suicides, but it may also be read as suggestive of allopathy's inevitable goal: death by drugs.

There are already so many conventional drugs that are toxic, even deadly, by "side effect"—"chemotherapeutic" is the euphemism—that now it is official: drugs may be used to kill directly.

The vast conglomerate of insurance companies, hospitals, physicians, pharmaceutical companies, and physician trade associations keep this philosophical domination institutionalized through an economic matrix in American society. One of the results is the awesome, untenable, unaffordable $900 billion a year medical services bill—the world's largest—which no agency in the U.S. can possibly pay for anymore. The burgeoning debate about health care reform and possible nationalization of health insurance coverage are bringing these underlying issues to light. Key questions will be forced to the surface: Why are we so sick? Why does medical care cost so much? Are there cheaper, more effective alternatives? One of this book's intentions is to provide a therapeutic and philosophical rationale for the optimistic "yes" to these questions.

References

Adams, E.K., and Zuckerman, S., "Variation in the Growth and Incidence of Medical Malpractice Claims," *Journal of Political Policy Law,* Vol. 9, No. 3, (Fall 1984).

Alternative Medicine, "Too Many M.D.s Don't Listen to Their Patients," Issue 6, (April 1995).

—"Patients Want Alternative Medicine," Issue 6, (April 1995).

—"The AMA—Looking After Medicine's Special Interests," Issue 7, (June 1995).

—"America's Medical Gulag," Issue 10, (January 1996).

—"69% of Americans Use Alternative Medicine," Issue 28, (March 1999): 89.

—"37% of Americans Use Herbal Supplements," Issue 25, (August/September 1998): 109.

—"81% Growth in Canadians' Alternative Medicine Use," Issue 24, (June/July 1998): 107.

—"Sales of Nutritional Supplements Up 19%—Medicinal Self-Care Emphasis Strong," Issue 27, (December 1998/January 1999): 106.

Angier, Natalie, "Bedside Manners Improve as More Women Enter Medicine," *New York Times*, (June 21, 1992).

Astin, John A., Ph.D., "Why Patients Use Alternative Medicine: Results of a National Study," *Journal of the American Medical Association* 279:19 (May 20, 1998): 1548-1553.

Ausubel, Ken, "Cancer Cures—An Outbreak of Controversy: The Silent Treatments," *New Age Journal*, (September/October 1989).

Beardsley, Tim, "Fads and Feds," *Scientific American*, (September 1993).

Begneaud, W.P., "Obstetric and Gynecologic Malpractice in Louisiana: Incidence and Impact," *Journal of the Louisiana State Medical Society*, Vol. 141, No. 9, (September 1989).

Belkin, Lisa, "On Their Own, More Parents Raise Funds to Fight Disease," *The New York Times*, (April 14, 1993).

Berlin, L., "Malpractice and Radiologists Update, 1986: an 11.5 Year Perspective," *American Journal of Roentgenology*, Vol. 147, No. 6, (December 1986).

Blevins, Sue. *The Medical Monopoly, Protecting Consumers or Limiting Competition?* Policy Analysis No. 246, December 15, 1995, Cato Institute, Washington, D.C.

Bloyd-Peshkin, Sharon, "The Health-Fraud Cops—Are the Quack Busters Consumer Advocates or Medical McCarthyites?" *Vegetarian Times*, (August 1991).

Booth, Michael. "State charges Springs dentist," *The Denver Post*, (August 30, 1995).

Blumberg, Daniel L., M.D., et al., "The Physician and Unconventional Medicine," *Alternative Therapies*, Vol. 1, No. 3, (July 1995).

Brimelow, Peter, and Spencer, Leslie, "The Plaintiff Attorneys' Great Honey Rush," *Forbes*, (October 16, 1989).

Brown, Donald. "SELF Magazine Surveys Readers on Use of Alternative Medicine," *Quarterly Review of Natural Medicine*, (Summer 1994).

Bruni, Frank. "Court Overtuns Ban in New York on Aided Suicides," *The New York Times*, (April 3, 1996).

Caldwell, Mark, "The Transplanted Self," *Discover,* (April 1992).

Callinan, Paul, "A Guide to Natural Drugless Systems of Medicine," *Australian Well-Being,* No. 47, (April 1992).

Chappell, L.J., et al., "A Survey of Obstetric Malpractice in Western Frontier States," *Family Medicine,* Vol. 22, No. 3, (May-June 1990).

Clark, Matt, "Headaches—New Drugs and Advancing Research Offer Hope for 45 Million Chronic Victims," *Newsweek,* (December 7, 1987).

Classe, J.G., "A Review of 50 Malpractice Claims," *Journal of the American Optometric Association,* Vol. 60, No. 9, (September 1989).

Competitive Enterprise Institute, *A National Survey of Oncologists Regarding the Food and Drug Administration,* (Washington, D.C., 1995).

Consumer Reports, "How is Your Doctor Treating You?" (February 1995).

Coulter, Harris L., *Divided Legacy: Twentieth Century Medicine—The Bacteriological Era. A History of the Schism in Medical Thought,* Vol. IV, North Atlantic Books and Center for Empirical Medicine, Berkeley, CA, 1994.

—*AIDS and Syphilis: The Hidden Link,* North Atlantic Books, Berkeley, 1987.

—*Divided Legacy: A History of the Schism in Medical Thought, Volume 1—The Patterns Emerge: Hippocrates to Paracelsus,* Wehawken Book Company, Washington D.C., 1975.

—*Divided Legacy: The Conflict Between Homoeopathy and the American Medical Association—Science and Ethics in American Medicine, 1800-1914,* North Atlantic Books, Richmond, 1973.

—*Divided Legacy: The Origins of Modern Western Medicine: J.B. Van Helmont to Claude Bernard,* Wehawken/North Atlantic Books, Berkeley, 1988.

—*The Controlled Clinical Trial,* Center for Empirical Medicine/Project Cure, Washington, D.C., 1991.

—*Vaccination, Social Violence, and Criminality: The Medical Assault on the American Brain,* North Atlantic Books, Berkeley, 1990.

—and Fisher, Barbara Loe, *A Shot in the Dark: Why the P in the DPT Vaccination May Be Hazardous to Your Child's Health,* Avery Publishing Group, Garden City Park, 1991.

Culbert, Michael L. D.Sc., *Medical Armageddon: Behind the Healthcare Calamity of the Western World and How to Fix It*, C and C Communications, San Diego, 1995.

"CPR's Effects are Glamorized on Television, a Study Says," *The New York Times,* (June 17, 1996).

"Doctor Forced Into Bankruptcy," *FDA Hotline,* Vol. 2, No. 11, (November 1995).

Driedger, Sharon Doyle, "Healthy Options: The Poll Finds Strong Support for Alternative Treatments," *Maclean's,* (December 29, 1997): 36.

Dwyer, John M., *The Body at War: The Miracle of the Immune System,* New American Library, New York, 1989.

Egan, Timothy. "Seattle Officials Seeking to Establish a Subsidized Natural Medicine Clinic," *The New York Times,* (January 3, 1996).

Eisenberg, David M., M.D., et al., "Unconventional Medicine in the United States—Prevalence, Costs, and Patterns of Use," *The New England Journal of Medicine,* (January 28, 1993): Vol. 238, No. 4: 246-252.

Fanning, Deirdre, "Rx for Medical Malpractice Suits," *Forbes,* (April 18, 1988).

Feuer, Elaine, *Innocent Casualties: The FDA's War Against Humanity,* Dorrance Publishing, (Pittsburgh, 1995).

Findlay, Steven, Podolsky, Doug, and Silberner, Joanne, "Wonder Cures from the Fringe," *U.S. News and World Report,* (September 23, 1991).

Firshein, Janet. "Picture Alternative Medicine in the Mainstream," *Business and Health,* (April 1995).

Fisher, Peter, and Ward, Adam. "Complementary Medicine in Europe," *British Medical Journal,* Vol. 309, (July 9, 1994).

Freudenheim, Milt, "Dealing in Myths on Malpractice," *The New York Times,* (October 13, 1992).

—"People Want More Information for Health Choices, Survey Finds," *The New York Times,* (September 18, 1995).

Gaby, Alan R., M.D., "NIH and Alternative Medicine," *Townsend Letter for Doctors,* (February/March 1993).

Garelik, Glenn, "Exorcising a Damnable Disease," *Discover,* (December 1986).

Garr, D.R., and Marsh, F.J., "Medical Malpractice and the Primary Care Physician: Lowering the Risks," *Southern Medical Journal*, Vol. 79, No. 10, (October 1986).

Geisel, Jerry, "Malpractice Costs Rapidly Rising: GAO," *Business Insurance*, (September 29, 1986).

Gelman, David, "Depression," *Newsweek*, (May 4, 1987).

Goldberg, R.J., et al, "A Review of Prehospital Care Litigation in a Large Metropolitan EMS System," *Annals of Emergency Medicine*, Vol. 19, No. 5, (May 1990).

Goldman, Erik L., "Dissatisfied Patients Embracing 'Alternative' Therapy," *Internal Medicine News and Cardiology News*, Vol. 25, No. 11, (June 1, 1992).

Golub, Edward S., and Green, Douglas R., *Immunology: A Synthesis*, Second Edition, Sinauer Associates, Sunderland, 1991.

Gordon, R.J., "The Effects of Malpractice Insurance on Certified Nurse-Midwives," *Journal of Nurse Midwifery*, (March-April 1990).

Gorman, Christine, "New Ally Against Heart Disease," *Time*, (September 14, 1987).

—"New Clues to Detecting a Killer," *Time*, (August 24, 1987).

Grady, Denise, "The Ticking of a Time Bomb in the Genes," *Discover*, (June 1987).

Grossinger, Richard. *Planet Medicine: Origins*. North Atlantic Books, Berkeley, 1995.

Grünwald, Jörg, Ph.D., "The European Phytomedicines Market, Figures, Trends, Analyses," *HerbalGram*, (Summer 1995).

Harvard Medical Practice Study, *Patients, Doctors, and Lawyers: Medical Injury Malpractice Litigation, and Patient Compensation in New York*, Boston, 1990.

Health, "Communication Breakdown: Who's to Blame?" (November/December 1995).

Hollabaugh, E.S., et al, "Patient Personal Injury Litigation Against Dermatology Residency Programs in the United States, 1964-1988," *Archives of Dermatology*, Vol. 126, No. 5, (May 1990).

Illich, Ivan. *Medical Nemesis. The Expropriation of Health*, Pantheon Books, New York, 1976.

Inlander, Charles B., Levin, Lowell S., and Weiner, Ed, *Medicine on Trial: The Appalling Story of Ineptitude, Malfeasance, Neglect, and Arrogance,* Prentice Hall Press, Englewood Cliffs, 1988.

James, Walene, *Immunization: The Reality Behind the Myth,* Bergin and Garvey, South Hadley, 1988.

Jaroff, Leon, "Allergies—Nothing to Sneeze At," *Time,* (June 22, 1992).

—"Steps Towards a Brave New World," *Time,* (July 13, 1987).

—"Stop That Germ!" *Time,* (May 23, 1988).

"Jury Indicts Texas Doctor on 75 Counts," *The New York Times,* (October 26, 1995).

Kelly, Michael, "The Road to Paranoia," *The New Yorker,* (June 19, 1995).

Kirchfeld, Friedhelm, and Boyle, Wade. *Nature Doctors. Pioneers in Naturopathic Medicine.* Medicina Biologica, Portland (Oregon), 1994.

Kolata, Gina, "Lorenzo's Oil: A Movie Outruns Science," *The New York Times,* (February 9, 1993).

—"On Fringes of Health Care, Untested Therapies Thrive," *The New York Times,* (June 17, 1996).

Levine, Joe, "Viruses—AIDS Research Spurs New Interest in Some Ancient Enemies," *Time,* (November 3, 1986).

Leviton, Richard, "The Body Battlefield," *East West,* (July 1989).

—"The Malpractice Dilemma," *East West,* (March 1991).

—"America's Medical Gulag—Attacking Doctors," *Alternative Medicine Digest,* No. 10, (January 1996).

Lewin, Tamar, "Philadelphia Doctors to be Offered Data on Patients Who Have Sued," *The New York Times,* (August 27, 1993).

Lisa, P. Joseph, *The Assault on Medical Freedom.* Hampton Roads, Norfolk, Virginia, 1994.

Mendelsohn, Robert S., M.D., *Male Practice—How Doctors Manipulate Women,* Contemporary Books, Chicago, 1981.

Milner, Martin, N.D., and Bergner, Paul, "Insurance Reimbursement in Oregon," *AANP Quarterly Newsletter,* Vol. 5, No. 2., (1990).

Monmaney, Terence, "Preying on AIDS Patients," *Newsweek,* (June 1, 1987).

—"Vaccines for Adult Diseases," *Newsweek,* (October 12, 1987).

—"Young Survivors in a Deadly War," *Newsweek,* (July 18, 1988).

Nelkin, Dorothy, and Tancredi, Laurence, *Dangerous Diagnostics: The Social Power of Biological Information,* Basic Books, New York, 1989

Park, Robert L., and Goodenough, Ursula, "Buying Snake Oil with Tax Dollars," *The New York Times,* (January 3, 1996).

Pear, Robert, "Medical Malpractice Study Finds Unjust Payments are Rare," *The New York Times,* (November 1, 1992).

Procter, Robert N., *Cancer Wars: How Politics Shapes What We Know and Don't Know About Cancer,* Basic Books, New York, 1995.

Raterman, Karen, et al., "NFM's 17th Annual Market Overview '97," *Natural Foods Merchandiser* XIX:6, (June 1998).

Reynolds, R.A., Rizzo, J.A., and Gonzalez, M.L., "The Cost of Medical Professional Liability," *Journal of the American Medical Association,* Vol. 257, No. 20, (May 22-29, 1987).

Roach, Marion, "Reflection in a Fatal Mirror," *Discover,* (August 1985).

Sagan, Leonard A. *The Health of Nations. True Causes of Sickness and Well-Being.* Basic Books, New York, 1987.

Sale, David M. J.D., LL.M., *Overview of Legislative Developments Concerning Alternative Health Care in the United States,* Fetzer Institute, Kalamazoo, Michigan, 1995.

Schilcher, Prof. Dr. Heinz, "The Significance of Phytotherapy in Europe," *Quarterly Review of Natural Medicine,* Spring 1995.

Sibbison, Jim, "Covering Medical 'Breakthroughs,'" *Columbia Journalism Review,* (July/August 1988).

Sloan, F.A., et al., "Medical Malpractice Experience of Physicians: Predictable or Haphazard?" *Journal of the American Medical Association,* Vol. 262, No. 23, (December 15, 1989).

Sportelli, Louis, D.C., *Risk Management, Malpractice and Chiropractic,* Health Services Ltd., Palmerton, 1990.

Staff writer, "1989 Physician Survey Examines Attitudes, Professional Needs," *Texas Medicine,* Vol. 85, No. 5, (May 1989).

Starr, Paul, *The Social Transformation of American Medicine,* Basic Books, New York, 1983.

Sykes, Charles J., *A Nation of Victims: The Decay of the American Character*, St. Martin's Press, New York, 1992.

—"I Hear America Whining," *The New York Times*, (November 2, 1992).

"The Conspiracy Against Chiropractic May Have Failed, But It's Not Over Yet, Other Targets Remain," *Alternative Medicine Digest*, Issue 14, (September 1996).

Toufexis, Anastasia, "They Just Don't Understand," *Time*, (June 1, 1992).

The Landmark Report on Public Perceptions of Alternative Care, Landmark Healthcare, Sacramento, CA, 1998.

Ullman, Dana, "Getting Beyond Wellness Macho: The Promise and Pitfalls of Holistic Health," *Utne Reader*, (Jan/Feb 1988).

Wallis, Claudia, "Why New Age Medicine is Catching On," *Time*, (November 4, 1991).

—and Willwerth, James, "Awakenings, Schizophrenia: A New Drug Brings Patients Back to Life," *Time*, (July 6, 1992).

Warner, Glenn, M.D., "Dr. Warner's License Revocation," *Townsend Letter for Doctors*, (August/September 1995): 10-12.

Weisman, C.S., et al., "Practice Changes in Response to the Malpractice Litigation Climate: Results of a Maryland Physician Survey," *Medical Care*, Vol. 27, No. 1, (January 1989).

Weeks, John, "Charting the Mainstream: A Review of Trends in the Dominant Medical System," *Townsend Letter for Doctors and Patients*, (January 1996): 26.

Wilk, Chester, D.C. *Medicine, Monopolies, and Malice: How the Medical Establishment Tried to Destroy Chiropractic in the U.S.*, Avery Publishing Group, NY, 1996.

Wolinsky, Howard, and Brune, Tom, *The Serpent on the Staff: The Unhealthy Politics of the American Medical Association*, Jeremy P. Tarcher/G.P. Putnam's Sons, New York, 1994.

CHAPTER 2

Priestly Death Rites: The Inner Orientation of Conventional Medicine

Physician: Doctor as Priest of the *Physis*

In case you occasionally have the sense that contemporary doctors act as if they were the elect in a medical priesthood, there is a historical justification for this observation. In the Greek classical period, and before, the physicians of the day were in fact priests or spiritual guides for the medically uninitiated. Medicine then was an integral part of the *mystery* tradition, such that medical knowledge was initiate wisdom.

In the mystery initiation temples at places such as Ephesus and Eleusis, for example, the person undergoing initiation—which is to say, the gradual acquaintance (or *gnosis*) with larger spiritual realities of mind, body, soul, spirit, and world—the psychopomp was a master of both philosophy and medicine, of ontology and therapeutics. In fact, the concepts were not separate but integral to the same initiatory knowledge.

A person's destiny, likely to be glimpsed in a mystery initiation, would reveal information (potentially shocking) about their medical and spiritual health. An illness might be a gift of the gods, a means of spiritual illumination; all bodily, physical events were material reflections of etheric and spiritual processes in the life of the human soul. "Through their contacts with illnesses, physicians are placed in the center of spiritual activities," comments Holtzapfel. For physicians, medicine can serve as a path toward initiation and illumination.

"Illness and healing had to do with endangering and restoring the human image, which people knew originated with the gods," explains Walter Holtzapfel in *Medicine and the Mysteries*. In this ancient view, the human being (and its idea or "image") was regarded as the creation of high spiritual beings or intelligences; the physician's lawful role in this cosmology of the human was to complement and preserve this original pure creation. Even as recently as the time of Hippocrates, the putative "father" of Western medicine, a physician who was versed in philosophy was godlike.

Traces of the physician's theocratic imprimatur and spiritual responsibility for the welfare of the human soul could still be encountered in the nineteenth century in the writings of German physician Dr. Christoph Wilhelm Hufeland (1762-1836), a contemporary of Wolfgang Goethe. In his memoirs recounting fifty years of medical practice (Enchiridion Medicum, 1836), Dr. Hufeland summarized his principles of "Physiatric" for doctors: "All cures of diseases are caused by Nature; the medical art is only Nature's servant and cures through her."

Do little and leave everything to nature, he exhorted his fellow physicians. Dr. Hufeland encouraged them to remember their charge: "You are god's priests, ordained to look after the holy flame of life and to administer his greatest gifts, which are health, life, and the mysterious forces he bestowed on nature for our benefit." Guarding the human *physis* ("the holy flame of life") is a "lofty, sacred undertaking," Dr. Hufeland added. As if anticipating our own medically aberrated age, Dr. Hufeland warned: "A time will come when you have to account for your actions."

Holtzapfel's remarkable observation that medicine, through its practitioner's constant encounter with illness and infirmity, could be a path of initiation is slowly dawning in the awareness of a few late-twentieth-century physicians specializing in holistic, alternative medicine. Among the more prominent exponents of a soul perspective in medicine, and the revived role model of doctors as gurus, are Larry Dossey, M.D., who writes convincingly about the "meaning" of illness and the "healing" power of prayers, and Deepak Chopra, M.D., who uses a Hindu meditational context to highlight the "unconditional" and "quantum" aspects of life, consciousness, illness, and healing.

Today's medical savant is a coexplorer with the patient in the perils of self-generated illness and health. The exploration is perilous because of what it implies. What if the universe, human life, and health are participatory and consciousness-dependent, as the mystics have perennially told us? Success in healing could change the way we regard the human experience itself. We might have to unconditionally accept responsibility for our well-being and life, knowing we already have the means within for this staggering task.

For Dossey, the most prominent possibility is finding meaning in the experience of illness. Allopathy long ago outlawed meaning in pathology: if the human body is a machine, then illness is simply a loose screw or defective motor. These are facts; meaning is not required. Allopathic medicine disregards the patient's interpretation of the significance of an illness as bad science and etiologically irrelevant. But for Dossey the way in which a patient perceives meaning in the illness experience is crucial to its outcome.

That's because meaning is inseparable from the actual thoughts, feelings, and emotions of the patient, the human who has an illness. A patient's meanings enter the body and change it on the atomic and molecular level. Illness for many is often the pivotal life experience in which the issue of meaning is first articulated. In this life-questioning moment, the patient witnesses the dramatic interaction of mind, meaning, and matter. Understanding this "must involve going beyond science to a fundamental shift in consciousness." Meaning is being, Dossey argues; therefore, healing requires "a fundamental change in our own being."

"Genuine healing is frequently unexpected and radical, seemingly out of the blue, and often depends not on what we *do* but on how we choose to *be*," says Chopra. His therapeutic concern is for more than our physical or psychoemotional health; he wants to provoke healing in the metaphysical foundations of our existence. "Disease is no way to solve the core issues of life. People have to be transformed *before* the crisis." Chopra wants to help heal our "hurt awareness," by which he means prime errors of cognition. Reality is a subjective, personalized field of experience, comments Chopra. The forces that shape our personal reality are unconscious beliefs, attitudes, perceptions, the boundaries of subjective conditioning—the ancient Hindu sages called them "mistakes of the intellect."

We suppose, mistakenly, that the world is solid, material, static, and formidable, yet the *rishis* assure us it's really a mirage of molecules, a mask of *maya,* a "layer of trick effects." If reality is malleable, who's in charge? The self, answers Chopra, the "potentiality of untold possibilities" and the "field of pure awareness" at the heart of atoms, molecules, human bodies, and galaxies. If he's right, then health is negotiable, psychopomps are the best deal makers, and better health means better metaphysics.

Representing the patient's experience of serious illness as initiation, Barbara Stone, Ph.D., who developed breast cancer at age forty-two, likens the ordeal as akin to a Native American vision quest. The experience challenged her to grow and "threw me into an emotional wilderness filled with many physical dangers" yet revealed her destiny, that "the reason I came to Earth was to learn secrets of healing."

Stone's journey through the allopathic wasteland of cancer treatment had many of the hallmarks of traditional initiation rituals, she notes, "an initiation into the 'Wise Woman' stage of life." For Stone, the experience of cancer initiated a soul process of "peeling away the layers of emotional wounds barricading my heart"; in the end, after surviving, Stone could see that initiation by cancer had brought her not death but new life.

Mystery Initiations into the "Most Frightful Magical Arts"

The insights of Dossey, Chopra, and Stone represent the positive side of this re-emergence of doctor as medical savant and patient as courageous novice. But there is a dark side as well. In fact, one can make the case that nearly all of contemporary allopathic medicine adheres to the darker expression of physician as inimical priest.

Psychiatrist Thomas Szasz, M.D., devoted many of his essays to charting the ceremonial or religious aspects of medical practice and what he called the theology of medicine. "Formerly, people victimized themselves by attributing medical powers to their priests; now, they victimize themselves by attributing magical powers to their physicians." Formerly, priests mediated on the laity's behalf regarding the problem of sin, says Szasz; now, physician-priests intercede on behalf of pain and suffering. The result is that men, women, and children—the entire health care consuming class—become "the patient-penitents of their physician-priests" over which presides the "Church of Medicine."

Szasz' critique of contemporary medicine faults it for an abuse of power masquerading as theological authority and canonical conformity. This is a benign analysis of allopathy, requiring a mild corrective; here, the democratic rights of individuals are infringed by an overarching physician class. But physician-priests can also stray into the domain of magic, of soul manipulations and transgressions—and the magic is not always white.

"Medical procedures turn into *black magic* when, instead of mobilizing self-healing powers, they transform the sick man into a limp and mystified voyeur of his own treatment," writes Ivan Illich. We are not accustomed to thinking of modern medicine in terms of magic, which tends to be a dismissive pejorative term for ineffectuality; to suggest a link between contemporary medicine and black magic opens an unexpected, probably unwanted, and certainly shocking door into the occult, and the unconscious. Unconscious in the sense that doctors, as agents of allopathy, may have no inkling of the forces (purposefully occulted) driving this paradigm. Before we dismiss Illich' s connection as nothing more than metaphorical (or paranoid), let us pause to consider Rudolf Steiner's observations on the relationship between medicine and magic among the ancient Mexican priests.

In the course of a lecture series at Dornach, Switzerland, in 1916, the Austrian spiritual scientist and clairvoyant Rudolf Steiner (1861-1925) sketched a picture of the bizarre mindset of the ancient Mexican priest initiates; shortly, we will see how it uncannily evokes aspects of the state of mind of allopathy today. Long before the European discovery of the North American continent, there were mystery initiations and traditions under way in Mexico that were both "grisly" and "revolting," Steiner says. A deity known as *Toatl* was the focus of a highly materialistic ritual and "the most frightful magical arts."

Initiates of Toatl had to perform ritual murders by excising the stomachs (or hearts) of victims and offering them up to Toatl; only then could they advance further in this fraternity and receive the secrets and mysteries it safeguarded. The circumstances surrounding the ritual murder of the victim were designed to produce a specific mood of soul, sensations, and feelings in the apprentice. Primarily, this meant obtaining "the wisdom to mould this earthly world in such a way that souls would be driven out of it." Highest among the initiates of this Central American priesthood of Toatl was one of the most formidable black magicians ever to walk the face of Earth, says Steiner. He possessed "the greatest secrets that are to be acquired on this path" and if he had not been stopped, his inimical works could have radically set the course of human evolution into a time of "terrible darkness."

The Toatl fraternity had an occult purpose, Steiner explained. This was to "rigidify and mechanize all earthly life, to make the whole earth a realm of death, in which everything possible would be done to kill out independence and every inner impulse of the soul." They sought to gain control over all the forces of death so that the physical world and humanity could become "a purely mechanistic, great dead realm" in which the soul of humanity would have no lawful place; the priests would have mechanistic control over all of life and its processes.

The rites of Toatl mobilized "actual powers of black magic" with the ultimate goal of preventing the soul and spiritual parts of humankind (Steiner called this the Ego) from finding a place in the human organization—from incarnating in the body. The Toatl priesthood wanted to render men and women soulless automatons from which the Ego had departed. For this priesthood, the soul was the enemy, or the object of their magical aggression: its eradication in the material world was their goal.

The Toatl mysteries may have particularly developed on Mexican soil, but over time they spread across a large part of the North American continent, Steiner said. Eventually, this priesthood was defeated in A.D. 33 with the crucifixion of their black magician (paralleling, in reverse, Christ's crucifixion on Golgotha), but the energies, ideas, and forces left over from the Toatl impulse survived in the etheric world, in the energy aura of the North American landscape. "They still exist subsensibly," still present under the covering of ordinary life, Steiner said.

Steiner's perception of the Mexican mysteries also rudely opens our eyes to a possibility not ordinarily credited in Western public discourse. "You must realize that there is a plan in world history in which the evil powers also come into the picture." This "plan" would seize upon medicine and its allopathic expression in the United States specifically as its prime theater. Its apocalyptic crisis would play out in the final years of the twentieth century.

Geographic Medicine:
The *American* Style of Doctoring

Is there any evidence that the North American *landscape,* with its subsensible residue of the Toatl black magic priesthood, has left an imprint on the face that American medicine has formed? In *Medicine and Culture,* Lynn Payer explores the role of cultural bias in doctoring. She shows how in a given Western country—England, France, Germany, and the United States—there is a distinct approach to and implicit philosophy of allopathic medicine.

If there is a single word with which to describe American medicine, it is *aggressive.* American doctors always want to *do something,* Payer explains. All illness has an external cause—an infection, an organ defect, a germ, a virus—that can be conquered, killed, or cut out. To do nothing, to wait and allow the healing forces of nature to set things right—this kind of restraint is unthinkable for this "can do" attitude. Further, in the war against disease, American physicians expect *immediate,* unequivocally positive results; failing this—as evidenced in the putative "war against cancer," which doctors are steadily losing—ever stronger, more toxic chemotherapeutic approaches are deployed.

The goal is to wipe out the disease quickly and thoroughly, marshaling the same "heroic" approach by which Americans conquered—some would say raped and pillaged—their own interior frontier in the eighteenth and nineteenth centuries, claiming a broad swath of the North American continent between the two oceans as their rightful manifest destiny. Not only is American medicine aggressive, but more is always better: more doses, stronger doses, more surgery, more interventions, technology, tests, screens, procedures. Nature—what the French physicians call the "terrain" or encompassing environment—is not expected or trusted to heal the body on its own.

American allopathy has more than a distrust of nature: it holds a Puritanical abhorrence of natural processes. They are messy, unreliable, inchoate at best. What witches were to some Christian societies, germs are to American doctors. They are dangerous heretics, best burned at the stake in a sanitizing *auto-da-fé*. In this struggle against invading germs, antibiotics—agents for killing life—are the physicians' preferred weapon. Even the possibility of bacterial activity sends the doctor running for the penicillin.

Thus "the imperative to intervene was critical to American physicians' professional identity," says Payer. The physician's careful examination of a patient and detailed case taking is not valued in American medicine; rather, the results of a diagnostic test are of paramount value in charting the outcome of a case. As Payer sees it, this approach "gives primacy to the idea that disease is some wild and hairy monster that can be locked up with diagnosis." In American medicine, the body is a machine with plumbing; the heart, for example, is a mechanical pump; if it "breaks" or becomes defective, then first you try to fix it with bypass surgery, then you replace it with somebody else's heart, or you install an artificial heart altogether.

Psychiatrists tend to view the human mind as a machine with plumbing as well, leading to what one observer calls the "Saniflush" concept of psychiatry. The role of the therapist is to flush out the inhibitions and psychological complexes from a person, thereby freeing them for greatness. Whatever soul or spiritual quality Sigmund Freud's model of psychoanalysis may have once possessed in his original German context, all that was lost in the translation into American. "This denial of soul, or indeed of the less mystical emotions, has taken its toll on American medicine," Payer says. What doesn't conform to this mechanistic, quantifying model is excluded, even denied existence.

Payer's analysis of American-style medicine is instructive, yet we need to probe deeper into the unique temperament of expression of allopathic medicine as conditioned by landscape and culture. Why is American medicine so aggressive, so fixated on diagnosis and invasive biological problem solving? Why is the American allopathic establishment so stridently, even militantly, opposed to the open marketplace competition of alternative, empiric therapies that work *with* the body, not against? Why is the battle between the therapeutic paradigms of empiric/holistic and rational/allopathic being waged primarily on American soil (with secondary skirmishes under way elsewhere, such as Canada, England, and Australia) with the American (soulless) body as the spoils of war?

We might answer it's the *mood* of the American people, but where does this mood come from? Steiner's observations about the soul mood of the ancient Mexican Toatl priests and their residuals in the etheric field of the continent induces us to ask if the North American *landscape* itself might contribute to the American style of doctoring. Might the American *environment* exert an influence on the style of doctoring? Steiner called this factor "geographic medicine," that is, a therapeutic style informed, even determined by, the geomantic energy of a landscape. "In accordance with geographical differentiations, the most varied forces stream up out of the various territories," Steiner wrote in 1917.

According to Steiner, who was widely regarded by his peers as a master initiate-clairvoyant, Europeans actually knew about the American continent for many centuries before its official discovery in 1492. Norwegian ships had "continually" made trading missions with America up until about the ninth century A.D. At that time, the Roman Catholic Church decided it was necessary to cut off all trade relations with America and to expunge all cultural record and memory that there had ever been any. The purity and unfettered evolution of the European soul was literally at stake and must be safeguarded against inimical influences. The Church elders, taking counsel from Irish monks who represented a pure form of Christianity, saw the necessity for erecting "spiritual walls" around Europe so that the "tender plant of Christianity" could spread across the continent, protected from the influences of the American continent.

"Behind the processes of world history lie deep mysteries filled with significance," Steiner explained, adding, "Things have deep foundations." The harmful influences associated with the American continent pertained to a certain pressure of awareness of an aspect of the human organization that had previously been known only to the occult brotherhoods in Europe; premature knowledge of and exposure to this aspect could literally injure the European soul. Steiner called this influence the human double. In Steiner's complex model of cosmology and humanity, numerous spiritual beings and intelligences have helped to create, continue to maintain, and actually reside, in different ways, in the human being. Their presence and influence within us is dialectical: some favor our spiritual unfolding, others oppose or thwart it.

This struggle between two fundamental opposing forces is played out in all spheres of human life, from our notions of cosmology to the processes of consciousness and the body. Steiner borrowed the term "Ahriman" from the ancient Zoroastrian philosophy to indicate a hardening, densifying, materializing energy, an energy that, unchecked, can prove to be inimical to human evolution. Let this be our first introduction to the unavoidably spiritual, even occult, side of medicine, a theme that will emerge more fully as the book progresses.

In this archetypal dialectic, one kind of being (Steiner called it "Ahrimanic") takes "possession of us before our birth and always remains there, always creating a figure around us in our subconscious." Another name for this spiritual being of ambiguous intent is the *double* (in German, *Doppelgänger*). As such, it is an exceedingly complex reality, unfamiliar to most people. In general terms, think of the double as something akin to conventional notions indicated by such terms as *alter ego, phantom, shadow, mirror image of the self;* it's the darker, unacknowledged aspects of the self, or the deceptive image of one's own shape—another you, if somewhat distorted.

This double is the "creator of all physical illnesses that emerge spontaneously from within; and to know him fully is organic medicine." All organic illnesses that arise spontaneously within us, Steiner says, come not through outer injuries or from the soul, but from this Ahrimanic being. The Ahrimanic being makes use of the human being in order to profit from the relationship. It enters at birth and leaves just before death. "Illnesses emerge because this being works in the human being." The double accompanies humans under the threshold of consciousness, subliminally; though we encounter it every night during sleep, during our waking daytime consciousness, we are oblivious of the double.

In a curious sense, this veiled quality makes the double our benefactor, with respect to maintaining the parameters of conventional consciousness and identity. "Shame or fear, and partly also doubt, inhibit us from encountering this double, who in the last analysis mirrors our total being and our past karma," explains Werner Priever, M.D., in his monograph, *Illness and the Double*. In the old initiation tradition (and its twentieth-century revival in the form of anthroposophy, as formulated by Rudolf Steiner), encountering the double is another term for meeting the Lesser Guardian of the Threshold.

To dip into more familiar Western terms, we might say this encounter is similar to C. G. Jung's formulation of meeting the *shadow*—all the rejected, denied, forgotten, unassimilated, and unconscious elements of a person's total identity. Jung's concept of the shadow encompasses a single lifetime, but Steiner's is multilifetime, an accumulation of rejected, unacknowledged debris from potentially thousands of incarnations. Either way, it's not the kind of meeting you'd want to entertain in the dark—that is, without initiate supervision.

The "threshold" in question is the lintel of the *other world,* the authentic spiritual realms as distinct from the torturously distorted simulacrum that is the unwise apprentice's who tries to enter without undergoing the painful, possibly apocalyptic, purgation in the hands of the guardian.

What are the potential liabilities of a freer, more wakeful contact with one's double? It would be an experience, probably frightful, approaching the nature of a mystery initiation, but with rather the quality of a house of horrors made of mirrors full of terrible images. Encountering the Double without inner preparation could sunder the personality into its component parts, with the moral, will, and emotional aspects proceeding in different, somewhat autonomous directions. Further, the experience could lead to a densification of consciousness, to a tightening of the bonds of materialism, of construing the world as purely what is limited to sense impressions, of focusing exclusively on genetic, hereditary, and blood mechanisms for the etiology of illness and the basis of therapy. It could lead to the soulless and soul-killing state of mind of allopathy.

The Double, in its influence on the disease process, is bivalent: it can exert an inflammatory (expansive, producing fever) or sclerotizing (hardening, producing cancer) influence. But it does not willingly brook a third mediating pole. "Only consciously and deliberately, after adequate preparation and conditionless self-knowledge, can the encounter with the Double proceed without danger," Priever counsels.

Thus a companion spiritual being creates all psychological or nervous system illnesses in us with our *unconscious* complicity. To be more precise, perhaps we should say it helps to generate these illnesses out of our karmic residues, almost always unknown to us. But not unknowable, for the wakeful knowing of these illness-producing karmic residues was an element of the ancient mystery initiation. This wakeful knowing in itself goes a long way toward weakening the Ahrimanic influence, which thrives in states of spiritual ignorance. We are not helpless victims in this illness etiology, but we live unaware of the *terms* of physical embodiment; hence, illness often seems an irrational ambush of our orderly life. Conscious, wide-awake effort is required to change the scales.

To an extent, where we live on the North American continent makes a difference in how the Ahrimanic Double insinuates itself into life and consciousness. The Ahrimanic beings are especially sensitive to the forces or magnetic radiations that stream up out of the Earth such that there is a specific connection between the illness-producing being in the human with the local geography or geomantic terrain. "A certain portion of the Earth's surface shows the closest kinship to these forces. If a person goes to this place, he enters their realm," Steiner said.

At the time when Norwegian trade ships were regularly plying the routes between Europe and America, the latter was known to be "the region where the magnetic forces particularly arose that brought the human being into relation with this Double." The esoteric fraternities in Europe, like medical anthropologists, found this interesting: "The illnesses in America brought about under the influence of earthly magnetism were studied by Europe," Steiner explained.

The unique character of American illnesses actually contributed formatively to the development of European medicine. Like anthropologists, they studied these elemental-produced disease products. The European physicians also appreciated the mercantile envoi to America because it provided them with information on the role the Double played in the constitution of the Native Americans. Notwithstanding, as the finer spiritual sensitivity of Europeans had to be protected from this strong influence for at least 500 years, so knowledge of America and its landscape's ability to precipitate awareness of the Double and a materialistic densification of consciousness was eclipsed from knowledge and history for centuries.

Teaching Doctors
the Allopathic Paradigm

Keeping Steiner's disquieting scenario of Mexican black magic and mystery knowledge, and the initiatic quality of the American environment in mind, let's peruse a sampling of modern accounts of the training of allopathic doctors on American soil. We should pay particular attention to Steiner's warning that the bizarre, frightful magical arts of the ancient Mexican Toatl priesthood may still linger in the subconscious ethers of the landscape and its inhabitants.

Let's begin with *Surgeon: The View from Behind the Mask* by Richard S. Weeder, M.D. This is a shocking tableau (italics added for emphasis), as if the general surgeon is unconsciously posing as a kind of modern day Mexican-Aztec priest about to make the stomach incision. It's as if the two realities were overlaid like filo dough. "I think we're going to have to *do him,*" a mild-mannered M.D. says about this patient with a stomach cancer, requiring immediate surgery. First he would put his patient to sleep with anesthesia, "Then, having gained command of the patient's mind, Cooper would *open his belly widely, with a knife.* On the face of it, it was *a brutal act, like a bayonet stab*—warlike, something done in rage or the panic of self-defense. In ancient times, such things were done in *sacrificial rites,* a carefully considered *holy act.*"

It's astonishing that at some level, at least metaphorical, Weeder is actually tuning in to this antecedent negative version of stomach surgery. Remember that Steiner insisted residuals of the Mexican mysteries lingered in the etheric aura of the landscape. Then the priest deliberately killed the victim while awake; now they try to save the patient while he's asleep; either way they incise his stomach while he—the victim/patient—lies on his back on a steel (stone) table in the "operating theater."

In Weeder's example, the patient has a heart attack and dies during the stomach (vascular) surgery. Weeder evokes the ritualistic aspect of surgery/initiation in reference to the presurgical hand-scrubbing routine. "He'd been doing this, rubbing his arms and hands until they hurt, since he was a kid . . . It was a *ritual,* like grace before a meal, or *holy water before mass.* It had set him up for work, *preparing his spirit* as it purified his hands."

Weeder finds that the experiences of his four years of medical training gave him an almost palpable sense of "playing God" that in its responsibility over life and death was both "outrageous and blasphemous." Just as, according to Steiner, the Mexican apprentice developed a certain mood of soul through his ritual murder of victims, so Weeder found that playing God in the hospital has an insidious way of changing his state of mind in all aspects of his life. "He was becoming an expert on everything."

Weeder is self-conscious of his anonymity as mandated by peer standards: *"Only his eyes are visible,* the rest of him hidden. His hands, the tools of his craft, are *distanced* from the patient by gloves; less infection, less intimate, more comfortable." During surgery, he holds the heart in his hands: "But Cooper *could feel the heart beating against his hand,* transmitted through the diaphragm." When the patient dies on the table, the surgeon removes his mask, because up until now, only his eyes were visible. "But taking down the mask was also a gesture of respect. Cooper's face was bare now before the patient." That is, only when he's dead. The patient's face had been hidden also.

"Cooper would not see the patient's face again until the operation was over . . . . The gowns, gloves, and drapes distance us emotionally as well as bacteriologically. *We don't see the patient; he doesn't see us."* Of a woman whose cancerous breast he surgically removed, Weeder reflects on the ritualized act of medical killing his team has colluded in. The surgeon had taken her breast, the chemotherapist had taken her long red hair [chemotherapy commonly makes the hair fall out], then the three of them [including a radiologist] "would take the radiance from her face, dooming her to a life of apprehension."

Reading *A Year Long Night: Tales of a Medical Internship* by Robert Klitzman, you gain the impression that in many cases the hospital can do little to arrest the progress of a pathology. It's more a matter of dispensing high-tech chemicals ("chemo and meds"), tests, and procedures until the inevitable death arrives. The hospital becomes a holding pen for terminal cases. "When I was a medical student, my first sight of the day each morning . . . had been a row of six-foot-long black boxes being rolled out from the freight elevators into the icy daylight," writes Klitzman. "Few things in a hospital are painted pitch black. A special forklift lowered one box at a time into the back of a waiting station wagon."

Klitzman sees there is little M.D.s can do most of the time. "I *had no life-affirming inspirations to offer her* in dealing with her illness . . . The only symbols of hope I offered were medicine and drugs, which were necessary but not sufficient . . . Much of what I did as an intern was medical hand-holding, making someone more comfortable as he or she waited to die."

Next we look at *First Do No Harm: Reflections on Becoming a Neurosurgeon* by J. Kenyon Rainer, paying close attention to word choice and nuance (emphasis added). "The last four years had given me volumes of medical knowledge but little medical training: facts, but few skills . . . I was a *thoroughly programmed* medical textbook." Rainer indicates the high degree of theoretical content of M.D. training which is based primarily on dissecting corpses: "rows of men and women pickled in formalin, lying naked on stainless steel tables with white neon light flooding their bodies."

The individuality of the patient isn't important; the pathology is everything; deformed biology is accorded more ontological importance than the individual human bearing, presenting, or creating it. "'What are their names?' I asked. 'I don't know. It's *the disease that's important,*' he answered."

Of a training doctor making his rounds, Rainer observes: "He knew no patient's name or occupation. To him they were simply diseases." As pathology is the crux of medical work, it's also the central part of training and skill refinement. "I never enjoyed visiting the psychiatric ward, but *I needed to find brain tumors* for more surgical practice, so I ignored my fear and walked through the room."

Psychiatric cases are not so amenable to surgical fixing (as lobotomies have gone out of fashion), so something unfixable and aberrantly human as opposed to aberrantly biological is dismissed as irrelevant: "neurosurgeons spend so little time with medical diseases because *they are boring,* difficult to treat, and often impossible to cure."

An Inventory of Allopathic Medical Perception

Let's go deeper into the subject of physician training as revealed in popular accounts by the doctors themselves by organizing their observations into categories. Keep in mind Steiner's observation that the state of mind of the ancient Mexican medicine mysteries are still in the subconscious ethers. Italics are added to emphasize key expressions.

Keep also in mind that the physicians quoted have reported their observations in good faith, according to the standards of their medical practice. The possibility that their well-meaning doctorly observations would be construed as evidence of an allopathic distortion of human incarnation is surely something that would never occur to them. In a curious way, they are blameless, even though their words embody the allopathic paradigm, or thought field, if you will, and *that* is the focus of this analysis.

- **Diagnosis.** The crux of allopathic practice is making the diagnosis, naming the pathology; this is the challenge, like a detective seeking the criminal. "Everyone else had drawn a blank on this lady; by damn, he was going to make a diagnosis," says Weeder. "The good diagnostician is a detective; the disease is the criminal."

- **The anathema of diseased flesh.** A surgeon says: "What bothers me would be touching the patient. I like gloves. *I don't want to touch that stuff*—that disease."

- **Nature is inimical, the physician's enemy.** A surgeon quoted in *Invasive Procedures* says: "'When the trouble is big enough to *attack with a knife*, I do all I can.' It was a candid and striking assertion, a surgeon's explanation of his sense of mission, a heady conjunction of *out-and-out aggression* and saintliness— 'attack with a knife' meets 'do all I can.'" Elsewhere we learn: "The unfairness of disease—which may triumph in spite of efforts to eradicate it—helps shape the transaction on both sides . . . we seem to need sworn enemies of death . . . we have allowed them [physicians] to take on power and privilege and prejudice, in return, perhaps, for both their practical and *ceremonial chores.*"

- **The nonhuman face of pathology.** The pathology itself— especially malignant tumors—has a face, a kind of beingness. Tumors are strange, alien, frightening, inimical aberrations of biology. "It looked like a gray tennis ball with rough, irregular ridges resembling fish scales on its surface . . . Malignant tumors usually spread into the brain and you can't tell where they start or stop." The tumors get the body to feed them through its arteries. The surgeon "tracked the tumor through a tunnel it had formed as it grew into the brain . . . I carefully teased arteries off the surface of the tumor before delivering the mass from the center of the brain. At 2:15 I lifted the meningioma out of the brain."

It's as if the bad fruit of the patient's destiny (or spiritual karma) were materially present in the surgeon's hands after excision from the body. From the surgeon's view, the tumor is an inexplicable biological aberration that has hijacked the patient's body for its own dark purposes: "the tumor was clearly visible . . . it was growing inside the (spinal) cord and had burrowed a tunnel into it like a mole. The tumor was rubbery and would not suck away from the spinal cord and nerves." The surgeon spends eight hours "disintegrating about 75% of the tumor by burning it with the laser." Of an aneurysm: "It looked like a cherry-red plum, although slightly bigger, and I could see blood swirling within it, pulsating and bulging the dome of the aneurysm and threatening to explode it at any second."

In the spirit of Steiner's remark that the Mexican mysteries wanted to exert control over all the mechanistic aspects of biology, we read: *"We made the child a new skull* out of acrylic since much of hers had been destroyed by the injury." On seeing a lung cancer, a physician in *Invasive Procedures* says: "It's smog yellow, and it lurks just under the surface of the lung, smeared around in patches, like skin-covered cottage cheese."

- **Organs are dispensable.** To a surgeon, internal organs are not inviolate; they are usually fixable, often dispensable, and subject to radical excision, even replacement. If the diagnosis is uncertain, or drugs fail to work, removal is an obvious choice. "Removing the gall bladder always cures the pain," says Weeder. He makes a presumptive diagnosis of an obscure gall bladder pathology, but he can only verify it by removing the gall bladder. "We won't know if it was the right diagnosis until the pathologist examines the tissue."

The doctor is trained to be able to fix organs and repair their function, like a good technician. "Cooper recognized in himself that he was, *like most surgeons, a Mr. Fixit* . . . And it remained important to his ego that he could 'make all better.'" Organs have no feelings or value once they're moved from the patient. "It would be fun—one last gall bladder—God, that's a satisfying operation! . . . Finally he pulled the gall bladder free and dropped it into a stainless steel basin held by the nurse. 'Another nasty gall bag bites the dust.'"

- **Soulless organology.** For the purposes of autopsy, dissection, and teaching, human bodies are reduced to a collection of disembodied organs, what Klitzman calls "the man in the pan."

After one of Klitzman's patients died, his organs were removed and displayed in a stainless steel pan for the medical students in the hospital. "The man I knew to be Mr. Draper and 'the man in the pan' were materially the same, yet different—entities related by mere fact . . . Now *he was a pile of organs on bakery sheets.*"

Klitzman working as an intern in the operating room, confronted by a patient's body part: "I began to see it only as 'tissue' and not as something human . . . In surgery, *blood seems of little consequence. It's like money* in the middle of a poker game. One's notion of its value changes, excitingly." Klitzman describes the gallery of CAT scans hung on the walls in a consultation room: "The effect of these many small panels lined across the walls, with patterns of variegated shades illuminated from behind, was that of entering *a medieval chapel* where light seeps through translucent stained-glass windows . . . In the CAT scan suite, the walls were decorated with images of the human brain, now believed to be the seat of the human soul and man's highest capacities. Though windowless, this room was ethereal and light, a *modern sanctuary* of the mind."

- **Organological reductionism.** At best the human presence is located within specific organs as a kind of mechanical homunculus, as Rainer writes: "'And that,' Walker said, pointing to an area of brain deep between the two cerebral hemispheres, 'is where he lives. That's the hypothalamus. Mess that up and your patient remains in a coma or dies.'"

- **The body as soulless machine.** "The steps a surgeon takes are as orderly, as procedural, as physically explicable, as the steps of *disassembling an engine,*" we read in Kramer. A surgeon says: "I never cut my patients. I operate. I *fix* people." The physician is Dr. Fix-It: "Patient after patient comes to him, betrayed by ill luck and an unreliable body . . . He observes symptoms, formulates diagnoses, plans the tactics of treatment. His interest is no broader than that." The human body is a traitor to the patient's well-being; it is the cause of the patient's vulnerability.

"He [the physician] has been confronted each day for decades with a few dozen reminders of the unreliability of the body—and therefore of *his body*—of its mechanicalness, and therefore its *funda-*

mental vulnerability." Sometimes the surgeon has to slap the parts around, the way he might discipline truculent teenagers. "We took that diseased artery, tore hell out of it, beat it up, sewed it up, and it works better than ever." A surgeon says: "I thought you were a medical insider now. Don't you know *the body's just a machine* and it breaks down every once in a while?"

- **The depersonalization of surgery and interventions.** The nature of surgery is inherently soulless, in that the patient (victim) is unconscious, absent, not individually a factor, and his body is mechanically worked on by the surgeon. "Heat from the saw burned the bone, and wisps of smoke drifted up from the head . . . the entire beveled skull of the forehead was lifted free from the rest of the head, *like taking the top off of a teapot."* Pathologies and injuries are regarded, not in the context of a living person, but as evidence of damaged physical merchandise: "Instead of its normal, pulsating, pale yellow appearance, it [the brain] was swollen, discolored, and mottled red from the hemorrhage. *'It's an angry brain,'* Dr. Clark said as he stared at the tight red brain."

Bodily organs have a life of their own but no human soulness; they are severed from the central human individuality; they are merely reactive tissues, manipulable according to mechanistic laws of biology. "Suddenly, without warning, the brain began swelling so violently that I had to hold it with the palm of my hand to keep it inside her head . . . Still the brain continued to swell like a balloon filling under a faucet." Or: "Pete cut the dural covering of the brain and pulled it up like a veil, *exposing the yellow, pulsating face of the brain."* Or: "Red arteries throbbed on the brain's surface and the crystal-clear spinal fluid surrounding the brain continuously bubbled up like a spring." Or: "I stared at the hemorrhagic, swollen brain; fiery red instead of its normal pale yellow color . . . I hesitated and continued to look at *the angry, throbbing artery* in front of me."

These descriptions suggest an autonomous but nonhuman source of the emotional qualities of anger, threat, and energetic throbbing—again, the surgeon is construing a mechanistic, Egoless biology. It's all performed at extreme risk: for the patient, it's dying; for the physician, it's malpractice lawsuits. "The microscopic work was exhausting, the danger of paralyzing the girl present every second of every minute for eight hours."

Pathologies have their own arcane agenda, timing, and course of action, independent of the human recipient; the goal is death, and death defeats, renounces, and repudiates the surgeon who expects to be the provider of a longer life span. "Eula's medical treatment was carefully planned, meticulously delivered; a product of scientific thinking and medical technology. Yet she had died . . . in the end it was the disease, not I, that determined the length of her life."

The physician is hired entirely for his *technical* skills. "It seems unregenerate but also unexceptional for him to wish to forget the personhood, and the vulnerability, that he shares with every patient," cites Mark Kramer in *Invasive Procedures.*

- **The primacy of technology.** Doctors accord a degree of faith and trust in their technological extensions that ancient priests once bestowed upon their gods of healing. "Radiologists *trust* their machines' power," writes Klitzman. "Dr Flint had an *implicit faith* that he could follow the progression of a disease and know a patient's clinical course and fate better than the treating doctors who examined the patient daily . . . A *calm confidence* prevails in the radiology suite, removed from nurses and patients." Of a man on mechanical life-support systems, Klitzman writes: "There, *the parts of his body communicated to me* without mediation through him . . . Several times each day, I performed the duties of an integrating mind for his failing body . . . *He was a crucible in which I tinkered.*"

- **The veiled anonymity but physical intimacy of the surgeon.** "The drapes on the operating table have the contour of a chain of old mountains," we read in Kramer's *Invasive Procedures.* "*No hint of what lies underneath;* it could be a goat or a large sheep. The face is draped, too, like the face of some veiled Moslem bride, hooded in tribute to its power to contaminate. The surgery will be an exercise performed upon some *abstract sick creature, not on anyone in particular.* Andersson . . . never refers to the patient, but only to the parts encountered." A surgeon says: "'They don't delve deeply into the patients because they don't want to—or are afraid to . . . But surgery—that's where you can really change things, make things better, save lives, prevent heart attacks, strokes.'"

A point is reached when the patient no longer has an aorta and the physician has achieved maximum invasion of the patient's body: "Andersson is in the patient as far as he can go." A doctor reflects on the bizarre paradox of the alienated, abstracted physical intimacy that is surgery: "this odd life, whose functional moments take place inside other, sleeping, trusting people . . . the touching of the sick places where life is hidden, held, and lost."

- **Allopathic medicine is life-destructive.** The "meds" are biologically devastating, such as chemotherapy, which destroys blood cells. Klitzman writes: "His marrow was then *blasted* further with chemo to *wipe it out* altogether . . . he was 'nadir,' meaning that he had almost no cells left in his blood supply. The physician obliterates and restores life at the cellular level: "I gave him back his own marrow, to try to reseed his now vacant trabeculae . . . but the sowing failed to germinate . . . This drug of last resort was potent but *destructive,* inflicting many side effects . . . The drug *slashed* even further the numbers of Mr. Vier's white blood cells and platelets, *decimating* these troops."

For the heroic physician, there's little difference between dispatching Patriot missiles in the Gulf War and sending in chemotherapeutic troops to decimate hostile platelets. "The body was *weakened* before becoming stronger. In an effort to *fight* disease, it was first rendered *defenseless."* The agent of death seeks also to be the agent of life, *sowing* new cells in the bone marrow.

- **Humans are dispensable objects for experimentation.** Of a young girl with a liver transplant, Klitzman says: "Her doctors had undertaken this costly investment as a carefully monitored trial. They *chose as their laboratory the body* of this beautiful and innocent little girl."

- **The hospital is a house of the dead.** This excerpt from Klitzman evokes the hospital's mechanistic and soulless theater-of-death aspect. "Sixty-four operating rooms stretched along the third floor of the Thomas Wing like an *ancient Roman catacomb.* The halls and rooms were *cold* and smelled of disinfectant." Surgeons make life-and-death decisions constantly, in a shadow play reenactment of the rites of the Mexican priests: *"Surgeons decide* every day who lives and who doesn't."

Here's Klitzman on working with dead bodies as a training foundation in the Gross Anatomy Suite: "yet the corpses were cut up each semester, *their amputated parts pitched into wastebaskets* till all that remained was *flesh clinging to bones, reminiscent of a roasted turkey* the day after Thanksgiving . . . One had to *master the dead* before handling the living."

After all, the students' medical education begins with learning from the dead in anatomy class; then, during internship, from the dying and the sickest, Klitzman writes. The rituals of crucifixion are reiterated every day in the surgical room, Kramer reminds us. "The modern operating table is *cruciform:* armrests extend from it at right angles. This keeps the arms out of the action and offers the wrists. Masked, a nurse and the surgical resident work rapidly, *binding Mr. Luskin's hands* to the table, palms up, then installing long *intravenous spikes in both wrists.*"

Providing the patient survives the experience, surgery becomes spiritually redemptive, again in a strange soulless dimension. Allopathic medicine is a purgative hallowing. "Sealed, clean, cancer-free, the patient is again topologically identical to healthy persons," writes Kramer.

- **Medicine's cyborgian ideal.** Where is medicine headed? In what ways does it yearn to transform human biology? Here is one physician's answer, as reported by Kramer: "a graft, a section of aorta woven of Dacron . . . The graft is complete, *a headless homunculus* pulsing inside the veiled patient . . . the replumbed and still groaning Mr. Lazarus in the recovery room." The postsurgical patient is a patchwork of medical interventions: "His body is welted with surgical scars, and with the wales of arterial prostheses already in place. He's in his fifties; he's had one leg replumbed and has an artificial aorta."

Pacemakers are a lifesaving technological insult to a man's humanness: "But for a very few, dependence on a *machine,* on something chancy, manufactured, not really part of themselves, turns out to be an unbearable burden, a metaphor, perhaps, for the *impositions of the age of technology upon private being.*" In a bizarre reversal of the Mexican mystery murders in which the priest would exultantly hold aloft the extricated stomach or heart, here a surgeon contemplates a pacemaker before installing it in the chest cavity: "now it all fits in the palm of my hand as I install it in a patient."

Whether you excise the heart and control the body by killing its circulatory core or install an artificial heart control, either way, the medical priesthood has colonized the body. But allopathy's invincible desire to thoroughly control the human organism has already gone another level deeper—into the molecular heart of the immune system. Here the weapon for conquest has been vaccinations and selfhood has been its prize.

Immunizations against Selfhood: The Politicization of the Immune System

With the subject of vaccinations, we confront what allopathy considers one of its most significant achievements. This is the ability to inoculate, and generally protect us against a variety of infectious diseases. Founded on the germ theory of disease, in which pathogens invade the body from outside and produce illness inside, vaccinations represent medicine's ability to manipulate the immune system at the molecular level, presumably for better health.

Infectious pathogens cause illness, says allopathy, especially childhood illnesses like diphtheria, measles, mumps, rubella, and whooping cough; therefore, physicians use immunizations to pre-empt these sometimes dangerous and always inconvenient infections. Modern medicine regards vaccinations against infectious disease as incontestably a public good, but might there be a dangerous flaw—an intellectual pathogen—in allopathy's logic?

The operating theater for vaccinations is the human immune system. The Western medical tradition in its early days used the term *physis* to describe the natural vitality of the immune system that could homeostatically respond to environmental factors; the physician is the one who expertly guides, coaches, and benignly manages the response of the *physis*. The immunological theater involves the molecular basis of our identity, the deployment of our body's innate healing response, and the struggle to maintain and evolve an integrated individuality. Immunology is at the molecular heart of healing. Allopathic practices have direct and long-term consequences for our immune function.

The largely unquestioned practice of mandatory childhood immunizations may have long-term *developmental* consequences for the immune system and its correlate—identity, both biological and psychological. There may also be a political dimension to immunizations as well, a matter of democratic rights. When identity is compromised at the molecular, immunological level, then democratic rights are in jeopardy, specifically, meaning, the right for self-determination, self-fulfillment, and individual personhood. On a molecular level, that's what our immune system provides.

The human immune system of an entire generation—the 70 million Baby Boomers—has been taken over by the antigen-filled syringes of allopathy. Since 1945, a major public health effort has sought to build disease-immunity in American children against a host of presumed microbial scourges. It hasn't let up since. The intention of this arsenal of vaccines is to artificially generate maximum protection against the infectious childhood diseases through early, controlled exposure to pathogens injected into the body through inoculations. The immune system then wages a mini-campaign against the foreign materials (called antigens) and develops antibodies specifically tailored for that disease organism for future reference. The result is what immunologists call specific or adaptive immunity.

Ever since Edward Jenner's discovery in 1798 that childhood cowpox inoculation prevented later infection through developing immunity, Western medicine has inundated the world with new, always stronger, vaccines against rabies, typhoid, tuberculosis, yellow fever, influenza, measles, mumps, meningitis, and, before too long, against AIDS, melanoma, lung, kidney, colon cancer, leukemia, even pregnancy. It's estimated that every week physicians inoculate about 57,000 young Americans, such that today about 97% of young American children have been inoculated with at least seven vaccines—typically a total of twenty-seven different disease antigens in nine shots by age eighteen months—by the time they enter first grade at age five.

By 1988, there were nineteen licensed vaccines in America, seven of which were legally required for schoolchildren in nearly all fifty states. Increasingly children get most of their immune-boosting shots while still infants, generally between the ages of two months and two years. The result is "the most immunized child in history," as allopaths like to boast. However, the historical record contradicts allopathy's boosterism about the efficacy of vaccinations.

With tuberculosis, in 1812, the death rate was about 700 per 10,000 infected; by 1882, when Koch first isolated the TB bacillus, the mortality rate had dropped to 370 per 10,000; by 1910, when the first sanatoriums opened, it had dropped to 180; and by the mid-1940s, before antibiotics became routine, TB mortality was even lower at 48. "Cholera, dysentery, and typhoid similarly peaked and dwindled outside the physician's control," writes Ivan Illich. "By the time their etiology was understood and their therapy had become specific, these diseases had lost much of their virulence and hence their social importance." Illich contends that the combined death rate from scarlet fever, diphtheria, whooping cough, and measles among children up to fifteen shows that "nearly 90% of the total decline in mortality between 1860 and 1965 had occurred before the introduction of antibiotics and widespread immunization."

According to Richard Moskowitz, M.D., a homeopathic physician and outspoken critic of vaccinations, immunizations may not produce the immunity doctors expect, and instead, make the infant susceptible from birth to chronic illness. Based on his clinical experience, Dr. Moskowitz argues that vaccines make the child less likely to respond acutely—with a fully symptomatic episode—to a childhood illness such as measles or to other foreign or infectious agents as well. The trouble is, children inoculated against measles "are less likely to come down with the typical acute case of measles because they already have *chronic* measles, so to speak, and have also been reprogrammed to respond *chronically* to other such threats in the future" [emphasis added].

As Moskowitz sees it, vaccinate a child against measles today and perhaps she won't have a bad (acute) case of measles, but she will become susceptible to a lifetime of chronic illnesses against which her weakened immune system cannot wage a proper defense. Immunity conferred by vaccines is "inherently counterfeit," says Moskowitz. All you're doing is substituting a chronic illness later in life for an acute illness in childhood. Mandatory vaccination—increasingly, more vaccines for different illnesses are given either simultaneously or close together in infancy—is a kind of ill-advised genetic engineering. "I fear that we are like the sorcerer's apprentice, unknowingly precipitating an evolutionary crisis of major proportions."

For the most part, childhood vaccinations are legally mandatory in the U.S. Choice isn't part of the picture because the paradigm is politically enforced—that's the key point. There is little opportunity for exemption and allopathic medicine—characterized by invasive procedures, surgery, transplants, drugs, antibiotics, and vaccines—is the order of the day, as far as most doctors, hospitals, and insurance companies go. In other words the rationalists have legislated the nature of our immune response, putting the *physis* in thrall to the "contraries." But if our immune freedom is compromised, this really means allopathy now controls the molecular elaboration of our individuality.

Profound matters are at stake—most concisely put, immunological freedom. This means our right to uniquely, individually respond to a disease process and establish health in our own terms, to develop immunity out of the innate vitality of our organism, to exercise biological self-determination through immune response, and the freedom to choose the type of therapeutics we judge will best enhance our health. This is freedom at the molecular level. But medical laws, the monopolistic practices of conventional medicine, and vaccination requirements all prevent this—and that's political. Immunological freedom, which should be our inalienable right as citizens of a democracy, is jeopardized by the ways of modern medicine.

The immune system, after all, is the physiological theater whereby the body negotiates on a biochemical level what is self and not self. These antigens are okay; these are "outta here"—and the net balance is *me*. That's essentially how immunology works, according to modern science. In other words, immune response involves a determination of identity. The *physis* reacts flexibly to a constant barrage of possibly inimical influences, yet always in accordance with a reference point: an integral biological sense of self. The antibiotics, cortisones, and vaccines get rid of the symptoms in the given moment, but down the road, the patient is progressively weakened, the *physis* staggers.

Maybe the "immune system" itself is an allopathic abstraction, suggests Coulter. Maybe it's a misleading compartmentalization of the innate, diffuse *physis* into one organic subsystem. The early Greek empirics did not distinguish between digestion and the body's ability to deal with pathology, germs, or morbific outside influences. To them, the unilateral organismic response was just "coction" (cooking); immunology was coction, too. They always said the way the body deals with disease is by digesting it; body temperature rises because it is cooking, or digesting.

In contrast, the empiric homeopaths emphasize the immune reaction of the whole body, not just the glandular and lymphatic system. It's all one response to them, not fragmented into systems: the integral response of the individual, all the systems "cooking" together flexibly as one.

The rationalists can't get around this concept of flexibility, notes medical historian Harris Coulter. "To them the immune system is like a billiard table covered with balls, one ball hitting the next in an intricate chain of causality. There's never any sense that these blood proteins act in response to some higher force, the body's vitality, which compels, governs, steers, or dominates them. They think there is an on/off switch, that something fires or doesn't fire. The idea that new switches can be produced at will, that the body can deal with new morbific threats as they arise—that's alien to the allopaths."

Vaccinating the Soul
out of the Human Body

The empirics are sufficiently emboldened to propose that certain of these early morbific threats might actually be salutary for children because through them they help the child's organism develop natural, permanent immunity. "Worth considering is the idea, quite heretical in the context of late Twentieth Century industrial medicine, that childhood diseases actually *benefit* the child." suggests Harris Coulter. Physicians familiar with these diseases in the past often noted a spurt in growth and development after a bout of measles, mumps, or whooping cough. "That wisdom has been forgotten today."

Perhaps not entirely. Another group of Twentieth-Century empirics—all M.D.s, incidentally, practicing anthroposophical medicine—strongly advocate abstention from most standard childhood vaccinations. The subtleties of immunology and the spiritual liabilities of vaccinations are not unknown to them.

Anthroposophic medicine, which took its inspiration from the Austrian polymath and spiritual scientist, Rudolf Steiner (1861-1925), contends that the inflammatory, fever illnesses of childhood shouldn't be circumvented by immunizations. Rather, they are best interpreted as benign healing crises in which an immature immune system struggles to remodel the body from the experience of responding to disease influences. According to this view, childhood infections like measles, mumps, or chickenpox, are immunological exercises, healthful experiences ultimately. An immunization diverts a child's inherent health and vigor (*physis*) into developing chronic medical problems such as cancer or immune dysfunctional illnesses later in life. The immune suppressions of the 1960s are revisited as the immune dysfunctions of the 1980s.

But there may be a still darker side to immunizations, something worse than chronic immune suppression. Rudolf Steiner indicated as much in 1917. Steiner made an unsettling prediction about the future of Western medicine, just six years after the development of the typhoid vaccine. "The soul will be abolished by means of a medicament in the form of a vaccine which will be injected into the human organism in earliest infancy, if possible, immediately after birth, to ensure that this human body never has the idea that a soul and a spirit exist. Materialistic doctors will be entrusted with the task of driving souls out of human beings."

Many will find Steiner's analysis bleak, possibly paranoid, but his argument was based on a complex spiritual model of the human organism. Essentially when he says vaccines will drive the soul out of the body it's the same as our saying vaccines suppress the immunological elaboration of identity, that they prohibit the freedom of a unique immunological response. Anything that impinges on our immune system touches a profound aspect of our being.

The prolonged Western medical schism may involve nothing less than control over human individuality through the roots of our biological reality. The *physis* is uniquely individual; that's the empiric's powerful message. The *physis* is the total expression of biological selfhood, from the molecular to the organismic level—our immunological identity, in short. That directly implicates our psychological sense of self, too, because anything that circumvents or suppresses immunity interferes with our democratic freedom to be unique individuals, even if that means getting sick. Further, driving souls out of human bodies through medicine is a strategic, though occult, element in Ahrimanic landscape-mediated American allopathy.

In this new interpretation, the roots of democracy are immunological. Immunological democracy means the freedom of an individualized immune response; the inalienable, immedicable right of the *physis* to respond uniquely, appropriately, and without coercion to environmental influences; and the biological right to conduct one's own molecular identity negotiations. Quite a lot is at stake in the life of our T-cells.

So when Harris Coulter contends that vaccinations represent the rationalist "medical assault on the American brain," maybe that's not saying enough. Maybe the contention is better put as the medical assault on the American individuality. "It's ironic because Americans think of themselves as individualistic but really they're possessed by a herd mentality," Coulter speculates. "Maybe the American instinct for conformity is caused by childhood vaccinations."

Is Modern Medicine Now in the Domain of the Criminally Insane?

The project to vaccinate against selfhood is not allopathy's final play to control the human organism, although it's a strong one. From the vantage point of a strategic ploy to capture the human body, defeat the *physis,* and expel the soul from the body, the enforced use of vaccinations is a brilliantly effective move. Ultimately, it's as if allopathy yearns not only to control the mutable biological body, but to replace it with an immutable, synthetic, and perfectly manipulable one—a nanotechnological golem.

It is but a continuum, and not a marked threshold, between the acceptable medical logic of rationalist medicine and the unacceptable medical illogic of an unregulated allopathy that has entered the domain of the criminally (and spiritually) insane. Arguably— certainly from an empiric viewpoint—there are strange developments under way in conventional Western medicine. Counterpointing these developments with practices in seemingly unrelated fields might help tease out the element of insanity, otherwise unacknowledged by contemporary assumptions. A brief annotated inventory paints the gruesome picture.

- **When evil takes the Hippocratic oath.** The suspicion that modern allopathy may have crossed the "line pass not" from healing into black magic is increasingly sounded in mainstream popular fiction. Consider the recent "novel of medical suspense" *Lifebank,* by Howard Olgin, M.D., a leading exponent of laser surgery (called laparoscopy). Here a physician uses his own prestigious reputation and that of a prominent medical research organization called Med-Tek as a cover to steal human organs by way of laparoscopic surgery; as he builds his inventory of "harvested" organs, he discovers a way to preserve them indefinitely in a laser-treated "fluocil" solution.

Even better, he finds a way to inoculate this tissue such that it becomes immune to nuclear radiation and the bacterial strains used in germ warfare; he proposes to sell this information to a Middle Eastern government for a billion dollars. It's almost uncanny the way even the copywriter of the expected purple prose singing the book's wonders catches the black magic drift of Olgin's "novelistic" proposition. Med-Tek offers all surgeons a new technique by which they can discharge patients in a day, triple their profits, and cut their risks: "The only hidden cost is your soul."

- **Genetic nihilism.** The Human Genome Project is a massive, $3 billion federally funded project to map the presumed 100,000 genes constituting the genetic human. Along the way, it is generating refinements in allopathy's way of regarding health, illness, and destiny. Every illness is caused by a defective gene; identify the aberrant gene, fix it with gene therapy, and the illness should go away. You can identify an infant's susceptibility to disease that may not manifest for fifty years in that body. "The oncoming tidal wave of genetic data has not yet affected most people," writes Tim Beardsley in *Scientific American.* "That will change."

Except the proposition of a hugely detailed roadmap of human molecular destiny has its downside. It generates a highly pessimistic, mechanistic, deterministic, and nihilistic view: our destiny is written in gene codons. Illness has nothing personal to do with us: it's a gene flaw, a bad luck roll of the dice. Knowing the DNA "we've been dealt" can be toxic knowledge, writes journalist Charles Siebert.

Physicians are coming ever closer to being able to give a patient a personal genetic report outlining their genetic predisposition to a variety of chronic or potentially mortal illnesses. If everything is determined by genes, then the once elusive concept of fate or destiny is now biologically measurable—and, if you are a subject of allopathy, chances are, it's bad news. Genetic self-knowledge, to Siebert, represents the "world's most high-tech fortunetelling tent." Seeking knowledge he feared he would regret knowing once he had it, "I came to think of my journey as a kind of personal reconnaissance mission to find out what genetics could tell me." The genomist is today's seer of Delphi, but the oracular pronouncements of high-tech gene therapy leave no room for the *human* in the physical being. Destiny is now a mathematical formula, a sequence of codons.

Siebert is not to blame for his unconscious immersion in the nihilism implicit in genome technology, but insofar as his article represents a forum for prevailing views, it is deeply immoral. Using mainstream media, it fosters a delusionary, pessimistic, mechanistic soulless new role model for the patient; as such he choreographs a new gesture for the death dance of patient victimology. It could also produce a new subclass of genetic untouchables; families marginalized and uninsurable because of demonstrable genetic tendencies to certain expensive diseases.

Now allopathic medicine has figured out a new way to kill patients before they are even palpably sick; the presymptomatic ill are hereby instructed to self-destruct their immune system, using the toxic knowledge that their DNA carries misspellings, typographical errors in the script, mechanical glitches—time bombs scheduled to blow them away from inside.

In this emerging model of genetic determinism, the gene disturbance is not secondary, but the primary determinant of illness, notes Paul W. Scharff, M.D., a physician schooled in Rudolf Steiner's anthroposophical medicine. "In this world-wide search for the genetic disturbances of chronic and metabolic illness, we come to an absolute elimination of the human soul and spirit. The gene becomes the all-powerful demon of man's struggle with chronic illness, but here the demon is not a being but a chemically disordered configuration."

This becomes a body without soul or absolution, or even a venue for interaction, other than another mechanistic manipulation, gene therapy. No room is allowed for conscious, willed human interaction with this supposedly predetermined genetic destiny. It is the Double's vindication, Toatl's validation: the absolute genocidal dead end of allopathic anticonsciousness thinking. The soul in the body is dead: long live the soul!

- ***Disembodied diagnosis.*** Since the advent of chemicalized medicine in 1945, the allopathic physician's bedside manner has become increasingly cold and impersonal. Now the allopath's attitudinal aloofness can be matched by his literal physical nonpresence in the diagnostic process. It's called telemedicine or whimsically, the "300-mile stethoscope."

The idea is that doctors can examine patients using closed-circuit two-way televisions, interactive video hookups, electronic stethoscopes, long-distance x-ray transmissions. The new house call is made by the doctor's electronic double, a cybernetic *Doppelgänger*. According to one supporter of the approach, telemedicine is "the perfect use of the technology" because patients "get the same kind of care they'd get if they were sitting next to me"—minimal, disinterested, technologized. If the doctor has any intangible healing presence (once called, pejoratively, the placebo effect), it is now conveyed by pixels and bytes and mediated by a mechanical (Ahrimanic) contrivance.

- *Molecular engines.* To its supporters, nanotechnology is the ultimate in the technological conquest of nature. Now scientists can manipulate and control matter at the smallest (hence, "nano") level of molecules; they can rearrange atoms as if they were bricks, building living molecular structures or substances at will. Conceived by physicist Richard Feynman and articulated and developed by MIT graduate K. Eric Drexler, nanotechnology's goal is to remake the world, molecule by molecule, using atom-sized robotic assemblers.

You could make a meat machine, obviating the cow yet ending up with edible meat, "absolutely indistinguishable" from the cow. It would be a mechanical cow, a meat factory at the atomic level, as billions of robotic assemblers work mechanically in parallel, pushing individual molecules into place, synthesizing beef. The crowning feature of nanotechnology, as Drexler sees it, is this mechanical, robotic aspect: objects, molecules, even DNA, could be manufactured "automatically, effortlessly, without human hands or labor, by a fleet of tiny, invisible robots," explains Ed Regis in Nano.

Molecular nanotechnology is admittedly a "radical" concept, Regis says, "but one thing complete control of the structure of matter meant was *complete control of human biology*, and that in turn meant the eradication of disease and aging." Nanotechnology will make gene therapy a practical reality; if Parkinson's disease is a flaw in the genetic code, send in a nanoassembler to fix it; if sickle-cell anemia is the result of a single misplaced amino acid, then send in a nanomachine to remove the valine and install the correct glutamic acid instead. By the mid-1990s, Regis says, nanotechnology was advancing steadily toward its goal; already there were atomic switches, self-replicating molecules, molecular shuttles and trains, even artificial atoms.

- **Transplant frenzy.** For conventional medicine, increasingly the master of ever more technologically heroic procedures, the human has become a body parts shop. Organs—kidneys, lungs, livers, hearts, eyes, pancreases—are expendable, exchangeable, transplantable. A 1990 report by the U.S. Public Health Service documented the success of transplant technology at 261 hospitals involving 60,100 transplant procedures performed on 57,457 patients. One-year survival rates range from 57% (heart-lung) to 93.8% (kidney), with 38,000 Americans on the waiting list for other people's spare parts. In one year alone (1989), 1,673 heart transplants were performed in the U.S.; 8,886 kidney, 2,160 liver, 412 pancreas, 89 lung, 70 heart-lung. If humanity is one composite creature, then medicine is enabling a high degree of organological promiscuity.

The end result may be "puzzle people," according to Thomas E. Starzl, M.D., director of the Transplantation Institute of the University of Pittsburgh Medical Center. A "puzzle man," Starzl says in his memoirs of a transplant pioneer, may have multiple organ endowments from different donors: a heart and kidney, pancreas and kidney, heart and lungs, liver and heart. Transplantation is "a very large miracle, perhaps the least anticipated and potentially the most important one in the history of medicine," Starzl writes.

Energizing the transplant "boom," "explosion," and "gold rush," was the introduction in the 1980s of cyclosporine, a fungal metabolite that suppressed the human immune system's natural shock-and-destroy reaction to foreign tissue—somebody else's organ. Cyclosporine and subsequent immunosuppressive drugs (such as FK-506) enabled organ transplantation to flourish by biochemically strong-arming the immune system into an unnatural submission. Of the numerous toxic side effects produced by the denial of the body of its own protective *response*-ability, doctors described them as "unforeseen" and "surprising."

But at least some medical ethicists regard this science fiction vista of rebuilt people, man-machine unions, and the "array of extracorporeal and implanted devices" with alarm. "It is the 'spare parts' pragmatism, the vision of the 'replaceable body' and limitless medical progress, and the escalating ardor about the life-saving goodness of repairing and remaking people in this fashion that we have found especially disturbing," write Renee C. Fox, Ph.D., and Judith P. Swazey, Ph.D. This is still a technical question; but what of the personality and energy residues of transplanted organs? Does my liver have anything to do with who I am?

If you ask a doctor of Chinese medicine, the answer will be yes: my liver carries a definite signature of my energy, my style of Qi. Perhaps it is "rebellious Qi," in which the fire (or *yang* quality) of the liver energy is usually banked down but subject to sudden, unpredictable flare-ups. Ask an esotericist, such as a doctor practicing anthroposophical medicine, and the answer will also be yes: the energy contours and functionality of my liver are a direct result of my soul destiny and the subtle input of macrocosmic stellar bodies.

"There lies in every organ a more or less unconscious soul-spiritual relationship, which in olden times was directly experienced as a reality," observes Otto Wolff, M.D., an anthroposophical physician. The liver mediates a human's physical life, Wolff says. "It allows him to incarnate on earth, that is, to immerse himself with his ego into living substance." Can cyclosporine completely suppress this soul-necessity if my liver ends up in your vascular cavity? Transplanted humans are a bizarre cadre of the surgically mediated organologically possessed.

- **Technovampirism.** The FDA has approved a new mechanical device called the Liposorber to take cholesterol out of human blood in patients whose serum cholesterol is severely high. During a three-hour process, the machine slowly extracts the patient's blood and separates out the low-density lipoprotein (LDL) portions (the so-called "bad cholesterol"), which accumulates as a yellowish gunk; the cleansed blood is pumped back into the patient, on the average 73% to 83% purified.

Obviously, this procedure evokes classic images of vampirism, of malevolent astral beings sucking the blood out of a person's jugular vein. Even more engaging is the nuance of ectoplasm, an amorphous, semi-physical gelatinous material extruded out of the ethers by nine-teenth-century occultists. If the condition of one's blood reflects both how one has lived (dietary choices, exercise) and what one has inherited (genetic matrix, soul destiny), then the Liposorber is the ultimate mechanization of absolution: it will literally suck out the materialized residue of these ill-advised choices from your blood and mechanically constitute (absolve) your plasma.

- **Undead corpses.** Western technological medicine has so advanced in the questionable practice of artificial life-support systems that people are not allowed to die, or to be classified dead. The parents of a five-year-old child whom doctors declared brain dead, unrevivable, and legally a corpse, insisted on keeping their daughter on artificial life support. Western medicine now has the technical means (and insurers seem willing to pay the bill out of some unfathomable reckless giddiness that such medical bravado ought to be supported) to maintain a brain-dead body for months, even years, however bizarre this practice might be.

What is unsettling is that what passes for a high-tech bravura performance in the West, is the basis for necrophilic black magic elsewhere. A German traveler in the Tibetan outback of the 1930s reported encountering a spectral community of the walking dead; Tibetan black magicians has resuscitated the clinically dead and like puppet masters, set them to work as soulless automatons. In a sense, this is an aspect of the allopathic ideal: total control over all materialized physical processes of the human form, regardless of whether the person is "home."

- **Transgenic baconology.** Allopathic medicine is now working on ways to intermix animal and human organs or "beast machines" as Andrew Kimbrell writes in *The Human Body Shop*. Biotechnologists have revived the practice of creating chimeras that cross species boundaries, writes Kimbrell. "They are real-life *transgenic* animals—animals engineered to contain the genetic traits of humans and other species." Human ears are grown on the backs of laboratory mice as animals and pig livers are harvested for human transplantation as animals become biofactories "for the production of valuable human body materials," says Kimbrell.

Already four American biotechnology companies are racing to develop (patent) pigs that could serve as organ donors for human transplant operations. It's a huge market, worth at least $1 billion: while 18,000 organ transplants are performed annually in the U.S., 40,000 more patients wait for donor organs to become available. Were there enough organs, transplants could increase tenfold, industry specialists speculate. Thus genetically altered pigs will be bred for human organ "xenografts," with pig organs going for about $10,000 each. Human recipients will be pretreated with a small amount of pig donor tissue in advance of the transplant, to school its immune system in nonrejection of otherwise inimical porcine DNA. As pigs supply hearts and valves, a baboon supplies livers, and an AIDS patient gets a baboon's bone marrow, "Surgery gives man new best friends," quips health policy analyst Jeff Stryker.

Can baboon immunity rescue a ravaged human immune system? In December 1995, a thirty-eight-year-old AIDS patient received an injection of baboon bone marrow with the expectation that the bone marrow cells from an animal not susceptible to AIDS might proliferate in the patient's body and restore his highly compromised immune system. The paradox of suppressing the patient's immune system to not reject the foreign protein so that this could stimulate the immune system to respond better to foreign viruses and proteins was lost on the physicians and journalists covering the story. Ironically, two months after the experimental interspecies transplant, the baboon cells had failed to thrive but the patient had improved—a transgenic placebo effect, perhaps.

- *Lupus redivivus.* You need to step *way* back from this proliferation of bravura "heroic" medicine to see, shockingly, what is going on, what kind of writing is on the wall. In the film *Wolf* (1994), Jack Nicholson portrays a book editor literally bitten by a wolf; the wolf DNA takes hold in Nicholson and he begins a torturous transformation from human to human-wolf. At first, his lupus mode is activated only at night, but soon he is as wolf as a human can become, and he bounds off, feral, into the wilds, never to return to human society. This movie summarizes, inconically, the multiple transgressions of Western allopathic medicine against human morality, against humanness itself. The animal components of the human being, divinity's superior evolutionary creation, begin to come out of the human matrix.

Rudolf Steiner claimed that the human being comprises the entirety of the mineral kingdom (in our skeleton and body mass), the plant kingdom (in our etheric or energy body), and the animal kingdom (in our organs and emotions—called the "astral" body). In *Wolf*, it's as if the spiritual glue that has held the transpecies, transkindgom composite of the human together has become water, releasing the constituent parts to their evolutionary recidivistic domains. The soul—Steiner used the term *Ego*—in the human being (Nicholson's character) is no longer strong enough, or fully incarnate enough, to hold the human organization together. Thus, the feral triumphs.

As another twist on this emerging deconstruction of the spiritual integrity of the human being, scientists recently announced their discovery of a way to preserve sperm cells of individual members of a species (not just human) and to implant human spermatogonial stem cells (the virtually and potentially immortal source of sperm cells) into the testes of other male animals, such as mice and rats. Once in the mouse testes, the human stem cells could mature into human sperm cells, then be harvested, and reimplanted in the male or female human.

The scientists—truly mad as mercury-poisoned hatters—can't see beyond the "thrill" of their discovery—one bemused scientist called the news "staggering and flabbergasting and amazing"—to appreciate the profound genetic and spiritual deconstruction process they have set in motion, downbreeding, as it were, the human organism back into its constituent animal parts.

The magnetic center holding the human organization together around the core of the soul loses its force and the individual strands of mice, wolf, pig, baboon, and others assert themselves, precipitating transgenic chaos. The human astral body goes wolf as baboons and pigs take up residence in our organs. At least twenty-four human genes have been disseminated wantonly throughout the animal kingdom in experimental xenografts; the integrity of the human biological organization is being abrogated and deconstructed. Ahrimanic America, inheritor of the medical rites of Toatl, "remains the undisputed leader in the genetic engineering of animals," says Kimbrell.

Environmental Estrogens: Ahrimanic Elementals Commandeer the Human Endocrine System

There are other human-made but Ahrimanically influenced agents that are also taking the human organism apart, at the molecular level of hormones. Hormones are the chemical messengers of the endocrine system that impose order through an integrated communication system among the body's estimated fifty trillion cells.

Endocrine glands, including the testicles, ovaries, pancreas, adrenals, thyroid, parathyroid, and thymus, are central to the regulation and normalization of all the body's complex, interconnected systems, from metabolism and heat production to spermatogenesis and uterine preparations for pregnancy. Even more crucially, hormones organize or program the cells, organs, and brain before birth, when the fetus is still growing and becoming human, in effect, controlling the way the individual's genetic blueprint will be expressed during a lifetime.

When it comes to hormones, a very little goes a long way: hormone concentrations are typically only a few parts per trillion in the blood, indicating what Theo Colborn, Ph.D., a senior scientist with World Wildlife Fund and co-author of *Our Stolen Future,* calls an exquisite sensitivity. "If such exquisite sensitivity provides rich opportunities for varied offspring from the same genetic stock, this same characteristic also makes the system vulnerable to serious disruption if something interferes with normal hormone levels."

Something is seriously interfering with normal human endocrinal functioning: many thousands of human-made, synthetic chemicals (such as DDT, DES, PCBs, dioxin, among many others) that have been released into our air, water, soil, food, and body since 1945. At least fifty-one of these have been conclusively shown to disrupt the human endocrine system, and proper testing has barely begun. Each year, an estimated 1,000 new synthetic chemicals enter the world market, swelling the planetary total to well over 100,000. All of these are new, exotic, completely foreign, and potentially harmful to the human endocrine system; almost none have been thoroughly tested for long-term, transgenerational health effects.

The scientists who can read the writing on the wall (instead of denying the validity of the relationship) refer to these endocrine-disrupting chemicals as environmental estrogens, acknowledging the way synthetic chemicals can *mimic* the structure and activity of natural hormones such as estrogen inside the body. "Man-made chemicals scramble all sorts of hormone messages," says Dr. Colborn. Polychlorinated biphenyls, or PCBs, were introduced in 1929 as a wonder substance and remained on the market for thirty-six years before scientists began to suspect they might have harmful health effects. When the U.S. finally banned PCBs in 1976, the worldwide synthetic chemical industry had already dumped about 3.4 billion pounds of PCBs into the world environment.

Today, they are ubiquitous: in all nooks and crannies of the outer and inner environment, especially human body fat. They are persistent and don't go away; degradation takes a very long time. "Virtually anyone willing to put up the $2,000 for the tests will find at least 250 chemical contaminants in his or her body fat, regardless of whether he or she lives in Gary, Indiana, or on a remote island in the South Pacific," says Colborn. "There is no safe, uncontaminated place." When a mother breast-feeds her new baby, she gives it more than love and nourishment, says Colborn: "she is passing on high doses of persistent chemicals as well."

The awesome increases in the rates of specifically breast and prostate cancer and of most cancers in general in the last several decades is attributed by a growing number of scientists to the proliferation of inadequately tested human-made industrial chemicals. But evidence is accumulating that these chemicals, even at very low concentrations and exposures, can cause more than cancer; by disrupting the endocrine system, they can cause "hormone havoc:" autoimmune diseases, clinical depression, genital and reproductive system defects (such as infertility), and long-term, delayed developmental effects across the generations.

A mother's exposure can have a negative impact on the health of her fetus, producing effects that impair function but that do not become apparent until years after birth. Hormone-disrupting chemicals can impair function, diminishing humans without making them overtly sick. The danger endocrine-disrupting chemicals pose is more than disease and death. "By disrupting hormones and development, these synthetic hormones may be changing who we become," warns Colborn. "They may be altering our destinies."

The result is that it is no longer possible to "define a normal, unaltered human physiology." Every human living today has been affected; every aspect of the global ecosystem is contaminated. There is no longer any clean, unpolluted place nor any human body that isn't carrying a "considerable load" of these long-life, fat-stored synthetic chemicals. Fundamental changes in the systems that support life and in the chemistry of the human body are the grim results of this uncontrolled onslaught against the lawful, endocrinal order of the human organism.

In Colborn's view, the broadscale use of synthetic chemicals has been a "reckless experiment"; human beings have been the unwitting guinea pigs in this multigenerational "scientific" study conducted without an unexposed, double-blind control group.

While we cannot blame conventional medicine for this proliferation of endocrine-disrupting chemicals, the net effect does support the hidden (or occult) goals of allopathy. In the fat tissues of the bodies of nearly all living human beings today dwell foreign, synthetic chemical molecules whose activity, in this context, consists of disrupting communication between hormones and their rightful receptors, whether it be organs, blood, or the brain.

To disrupt is to control, or at least it is the first step toward gaining control, of a biological organism. Once seized, it will be a control that encompasses generations: the mother and her fetus, the fetus and its future life as a mature adult. To see how this proliferation supports the allopathic agenda, we need to deepen our understanding of what Rudolf Steiner called Ahrimanic elementals.

Steiner's model of elementals is part of a very large concept, in fact, a description of the cosmos and its relationship to the planet and all life forms. As the book proceeds and our argument deepens, more of this world-view will be brought forward; for the present, we will limit our attention to a brief synopsis of Steiner's model of elementals. Consider these subtle energies or the unseen intelligences of nature, even "nature spirits," in the old European sense. "The world ether is made of the same substance as one finds in the human etheric body," Rudolf Steiner said. "Man's etheric body is connected with the entire sphere of nature spirits in our environment."

The task of these elemental beings is to create the etheric bodies of all living organisms on Earth, including the human being. The etheric body will be defined and portrayed in greater detail later, but for the moment what we need to understand about this concept is that it is a complex, intelligently organized energy field surrounding and permeating the physical organism and is believed to contain the organizing principles, energies, and memories of the physical body. The etheric body is the energy blueprint of all that is to be in an individual human physical organism; it shares its substance with a similar energy blueprint or field that surrounds and permeates the planet.

Elemental beings, according to Steiner, are the (generally) unseen intelligences that create, work in, and maintain the individual etheric bodies of humans and of nature. Like everything else, the nature of elemental, etheric beings is dialectical: there are "good" ones that support the healthy unfoldment and development of the individual, and there are "bad" ones that oppose it. Let's deepen this a little: this unfoldment also involves the full flowering of the soul within the physical organism and its matrix of consciousness. When it comes to synthetic, laboratory-concocted endocrine-disrupting chemicals, we are dealing with the "bad" or negative elementals. Steiner called these the Ahrimanic elementals.

Ahrimanic elementals seek to hold human beings spellbound to the material world and to conceal all evidence of a spiritual, intangible world lying beneath or beyond the veil of matter, Steiner explained. Ahrimanic elementals work through our concepts of genetic destiny. The goal of Ahrimanic elementals is complete rigidification, to darken human perception so that it cannot see through the material world into its true, spiritual foundations. They will use "subtle scientific means of every kind to achieve this," Steiner said, so that humans will regard themselves as nothing but "completely developed animals." They strive to "kill out in him the consciousness of his own spirituality," that is, of any soul awareness.

Machines and all forms of mechanisms (including nanotechnology and artificial organs and synthetic blood) are points of attachment and insertion for these energies. Modern vaccinations not only compromise the immune system; they infiltrate the body's organs, tissues, cells, and consciousness with nonhuman inimical elementals, with Ahrimanic protein products that do not belong in the human bloodstream and, once there, engage in a seek-and-destroy mission against the human soul.

Ahrimanic elemental beings dive down deep into human nature and consciousness, seeking to deprive us of our individuality and volition. They want to fasten humans permanently to the physical

Earth, mechanizing their thoughts and organic processes. Their goal is to dominate and control the physical plane and to darken our perception of everything else, to heighten intelligence, but to obscure its spiritual referents, "to make [a human] into a sheer automaton of cleverness."

As nanotechnology illustrates, the goal is complete *mechanical control* (by automatic robots) of human biology and matter. The influence of Ahrimanic elementals is "as a cold and freezing, soulless cosmic impulse," icy logic without love or compassion that "strangles men's individual intelligence" and appropriates it for themselves.

The myriad of synthetic chemicals, pesticides, and herbicides released into the world environment since 1945 can be seen, in Steiner's perspective, as a spectral legion of Ahrimanic negative or "demonic" elementals out to conquer and deaden the world. These inimical beings work through the entire pharmacopoeia of allopathy: its antibiotics, magic bullets, vaccinations, gene therapies, nanotechnologies, and immune-suppressing drugs. Insofar as these beings can now work at the level of the endocrine system, which coordinates the expression of one's genetic blueprint, you can see how deeply they have wormed their way into the human organism in the service of the allopathic agenda.

Yet strictly speaking, the reverse is the deeper truth. The visible activities of allopathy serve the occulted agenda of the Ahrimanic elementals. Why stop with the body and its processes? Why not take colonize the mind and its activities of consciousness as well? Not to worry, the allopathic logic is already seeing to it. It's under way, thanks to the Ahrimanic Trojan Horse called Prozac and other selfhood-altering mind drugs.

Listening to Elementals:
The Pharmacology of Selfhood

Since 1987, the antidepressant Prozac has been prescribed to well over 5 million Americans; in fact, as a popular term for a quick fix for nagging depression, Prozac has entered the American lexicon. Psychiatrist Peter Kramer, M.D., certainly helped Prozac's assimilation into mainstream psychiatric practice and public parlance with his best-selling *Listening to Prozac*. It changed his way of thinking about psychological change. He had been used to watching the personalities of patients change slowly as a result of painfully acquired insight and plodding implementation in daily life. Prozac showed him the fast lane to personality alteration, the power of biology, biochemically manipulated, to bring peace of mind and an end to depression, superseding the classical talking-cure and cognitive route.

Prozac has rapidly become allopathy's magic mental bullet, the state-of-the-art psychological quick fixer. The phenomenon of learning about yourself while under the influence of Prozac Kramer aptly coined "listening." Kramer's own listening to Prozac schooled him in what a drug could do and how it could change his professional sense of "what makes people the way they are." If personality is almost entirely determined by biochemistry ("inborn, biologically determined temperament"), who needs to spend much time dredging the psychic depths to reveal the formative layers of personal biography and experience? It's so much easier to let Prozac "catapult people into new ways of behaving," says Kramer.

The trouble is, are these "new ways" of behaving truly *human* ways? If the self is mutable under the influence of powerful neurotropic medications, has human self-awareness and consciousness made a Faustian bargain, allowing an infiltration by Ahrimanic elementals in exchange for a simulacrum of peace of mind? Prozac is a designer drug, "sleek and high-tech," says Kramer, engineered specifically to alter brain biochemistry and neurotransmitter interactions. It plays perfectly into the authoritarian allopathic agenda of control of all bodily and now consciousness processes. "To the extent that medications are important agents of personal transformation, change becomes ever less a matter of self-understanding and ever more a matter of being understood by an expert," Kramer notes. The effort to understand one's labyrinthine biography and to return, like Theseus, from its innermost core bearing the gold of insight, is obviated with the advent of sleek, high-tech, personality-altering Prozac.

Why make an effort of will when a pharmacological expert can prescribe a pill that will magically alter the chemistry of behavior along more socially and personally preferable lines? Kramer seems to agree with the notion that the quality of psychological change produced by Prozac is a simulacrum when he says, "Patients who do well on medication quickly take on positive beliefs about the self. The new valuation of self seems to come from nowhere."

It only seems like "nowhere" when you are not crediting the occulted intelligences working behind the scenes, namely, the

Ahrimanic elementals of medicine. For them, Prozac is another ripe opportunity to invisibly infiltrate the human organism (in this case, the biological supports for consciousness) and claim it for their own. Prozac may be the most popular of the new psychotherapeutic drugs, but there are many other antidepressants, such as Tofranil, Pamelor, and Elavil, and patients everywhere are listening to their biochemical messages as well.

Margaret, aged sixty, describes her four-year experience on Tofranil, then Anafranil, both tricyclic antidepressants. They completely changed her life, giving her "well feelings," making her into what her friends describe as a "different" person having a "wonderful" life. "The side effects of antidepressants [in her case, weight gain, dry mouth, bloating, constipation] are very minimal compared to the tranquillity and peace of mind they've brought me," she explains. On occasion, stress brings her old symptoms back to the surface, so she reaches for more Anafranil, knowing "the medicine will kick in and I'm all right!" She expects to take antidepressants for the rest of her life. Margaret may experience minimal side effects on her tricyclics, but she's looking in the wrong place to assess the drugs' true effects.

Paradoxically, her tricyclics actually prevent her from seeing this because they are an artificial buffer inserted into the stratigraphy of her psyche. Problems lie below this biochemical buffer, coping mechanisms and "sunniness" lie above. What Margaret doesn't see, because her consciousness is now chemically colonized, is that she has an invisible co-dweller in her stream of consciousness; she has a variant of what Colin Wilson once called a "mind parasite," or what we might describe as a "mole," borrowing the term from the world of espionage.

The integrity of Margaret's sense of self—Rudolf Steiner calls it the "I" or Ego—is compromised, occupied, infiltrated. Something—an Ahrimanic elemental—is dwelling in consciousness that has no right to be there. Its task is to modulate a distressed psyche into a *simulacrum* of normalcy and integration. As it blocks entry of the disturbing mental contents that precipitated the need for medication, this "something" blocks the activity and expression of the soul in the medicated patient's life, and it keeps her from even noticing or caring that this soul participation has been obstructed.

Such a drug-induced modulation of consciousness has profound *spiritual* effects, which thoroughly serve the allopathic agenda and strive to defeat the empiric's defense of the *physis*.

The Genocidal Goal of Allopathic Rationality: No Body, Only Artificial Intelligence

At a certain crazed level of extrapolation, allopathy yearns for genocide. It desires the destruction of the wonderful organic mutability of the human organism. The vanguard of science fiction can illuminate the logical genocidal end of rationalist medicine.

The Modular Man by Roger MacBride Allen is about a disembodied human soul transplanted into a cybernetic machine of steel and plastic. The story is an extrapolation of the medical logic of organ transplantation upgraded with artificial, cybernetic intelligence. It's rationalist allopathy taken to its necessary, teleological extreme: artificial intelligence without a body, totally programmable, manipulable, controllable.

Suzanne Jantille is a cyborg: she's a paraplegic literally without limbs, who lies in bed wearing a virtual-reality helmet and operates a remote humanoid robot on her behalf out in the world, as a perpetual out-of-body experience and human simulacrum. She is a *remote person*. "This is how she sees and hears, through a machine. All of her world is far away from her body. All she can see and hear and do, she must do through a cold machine like the one in front of you . . . So the remote unit goes out into the world to walk and talk and carry for her, while her inert, motionless body lies at home, vision goggles over its eyes, earphones stuck on its ears. And I say 'it' and not 'her' because that is all her body is by now—an *it*, a thing, an encumbrance Suzanne Jantille must endure. In a very real sense she does not occupy that body. Instead her soul is in a machine. Her entire life, day after day, is an out-of-body experience."

Allen gives us an image of a mechanical Ahrimanic *Doppelgänger,* the soul navigating the world through a technological device, a Double made of steel and plastic, an Ahrimanic etheric body. She has moments of startling self-reflexivity, seeing her "biobody" as foreign, independent while viewing it from the remote as she tends herself. "Her living eyes saw what her robot eyes sent them, showed her the image of her own inert body . . . Every morning she found herself caught by the strangeness of seeing herself from the outside, and every morning her imprisoned living eyes tried to look toward the very robot eyes they were seeing through."

Her artificial visage is shocking: "The head englobed in the black, beetle-like teleoperator helmet, thick black cables trailing off from it into the forest of machinery discreetly hidden away in the next room . . . And between the two sets of tubes and machinery, the pallid white torso, all that was left of her natural self, all that still functioned on its own . . . Only the helmeted head was outside the sheets and her body looked like a deformed corpse . . . Stepping out of that room, she immediately lost the very disturbing feeling that there were two of her. Outside that room, she no longer wondered which was her body, or who, exactly, she was." Suzanne says: "I can forget my own living body so completely, become so involved in the job of controlling this *robot* body, that I begin to think of *myself* as a machine."

David Bailey, her husband, also a paraplegic, is the other cyborg. He tried to download his mental contents into a nonhumanoid robot, but this partially failed, such that he was rendered mutely sentient within this machine until another robotics expert wired him to another humanoid robot, literally with an umbilicus, so that Bailey, resident within the robot called Herbert, operates a remote called Clancy, and this becomes his vehicle in the world. Philippe, the robotics expert, after great mechanical struggle, midwifes Bailey's oxymoronic return to his senses, using the Clancy robot as his remote Double. Bailey's consciousness, or disembodied selfhood, was trapped gnostically within Herbert the now mute robot after the flawed download. Using intelligently engineered devices, Phillipe wires David's living mind to the world through video cameras and voicebox. "I am growing used to who I am, a soul divided into two metal vessels." This is a simulacrum of human selfhood borne regressively through the mineral-metal world.

In this vision, the rich, wishing to be immortal, transform themselves into cyborgs, cheating death and also inheritance taxes, as they don't die. The authorities fear "a world overrun by the rich who refused to die, encased in their flawless mechanical bodies . . . Sooner or later dead minds *would* be fully and accurately recorded into bodies of metal and plastic. And those bodies would never have to die. [They would be] the mechanical survivors of death . . . "

What Bailey accomplished was a mind transplant of only the neuronal contents without touching the physical brain, so it's not a brain transplant. Mindloads are like "quotes from a book—they should be complete and meaningful by themselves, but they are only the tiniest part of the book itself . . . It's just a little tiny part of a person, a tiny shred."

In an afterword, the late science fiction magus Isaac Asimov reflected on what the line between cyborg and humans might be. An artificial brain means you are a cyborg, not human. "We can imagine, little by little, this part and that part of the human being replaced by inorganic materials and engineering devices." We could have a robotic brain in a human body or a human brain in a robotic body. The visible fleshiness of the human is the distinguishing feature in this crucial definition, said Asimov: "a cyborg with a robotic brain in a human body is going to be accepted by most, if not all, people as a human being; while a cyborg with a human brain in a robotic body is going to be accepted by most, if not all, people as a robot."

The Modular Man is a clever, engaging story about the definition of humanness and agency, but it's based on a flawed premise. As the empiric pole of medical thinking postulates, consciousness and ensouled selfhood are neither dependent on matter nor mechanically or electronically transferable. Human selfhood and intelligence inhabits and permeates the physical brain as an etheric force; you can't mechanically extract selfhood from millions of brain neurons and convey it into another, inorganic container.

Yet as an Ahrimanic propagandistic icon, *The Modular Man* is worthy of the allopathic priests of Toatl. Out-of-body experiences in the pseudosentient Double are possible only through working a robotic remote. Allen's story is about the deconstruction of body-based consciousness. It implies that living matter cannot be re-created by human intelligence or focused spirituality, but only through inorganic contrivance. It also tacitly works from the assumption that individual consciousness is a quantifiable, movable commodity, a neuronal sum, that Bailey's neuronal identity can be mindloaded from living biobody to inert mechanical robot. The ultimate result is a *Doppelgänger* without the human referent, a technological golem.

Allopathy Faces a Conceptual Dead End Called AIDS

Nowhere is the inner orientation of allopathic medicine more evident than in the way it relates to AIDS. As AIDS emerges as an apparently invincible disease, Western conventional medicine finds itself at the end of its therapeutic tether. After almost twenty years marked by the steady proliferation of AIDS, the adversarial, antibiotic, mechanistic reflex, which is the hallmark of the allopathic model, has failed to produce any therapeutic inroads against AIDS. Allopathic rationality is imploding and collapsing in the face of AIDS. Medicine's prevailing model of immunology, because it insists on single causal factoriality in disease origin and because it discounts the presence or efficacy of active, willed human consciousness in physiological events in the body, cannot comprehend and thus cannot act effectively regarding AIDS.

The allopathic view may have carried the day in terms of enforcing its ways (therapeutically, with vaccinations; and ideologically, with conventional medical reporting), but it has hit a brick wall named AIDS. It is now stunned from the sheer force of its own momentum hitting this immovable wall. In AIDS, we see the end game of *self versus environment,* the dead end of the politics of allopathy. For allopathic physicians, AIDS is a cul-de-sac, yet for empiric physicians, AIDS is a swinging doorway providing glimpses of an awesomely mutable terrain of biology and medical practice.

What's crucial here is what the *fact* of an AIDS epidemic says about the therapeutic deficits of the prevailing medical model and what it shows us about the nature of environment—in this instance, its inner, immunological domain. AIDS is a systemic, frequently mortal disease, of the human bodily environment. It does not affect individual organs, but rather the entire terrain, the complete molecular environment.

Under the tutelage of Western medical thinking, doctors have outlawed consciousness from this environment. The human body and its interdependent systems (including its immune response) is now conventionally regarded as a machine essentially preprogrammed through genetics, its operation subject to apparently inexorable biochemical equations.

AIDS is the cul-de-sac at the end of the allopathic paradigm. Its message couldn't be written more clearly throughout the human immune system: the old way of thinking won't get us out of this. Immunology is our inner environment and we have positioned it wrongly. We are desperate, as patients, physicians, and compassionate bystanders, before the AIDS onslaught. We're desperate because, astonishingly, hardly anyone in the medical mainstream is asking the right questions or drawing the irrepressibly obvious conclusions—that the dominant allopathic paradigm fails to account for the situation before us and that its methodologies are inadequate to the therapeutic need.

The implications of AIDS stare us in the face through their organic ravages; Kaposi's sarcoma, Pneumocystis carinii pneumonia, cytomegaloviral infections, cryptococcal meningitis, rampant candidiasis, are telling us something more, much bigger and profounder than the undeniable fact that palliation and cure are needed. They are telling us that we have misconstrued the fundamental nature of immunology itself, how it works, how it's part of us, how it can heal.

Scientists were alarmed to learn of thirty cases of AIDS-like symptoms without any detectable HIV infection, a development that could potentially pull the rug out from the scientists' presumption of specific viral causality. Ironically, the possibility of a non-HIV infection vector might be the breakthrough allopathic scientists have struggled for during the last decade: the doorway of multifactoriality. The unfortunate paradox is that their medical view itself precludes acceptance of this probability. Allopathy is alert for single magic bullets of causality; the possibility of a shower of bullets from all directions is something altogether unexpected from this perspective.

Multifactoriality in AIDS may contribute to the collapse of the allopathic edifice, making it possible for physicians to perceive the data afresh: it's not a question of which specific virus triggers what condition, but that the immune system as the heart of human organic integrity is radically compromised. AIDS is the gross symptom of systemic immunological failure; to blame this kind of unilateral decommissioning of organic integrity on a single probable viral agent misses the point and may in fact be tautological. After all, the biological nature of viruses in general is still uncertain and under debate.

Throughout the 1980s, scientists boasted and patients came to expect a quick technological medical fix on AIDS, a swift and decisive immunological Desert Storm in the form of a miracle vaccine and a powerful palliative drug. After all, with the world's foremost medical establishment, both in terms of research and health care delivery (for those who can afford it), it shouldn't be that hard. The perennial allopathic fixation on finding the "magic bullet" and "miracle cure" only intensified in the wake of the AIDS mystery. AIDS patients demanded more drugs faster and scientists developed more powerful biotoxic drugs. The whole scenario was the allopathic habit speeded up, made frantic by physicians and patients as a demand for stronger drugs that worked faster, that were available immediately.

AIDS heralds the end of the allopathic paradigm. The premise of allopathic therapeutics is to assault the presumed causative agent with toxic antibiotic interventions and/or surgical excisions. Considerable populations of beneficial microbes and general systemic vitality are readily sacrificed in the effort to hammer the single terrorist microbe.

But with AIDS, in which the immune system is by definition severely compromised, to employ drugs and practices that indiscriminately, prodigiously damage immune function as a "side effect," is a *reductio ad absurdam.* Two immunological onslaughts cancel each other out; they implode the system, defeat the physicians, and kill the patients. Surely to deal rationally with AIDS we must *enhance* immunity, not further ravage it; to do this means we must radically reposition our concept of environment.

Penetrating the Enigma
of Identity at the Heart of Biology

AIDS is the medium and immunology is the message—that is, our model of immunology is terribly flawed. As a disease, AIDS operates in the deepest layer of human biochemical individuality, the immune system that negotiates the biological boundaries between self and nonself, that discriminates between inner and outer environment. Environmental boundaries are decided at the immunological level. Within the immunological environment, molecular constituency decisions are constantly made: "these microbes I can live with these I can't; these can reasonably become part of me, these are antithetical to who I am."

AIDS deactivates this immunological border function, the molecular voice of "I" and "me," making our system permeable, nondiscriminatory, chronically unresponsive, even passively paralytic, to everything that enters our interior biochemical milieu or lives there in latent, benign inactivity. The origin and propagation of the HIV retrovirus, still believed by most scientists to be responsible for AIDS, remains mysterious and largely unknown, Merely to correctly explicate its epidemiological vector will radically widen our medical parameters, so the physicians believe.

Something has gone awry—human identity at the immunological, molecular level—and AIDS is here to unrelentingly demonstrate this until we understand. The immunological environment of a person with AIDS is chaotic and undifferentiated, lacking the cohesive force of a strong (immunological) sense of self.

The early descriptions of AIDS-precipitated deaths are awesome portraits of bodies tortured, battered, and abandoned to unimpeded microbial digestion. It seemed that as the "horrifying" symptoms moved in, the human identity and soul presence departed. AIDS patients were so emaciated "they looked as though they had been dragged out of a some sadistic concentration camp," one physician observed. Of another patient, Shilts writes, "Never before had (Jim) Groundwater seen anybody so consumed by any disease": chronic 102°F fever, blindness from cytomegalovirus, herpes infections, signs of incipient dementia, Kaposi's sarcoma (KS) lesions on his skin, mouth, internal organs, and lymph and adrenal glands. Of another patient: lymph cancer of the brain, rampant diarrhea, KS lesions disfiguring his face, his body swollen by toxic medications—"Simon had taken on the appearance of the bloated and scarred Elephant Man."

If they can figure it out, scientists will readily use AIDS vaccines, synthetic blood transfusions, transferals of trained, "killer" T-cells from HIV-negative patients to HIV-positives, or gene therapy that injects the gene for interleukin 2, a hormone that stimulates the growth of immune cells. These are not science fiction speculations, but actual developments, in progress in the 1990s. The intention to develop an effective AIDS vaccine was among the first (predictable) reactions in the 1980s to the belated scientific acknowledgment of the AIDS proliferation

So the scientists plod on with other futuristic medical schemes. Scientists would transplant an entire healthy immune system if it were technically possible, so reductionist is their thinking. But this is precisely where AIDS shows allopathy its inevitable dead end: immunity isn't transplantable. AIDS signals the end of the line for allopathic logic, because to transplant an entire immune system (which has no centralized organs other than the lymph nodes) is tantamount to transplanting a human identity, a self—a person. You can't transplant a person.

Can allopathy, a paradigmatic view based on contraries, dialectics, and automatic mechanisms in self, environment, and in the quality of interactions between the two, ever divine the nature of immunology and "devise treatments"? What is the biochemical treatment for an organism whose human self-identity is in shambles? Can identity be biologically imparted, or will it require an exertion of human consciousness?

This is why I stated at the outset that the message of AIDS is that we've reached the end of the allopathic paradigm. For centuries the prevailing Western philosophical paradigm, which has informed our relationship to the inner immunological and outer ecological environment, has been characterized by what Owen Barfield once called "the Cartesian guillotine." Descartes, the great head chopper, gave Western culture the philosophical rationale for severing the mind from the body. Newton gave us linear causality and a rigid, predetermined clockwork universe. Between the two, Western culture has nurtured a mechanistic, reductionist, materialist model of life—in effect, an antilife paradigm whose biases and assumptions have permeated everything, from politics to medicine. Our thinking about medicine and our therapeutic practices have emerged as expressions of this *allopathic* paradigm (from *allos,* "other" and *pathos* "suffering").

Allopathy is more than a style of medicine, a therapeutic strategy of using contraries (or opposites) to cure bodily suffering. It's an ideology of matter, a politics of the body, an orthodoxy of self, and, however oxymoronic it sounds, a metaphysics, a presumptive model of reality. Worse still, it is in America a politically enforced ideology, dominating by legal fiat our health care practices and, by clever media-generated propaganda, our thinking. While allopathy's microbiological standards and technical competence have much to recommend it, as an ideology it prohibits the useful exploration and exploitation of complementary alternatives—extraparadigmatic therapies such as homeopathy, naturopathy, and acupuncture, among the most notable.

Penetrating still deeper, we must consider how closely medical care cuts to the pith of who we are, how great an impact a style of therapeutics can have on our health, well-being, longevity, our biological viability, our philosophy, our sense of self, our molecular identity. Ultimately, medicine is a philosophy of matter, a cosmology of identity; allopathy may be fixated on studying parts, fragments, linear pathways, isolated systems, specific microbes, but it affects the whole human.

Allopathy is a litany of schisms, a catechism of confrontations: mind versus matter, soul versus flesh, self versus environment, antibodies versus antigens, medicine versus disease, disease versus personality, antibiotics versus microbes, health versus illness, invasion versus repulsion, heredity versus environment. In short, allopathy is *antibiotic,* against life, against ecology, and *cytotoxic,* cell-killing; its practices qualify its essence. Allopathy is implicitly about war in the environment. Nature is ambivalent, dangerous, even inimical to humanity, says allopathy; it must be controlled, manipulated, and aggressively combated.

Reality is a clockwork that operates according to linear, causal, etiological, minutely detailed, and programmable principles: one cause mechanically, inevitably produces one traceable, demonstrable, and measurable effect. Allopathy construes events according to a quantifiable causality. In this view, AIDS is caused by one mutable retrovirus that deactivates the CD4 helper T-cells in the human immune system and commandeers its genetic mechanism. That's how AIDS works, says allopathy; to stop AIDS, decommission HIV at any step in its biochemical pathway.

This is the style of precision with which allopathic perception narrowly positions environmental effects—*in vitro,* as it were, disembodied, out of the living context.

You Can't Transplant an Entire Immune System

The issue of identity is a swinging door between the paradigms. AIDS is the doorman, the momentum that keeps the interparadigmatic door perpetually swinging. Allopathic scientists are about to discover that a person is more than the organic material they've been studying and manipulating so assiduously. AIDS is about to upgrade human identity from "meat" to spirit.

Identity is more than molecular configurations. So the transplant habit is now a logical and technical impossibility, a biological double negative. It might be better, really, to attempt a clone of the entire person from uncontaminated, pre-HIV infected genetic material. Allopathically, this is logical; humanistically, it's absurd. It's a utilitarian value system of plumbing at work here: if a pipe or valve is defective, replace it; if the kidney, heart, or liver are dysfunctional, put in a replacement, human-donated, animal-donated, or synthetic one, then suppress the immune system so it won't reject the foreign organ.

The allopathic M.D. is the master technician for whom everything, given enough time, equipment, and money, is possible. You don't have to extrapolate the logic of allopathy too far—science fiction has done this for decades, anticipating allopathic developments—to get the bionic, cyborgic human, a semisynthetic being, half-technology, half-nature—Roger Allen's modular man—in which consciousness and reflexive self-awareness, the roots of the human identity-making activity, are at best a manipulable epiphenomenon of the physical brain controlled by a medical dimmer switch.

We're not quite there yet, but if a philosophical paradigm has an aspiration, surely allopathy as a collective thought form has a scenario something in the spirit of *Robocop* or *Terminator* in mind. However, a moment comes when logic collides with reality, when the difference between *in vitro* and *in utero* becomes startlingly clear. The trouble is, if you're an allopath and think about it, killer T-cell-mediated immunology can't be transferable from one human to another. An organ transplant recipient must receive huge, continual amounts of immune-suppressant drugs (such as cyclosporine or FK-506) to keep the immune system from rejecting the foreign organ; the larger, more precious the organ (such as the liver), the stronger the dose required.

Now, if you transfuse billions of healthy bone-marrow-generated white blood cells (containing killer T-cells, trained to respond to cytomegalovirus) into a leukemia, cancer, or AIDS patient, allopathic logic itself argues that you'll need to inject antirejection, immune-suppressant drugs at the same time, to prevent the recipient's immune system from rejecting the foreign T-cells. You have to suppress the recipient's immune response so his immune system can receive an immune enhancer—no gain is possible. Again the double negative collapses the medical logic and negates any therapeutic value. AIDS demonstrates the extrapolated futility of allopathic therapeutic logic; when it hits AIDS, the allopathic syllogism collapses in a heap of contradictions.

Allopathy will end up destroying the immune system even faster than AIDS. That's because when we're dealing with the nature of immunology, we must acknowledge we have reached the threshold of the mystery of being human. Dynamic, interactive, defensive identity is more than competent killer T-cells. You can't transplant a person. Immunology brings us right up against the mystery of human identity. It's no different than the final surprise awaiting particle physicists and their multibillion-dollar supercolliders: the ultimate particle, as Deepak Chopra argues, is consciousness itself.

You don't need to spend $10 billion to find that out. Physicists will discover this the minute they accept the primacy of self-reflexive consciousness, when they comprehend that the physicist makes particles, that physical reality participates in the mind of the physicist. They even have a term for it: the observer effect.

Qualitatively, the same revelation awaits the immunologists at the threshold between matter and mind. With a shock—and relief—we'll realize we've been looking in the mirror all along: all those gestures and movements that we thought were somebody else's—our lymphocytes—are our own, starkly reflected back to us. Thinking happens at the level of DNA, says Chopra. "You may not think that you can 'talk' to your DNA (another prejudice that comes from seeing DNA as only a material blueprint) but in fact you do continually."

Beholding the Mystery of Consciousness at the End of Immunology

Allopathy represents the conventional way science have *positioned* environment in the standard medical model. We have structured our perceptions and developed our conceptions of environment under the influence of allopathic rationality; having created and shaped it, we've placed, or positioned, environment as a category of reality in precisely *this,* not that, place.

This is an active, cultural process of cognition; it didn't just happen on its own. But now we must ask in light of our medical *cul-de-sac:* With AIDS as our inspiration, is there an alternative way of positioning environment? Is it possible that consciousness can directly effect the environment, both inner and outer, at its formative, energy level, and become a new player in the game of immunity?

Consider the problem from an existential point of view. Consciousness finds itself in an environment—the body and the world. Everything follows from how we position, or construe, our relationship with each environment. Are we separate, related, integral, or identical with this environment? Is the mind a secondary product of the body or is the mind-body a seamless whole? Does consciousness permeate matter? Do we live in a spiritually animate material world? Are consciousness and matter ultimately the same?

These are crucial, perennial questions of philosophical depth and practical import. And they are in need of our reconsideration, because if the twin crises of AIDS (inner environment) and global ecology (outer environment) are any measure, we've positioned things wrongly. We act as if the human were one thing, the body another; as if our sense of self were one thing, the immunological domain another; as if human intellect were one thing and the consequences of its machinations another; as if people were one thing, the ecosystem around us another—and as if the only benefit to any relationship across the gap is limitless pleasure and profit.

The environment exists for our use, whether it is body or world. Because we've positioned the environment, both inner immunological and outer ecological, as if it were something separate from our human self, we have created a world in which our immunological milieu threatens to destroy us from within and our exterior ecological milieu threatens to bury us in its collapse. It's a desperate time, yet it needn't be this dire. The future *is* redeemable from its apparent apocalyptic trajectory.

In all of allopathy's positionings of self and environment, one key element has been omitted: *consciousness.* Let's provisionally consider consciousness to mean willed, active, penetrative awareness, self-aware presence aware of its awareness, temporarily empty of arbitrary or random content. The consequences of our mistaken positioning of immunology and ecology follow directly from our refusal to posit consciousness as the fundamental characteristic that informs both domains, providing for us the creative interface with which to constructively re-create our world. Conventional immunology and ecology both tell us that we as human wielders of consciousness stand essentially outside environment, as feckless bystanders; we may mechanically shape environment with our hands and our technological extensions, but not with our minds, not with consciousness alone.

The way to rectify our mistaken positioning of self and environment is first to become aware that it is dictated by this paradigmatic view of the world, a unilateral positioning of self and environment that pervades everything, our thoughts, concepts, and actions. Our medical paradigm is a philosophy of life, an ontology of matter. A paradigm is a total, tacit, politically enforced ideology of life—a colonialization of the mind, if you like, the allopathic cosmology, the progenitor of schisms.

AIDS brings us to the mystery at the end of immunology. Can consciousness manipulate AIDS? Allopathy thrives on little mysteries but avoids mystery itself—for these questions nip at the heels of mystery—and would quantitatively demystify every aspect of the human, given enough time, money, and personnel, to proudly display the revealed clockwork of the human organism like a desiccated butterfly collection.

But the message of AIDS is that we must transform our vocabulary and concepts and begin thinking qualitatively differently. Organic disease has established itself at the deepest layer of our physical being: at the threshold between identity and biology, at the interface between intangible self and tangible organicity.

The allopathic world-view prefers to deny this, but it's now an irrepressible factor—the key to the "spectacular scientific breakthrough" everyone expects. Allopathy wants to suppress, destroy, or at least palliate the effects of the AIDS-related pathologies, but what antibiotic is there for a dysfunctional sense of self? Will chemotherapy remedy an identity in molecular shambles? In the early 1980s, allopaths recommended chemotherapy to treat Kaposi's sarcoma, but since the presence of Kaposi's indicates the inactivity of immune function and as chemotherapy deactivates all cell reproduction, including lymphocytic, the doctors gradually realized the approach was pointless.

Allopathic logic tells us that the only antibiotic possible for a confused, nondiscriminatory sense of self at the biological level is death. Death to HIV-mediated immune dysfunction. After all, antibiotic means "against life." That's where the logic of allopathy inexorably leads us—to the inert realm of death. The allopathic medical strategy of contraries is based on overpowering infectious organisms with something stronger, like supertoxic chemotherapy for toxic cancer; if you don't succumb to the treatment, you might survive long enough for another one.

To overpower AIDS, you might have to destroy the entire AIDS-infiltrated immune system; after all, antibiotics, in their attempt to destroy a single specific microbe, indiscriminately kill *everything*, including resident friendly bacteria. But if you destroy the immune system, you've killed the patient faster, even more efficiently than

AIDS. If you go after the secondary, opportunistic infections (KS, CMV, *Pneumocystis carinii*) with strong antibiotics and chemotherapeutics, you may destroy a radically underachieving immune system and the patient as well.

So the only allopathic intervention for AIDS that's stronger than a nonworking immune system (a dysfunctional molecular identity) is inescapably deadly to that identity. The only allopathic medicine possible for AIDS is one that ends life and identity. As the scientist quoted earlier said, the reason we haven't figured AIDS out yet is because it's something that's not too obvious. AIDS is a permeable membrane through which we can pass from a biomechanically mediated view of identity to a spiritually malleable experience of self.

The real scientific breakthrough in AIDS treatment would be to impart something contrary and opposite to immune incompetency—something truly, authentically allopathic to oppose the AIDS shutdown of immune function. If AIDS curtails immune response, let's add something that restores immune competency. We need to think deeply about what immunology accomplishes. It negotiates boundaries; it maintains the molecular integrity of the individual; it chaperones the individuality in its material context. So, to restore an inactive immune system that has ceased making identity decisions, surely we must add: *identity*.

Allopathy could "cure" AIDS by imparting its contrary—self-cohesion, molecularly competent identity, a self-reflexively aware coherency, a pattern of individuality, a center of gravity. The contrary to AIDS is identity. Allopathic logic can take us this far, to the theoretical indication of a cure—in spite of itself. But allopathy cannot deliver the cure because of its own ideological limitations.

Ironically, the allopathic breakthrough that could perceive identity as the effective cure for AIDS will also decommission allopathy as a therapeutic paradigm. Allopathy cannot deliver the miracle cure of identity because this contradicts its logical, theoretical foundations. It cannot accept the fact that identity originates in consciousness, not in matter. Too bad, because as allopathy has legislated consciousness out of its materialist framework, so has it legislated itself out of therapeutic efficacy with AIDS. And, so will AIDS legislate allopathy out of its dominant position.

Identity is not, as allopaths would have us believe, the product of automatic, mechanistic, preprogrammed molecular negotiations in the diffused "immune system." Consciousness is not made of the fortuitous exhalations of the physical processes in our organs. Identity is compounded not of molecules but consciousness, reflexive, self-aware human consciousness, the lifeblood of our *human* being-ness, the *life* within the human *bios*. But human consciousness has no role to play in immunological, environmental interactions, says antibiotic allopathy.

Consciousness emerges secondarily, incidentally, coincidentally, as a feckless, impotent attribute, observant but paralytic, without any power to interact with, influence, or shape matter. Consciousness, decrees allopathy, is a little spark of matter-borne intelligence held hostage and tortured in the body until death, when it vanishes into oblivion.

The Cure for AIDS Is, Literally, a New Person, Re-Created through Consciousness

In the preceding discussion, we've characterized the allopathic positioning of AIDS. But in saying this, we are up against the ultimate oxymoron of allopathic logic: allopathy cannot position AIDS, except incorrectly, because AIDS shatters all of allopathy's positional categories. It doesn't fit; it's too large; it's too vexingly multifactorial, too demanding of a new conceptual framework. AIDS transfigures our perception of the inner environment. AIDS repositions our understanding of environment.

AIDS forces us to reposition therapeutics in light of the true bedrock of immunology: consciousness. Consciousness is the life blood of identity, the underpinning of immunology. Killer T-cells and CD4 lymphocytes are *agents* of consciousness, factotums of identity, not kingmakers. If anything, HIV is our molecular golem, fabricated from our inattentive, unconscious immunological black magic. We projected it, so we can reabsorb it. AIDS is an enigmatic explosion of meaning from the pith of our being.

What lurks behind the immunological facade of HIV immune-suppressant activity is self-identity, consciousness, the immateriality of spiritual existence. For allopathy, this is ideologically prohibited terrain, anathema to its materialist paradigm. If it could, allopathic logic would prohibit self-reflexive consciousness from all rights of existence, declaring it theoretically impossible in all domains of life, attributing self-awareness to the simultaneous automatic firings of multiple neurological homuncular hordes in the brain, as Tufts University brain maven Daniel C. Dennett supposes in his much-acclaimed but deadly nihilistic *Consciousness Explained*.

Dennett, the ultimate reductionist, hypothesizes that the master controller in the brain (or mental operating system) is not, as George Johnson explains in *The New York Times Book Review,* a "fully cognizant marionette but a 'virtual machine,' created on the fly from temporary coalitions of stupid homunculi." Dennett explains consciousness as the result of unconscious, purely physical processes, a "Center of Narrative Gravity" compounded of a hodgepodge of neurological events. For Dennett, who is director of the Center for Cognitive Studies at Tufts, to think there is an ego inside each human peering out through ocular peepholes, is tantamount to "lapsing into a deeply grooved mental habit"—a scientifically imprecise and incorrect assumption.

Here is a state-of-the-art expression of allopathic antibiotics, a theoretical exposition of how AIDS works as a mental process. AIDS suppresses immune identity at the molecular identity; Dennett would suppress coherent identity at the conscious level. It's not preposterous to contend that this style of antihuman reductionism is an HIV infection vector itself, the intellectual expression of AIDS. Dennett deconstructs the cohesion of human identity as swiftly and inexorably as HIV does.

Paradoxically, Dennett's nihilistic reductionism actually demonstrates—proves, as allopaths would say—the immaterial etiology of an organic infection. But this is a contradiction in logic and a theoretical impossibility within the allopathic framework. Dennett's explanation of consciousness shows us how HIV begins in the mind, in consciousness, in an amazing autocidal act of self-denial. When this reductionist antihuman stance becomes a habit of mind—a transmission mainstream culture greatly aids—it effectively undermines and suppresses our belief (our empirical experience) in a coherent, egoic self-identity. Mental autocide ("self-killing") precipitates organic HIV and its immunocide—here is an etiological pathway worth contemplating.

When we don't know who we are psychologically (because, as Dennett tells us, the consciousness of "I" is a compilation of homuncular attention), and when an egoic center of gravity has been rendered theoretically impossible, surely this is the suitable environment in which HIV can begin effecting the same agenda in the organic context. As Chopra says, if we give our DNA a nihilistic message, that's the world-view it will act on. Dennett's reductionist arguments, which he presents on behalf of two centuries of "I"-killing allopathic thinking, embody the entropic, immune-suppressant energy of AIDS at work in the intellectual sphere masquerading as allopathic brilliance. Dennett deconstructs human identity at the mental level; HIV deconstructs identity at the molecular level: either way, it's AIDS.

An inversion of allopathic medical logic, however, reveals to us the only cure for AIDS: *consciousness*—active, engaged, focused, enriched, identity-making human consciousness, the true "lifeblood" of immunology and its biological expression of self-identity. If you want to call it a drug, call it *autopoiesis,* self-making power. More consciousness will cure AIDS because a transfusion of more consciousness will literally re-create human identity at its biological foundations.

The cure for AIDS is, literally, a new person, re-created through consciousness, transformed at the molecular level as an act of quantum healing. In a paradoxical sense, that's the allopathic dream of transplanting an entire immune system, except here it's accomplished in a radically different way: from within, working from the roots upward to transfigure identity. The cure for AIDS is a transfiguration of identity, an act of self-re-creation and reidentification using the only nontoxic therapy ever devised: focused human consciousness.

In this way we may invert that ominous hourglass filled with T-cells and regain our rightful allotment of time, perhaps even gain more time. The metamessage of AIDS is this: we must reposition environment; "oxygenate" the immunological milieu with consciousness; believe, know, and act as if matter follows mind until it does; acknowledge that consciousness is creative, reconstructive, restorative, regenerative, the long-sought foundation of a "solid understanding" of immunology.

The biochemical intricacies of immunology are the grammar of self-identity in a script written by human consciousness. T-cells, B-cells, macrophages, monoclonal antibodies, immunoglobulins—these are *agents*—not initiators—of immune response, biological *mirrors* of our psychological self-conception, *cognitive* factotums for our experienced, historical sense of self.

The immune system is a cognitive network, argues Francisco Varela, professor at the Institut de Neurosciences at the University of Paris. Varela is an immunologist pioneering a new metaphorical understanding of human immunology—"Immu-knowledge." Varela says, as co-author of *Immu-Knowledge: The Process of Somatic Individuation,* that the immune system, similar to brain and nervous system function, involves recognition, learning, and memory. "We want to show that this network view naturally leads to the notion of an autonomous 'cognitive' self at the molecular level as the proper view of immune events."

What Varela describes as an autonomous cognitive self is very likely the same as our indication that immune cells are empowered agents of our conscious intent, executing identity decisions at the molecular level on our behalf. The logical implication of Varela's immune cognitive network is that to recognize nonself requires knowing what self is, which is a function of cognition—the discriminatory activity of consciousness.

Somehow universal knowledge of identity is distributed throughout the immunological network creating a cognitively alert web. Immunity isn't so much about defense as it is about "being alive with flexibility" and how to "think with our entire body," says Varela. Immunology is about to emerge from a long dominance by the "original sin" of having been formulated out of the exigencies of infectious disease, which held vaccinations as its main paradigm, says Varela. Cognitive science, too, is about to transfigure itself and abandon its original paradigm of the digital computer as dominant metaphor.

In Varela's model, cognitive theory and immunological discovery come together on behalf of identity. "If we are willing to follow the central importance of the autonomy of process in both these biological networks, neural and immune, they can teach us how we think with our body."

The Transfiguration of Identity on the Cross of AIDS

Lives undermined by AIDS are saved and transformed. That's another crucial point; as ACT-Up's Tom Lorango insisted, we must "get to the real issue, which is saving lives." But saving the lives of people with AIDS has a unique price; in fact, the cure is the price: more consciousness paid in the currency of self-transformation. The life, to be saved, must be psychologically transfigured at the molecular level of identity. A new person must emerge from the ashes of AIDS.

Surviving AIDS is possible and it will cost your life, as self-transformation always does, but what dies is not your body but your old way of living. "I will always be grateful to my doctor for admitting there was nothing he could do, because his honesty forced me to take responsibility for my own life," admits former HIV-positive Niro Markoff Asistent in her account of AIDS recovery, *Why I Survive AIDS.*

Asistent's story is a chronicle of self-investigation and transformation that will stun the allopaths because it should not have happened; it's not theoretically possible. But it did happen, it is possible, and it's not even that rare; the allopathic theories are faulty—the therapeutic experience is accurate. In fact, says Asistent, who now works full time with AIDS patients as a therapist under the auspices of SHARE (The Foundation for Self Healing AIDS Related Experiment, which she founded in New York City), AIDS is no longer 100% fatal, as evidenced by the hundreds of long-term survivors "living full, valuable, and inspirational lives." The secret? AIDS, says Asistent, became her greatest teacher.

In November 1985, Asistent, a middle-aged heterosexual woman, was diagnosed as HIV-positive and as having AIDS-related complex (ARC); presumably, she was infected by her bisexual male lover. When she received her diagnosis, Asistent felt deep numbness and extreme rage and vacillated strenuously between the two positions; then she surrendered and accepted the inevitability of her death from AIDS. Paradoxically, accepting her death was the doorway to her eventual recovery. "In that instant, I recognized that I could no longer pretend that I was not personally accountable for my physical condition. It is my belief that it is because I totally accepted that I would die, and began living in the moment, that I am still alive today." In May 1986, she tested HIV-negative, asymptomatic, in full remission from ARC. What cured her?

Figuring she had 500 days left to live, Asistent rearranged her priorities, putting herself at the top of the list, no longer suffocating her vital needs in unending service to others. "Having nothing left to lose, I decided to use my disease as a final opportunity for learning and growth, instead of being victimized by it. I embarked on a journey to discover who I am, not in relation to the world outside, but in terms of my true essence within." In a way she could never forget and never cease acting from this essence. Asistent discovered that she is not a soul in a body, but as physicist Gary Zukav phrases it, "a body in a soul." Underneath the innovative psychological and medicinal strategies she undertook, what really cured Asistent? Identity—more consciousness.

Inevitably someone who has faced death and experienced a remarkable remission or cure from a life-threatening disease comes to reflect on larger purposes. Deeply provocative questions get asked: What have I been saved for? To what useful end can I devote my remission? To what end have I been cured of AIDS? And if, like Asistent, you're especially insightful, it may become apparent that the timing, intensity, and style of your disease is utterly appropriate and unsettlingly meaningful; you intuit that in some strange, coincidental way, it came to you specifically with a purpose, not as a judgment, but as a revelation. Your life-threatening organic malady has heuristic value.

That's called teleology, an old-fashioned way of construing events in terms of their intended final ends, as purposeful, not meaningless, events, as if they were elements in an overall intelligent pattern evolving inexorably according to an immanent logic.

Is AIDS teleological? Yes, says Asistent. AIDS erupted like a bomb under the complacent surface of society, precipitating a healing momentum on the planet, affecting us on every level. "It is the beginning of the drastic change that needs to happen on our planet. I believe that AIDS is the most powerful transformational tool that has ever been available to us on a mass level. It is forcing us to reevaluate the entire foundation of life as we know it." The detonation of AIDS at our deepest, molecular level of self, says Asistent, is shaking the medical community, jolting the educational and judicial systems, and forcing us to question everything—our values, morals, identities—and to seek a deeper stream of understanding and compassion.

The AIDS time bomb is ticking, "and it is literally our wake-up call," Asistent advises. AIDS comes as a corrective for the ravages of allopathy, as a miracle cure and *coup de grâce* for an incompetent, destructive ideology; and AIDS comes as a stunning personal initiation into the molecular mystery of being, as a spark with which to newly ignite identity, an incentive for more consciousness, a request to respiritualize nature, to oxygenate environment with the out-breathing of human awareness. AIDS requires us to reposition environment—our immunological identity—and to reposition ourselves within the environment, where we are an antibiotic energy.

AIDS demands we stop destroying the ecological, immunological web of the planet. However, this destruction may not be accidental, in which AIDS is a frightful aberration of nature, but deliberate, in which AIDS is yet another product of the allopathic regime.

Designer Viruses: AIDS and Ebola as Genocidal Germ Warfare?

Paracelsus, the sixteenth-century Swiss alchemist-physician, wrote: "God has not permitted any disease without providing a remedy. Only ignoramuses allege that Nature has not provided a remedy against every disease." This Paracelsian maxim gets a bizarre confirmation in the widely held suspicion that AIDS may have been developed in a government laboratory for the purposes of selective population control. If so, then the cure or antidote for AIDS also exists because not even insane scientists would release a killer virus without providing the means for protection of selected personnel.

AIDS and Ebola, two of this century's most virulent diseases, may not be the deadly aberrations of an indifferent nature nor the revenge of a moralistic, disapproving deity, but government-financed, human-made toxins possibly designed to reduce world population. That's the considered view of Leonard G. Horowitz, D.M.D., a Harvard graduate, independent researcher, lecturer, and author of *Emerging Viruses*.

"A mass of circumstantial and scientific evidence presented in this book supports the theory that black Africans and American homosexuals may have been targeted for genocide by agents for the CIA and activists in America's military-medical-industrial complex" says Dr. Horowitz, who devotes 500 pages to making his case. Dr. Horowitz claims that beginning in the late 1960s, the U.S. government developed and expected to use immuno-suppressive agents such as HIV and Ebola viruses as biological weapons "to effect military, economic, and 'national security' objectives," including population control and the elimination of radical, subversive, or unsavory elements (such as black radicalism) as judged necessary by the U.S. intelligence community.

Horowitz documents a complex network of U.S. government officials and departments, drug companies, international agencies, and well-known scientists that in the last fifty years has vigorously pursued biological warfare as a defense alternative to nuclear war. According to Dr. Horowitz, one of the prime players was Henry Kissinger, former U.S. secretary of state, who in 1969 allocated $10 million of congressional dollars for the development of AIDS-like viruses by the U.S. military. Kissinger also allegedly instructed the CIA to stockpile a Pandora's box of deadly viruses for a secret germ-warfare project code named MKNAOMI. By 1969, 592 virus laboratories in thirty-five countries were developing and sharing deadly virus strains.

Dr. Horowitz also implicates AIDS researcher Robert Gallo, M.D.; the National Cancer Institute; the Centers for Disease Control; the World Health Organization; and various major pharmaceutical corporations in this grim—one might reasonably say, evil—scenario ten to twenty years before the public heard of AIDS. Even more shocking, Dr. Horowitz reveals the early Nazi roots of biological warfare research.

Beginning in 1945, the U.S. Army's Project Paperclip recruited, protected, and financed more than 2,000 Nazi war criminals and "mad scientists" for work in the U.S. defense and intelligence industries. Dr. Horowitz's research also unveiled a secret agreement among NATO, NASA, and a Nazi-linked West German company called OTRAG to lease 29,000 square miles of eastern Zaire (inhabited by 760,000 people) for military purposes. This area is very close to what is now known as "The AIDS Highway" and the eruption point for Ebola virus. This Zairian site might have been ground zero for both diseases, says Dr. Horowitz.

In the 1970s, the toxic AIDS virus may then have been inserted as a kind of biological Trojan horse into hepatitis B vaccine trials (and smallpox vaccine, to a lesser extent) in Zaire (mainly for children), New York City (in 1,083 gay men), and San Francisco (in 7,000 gay men).These areas soon became the prime epicenters of HIV outbreaks. Alternatively, argues Dr. Horowitz, experimental and production vaccines might have been accidentally contaminated by the deadly toxins, giving eventual rise to mutated virus strains that crossed the species barrier to infect humans.

Either way, if Horowitz is right, the U.S. government is to blame. "Perhaps now, as AIDS consumes the lives, liberties, and pursuits of an estimated 30 million HIV-positive people worldwide, the time has come to vanquish our delusions about it and its origin." Already, one can easily read the news in support of Horowitz's contention. As of July 1996, demographic data released by the Population Reference Bureau indicates that AIDS has effectively reduced by 100 million people the expected 2025 A.D. population of sub-Saharan Africa. The same may prove true of India, which is now the country with the largest population base infected with HIV: three million of its 950 million people. All told, as of July 1996, twenty-two million people worldwide were believed infected with HIV, with 8,500 new infections developing daily.

It's gruesome to say this, but in terms of the kind of population control Dr. Horowitz's germ warfare conspirators might have had in mind, AIDS is a highly successful technique. It is also a chance for pharmaceutical companies to clean up in market share once they figure out a "cure." At this same time, at least twelve new AIDS drugs were poised to enter the drug marketplace and their makers were starting to "get aggressive in pitching AIDS treatment," as *The New York Times* observed.

The drug companies involved are "battling" for market share with the same aggressive promotions that they employ for selling ulcer medications, said the *Times*. What finer business arrangement could there be: first you engineer an infectious disease, then after a proper amount of time has elapsed to cover your tracks, you start releasing palliative treatments, even "cures," assured of a gigantic, captive market.

The terrain is vexingly rife with paradox. If AIDS (and Ebola) is a deliberate germ-warfare project designed to reduce world population and as such, one hopes, the ultimate (and final) practical product of allopathic logic (a medically designed disease weapon), this may also serve to profoundly challenge our conventional understanding of bodily based consciousness.

Allopathy may have generated the very wedge that cracks open its own deadly and deadening edifice. If AIDS is human-made, this raises the stakes in the immunological struggle to incarnate an authentic human identity (Steiner's Ego) in the human organism, but it doesn't change the basic issue. That issue remains whether the soul and its agent, bodily based consciousness, will survive and flourish in its rightful environment, whether it be the inner immunological or outer ecological. AIDS and other possible designer viruses represent another front of the Ahrimanic elemental onslaught against humanity seeking to spiritualize its material life.

References

Aikman, Bonnie. "Organ Transplant Report Shows Continued High Success Rate," *Public Health Service Press Release*, (January 24, 1995).

Allen, Roger MacBride. *The Modular Man,* Bantam Books, New York, 1992.

Altman, Lawrence K. "Man Gets Baboon Marrow in Risky AIDS Treatment," *The New York Times,* (December 15, 1995).

Altman, Lawrence, "At AIDS Talks, Reality Weighs Down Hope," *The New York Times,* (July 26, 1992).

—"Conference Ends with Little Hope for AIDS Cure," *The New York Times,* (June 15, 1993).

—"Cost of Treating AIDS Patients is Soaring," *The New York Times,* (July 23, 1992).

—"Two Speak as One: Those With AIDS Reach for Constituency," *The New York Times,* (July 14, 1992).

—"U.S. Doctors Said to Deny AIDS Care," *The New York Times,* (July 19, 1992).

—"India Suddenly Leads in H.I.V., AIDS Meeting is Told," *The New York Times,* (July 8, 1996).

Anderson, Roy M., and May, Robert M., "Understanding the AIDS Pandemic," *Scientific American,* (May 1992).

Anderson, Roy, and May, Robert, "The Logic of Vaccination," *New Scientist,* (18 November 1982).

Annas, George J., "When Death is Not the End," *The New York Times,* (March 2, 1996).

Arno, Peter S., and Feiden, Karyn L., *Against The Odds: The Story of AIDS, Drug Development, Politics and Profits,* HarperCollins, New York, 1992.

Assistent, Niro Markoff, *Why I Survive AIDS,* Fireside, Simon and Schuster, New York, 1991.

Bazell, Robert, "Vaccination Market," *The New Republic,* (July 1, 1991).

Beardsley, Tim, "Vital Data," *Scientific American,* (March 1996).

Beck, Melinda, "'Good News, But No Cure,'" *Newsweek,* (June 14, 1991).

Bloom, Barry R., and Murray, Christopher J.L., "Tuberculosis: Commentary on a Reemergent Killer," *Science,* Vol. 257, (August 21, 1992).

Brody, Jane E., "Personal Health—Skipping Vaccinations Puts Children at Risk," *The New York Times,* (August 11, 1993).

Buttram, Harold E., M.D., and Hoffman, John Chris, *Vaccinations and Immune Malfunction,* The Humanitarian Publishing Company, Quakertown, 1985.

Callen, Michael, *Surviving AIDS,* Harper Collins, New York, 1990.

Cantekin, Erdem I., McGuire, Timothy W., and Griffith, Terri L., "Antimicrobial Therapy for Otitis Media with Effusion ('Secretory' Otitis Media)," *Journal of the American Medical Association,* Vol. 266, No. 23, (December 18, 1991).

Cherry, James D., 'Pertussis Vaccine Encephalopathy': It is Time to Recognize it as the Myth That it is," *Journal of the American Medical Association,* Vol. 263, No. 2, (March 23, 1990).

Chopra, Deepak, M.D., *Quantum Healing: Exploring the Frontiers of Mind/Body Medicine.* Bantam Books, New York, 1989.

—*Unconditional Life: Mastering the Forces that Shape Personal Reality,* Bantam, New York, 1991.

Cohen, Mitchell L., "Epidemiology of Drug Resistance: Implications for a Post-Antimicrobial Era," *Science,* Vol. 257, (August 21, 1992).

Colborn, Theo, Dumanoski, Dianne, and Myers, John Peterson. *Our Stolen Future: Are We Threatening Our Fertility, Intelligence and Survival?—A Scientific Detective Story.* Dutton/Penguin, New York, 1996.

Congdon, Robyanne, "Don't Overload My Child's Immune System," Letter to *The New York Times,* (July 17, 1993).

Coulter Harris L., *AIDS and Syphilis: The Hidden Link,* North Atlantic Books, Berkeley, 1987.

—and Fisher, Barbara Loe, *A Shot in the Dark: Why the P in the DPT Vaccination May Be Hazardous to Your Child's Health,* Avery Publishing Group, Garden City Park, 1991.

—*Divided Legacy: A History of the Schism in Medical Thought, Volume 1—The Patterns Emerge: Hippocrates to Paracelsus,* Wehawken Book Company, Washington D.C., 1975.

—*Divided Legacy: The Conflict Between Homoeopathy and the American Medical Association—Science and Ethics in American Medicine, 1800-1914*, North Atlantic Books, Richmond, 1973.

—*Divided Legacy: The Origins of Modern Western Medicine: J.B. Van Helmont to Claude Bernard*, Wehawken/North Atlantic Books, Berkeley, 1988.

—*The Controlled Clinical Trial*, Center for Empirical Medicine/Project Cure, Washington, D.C., 1991.

—*Vaccination, Social Violence, and Criminality: The Medical Assault on the American Brain*, North Atlantic Books, Berkeley, 1990.

Cowley, Geoffrey, "A Deadly Return," *Newsweek*, (March 16, 1992).

Day, Doris, "A Cancer Answer: The New Melanoma Vaccine," *Mademoiselle*, (January 1990).

Dennett, Daniel C., *Consciousness Explained*, Little Brown and Company, Boston, 1991.

Dossey, Larry, M.D., *Meaning and Medicine: A Doctor's Tales of Breakthrough and Healing*, Bantam, New York, 1991.

Dunlap, David W., and Fisher, Lawrence M., "Drug Makers Get Aggressive in Pitching AIDS Treatment," *The New York Times*, (July 5, 1996).

Eckholm, Erik, "AIDS, Fatally Steady in the U.S., Accelerates Worldwide," *The New York Times*, (June 28, 1992).

Edwards, S.S., "New Lung Cancer Vaccine May Double Survival Rates," *Science News*, (March 26, 1988).

Elfenbein, Debra, Editor. *Living with Tricyclic Antidepressants*, HarperSanFrancisco, San Francisco, 1996.

Emanuel, Ezekiel, J., "Politicizing Whooping Cough," *The Wall Street Journal*, (March 7, 1985).

Fackelmann, K.A., "Vaccine Confers Pertussis Protection," *Science News*, Vol. 136, (October 28, 1989).

Fauci, Anthony S., "Optimal Immunity to HIV—Natural Infection, Vaccination, or Both?" *Journal of the American Medical Association*, Vol. 266, No. 3, (June 13, 1991).

Fisher, Barbara Loe, "Vaccination, Public Education, and Freedom of Choice," *NVIC Mini-News Bulletin*, (Vienna, 1991).

Fisher, Lawrence M. "Down on the Farm, a Donor," *The New York Times,* (January 5, 1996).

Fox, Renee C., and Swazey, Judith P., *Spare Parts, Organ Replacement in American Society,* Oxford University Press, New York, 1992.

Gibbons, Ann, "Exploring New Strategies to Fight Drug-Resistant Microbes," *Science,* Vol. 257, (August 21, 1992).

Goldsmith, Marsha F., "Long Past Date Set for its U.S. Disappearance, Measles Remains a Threat to Many Children," *Journal of the American Medical Association,* Vol. 262, No.1, (September 1, 1989).

Golub, Edward S., and Green, Douglas R., *Immunology: A Synthesis,* Second Edition, Sinauer Associates, Sunderland, 1991.

Gore, Senator Al, *Earth in the Balance—Ecology and the Human Spirit,* Houghton Mifflin, Boston, 1992.

Gorman, Christine, "Invincible AIDS," *Time,* (August 3, 1992).

Graham, Mary, "Unprotected Children," *The Atlantic,* (March 1993).

Hagemann, Ernst. *World Ether, Elemental Beings, Kingdoms of Nature.* Mercury Press, Spring Valley (New York), 1993.

Hamilton, Joan O'C., "Vaccine Programs Need a Booster Shot," *Business Week,* (January 25, 1988).

Harriman, Ed, "Adverse Reactions to a Better Vaccine," *New Scientist,* (February 26, 1987).

Holt, Patricia, "Shedding Light on a Drug Controversy," *San Francisco Chronicle,* (February 8, 1985).

Holtzapfel, Walter, *Medicine and the Mysteries,* Mercury Press, Spring Valley, 1994.

Horowitz, Leonard, D.M.D., *Emerging Viruses, AIDS and Ebola—Nature, Accident or Genocide?* Tetrahedron, Inc., Rockport (Massachusetts), 1996.

Husemann, Friedrich, and Wolff, Otto. *The Anthroposophical Approach to Medicine: An Outline of a Spiritual Scientifically Oriented Medicine, Vol. 2,* Anthroposophic Press, Hudson, New York, 1987.

Illich, Ivan, *Medical Nemesis: The Expropriation of Health,* Pantheon Books, New York, 1976.

Johnson, George, "What Really Goes on in There," *The New York Times Book Review,* (November 10, 1991).

Kantrowitz, Barbara, "Teenagers and AIDS," *Newsweek,* (August 3, 1992).

Kimbrell, Andrew. *The Human Body Shop: The Engineering and Marketing of Life.* HarperSanFrancisco, San Francisco, 1993.

Kolata, Gina. "Study Finds Way to Produce Sperm Cells in Other Species," *The New York Times,* (May 30, 1996).

Kramer, Peter D., *Listening to Prozac,* Penguin Books, New York, 1993.

Krober, Marvin S., Stracener, Carl E., and Bass, James W., "Decreased Measles Antibody Response After Measles-Mumps-Rubella Vaccine in Infants with Colds," *Journal of the American Medical Association,* Vol. 265, No. 2, (April 24, 1991).

LaForce, F. Marc, M.D., "Immunizations, Immunoprophylaxis, and Chemoprophylaxis to Prevent Selected Infections," *Journal of the American Medical Association,* Vol. 257, No. 18, (May 8, 1987).

Leary, Warren E., "Mandatory AIDS Tests for Doctors Opposed," *The New York Times,* (July 31, 1992).

Levine, Art, "Return of the Old Childhood Scourges," *U.S. News and World Report,* (July 4, 1988).

Leviton, Richard, "Who Calls the Shots?" *East West,* (November 1988).

—"A Shot in the Dark," *Yoga Journal,* (May/June 1992).

Lunzer, Francesca, "Scared Shotless," *Forbes,* (November 18, 1985).

Marin Independent Journal, "FDA Clears Blood Filter that Skims Cholesterol," (February 23, 1996).

Marwick, Charles, "Secretary of Health, Human Services to Hear Recommendations for Improving Immunization," *Journal of the American Medical Association,* Vol. 264, No. 2, (October 17, 1990).

Marx, Jean L., "Cancer Vaccines Show Promise at Last," *Science,* Vol. 245, No. 3, (August 25, 1989).

McAuliffe, Kathleen, "A Shot in the Arm for Cancer Therapy," *U.S. News and World Report,* (April 4, 1988).

McMahon, Peggy O'Mara, editor, *Immunizations,* Mothering Magazine, Santa Fe, 1987.

McNeil, Donald G., Jr., "Once Again, the Disease Confounds Science," *The New York Times*, (July 26, 1992).

Monmaney, Terence, "Vaccines for Adult Diseases," *Newsweek*, (October 12, 1987).

Moskowitz, Richard, M.D., "Vacination Spcial—Experts' Forum," *Mothering*, No. 79, (Summer 1996).

Navarro, Mireya, "AIDS Patients, Facing TB, Now Fear Even the Hospital," *The New York Times*, (March 15, 1992).

Noble, Gary R., M.D., et al., "Acellular and Whole-Cell Pertussis Vaccines in Japan," *Journal of the American Medical Association*, Vol. 257, No. 10, (March 13, 1987).

Olgin, Howard, M.D., *Lifebank: A Novel of Medical Suspense:* Dell Publishing, New York, 1995.

Payer, Lynn, *Medicine and Culture: Varieties of Treatment in the United States, England, West Germany, and France*, Penguin Books, New York, 1988.

Priever, Werner, M.D., *Illness and the Double*, Mercury Press, Spring Valley, 1984.

Purvis, Andrew, "Forging a Shield Against AIDS," *Time*, (April 1, 1991).

Purvis, Andrew, "TB Takes a Deadly Turn," *Time*, (December 2, 1991).

Regis, Ed. Nano. *The Emerging Science of Nanotechnology: Remaking the World—Molecule by Molecule*. Little, Brown and Company, Boston, 1995.

Rennie, Drummond, M.D., "The Cantekin Affair," *Journal of the American Medical Association*, Vol. 266, No. 23, (December 18, 1991).

"Report Expects AIDS to Depress Africa's Fast Population Growth," *The New York Times*, (July 3, 1996).

Richards, Bill. "Hold the Phone: Doctors Can Diagnose Illnesses Long Distance, to the Dismay of Some," *The Wall St. Journal*, (January 17, 1996).

Richards, Evelleen, "The Politics of Therapeutic Evaluation: The Vitamin C and Cancer Controversy," *Special Studies of Science*, SAGE, London, Vol. 18, (1988).

Rosenthal, Elisabeth, "Drug-Resistant TB is Seen Spreading Within Hospitals," *The New York Times*, (August 1, 1992).

Ryan, Frank, M.D., *The Forgotten Plague: How the Battle Against Tuberculosis was Won—and Lost,* Little, Brown and Company, Boston, 1993.

Sattentau, Quentin, "AIDS: The Search for the Vaccine," *New Scientist,* (14 April 1988).

Scharff, Paul W., "Leonie Hoffman," March 26, 1996, Spring Valley, New York, unpublished monograph.

Schmalz, Jeffrey, "Riding AIDS Roller Coaster: Hope, Horror, Hope," *The New York Times,* (June 6, 1992).

Schwartz, Harry, "Shots or Not?" *The New York Times Book Review,* February 3, 1985.

Shepherd, Dorothy, "The Magic of the Minimum Dose: Experiences and Cases," *Health Science* Press/C.W. Daniel, Saffron Walden, 1938.

Shilts, Randy, *And the Band Played On: Politics, People, and the AIDS Epidemic,* St. Martin's Press, New York, 1987.

Siebert, Charles, "The DNA We've Been Dealt," *The New York Times Magazine,* (September 17, 1995).

Speight, Leslie J., *Homoeopathy and Immunization,* Health Science Press, Saffron Walden, 1982.

Standish, Leanna, N.D., Ph.D., Guiltinan, N.D., McMahon Elizabeth, Ph.D., and Lindstrom, Carol, "One Year Open Trial of Naturopathic Treatment of HIV Infection Class IV-A in Men," *The Journal of Naturopathic Medicine,* Vol. 3, No. 1, (1992).

Starzl, Thomas E, *The Puzzle People, Memoirs of a Transplant Surgeon.* University of Pittsburgh Press, Pittsburgh, 1992.

Steiner, Rudolf, *The Crumbling of the Earth and the Souls and Bodies of Men,* Mercury Press, Spring Valley, 1988.

—*Inner Impulses of Evolution. The Mexican Mysteries, The Knights Templar,* Anthroposophic Press, Spring Valley, 1984.

—*Geographic Medicine,* Mercury Press, Spring Valley, 1988.

Stone, Barbara. *Cancer as Initiation: Suviving the Fire,* Open Court, Chicago, 1994.

Stryker, Jeff, "Surgery Gives Man New Best Friends," *The New York Times,* (December 17, 1995).

Suro, Roberto, "The Cholera Watch," *The New York Times Sunday Magazine,* (March 22, 1992).

Szasz, Thomas, *The Theology of Medicine: The Political-Philosophical Foundations of Medical Ethics,* Syracuse University Press, Syracuse, 1977.

Taylor, Stuart Jr., "Court Eases Way to Sue U.S. For Safety Policy Violations," *The New York Times,* (June 14, 1988).

Toal, Jeanne, "Super Vaccines," *OMNI,* (July 1987).

Varela, Francisco J., and Anspach, Mark, "Immu-Knowledge, The Process of Somatic Individuation," in *Gaia 2, Emergence: The New Science of Becoming,* edited by William Irwin Thompson, Lindisfarne Press, Hudson, 1991.

Weeder, Richard S., M.D., *Surgeon: The View from Behind the Mask,* Contemporary Books, Chicago, 1988.

Wermiel, Stephen, "Court Says U.S. May Be Sued Over Vaccines," *The Wall Street Journal,* (June 14, 1988).

CHAPTER 3

Environmental Energies:
Forays between the Inner
and Outer Environments

The Collegiality of Holism: How Natural
Medicine Regards the Environment

Up to this point, I have characterized allopathy's refusal to credit the environment with intelligent, self-organizing life. Primarily, environment has meant the inner, immunological milieu, but allopathy's position is totalitarian and applies equally well to the outer, ecological domain. In effect, allopathy proposes that the individual human, as a focal point of consciousness, has no relationship with one's body and its natural processes other than to be the passive victim of its irrational aberrations.

Human consciousness, confronted with its body's internal biological terrain, says allopathy, has no efficacy. It is unable to effect any significant changes in the mechanistic, predetermined outcomes of an impersonal, soulless biology—its immediate material environment.

Allopathy officially alienates human consciousness from its bodily base and thereby sanctions a fundamental schism between body and soul, mind and matter, consciousnes and environment. As such, this schism lays us open to a host of opportunistic infections, of both thought and biology, as we have surrendered the immunological, discriminatory vitality of our thinking and blood processes.

When it comes to the greater, external environment of tangible, visible nature, allopathy similarly informs our conventional views of ecology. Nature and its processes may be mechanically manipulated by technological extensions of the scientist's will, but not by the mind itself. The realm of nature is intrinsically an "other." No longer universally threatening but only selectively so, kingdoms of nature (such as "wild" animals) are dispensable, and eventually the weather and geological events (such as unplanned earthquakes and floods) will be manipulable to our advantage. According to allopathic logic, eventually nature itself (and perhaps the planet, too) will be redundant and dispensable.

As humans, we are victims of weather, geology, and other environmental energies, says allopathy. Not so, say the philosophers of natural medicine. Implicit to the therapeutic view of all branches of natural (alternative) medicine—the empiric medical tradition—is the belief that the human organism and consciousness are mutably interconnected and interdependently related with forces and energies in the outer environment. There is a living feedback loop and mechanism for constructive interaction and change already in place. Allopathy denies such a connection and has schooled us vigorously in its nonexistence. In fact, the esoteric traditions of both Eastern and Western culture suggest even profounder links and equivalencies. Let's examine the empiric's case for our human connection—relatedness—with the energies of the "outer" environment, as put forward by Western science and natural medicine.

Embedded in an Environmental Web of Energies from Earth, Sky, and Technology

The human is embedded in an environment of energies, most of them fundamentally electromagnetic in nature. Whether it's the weather, the landscape, or the electrotechnologized intermediate zone of power lines, our environment enfolds us in a sea of electromagnetic influences. But these influences quite often are ambivalent, healthful in some cases, injurious in others, sometimes according to proximity, sometimes to degree of exposure.

The new science of biometeorology shows us the direct and subtle influences of weather, atmosphere, climate, and their seasonal, even daily fluctuations, on human psychological health and physiological stability. Ultimately our weather is dependent on planetary and extraterrestrial magnetic field influences and changes, themselves derivative of activities of the Sun.

Biometeorology may describe pure influences of electromagnetism, atmosphere, and weather, but these "natural" sources must be set into the human-made context of our electronic environment and its "side effect," electropollution. Electric power lines that thread the landscape like an electronic nervous system create massive, complex energy grids across the country—and, according to health researchers, in many cases release harmful electromagnetic radiations that may contribute to homeostatic imbalances, even degenerative disease, in humans living in their vicinity.

This is a highly problematic situation, considering our extreme cultural dependency on electric power and its advantages, to find that the very power transmission system that makes our lives comfortable may contribute to our ill health.

Completing this three-tiered system of electromagnetic influences are "geopathic" emanations from within Earth itself, according to research developed principally in Germany and confirmed by dowsers in America. Electromagnetic radiations presumably connected with geological fractures and subterranean water veins, when situated under domestic residences, can have remarkably deleterious, geopathological effects on the health of the occupants. We could appreciate geopathology as the medical aspect of the more comprehensive discipline called geobiology, which examines Earth's influence at precise locations on all life forms, plant, animal, and human.

In the case of both electromagnetic and telluric, geopathic emanations, we find the same puzzling paradox. In some cases the radiations are perilous, in others beneficial. Controlled, precise applications of electromagnetic fields and electrical currents have their health-promoting uses in medicine; the same Earth-emanations that are geopathic for long-term domestic residency are actually favorable for expansion of human consciousness at sacred sites and temples in the landscape when the exposure is brief.

The indications of these three fields of research—biometeorology, electropollution, and geopathology—while demonstrating yet new health hazards with which to acquaint ourselves with—on the positive side illustrate convincingly our high degree of systemic permeability to supposedly external environmental energies. Information of this kind certainly helps refute the allopathic adversarial model of reality, which pits self against environment. Instead we have a model describing perturbations and energy adjustments within a unified single system with many interdependent, holographically linked components.

But we needn't be overly surprised because these are but the logical ramifications of our status as *holographic* humans, whose lifeblood may well be the energies of the cosmos.

"He is a living barometer . . . irritability itself"

In his later years, the nineteenth-century German poet Johann Wolfgang von Goethe took to carrying a barometer with him. He wanted to foresee what "indispositions" he risked suffering from the day's weather. His contemporary, the French philosopher Maine de Biran, who was also meteorologically sensitive, wrote in his diary, "There is no atmospheric change, no matter how slight, which escapes my sensitive system."

It was worse still for Friedrich Nietzsche, the acutely weather-vulnerable German philosopher. "His whole body is a pressure gauge," observed biographer Stefan Zweig. "He is a living barometer. He is irritability itself. There may never have been an intellectual so sensitive to atmospheric conditions, or so acutely vulnerable to all the variations of meteorological phenomena. There seem to be occult electrical impulses between his pulse and the atmospheric pressure, between his nerves and the amount of humidity in the air."

Goethe, de Biran, and Nietzsche weren't the first weather sensitives to leave a record of their irritations. The anecdotal correlation of weather and well-being has long been acknowledged. Hippocrates, the Greek "father of medicine" (469-399 B.C.), in his "On Airs, Waters, and Places" described the essential bonds between human and weather and in his advice to physicians he helped to lay the foundation for a future science. "Whoever wishes to pursue the science of medicine properly must proceed thus," advised Hippocrates. "First, he ought to consider what effect each season of the year can produce, for the seasons are not alike but differ widely both in themselves and at their changes. Through these considerations and by learning the weather beforehand, the doctor will have available full knowledge to help him in each specific case."

Today that full knowledge is being collected by a new science of medicine called biometeorology. This is a multidisciplinary field that studies the effects of atmospheric phenomena *(meteoron)* on life *(bios),* including the human. Biometeorology is an expanding science that's making surprising biomedical connections between atmospheric effects and specific biological responses, such as the advent of winter and chronic depression, cold fronts and asthma attacks, hot weather and aggression, solar activity and the earth's magnetic field fluctuations and heart attacks.

Biometeorologists are finding that our behavior, mood, and health may be much more intimately connected to the vagaries of the weather than we suspected and that the weather itself may be highly responsive to solar, even cosmic, electromagnetic influences. We may be able to make practical adjustments in lifestyle, home environment, even psychological attitude that could prevent, for example, the cold season from becoming "the winter of our discontent."

The SAD Fact about
the Hibernation Response

In November 1982, this winter discontent and chronic depression, which engulfs many people in the Northern Hemisphere between September and April, got a name. Alfred Lewy, M.D., a clinical psychobiologist, and his colleagues at the National Institute of Mental Health (NIMH) in Bethesda, Maryland, labeled it Seasonal Affective Disorder, or SAD, thus removing this anomalous deep depression from the fold of psychiatry and delivering it to the barometers of biometeorology.

In a landmark article in the *American Journal of Psychiatry,* Lewy described the case of Larry Pressman, a sixty-three-year-old man suffering a seasonally related manic-depression syndrome. For half his life, Pressman had experienced a dramatic downturn in energy, mood, and functioning, accompanied by oversleeping and overeating, beginning with each midsummer, climaxing at Christmas, and turning into a manic cheerfulness in March. His doctors told

Pressman he had "Christmas depression syndrome" and prescribed antidepressants, which gave him unpleasant side effects and no relief to his depression.

What did lighten Pressman's seasonal depression, Lewy discovered, was light itself—specifically a longer photoperiod. Pressman's daily exposure to bright sunlight (his photoperiod) was artificially lengthened with bright lamps—about 2500 lux—to provide six more hours of sunlight daily, an amount comparable to a sun-drenched April day. Within four days, Pressman's depression lifted and he regained his energy and enthusiasm in the midst of winter for the first time in decades. The synthetic sunlight made the difference, Lewy theorized, because of its effect on melatonin, a pineal gland hormone which has a tranquilizing effect. The pineal gland is often called the seat of our "biological clock," "a gland that measures time," and "a gland for all seasons"; Descartes regarded it as the seat of the human soul.

Melatonin's purpose is to prepare the body for sleep, which is probably why its presence in the blood usually increases around dusk—scientists believe it is produced mainly at night, in the dark—especially in the short photoperiod winter months; bright sunlight suppresses melatonin activity which, phenomenologically, is why we typically find it easier to stay awake longer in the summer months than winter. "There is evidence for human seasonal rhythms in mania, depression, suicide, and various endocrine and neurotransmitter functions," noted psychiatrist Daniel Kripke of the University of California-San Diego in the journal *Biological Psychiatry*. "These results suggest that human seasonal responses may be sensitive to light of a particular bright intensity."

Melatonin acts as a time cue that influences numerous endocrine systems, which in turn regulate metabolism, appetite, and growth in response to seasonal changes, specifically to changes in the length of daylight in each twenty-four-hour photoperiod. Melatonin secretion follows the daily light/dark cycle with high levels at night and minuscule amounts in the daytime; during a long winter's night the plasma melatonin level remains high for much longer than in summer. When laboratory mammals are kept in complete darkness, the pineal rhythm of melatonin secretion takes on a circadian, or twenty-four-hour, rhythm called "free-run"; similar data have been observed with human subjects.

Under normal conditions the suprachiasmatic nuclei, a region within the brain's hypothalamus thought to generate this rhythm, "is entrained by neural input from the eye," explains Andrew Loudon in *New Scientist,* "and this in turn innervates the pineal gland so that the 24-hourly pattern of melatonin production follows daylength precisely.

"Light, therefore, would appear to have a suppressive effect." The reappraisal of the pineal-melatonin periodicity by neuroendocrinologists has generated major insights into the relationship of physiology to environment and the quality of our adaptation, notes Dr. Josephine Arendt, senior lecturer in biochemistry at the University of Surrey, writing in *New Scientist.* "A residual human sensitivity to photoperiod could conceivably link depression and neurosis to the incompatibility of our biology with our culturally imposed behavior."

Pressman's case clearly demonstrated the validity of biological responses to seasonal changes in sunlight. Before 1982 scientists had conservatively estimated the population incidence of seasonally related depression at only 5%, but by 1987 that estimate was radically revised at the American Psychiatric Association's annual meeting. As many as 25% of Americans are "troubled" by seasonal changes in photoperiod, the psychiatrists announced.

That "trouble," researchers now know, often takes the form of SAD, a condition with recognizable symptoms. SAD affects mostly women (86%), often beginning in their twenties, and, seasonally, in October, but with "anticipatory anxiety" as early as July. Most SAD sufferers experience carbohydrate craving, sleep about 17% longer, gain weight (10 to 15 pounds), lose interest in sex, feel irritable, sad, withdrawn, and fatigued; they can't concentrate and perform poorly at work—and for at least 60% SAD-inflicted people, it seems to grow worse with age.

A milder, probably more widespread version of SAD is the "Hibernation Response," a new clinical description put forth by Peter Whybrow, M.D., chairman of the psychiatry department at the University of Pennsylvania, and Robert Bahr, a medical-health journalist, in *The Hibernation Response.* Whybrow and Bahr describe what might be a natural, biological urge to hibernate in winter experienced by many people living in the colder regions of the Northern Hemisphere. Using the umbrella concept of the hibernation response, they explain why people tend to feel "fat, miserable, and depressed" from October to March, and they present a practical regime of "cheer-up strategies" for the legion of unhappy hibernators.

"We must begin by getting it clear in our minds that the urge to hibernate is a response of the human as animal," says Whybrow. "It's that conflict between the tendency to hibernate and the impossibility of doing so which makes autumn and winter a disastrous time for millions of us around the world." The hibernation response and SAD, adds Whybrow, are expressions of human adaptation in its oldest form to the periodicities of sunlight on the planet.

Whybrow couches his clinical formulations for the hibernation response in an anecdotal, almost bucolic context. In the 1970s he lived at Blow-Me-Down Farm in New Hampshire, where he noted firsthand the "New England soul in winter," with its characteristic cabin fever and "subjective tension." In 1977 Whybrow put his specialty in psychiatric endocrinology to good use in a lecture he gave at the nearby Dartmouth Medical School on the probable physiology of the winter doldrums; later, *Yankee Magazine* spread his observations nationally.

This made it possible in 1983 for Whybrow, in conjunction with NIMH colleagues in Washington, to undertake a study of seasonal behavior in normal—non-SAD—individuals. Whybrow instructed his 100 volunteers to keep daily records of their sleep, mood, energy, and appetite levels for fifteen months. The copious data produced unequivocally supported Whybrow's conclusion: "Normal people do have a markedly seasonal pattern in their activity. The variation in behavior through the year is very real."

The Psychological Effects of a Hot, Dry Wind

New clinical descriptions like Lewy's SAD and Whybrow's hibernation response put a great deal of other scientific, clinical, and anecdotal data on presumed biometeorological effects in rational perspective. Nobody yet has prepared a grand unified theory for biomedical/biometeorological correlations, but Dr. Michel Gauquelin, a Sorbonne-trained psychologist and statistician and director of the Laboratory for Cosmic and Psycho-Physiological Rhythms in Paris, has collected much of the clinical data and proposed some explanations in his numerous books, including *How Cosmic and Atmospheric Energies Influence Your Health*, first published in French in 1967. "Most of the physiological processes in the human body are constantly being modified by climate and weather," notes Gauquelin, "as the body's regulatory systems are overcome by atmospheric disturbances when fronts are passing."

Cold fronts are correlated with increased heart attacks, almost doubling their incidence, reports Gauquelin. Postoperative complications (60% to 90%) coincide with cold fronts (60%) and warm fronts (30%), while asthma and glaucoma episodes are frequently triggered by passing cold fronts. Cases of angina pectoris follow a marked seasonal pattern, peaking in autumn and winter, while a study of 1.6 million patients with circulatory ailments showed a peak in January and February, in the height of winter. Wind, too, can be especially troublesome, says Gauquelin.

"He who knows the origin of the winds, of thunder, and of the weather, also knows where diseases come from," observed the sixteenth-century Swiss physician and alchemist Paracelsus. Whether it's the *Santa Ana* in California, the *foehn* (Austria), *chinook* (Northwest and Rocky Mountains), *sirocco* (Italy's "father of depression"), Spain's *leveccio,* Egypt's *chamsin,* Argentina's *zonda,* the *autan* or *mistral* (France), or Israel's *sharav,* a hot, dry wind is bound to make many people feel awful. Typical symptoms of what the Central Europeans call *"foehn* psychosis" include physical weakness, irritability, headaches, anxiety, insomnia, nightmare, nausea, apathy, depression, dizziness, tension, panic, and a tendency to quarrel.

The injurious effects of "ill wind," say biometeorologists, seem to come from an overabundance of positive ions, electrically charged oxygen molecules in the atmosphere. Negative ions—commonly encountered at waterfalls, for example—seem to have a calming, healing effect on humans. The key factor linking ions and human comfort might be what's called serotonin hyperfunction syndrome. Serotonin, like melatonin, is a brain neurotransmitter and mood-altering substance, produced by the amino acid tryptophan, that instructs the brain cells to relax the body, to feel drowsy, even to sleep; apparently a high concentration of positive ions depresses serotonin levels. Bioclimatological researchers at the Hebrew University Medical School in Jerusalem found that unpleasant effects of the syndrome are felt even twelve hours before the *sharav* arrives, as the normal atmospheric ion ratio of 5 positive to 4 negative ions climbs to 132:4.

Many people find prolonged hot weather not only unpleasant but harmful on their health, and with the presumed heightening of the greenhouse effect, biometeorologists have made this a priority research question. In the U.S. biometeorological research began getting government backing in the 1980s and more recently, from the Environmental Protection Agency (EPA). In 1987 the EPA awarded forty the research contracts to assess the impact and implications of a possible global climate warming on environment and human health. Dr. Laurence Kalkstein's Center for Climatic Research at the University of Delaware at Newark received one of these grants and has been studying the impact of weather and climate on human mortality.

Kalkstein began by surveying the extensive scientific literature from forty-eight American cities to develop a weather stress index. "It's apparent that weather has a profound effect on human mortality and that the impact is differential on a seasonal and regional level," Kalkstein observed. He found that northern cities like Pittsburgh and Detroit, where excessively hot weather (90°F+) is uncommon, have a higher climate mortality rate in the summer than in consistently hot and steamy cities like New Orleans.

It's the sudden change in temperature and the difficulties in quick adaptation that kills people, says Kalkstein. "The population is unaccustomed and reacts in a stressful manner," and it's the elderly who are disproportionately stressed, with as much as a 50% increase in summer mortality. Further, the earlier in the summer the unaccustomed heat wave arrives, the higher the death rates attributable to the weather.

Not only are biometeorologists like Kalkstein developing a picture of medical geography, but others are formulating a kind of biometeorological criminality index. Hot temperatures are clearly correlated with aggressive, violent behavior, concludes Dr. Craig Anderson, psychologist at the University of Missouri. He published his exhaustive survey of about two centuries of scientific data on temperature-aggression connections in *Psychological Bulletin*.

Anderson catalogued incidence of homicide, assault, rape, riots, and beatings with high temperatures (exceeding 90°F) in nearly endless permutations of variables, clinical controls, and geographic regions. "The variety of supportive studies is suggestive of a strong, direct temperature-aggression relation." The hot and humid months of July and August are prolific times for murder, rape, and assault, says Anderson, and, generally speaking, hotter regions of the world regularly have a higher incidence of aggression, as do hotter years, seasons, months, even days.

The exhaustive literature survey led Anderson to make two conclusions. "First, temperature effects are direct; they operate at the individual level. Second, temperature effects are important; they influence the most antisocial behaviors imaginable." How significant an effect does temperature have on aggression? Anderson postulated two hypothetical cities of 600,000 population, drawing on 1980 crime rates from 260 "Standard Metropolitan Statistical Areas" similar in all respects except climate. "Assume that city A has 42 more hot days of 90°F+ temperatures per year than city B. The present results suggests that city A will experience about 7% more violent crimes than city B."

What seems to link hot weather with aggressive behavior is the body's thermoregulatory system situated in the brain's hypothalamus, a major endocrine gland, suggests Anderson. The unbearably hot weather apparently triggers the temperature-sensitive hypothalamus to release a series of body-cooling neurotransmitters, including norepinephrine, epinephrine; the neurotransmitters serotonin and acetecholine are involved in raising body temperature.

"All this is relevant to the temperature-aggression hypothesis in that many of the same neural and hormonal systems"—such as testosterone, cortisol, serotonin—"involved in temperature regulation are also implicated in aggression," although the links are not clear, says Anderson. Serotonin seems to inhibit aggression whereas acetecholine increases it. The "neural interconnectedness" of the hypothalamus, amygdala, and hippocampus, which are linked with aggression, emotion, and thermoregulation, may produce "the emotional and cognitive effects of temperature experienced by humans," says Anderson.

Most biometeorologists will grant a correlation specifically between heat and violent behavior and a more general link between some aspects of weather and human functioning. "The real debate these days, however, is what the *shape* of that relationship is," comments Dr. James Rotton, social psychologist at Florida International University in North Miami. "It sounds like a straightforward issue, but it's getting more complicated than we originally thought."

As a rule of thumb, Rotton estimates that about 20% of the population is weather sensitive, which, along with other discoveries of biometeorology, may not be surprising. "A lot of this is mop-up work in the sense of double-checking things your grandmother might have told you, but unlike her, we're trying to base this on some solid, empirical foundation. As we're talking about more than a dozen variables co-varying over time, it becomes really tedious to separate them out."

The multiplicity of variables is both an advantage and a stumbling block for biometeorology, says Dr. Michael Persinger, director of the Neurosciences Laboratory at Laurentian University in Sudbury, Ontario. Biometeorology is inherently cross-disciplinary, Persinger notes, requiring competence in such diverse fields as epidemiology, physiology, behavioral measurements, and weather forecasting. "In science today this happens to be a less than pleasing type of approach." Most scientists prefer a univariant or, at best, a bivariant approach to problem solving—but very few like to cope with potentially dozens of variables.

In this intellectually conservative stance, complex events are construed in terms of one or two variables alone, but this may be narrowing the picture too tightly, says Persinger. This attitude precludes the multivariant requirements of biometeorology "where a half dozen variables can all equally contribute to the same situation."

The confluence of weather variables meets in something Persinger calls the weather matrix. "This means not only do we look at the absolute measures—temperature, humidity, sunshine hours, wind speed, precipitation, and geomagnetic activity, which invariably couples them—but we also look at the *rate* of these changes over time." Weather matrix influences over a six-month period will account for about 20% to 30% of daily mood fluctuations, estimates Persinger.

The effect of a weather matrix on an individual may actually be the key to understanding its influence. "When you study weather, it's really the study of individual differences. The biggest limitation to biometeorology in the last century has been the failure to realize that individuals respond differently to the same meteorological stimuli."

The link may be neurophysiological, suggests Persinger, whose specialty is brain-behavior-environment relationships. "Mood or affect is probably one of the most powerful general features associated with the limbic and autonomic systems." Persinger's current research may provide deeper insight into our individualized mood responses to weather.

Beginning in 1989 Persinger began collating data on daily mood and sickness with personality type and cognitive style. He obtained the data through various standard psychological personality tests, including the Minnesota Multiphasic Personality Inventory and the Meyers-Briggs Type Indicator (based on the fourfold personality model of C. G. Jung). Persinger hypothesizes that personality type, or cognitive style, is related to temporal lobe sensitivity in the limbic system. "This may be the key and mediator of the effects of weather on mood."

But while the limbic system and personality type may mediate the influence of weather inside the human, it's the Sun that produces the outside influences, says Persinger. "Weather is basically a function of the Sun. Any perturbation in the Sun's output will certainly influence weather. Even the more conservative meteorologists now realize that when you change the irradiation output, or solar constant, by only a couple percent, you produce very clear changes in the weather and seasons."

Solar Winds, Geomagnetic Fields, and Life

The relations between the Sun, weather, and human functioning are complex but intriguing. When Persinger links weather to perturbations of the Sun, he's referring to the intimate, energetic connections between solar sunspot activity—an index of solar perturbations—and Earth's electromagnetic field (EMF), the recipient of solar perturbations. Scientists report that solar radiation is among our most important climatic elements and the primary source of atmospheric energy.

The Sun is subject to period energy discharges called sunspots— dramatic towering solar flares—which come in predictable cycles, each cycle with its peaks and troughs, of 11.1 years (with overlapping mini and maxi cycles of 27 days, 22.2 years, 80 years, 145, 205, and 290 years). In fact atmospheric scientists speculate there may be far greater sunspot cycles of 1265 years (postglacial), one of 40,000 or 80,000 years in the Würm glacial period, a 30-million-year Mesozoic cycle, and "an orogenic revolution cycle of about 400 million years, which may perhaps be linked in some way with the Galactic Cycle," comments astrogeologist D. J. Schove. Large solar flares, with momentary temperatures exceeding 20 million degrees Kelvin, generate energy equivalent to the explosion of 200 million hydrogen bombs in a few minutes; this is enough energy, if it could be harnessed, to satisfy humankind's energy needs for about 100 million years.

Periodicity of solar flares has more than passing scientific interest. The solar flare, note physicists Syun-Ichi Akasofu and Louis J. Lanzerotti in *Physics Today,* is "the most energetic transient process in the solar system." Solar fluctuations, sunspot activity, and prodigious ejections of corona gases, which generate the "solar wind," have a major, formative impact on Earth's magnetosphere, which is the outermost shell of the atmosphere (about 5,000 km above the planet). The magnetosphere is a kind of huge magnetic transfer zone, a comet-shaped, blunt-nosed cavity or bubble around Earth carved out by the solar wind.

On its sunward side, Earth's magnetosphere measures about 10 Earth radii, but on the downward side it resembles a luminous windsock (called the magnetotail) stretching out an estimated 1,000 Earth radii. Earth's geomagnetic field represents an obstacle to the solar wind, which is a supersonic plasma flow of hydrogen and helium ions blowing off from the Sun; as the solar winds flow around the magnetosphere, Earth and its magnetic field are confined within this long cylindrical cavity. (Magnetospheres also have been observed around Mercury, Jupiter, Saturn, Uranus, and Neptune.)

The solar wind carries the Sun's magnetic field far out into the solar system, an extension called the interplanetary magnetic field; through a process called magnetic reconnection, scientists believe, this magnetic field joins with geomagnetic field lines originating at Earth's polar regions. The magnetosphere is the part of Earth's atmosphere, which is influenced by the planet's magnetic field; conversely, changes in the magnetosphere may directly influence our weather.

The interaction between the solar wind and Earth's magnetosphere can generate tremendous amounts of energy—Akasofu and Lanzerotti call it a "gigantic natural magnetohydrodynamic dynamo"—producing a voltage drop of about 40 to 50 kilovolts across the magnetosphere and a current flow of a few tens of millions of amperes, "roughly the total electric power consumption in the U.S."

The "normal" velocity of the solar wind with respect to Earth is an estimated 400 km/sec. Sunspot activity augments the solar wind's kinetic energy, resulting in magnetic storms in Earth's atmosphere, which register as large fluctuations—initially a sudden increase in intensity, followed several hours later by a sharp depression, then a gradual recovery, in all usually lasting from thirty minutes to three hours—in the magnitude and direction of the geomagnetic field.

When solar flares erupt, these generate plasma shock waves that propagate within the solar wind such that it reaches speeds of 500 to 1,000 km/sec; when these shock waves collide with Earth's magnetosphere, it can generate power up to 10 million megawatts, a tremendous surge that produces geomagnetic storms. Astrophysicists report that magnetic storms can produce tremendous atmospheric disturbances, most notable of which is the aurora display in polar regions, including the Northern Lights. Magnetospheric substorms are less powerful and far more frequent, occurring four to five times daily.

The effects of magnetic storms on the planet's EMF strength, short-term weather, and long-term climate are pronounced, according to biometeorologists. Sudden, daily geomagnetic field fluctuations, which are preceded by solar eruptions by about two days, are actually predictive of major atmospheric storms, like blizzards, from Alaska to New England. Goesta Wollin, of the Lamont-Doherty Geological Observatory of Columbia University in New York State, who has been studying the links between geomagnetism, weather, and climate since 1970, is convinced he's identified a reliable short-term indicator of coming severe storms: they tend to be preceded by a sudden alteration in the geomagnetic field, often on the order of 45-50 gamma but sometimes jumping from -676 to -351 to -678 gamma in an hour (compared to the total background geomagnetic field of 25,000 gamma).

Wollin also found that planetary temperature changes over the last several hundred thousand years precisely mirror changes in the geomagnetic field intensity; when Earth's magnetic field is stronger, Wollin noted the world climate is colder. Wollin reasoned that the only agency that could produce these sudden changes in geomagnetic field intensity would be either changes in the strength of the Sun's magnetic field or in the strength of the solar wind, which Earth's magnetic field funnels down onto the magnetic poles. Through careful plotting and study of atmospheric and geomagnetic data, Wollin determined that changes in atmospheric pressure reliably occurred five days after magnetic field changes.

"But the most remarkable connection shown up by the study," wrote John Gribbin in *New Scientist*, "was the link between sudden, large changes in magnetic intensity and sudden, severe bouts of extreme weather." Wollin documented a similar kind of magnetic field-climatological correlation in three-year weather cycles. He found that the *rate* of change of geomagnetic field intensity from year to year apparently determined temperature variations, both annual and seasonal, one to three years in advance—again Wollin had discovered a biometeorological predictive scheme.

"The geomagnetic field," comments Wollin, "is constant only to the extent that it constantly varies and the rate of change itself is quite variable on a year-to-year basis."

The Feedback Loop of Planetary Magnetic Fields and Human Health

The magnetic activities of the Sun and its influences on Earth must be set into the larger context of the life of the solar system, suggests Theodore Landscheidt, director of the Schroeter Institute for Research in Cycles of Solar Activity in Belle Cote, Nova Scotia. Earth, its atmosphere, human life, the solar system, and its constituent parts are all components of one living organism, "a whole that embraces a complex web of holistic interrelations," says Landscheidt in his speculative treatise, *Sun-Earth-Man—A Mesh of Cosmic Oscillations.*

Landscheidt, a former West German High Court judge, began his unorthodox, interdisciplinary, and self-financed studies about twenty-five years ago in Bremen, West Germany. As a scientist, he's been sufficiently daring to know that to describe an entity as complex as the solar system, and to derive from this a predictive model for long-range solar activities that is allegedly 90% accurate, you have to be willing to cross a few academically proscribed boundaries—astrology, for one, the descriptive science of the subjective effect of astronomical alignments on human psychology and health.

Hardly antiquated, the premise of traditional astrology, says Landscheidt, "turns out to be trendsetting." Most scientists, he notes, "do not realize their findings confirm fundamental astrological ideas, and most astrologers do not see that creative scientists transgress the frontiers of traditional astrological knowledge." The Sun and planets function "like an intricate organism regulated by complex feed-back loops," says Landscheidt. The "tidal planets," Mercury, Venus, Earth, and Jupiter, cooperate to regulate and modulate the essential features of the Sun's activities; in fact, according to Landscheidt—his predictions are widely sought after by the scientific and business community—special Jupiter configurations may be among the predominant solar influences, affecting an astonishing range of activities: solar eruptions, geomagnetic storms, ozone column variations in Earth's atmosphere, rainfall, temperature, animal and human population changes, economic cycles, interest rates, phases of general instability, "and even historical periods of radical change and revolution."

Climate is a larger expression of weather, seen over time, and weather is a transient phase of climate, proposes Landscheidt. It's only a question of perceptual scale. Biometeorological cataclysms may turn out to be constructive. Consider the eruption of a medium-sized solar flare whose massive energy discharge destabilizes our planet's EMF, producing magnetic storms and weather perturbations.

This geomagnetic instability pattern propagates, influencing seasonal weather patterns, the human nervous system, even sociohistoric events. For example, on March 13, 1989, says Landscheidt, we underwent an energetic magnetic storm. "This was a chance to be creative. Instability is the precondition of creativity. There is less inertia, more freedom. Old structures crash and new patterns emerge." The results are not always instantaneous, but they are inevitable. By the end of 1989, the Berlin Wall had been taken down.

From the historical record, Landscheidt noted that the years following 1789, 1823, 1867, 1933, and 1968—years that witnessed "the special constellation of Sun and planets that makes the center of mass and the Sun's surface coalesce" or great magnetic upheavals and Jupiter conjunctions—were marked by radical change, revolution, a breakdown of old structures, and the emergence of new social forms and progressive ideas.

The next major instability period is expected between 2002 to 2011 A.D., says Landscheidt; it's an exceptionally long period as far as Sun/Jupiter-mediated geomagnetic cycles go—"a cosmic period of change"—but it's likely to be "another turning point, a period of instability, upheaval, agitation, and revolution, that ruins traditional structures, but favors the emergence of new patterns in society, economy, art, and science. If you have revolutionary ideas, this would be a fine time to spread them."

While independent scientists like Landscheidt extrapolate the broader picture of solar activity, geomagnetic storms, and their effects on major social and economic cycles, other researchers, like Russia's A. P. Dubrov, study the intricate impact magnetic fields have on biology and human life. Dubrov meticulously detailed his data on the biomedical geomagnetic link in his pioneering study,

The Geomagnetic Field and Life. Magnetics completes the connection between Sun, weather, and health, a connection that works through the subtle electromagnetic field of the body and its organs; it's a new field Dubrov calls "electromagnetic ecology."

Dubrov found that short-term variation of the geomagnetic field—"highly disturbed days"—directly effects the central nervous system and may trigger cardiovascular dysfunction, eclampsia, glaucoma, and epilepsy fits; increase road traffic accidents; affect blood pressure and plasma leukocyte count; generate DNA chromosomal inversions; and upset genetic homeostasis, among others. The evidence for a close relationship between blood serum and sunspot activities led one biologist to quip: "Man is a living sundial."

A famous American study from the 1960s published in *Nature* demonstrated the relationship between geomagnetic parameters and psychiatric hospital admissions. Scientists studied the admissions of 28,000 patients at eight hospitals against sixty-seven magnetic storms during a four-year period and found that significantly more people registered for psychiatric services just after magnetic disturbances than during times of geomagnetic field stability.

"Subtle changes in the intensity of the geomagnetic field can affect the nervous system by altering the living organism's own electromagnetic field," wrote Robert O. Becker, one of the study's principal researchers. The mass of data indicates "how closely the Earth is linked with the space surrounding it and how sensitively it reacts to changes in the parameters of the interplanetary magnetic field," says Dubrov. "Thus we see the apparently external, highly unusual, universal effect of the geomagnetic field on all indices and properties of living organisms."

Research emerging from the Madrid laboratory of Spanish neuroscientist Jose Delgado in the mid-1980s demonstrated how infinitesimal magnetic fields, often several hundred times below the voltage needed for an electrode to trigger a nerve to fire, when applied to animals produced "astoundingly diverse effects in virtually every species investigated," noted *OMNI's* Kathleen McAuliffe. Depending on the EMF strength—the "invisible energy pulses" that McAuliffe dubbed "mind fields"—one monkey would sleep while another became hyperactive.

Delgado's results highlight how weak electromagnetic fields may in fact represent "a potent biological force"; individual species may be characterizable as specific "biological wave bands." As Delgado remarks: "All the cells that make up living organisms are packed full of highly charged atoms and molecules that may change their orientation and movement in the presence of certain types of fields. This might in turn have an impact on innumerable chemical processes within the cells."

The high, if not acute, sensitivity of living organisms, including the human, to changes in geomagnetic field underlies the formative influence of biomagnetism itself. Changes in the EMF—through the interlinking web of sunspots, solar wind, geomagnetic storms, and transient EMF perturbations—can affect human life so profoundly because the basis of human physiology is apparently highly magnetics-dependent. "Life's geomagnetic coupling to heaven and earth is apparently more like a web than a simple cord and socket," notes Robert Becker in *The Body Electric*.

Magnetobiologists have found that living organisms emit their own magnetic field and electromagnetic oscillations in the low-frequency range. Weak magnetic fields (about 1×10^{-9} gauss, or about one-billionth Earth's magnetic field) have been detected in the human body and surrounding individual organs. Beginning in the late 1960s, scientists began documenting magnetic readings emanating from the central nervous system, the skull (with neuromagnetic waves of about 10^{-8} gauss measured at the scalp), heart (in normal subjects, about 1×10^{-6} gauss), and lung.

While Earth's EMF is about 0.5 gauss (a common horseshoe magnet is 200 to 300 gauss; a standard stick-on magnet is 1,000 gauss) the field about the human heart is 1 millionth of 1 gauss, and the brain field is 1 billionth of 1 gauss—little sparks perhaps but biologically significant. As David Cohen notes in *Physics Today*: "Fluctuating magnetic fields are produced by all the organs in the body that consist of or contain muscle or nerve."

In the 1980s, the development of nuclear magnetic resonance (NMR) imaging opened a "magnetic window into bodily functions," comments *New Scientist*'s Christine Sutton. This ultrasophisticated magnetic scanning technology has enabled biochemists to "observe the changing proportions of key substances during metabolic processes in the human body" while promising to explicate the metabolic processes underlying both disease and health.

Albert Roy Davis, investigating the "human biomagnetic aura" mapped out a "biological electronics" schematic for the human body in which the body's right side from ear to toe has a positive electrical potential, the left side negative in charge, while the spine has varying positive charges in front and negative in the back; Davis found two "magnetic equators" (at the sternum and pubic bone), where the voltages change valence. "The entire body of man is a field of continually flowing electromagnetic energy," concluded Davis.

Magnetic Field Sensors in the Human Brain

Not only are humans sensitive to magnetic fields on a cellular level, and not only do our internal organs produce extremely weak magnetic fields, but humans, as well as bacteria, bees, and birds—at least twenty-seven species so far in the "magnetic zoo"—apparently possess a special magnetic sensor in the form of magnetite crystals that enables us to orient ourselves with respect to the geomagnetic field.

Magnetite is such a powerful magnetic field receptor—it's also one of the hardest metals on Earth—it interacts one million times more strongly with external magnetic fields than any other biological material, even iron. Magnetite (or some distinct form of magnetic guidance system) has been found in dolphins, whales, rays, navigating birds like robins, warblers, indigo buntings, and blackcaps, homing pigeons, salmon, tuna, freshwater magnetotactic bacteria, honeybees, hornets, salamanders, mollusks, flies, snails, and humans.

That's the controversial contention of California Institute of Technology geobiologist Dr. Joseph Kirschvink, who proposes that human brain cells not only contain quantities of this highly magnetic mineral, but actually synthesize it. Kirschvink analyzed the brain-cell tissue from seven human corpses and found minuscule amounts of magnetite distributed throughout the brain, ranging from 5 million crystals/gram of tissue in most regions of the brain, to 100 million/gram in the dura mater, the tough membrane under the skull that lines the brain.

The average human brain, Kirschvink says, contains 7 billion magnetite particles weighing about one-millionth an ounce in total. In earlier experiments Kirschvink had detected ferromagnetic (magnetized iron) crystals in human adrenal glands (specifically, in the walls of the sphenoid-ethmoid complex) while other biologists discovered magnetic deposits of iron in the human sinuses, just behind the bridge of the nose, at nine times the background magnetic charge.

What had prompted Kirschvink's studies was the health controversy that brain cancer and childhood leukemia might be linked to electromagnetic fields emanated from high-voltage power lines (see below for a detailed discussion); he hypothesized that an indigenous magnetic material might mediate the interactions and his data seems to bear this out. But he's not quite ready to grant more extrasensory connections such as dowsing or ESP to a magnetite-rich brain, as he told *The New York Times* recently: "There's not a shred of evidence so far that these microscopic magnets mediate any sensory capability in humans."

"We live within a regularly oscillating energy environment"

The broad implications emerging from the research of scientists like Landscheidt, Dubrov, Davis, Becker, and Kirschvink is that all living organisms on Earth are intimately linked to and responsive to Earth's EMF, and to such an extent that daily, weekly, seasonal, and yearly fluctuations in EMF strength—what geologists call the planet's micropulsations—actually serve as a biological timepiece to coordinate fundamental bodily rhythms.

Earth's EMF is viewed as a kind of primal energy womb in which all living forms take their nourishment and continuing energetic sustenance and our body's biomagnetic centers may be the mediating interface between outer and inner magnetic domains. Dubrov postulated, for example, that the numerous human acupoints in the body might be ion exchange sites for the electrical and magnetic activities of Earth's EMF and the body's own biomagnetic field. That's a suggestion acupuncture scholar Stephen Birch willingly amplifies.

"From the classical Chinese view, we are the result of the interactions of Heaven and Earth," says Birch. "We are the product of the environment and cannot separate ourselves from this context. The processes that occur inside us are the result of often very subtle outside processes. This is especially true with the timing of biological rhythms." The periodicity of the Five Elements (earth, wood, metal, fire, and water) and the circulation of chi (vital life energy, dynamic life force) through the body's multiple meridians constantly express this biometeorological relationship.

"The human body's energy rhythms are modulated by variations in the environment," says Birch. The ancient Chinese knew this but couched their observations in what are to us confusing terms, like the Five Elements, the Ten Stems, and Twelve Celestial Branches. All biorhythms in the body are conditioned by fluctuations in the geomagnetic field. "Acupuncture meridians are simply lines of decreased electrical resistance to flow, channels in which the current flows easily. We grew up, both individually and evolutionarily, within this electromagnetic environment. We live within a regularly oscillating energy environment, one that provides the many regulating factors for the body, its timing mechanisms for integrating all its functions."

That's why acupuncture educator Caleb Gattegno coined the term "electromagnetic man" to suggest "a new grasp of human beings because we live in an electromagnetic environment." What the Chinese call meridians, Gattegno renames the human Faraday cage. In the early nineteenth century Michael Faraday invented what's now called the Faraday cage, a wire shield that operates like a continuously closed conductor that blocks off outside electrical influences.

Contemplating this device, Gattegno analogically understood that the Chinese model, which construes the human as a body wired with meridians, is in other terms "an electromagnetic shield that we need to help us live in the world we inhabit." The shield forms itself "as soon as we are born so that whatever happens electrically inside the soma is not affected by the electrical changes outside. There are many outside changes, yet nobody notices them, because of our shields." The insular human Faraday cage, says Gattegno, is a gift of nature that stays with us from birth to death, keeping us "immune to the changes in the environment." Otherwise, says Gattegno, we would be completely susceptible to all the "vagaries" of the surrounding electromagnetic fields.

As it is, obviously we are susceptible (even aware of, occasionally) to some of the more significant electromagnetic effects and cycles. Not only are there daily lunar-solar influences affecting the earth/human EMF, explains Stephen Birch, but there are longer range, more cosmic, variations as well. These include, for example, the daily axial rotation of Earth, the 28-day Moon cycle, the 365-day year, the 35-day solar axial rotation, the 8-day solar magnetic moment, the 12- and 60-year cycles of Jupiter and Saturn, and the 11.1- and 22.2-year sunspot cycles. The 22.2-year sunspot cycle is actually a magnetic cycle because at the mid-point of 11.1, the Sun reverses the polarity of its magnetic field.

This subtle though pervasive magnetic ecology has been interfered with and even functionally polluted by modern electrified Western civilization, says Birch. "We have changed the Earth's field recently, in geologic time. We have thereby interfered with the well-being of biological organisms, producing many undefined symptoms." Stiff shoulders, insomnia, unidentified chest pain, whole-body tiredness, and neck discomfort are some examples in which doctors cannot locate the origin of such complaints. This malady is what one leading Japanese biomagnetics researcher, Dr. Kyoichi Nakagawa, calls "magnetic deficiency syndrome."

Nakagawa published an influential study in 1976 in the *Japan Medical Journal* in which he described this syndrome and its remedy, magnetic treatment. Nakagawa first noted that the strength of Earth's EMF has decreased 50% in the last 500 years and continues to decline at 0.05% yearly. Moreover, contemporary styles of housing (steel- and iron-frame buildings), the prevalent use of enclosed, nearly airtight, cars, trains, buses, airplanes, and subways, all of which tend to absorb incoming magnetic energy, have tacitly conspired to shelter and deprive humans from necessary, wholesome, and regular exposure to EMFs.

The average urbanized human is thereby deficient in low-level EMF intake, and as the human biofield is interdependently linked with Earth's, various vague but chronic forms of disease have set in.

Orgone on My Mind: Atmospheric Energies Modulate Consciousness

Seeking that deeper context for biometeorology is what the research of James DeMeo, Ph.D.—director of the Orgone Biophysical Research Laboratory (OBRL) of El Cerrito, California, and editor/founder of the research journal *Pulse of the Planet*—is all about. DeMeo founded OBRL in 1978 to investigate the "bioenergetic, orgonomic basis of life and weather" based on earlier research by the controversial American scientist Wilhelm Reich (1897-1957).

Reich described a subtle energetic substance called orgone, which he contended is a fundamental atmospheric energy that charges or energizes life. "Orgone energy is probably the same as chi or prana, but it has a quantitative basis and its properties can be demonstrated experimentally," explains DeMeo. "Orgone is very plasmatic. It can expand or contract and exhibits pulsatory qualities. Reich's orgone is a spontaneously pulsatile, excitable, and negatively entropic energy. It is an active, creative principle which is tangible, real, measurable, and in the 'here and now.' Through experiment it was found that concentrated, excited orgone in high vacuum absorbs and diminishes electromagnetic excitations transmitted through it."

Reich's contention was that weather is basically a function of the pulsatory, atmospheric circulation of orgone. Reich observed that when the atmosphere is in a state of energetic expansion (a high-pressure system, bright sky, free of clouds) people on Earth feel expansive, buoyant, lively, and their energies expand outward. When the atmosphere is contracted from a low-pressure system (high moisture content, with rain, clouds, or cyclonic storms), the human orgone goes stagnant and people feel fatigued and depressed. The atmospheric expansion or contraction of orgone has immediate health consequences, says DeMeo.

Bioelectrically speaking, it's a function of atmospheric overcharge and undercharge with respect to an individual's energetic disposition. Undercharged cancer patients, for example, in this Reichian orgone model, have their symptoms exacerbated under low pressure, contracted atmospheric conditions, while overcharged hypertense individuals suffer when the atmosphere is expansive with orgone. Reich's research in America is still regarded as anathema and his reputation is beleaguered at best, admits DeMeo. "Today the biomedical community remains just as viciously hostile to Reich's findings as they were then in the 1950s," he says.

A Butterfly Stirring the Air in Peking Affects Manhattan's Weather

The conventional scientist would no doubt consider it beyond the limits of common sense were he presented with the speculative correlations of Buryl Payne, Ph.D., director of the Academy of Peace Research of Santa Cruz, California. Between 1984 and 1988 Payne, a physicist by training, studied the hypothesized human alteration on solar and geomagnetic activity achieved through meditation, visualization, or prayer.

As part of his Global Meditation Project, Payne coordinated meditators around the world to do their Sun-focused meditations at six yearly dates, including the two solstices and two equinoxes, with the intention of suppressing sunspot activity by thought suggestion. The effort culminated in June 1988, when the alignment of six planets close to the galactic center should have triggered a large increase in sunspot activity and, by connection, human aggressiveness. He had already established phenomenological connections between the onset of international battles with sunspot peaks during the last 200 years.

Payne accepted the standard biometeorological chain of influence—solar flares, solar winds, electron-proton sprays, magnetospheric perturbation, disturbances to the planet's EMF, human hormonal shifts, emotional mood changes, behavioral alterations—but he wanted to see if the system worked in reverse. Could human moods—focused attention through meditation—positively, creatively affect sunspot activity?

"Preliminary analysis of the data indicates that this is possible," declared Payne in 1989. "Although there was an increase in solar activity there was actually a dip around the time of the largest peace meditations. On the average, the effects of several million people meditating appears to have resulted in a decrease in solar activity of 30% for a period of 7 to 10 days following the meditations."

While Payne's report represents the far fringes of biometeorological speculation, the statistical conservatism of the majority of investigators doesn't keep them from proposing practical social applications for their conclusions. Weather data can be used to predict onset of aggressive behavior (says Rotton), to help reduce prison violence through summer environmental cooling (says Anderson), and to design future user-friendly cities (says Persinger). Research biologist Marsha Adams at the Time Research Institute in Woodside, California, found some personally practical applications for biometeorological data. Adams used a computerized weather station at home that collects data every thirty minutes on temperature, wind velocity, barometric pressure, chill factor, and EMF strength. Clients in the San Francisco Bay Area can have their emotional variability, anxiety attacks, even diabetic insulin fluctuations correlated—in a sense justified and rationalized, too—against Adams' "hard data."

Knowing about the weather and its probable biomagnetic influences is psychologically valuable, says Adams. "Ordinarily people are puzzled. How can they wake up one day feeling happy, then the next day depressed, while nothing has changed in their lives to account for such different feelings? They tend to internalize this disparity and conclude there is something wrong with them. The people I work with are extremely relieved to find out there is an external factor—something physical and measurable, like the weather—that causes at least some of the changes they experience."

Adams probably wouldn't find the grievances of weather sensitives like Goethe, Nietzsche, de Biran, or Pressman too hard to understand. Her own earlier professional work involved extensive work with "earthquake sensitives" and quake predictions through subtle human-registered, EMF-mediated signs. "Humans are constantly immersed in a changing environment," Adams comments. "Even though we can't sense these changes, they're real, and probably have an impact on our physiology. Nobody knows for sure what that is because biometeorology research is still in its infancy."

The result is that both biometeorologists and individual "weather consumers" are often left staring at the clouds and blue sky with a lot of unresolved puzzles. One puzzle is the Butterfly Effect. This was first demonstrated, somewhat inadvertently, in the 1960s by Edward Lorenz, an MIT global weather modeler working in Cambridge, Massachusetts. Lorenz was using an early-model mainframe computer to calculate future weather behavior based on a dozen variables. He expected the weather to proceed orderly, like clockwork, but it didn't. What happened instead helped establish the basis for a new paradigm that's gradually enveloping—in fact, intriguing—many sciences today: Chaos theory.

The Butterfly Effect in weather means a tiny, local, random perturbation of the weather system can have enormous, cumulative repercussions elsewhere in the world. "Tiny differences in input could quickly become overwhelming differences in output," explains James Gleick, who put the subject on America's intellectual map in his highly popular *Chaos: Making a New Science*. "A butterfly stirring the air today in Peking can transform storm systems next month in New York." No doubt Goethe, that human barometer, would have noted the wing colors on that distant butterfly as he sneezed in Weimar.

The Perils of Human-made Electromagnetic Energy

What we've been describing is a model of the pure effects of solar activity, planetary weather and climate, geomagnetic fields, and human health. The qualifying term "pure" becomes meaningful when we add to this natural electromagnetic matrix of energies the role of "impure" human-made electromagnetic influences, our ubiquitous electronic environment of power transmission cables and their toxic radiations—electropollution.

According to some health researchers, we may have a serious problem here. The unlimited, widespread, but unexamined use of electromagnetic energy in its many forms—microwave, radar, short-wave transmitters, television, radio, electric power lines, video display terminals, even electric blankets, the global commercial web of man-made electromagnetic energy, virtually the electronic nervous system of modern Western society—poses a grave danger for human, even planetary, health, contend Robert O. Becker, author of *Cross Currents*, and Paul Brodeur, author of *Currents of Death*.

According to Becker and Brodeur, considerable research now indicates that man-made electromagnetic energy can adversely affect such delicate human biological processes as bone growth, communication among cells, white blood cell activity, and the smooth functioning of the immune system. Video Display Terminals (VDTs) have been implicated in unusual clusters of fetal miscarriages among women operators. Power lines are linked with childhood leukemia, and microwave radar may be a cancer-promoting agent. Through unlimited use, according to Becker and Brodeur, we may have unwittingly put ourselves and Earth in peril. Commercially induced magnetic fields may not be user-friendly, Becker and Brodeur warn. The whole technological approach to electric energy must be reconsidered, and we had better do it very soon. "It's a compelling public health issue," cautions Becker. "We deny these problems at our peril," adds Brodeur.

Yet the news about electromagnetic energy isn't all grim. Almost in equal measure to its peril, electromagnetic energy, when appropriately used, promises remarkable innovations and therapeutic successes in healing (or at least causing to remit) such intractable diseases as cancer, and it may hold the key to the mystery of cellular, bone, and even limb regeneration. Becker documents numerous advances in the fields of electrotherapy, transcutaneous electrical nerve stimulation, electroacupuncture, pulsed magnetic fields, and nuclear magnetic resonance imaging, all of which produce positive effects through working with the body's subtle electric and magnetic fields. When something as fundamental to life as electromagnetic energy is both a killer and a healer, both peril and promise, then we are face to face with a basic paradox of nature.

Meanwhile, out on the front lines of controversy, their insurrection tends to pit Becker and Brodeur, and an expanding handful of committed scientists and colleagues around the country, against a formidable monolith. They're up against modern science, medicine, the military, and the electronics industry, for all of whom unlimited electromagnetic energy is as necessary and as taken for granted as water and sunlight.

But Becker and Brodeur have flown into the face of major opposition before. For more than thirty years, Becker's research into the electromagnetic basis of life has been eroding the reigning scientific paradigm, while Brodeur, in the last twenty-six years, has taken on the issues of asbestos, ozone depletion, and microwave radiation—and with considerable success.

The Electromagnetic Milieu and the New Plagues

Human and biological life on Earth, says Becker, originated and has been maintained within a fairly simple electromagnetic environment for several billions of years. These nourishing "fields of life" on Earth are interconnected with activities on the Sun, such as solar flares, and with events in Earth's atmosphere, such as magnetic storms.

This remained the case until the twentieth century. In the brief span of the last ninety years, and most acutely since the mid-1940s, Western technological society has created a unique situation of "global electromagnetic pollution of the environment, an electromagnetic jungle," says Becker. "Our unwise use of electromagnetic energy has produced environmental changes of unparalleled proportions." Unfortunately, what makes this situation unique also makes it extremely hazardous.

"Today we swim in a sea of energy that is almost totally manmade," explains Becker. "The evidence is clear that our unrestricted use of electromagnetic energy has produced a global environment that is more and more hazardous to life. We have now almost reached a state in which the normally empty portions of the natural electromagnetic spectrum have been completely filled in with large amounts of powerful man-made frequencies that never before existed on Earth. The global environmental alteration brought about by our use of electromagnetic energy has exposed all living organisms, from viruses to humans, to novel energetic fields that never before existed." And there's no place to hide.

Not even the remote snowclad mountains are free any more from this all-pervasive envelope of electromagnetic contamination, states Becker. Humans make good targets. "Magnetic fields," explains Brodeur, "are invisible lines of force that interact with magnets and certain metals, and readily penetrate almost anything that happens to stand in their way, including the human body."

This unintentional redesigning of our electromagnetic environment, continues Becker, may have a deleterious effect on Earth itself. It may be accelerating both the observed steady decline in the Earth's natural geomagnetic field strength and the arrival of the widely predicted geomagnetic field reversal of the planet, with the inescapable innuendo of possible species extinction. "The evidence indicates we are in the initial stages of a magnetic pole reversal," says Becker. However, this aspect of the problem may be academic.

Becker comments: "We may have unwittingly produced the equivalent of the greatest reversal ever through our global use of electromagnetic energy. Our artificial reversal is much greater in extent and has occurred in a much shorter period of time than any naturally occurring reversal. We're doing it in a span of only 90 years rather than the 2,000 years nature would take."

It's by no means out of the question that the species extinction possible with such a geomagnetic shift might include Homo sapiens—amateurish engineer of this designer evolutionary threshold, warns Becker. "Are we the ones who will start declining? Nobody really wants to hear about it." This doesn't daunt Becker, who takes the implications even further. "The exposure of living organisms to abnormal electromagnetic fields results in significant abnormalities in physiology and function."

A growing body of scientific research over the last three decades strongly suggests that a host of major biological, even genetic, effects, such as cancer and immune-system dysfunctions, may be attributable to occupational or residential exposure to abnormal electromagnetic fields. The unsuspected biological effects of electropollution, suggests Becker, may be among the most alarming issues of the 1990s. The documentation and discussion of these findings occupy Becker and Brodeur a great deal in their books.

The subtle interaction of magnetic fields with living organisms "appears to have been the origin of some new disease states and of a number of unexpected changes in the characteristics of some pre-existing disease states," says Becker, thinking, no doubt, of AIDS, childhood cancer, and other late-twentieth-century medical anomalies. Not without justification, he calls them "the new plagues."

Fortunately for us, a few scientists like Robert Becker have taken a hard, unprejudiced, and courageous look at the now voluminous data on the harmful effects of EMFs. Becker, for one, has reached certain striking conclusions. All abnormal man-made electromagnetic fields (EMFs), says Becker, regardless of their frequencies, produce the same biological effects. These include deleterious effects on growing and dividing cells (which can lead to cancer), embryonic abnormalities, neurochemical and genetic alterations, changes in biological cycles, and stress-mediated immune-system dysfunction.

Not only is it likely that EMF effects are cancer promoting, argues Becker, but "it's quite possible that chronic exposure to such fields is a competent cause for the origin of cancer." The multiple biological effects of abnormal EMFs on humans produce what Becker calls "a cascade of changes." The man-made electromagnetic milieu is challenging, if not assaulting, the human immune system on all fronts.

The overall incidence of cancer is slowly increasing each year. New, puzzling medical anomalies are appearing in the clinics, such as Electromagnetic Hypersensitivity Syndrome and Chronic Fatigue Syndrome. AIDS, autism, and Sudden Infant Death Syndrome remain pervasive and intractable. The incidence of earlier, "established" maladies such as Alzheimer's, Parkinson's, cutaneous malignant melanoma, mental disease, depression, and adolescent suicide, is growing alarmingly. All this may represent a sudden EMF-mediated mutation in the disease organism, suggests Becker. Clearly we are facing a crisis of major proportions, one that is all the more critical because it has not been recognized as such by the agencies responsible for dealing with it.

The groundbreaking clinical and field research in the last several decades on the hazards of electromagnetic energy has largely been the work of a small, "undeflectable" group of scientists and watchdogs, explains Brodeur. It's been the research of fearless, underfinanced, and ignored researchers like Nancy Wertheimer, a Harvard Ph.D. and University of Colorado epidemiologist.

Wertheimer established the link between common neighborhood electric power-distribution lines, carrying the standard 60-Hertz, 3-milligauss field strength current, and the increased incidence of childhood leukemia in children living in their vicinity. Wertheimer published her startling correlations in 1979. She noted that her mid-1970's field study of Denver, Colorado, suggested that "the homes of children who developed cancer were found unduly often near electric lines carrying high currents."

The electric utilities industry definitely didn't want to hear about this, says Brodeur. It was bad enough already that scientists had opened a controversy about the possible ill-health effects of the high-voltage metal giants that stand astride the countryside. Now Wertheimer was implying that the ordinary stepped-down, low-voltage power line that brought the electricity into individual homes might itself be a public health hazard. Data like this could put the entire electronic distribution edifice into question—which is why Wertheimer's report was "savagely discredited," says Brodeur.

Wertheimer's study is but one among many powerful scientific challenges to what Brodeur calls "the presumption of benignity" of electromagnetic energy, whether it's power lines, radar, microwave, or video display terminals. Brodeur's *Currents of Death* is a shattering sourcebook, meticulously reported, of all the watershed studies and their suppression by the electric utility industry. "The value of my book," says Brodeur, "is that I put all the research together in one place."

The clinical studies Brodeur describes speak alarmingly for themselves. In 1982 Dr. Lennart Tomenius, county medical officer in Stockholm, Sweden, surveyed more than 2,000 homes with proximity to power lines or substations. He found that the homes of children with cancer were located near the high-current, 200,000-volt power lines twice as often as the homes of non-cancerous children. In 1986, Dr. David Savitz of the University of North Carolina reported that 20% of childhood cancers appeared traceable to exposure to 3-milligauss fields, which had been generally regarded as a low, nonharming field strength.

Information released in 1986 from fifteen worldwide surveys of electric workers showed a link between exposure to "extremely low electric fields," magnetic fields and the development of cancer, says

Brodeur. Another study indicated that power-line workers in Texas are now developing brain cancer at a rate thirteen times that of the general population. A 1989 study links telephone line cable splicers with higher-than-average levels of all cancers. Numerous studies in the 1980s have linked unusual clusters of fetal abnormalities, birth defects, and miscarriages in women who use video display terminals (VDTs).

The U.S. military has installed massive radar/microwave systems, such as the notorious PAVE-PAWS of Cape Cod. This system emits a continuous magnetic field dangerously within the human brain wave frequency. PAVE-PAWS, explains Brodeur, began pulsing low-level microwave radiation "at a frequency and modulation that had been shown in repeated laboratory experiments to be capable of changing the brain chemistry of brain cells in living creatures." "Who is my enemy?" asked one outraged Cape Cod resident, living in one of the four towns within immediate irradiating range of PAVE-PAWS.

The ramifications of such unchecked expansion of electromagnetic energy into all domains of commerce and life are grim, says Brodeur. We now have a de facto situation in which "millions of human beings continue to be test animals in a vast long-term biological experiment whose consequences remain unknown but whose outcome looks pretty awful." The epidemiological data is starting to come in on the PAVE-PAWS "experiment." Already, the residents of Sandwich, Mashpee, Bourne, and Falmouth on Cape Cod, who have been exposed to the extremely low frequency (ELF) radiation for a decade, "have been found to be developing cancer at an unusually high rate," reports Brodeur.

Confronting the Crosscurrents of Electromagnetic Energy

What have our public health agencies and scientists been doing? How did we ever come to this perilous situation in the first place? These are indeed reasonable questions, says Becker. The answer is this: the scientists, technicians, regulators, and M.D.s were all looking at the wrong paradigm when they set up the twentieth-century electromagnetic edifice. That "wrong paradigm" Becker calls the "chemical-mechanistic" model, which sees the human as a machine aslosh with chemicals.

Around 1900 the prevailing scientific view saw the human as a chemical machine of low intelligence and sensitivity, as a composite of discrete parts that existed in isolation from any external effects of the geomagnetic field. "It was simply assumed that the laws of physics guaranteed there could be no interaction between unseen fields and living things," says Becker. "The decision of the body of science then was that there was no way an EMF, or an electrical current below the levels that produce shock or heat, could have any biological effects at all.

"The result was unlimited utilization of electromagnetic energy with no restrictions whatsoever." Medicine wanted its "magic bullet"—and industry wanted unlimited energy—and it never occurred to anyone back in the formative days of electric industry giants Thomas Edison and Nikola Tesla that the magic bullet of electromagnetic energy might start killing us only three generations later. Paradoxically, what awakened us to the perils of electropollution was the dawning discovery of the electromagnetic secrets of healing, says Becker who is refreshingly optimistic about current trends in medicine.

Becker's research, because it was original, and therefore unorthodox, led him to a frank confrontation with the crosscurrents of electromagnetic energy. He realized something had "gone wrong." It wasn't long before he was testifying against a major New York State power-line project, protesting the serious threat to human health it posed. During the 1970s Becker was "locked in a no-holds-barred struggle" against the electric utilities, the "target of savage criticism" and "an apparent vendetta," explains Brodeur. Becker's forthright convictions eventually cost him his job.

By 1990, Becker's understanding of the "two-edged sword" of electromagnetic energy was clearly formulated. "The new scientific paradigm of life, energy, and medicine has led us to reconsider many of our technological 'advances.'" We have put ourselves at peril from an unwise, indiscriminate deployment of abnormal forms of EMFs, Becker says, yet we are equally at an advantage by the newfound awareness of the healing potential of appropriate, low-strength EMFs.

But as to the troubling question as to how electromagnetic energy can both heal and harm us, Becker and his colleagues are still formulating their theories. Obviously the factors of field strength, duration of exposure, relative spectrum position, and physiological electromagnetic overload, if not toxicity, are important. It's likely that the present scale of electropollution somehow antidotes the body's innate electrical-magnetic balance, and thereby the immune system, and it may also hinder the full healing effects of various subtle-energy therapies. For the present, we'll have to wait for the theorists and researchers to resolve the paradox.

Of course if we're expecting the power industry to answer our questions, we'd better not hold our breath, says Brodeur. The last thing the "old boys network of epidemiologists" and the electric utilities industry magnates want to hear is cries for change, says Brodeur. He knows the pattern well. "I've been through this before," adds Brodeur, referring to his decade-long journalistic struggle against the massive but deadly American asbestos industry, whose involuntary juridical surrender he recounts in *Outrageous Misconduct*.

The public-relations program of the military is "specious," says Brodeur. The electric utility industry's public-relations program is "dishonest." And the collusion of the medical community with the EMF status quo is "shameful." Scientists who defend the energy establishment in the face of mounting contraindicatory evidence "perform an intricate dance of avoidance on the hot coals of this astonishing possibility," says Brodeur with panache.

"We have the orthodox scientific-medical community still laboring under the totally discredited assumption that the only harmful effects of low-level EMF radiation is the heat generated in tissues," he adds. "It's what I call the English muffin standard. If you don't turn brown and feel toasty, you're all right. That the American Medical Association goes along with this is absolutely absurd. They're dinosaurs. The medical and scientific community has simply fallen way behind, like the caboose at the end of a freight train."

The Geopathogenic Stress of Living

There are also significant mysteries about the energies emanated by our host planet, not all of which are favorable for human well-being. Geopathology is the name of a new science that studies harmful Earth radiations, but it's by no means as developed or as scientifically articulated as biometeorology—yet. On the other hand, its body of knowledge, investigative techniques, and palliative recommendations are growing fast. Information is being constantly gleaned by disparate researchers from forked-stick dowsers to biomagnetic field instrumentation designers.

The field of geopathology perhaps had its start, at least in our time, about sixty-five years ago in Germany. For a week in January 1929 Baron Gustav Freiherr von Pohl, Mayor Brandl, and a gendarme made a systematic tour of the Bavarian community of Vilsbiburg. This was a small town in southern Germany with 565 houses, 3,300 residents, and an unusually high rate of cancer. Von Pohl was acting on a hunch inspired from the earlier Winzer-Melzer survey of Stuttgart in the 1920s, which had determined that major geological faults in that city traversed the districts that had the highest cancer mortality rates. The tentative conclusion was that an unknown but noxious radiation emanating from the earth faults might be an important and overlooked contributory cause of the cancers.

Through dowsing, von Pohl located all the major subterranean water veins (lying at a depth of forty-four to fifty meters with a width of three to four meters) under Vilsbiburg, then mapped their courses onto the city street plan. Next he cross-checked this with the residences of the fifty-four recent cancer fatalities and arrived at a startling conclusion. "The completed check of my map confirmed all the beds of the fifty-four cancer deaths were where I had drawn the radiation currents," von Pohl wrote in 1932 in his now classic *Earth Currents: Causative Factor of Cancer and Other Diseases.* Eighteen months later von Pohl returned to Vilsbiburg and found that the beds of another ten cancer mortalities were situated directly over crossing underground streams.

Von Pohl's empirical discoveries at Vilsbiburg of a kind of noxious earth ray birthed a new field of inquiry now called geopathology. This evolving science deals with the possible causal relationship of geological factors such as underground water veins and radiational currents with human health and cancer etiology. The beds in these "cancer houses" were situated over what von Pohl characterized as geopathic zones marked by "dangerous radiation lines." Geopathology is still essentially unknown in America, but since von Pohl's day it's been the subject of considerable research, empirical investigation, and even medical recognition in his native Germany.

In a sense, geopathology is the medicalized, therapeutic aspect of a larger discipline called geobiology, which studies Earth's influence at precise locations on all life forms: plant, animal, and human. In America, geopathology has largely been the province of the dowsing community and electroacupuncture practitioners. Von

Pohl was confident about his discoveries, but tended to take a conservative stance regarding developing a hypothetical model. "My observations set down in this book about negative electrical earth currents are in the main virgin territory for medical science. We not only hope but expect that more doctors will research and advance this new knowledge for the benefit of mankind."

Don't Place Your Bed above a Strong Underground Current

In the sixty-five years since von Pohl's pioneering research in Vilsbiburg, it's been primarily the dowsers, not the physicians or academic scientists, who have continued his research indications and enriched his explanatory model. Von Pohl himself presented dozens of cases in which rapid, perhaps miraculous, cures of numerous complaints, from insomnia to heart spasm, were achieved simply by moving the sleeper's bed out of the geopathic zone situated underneath the house. In the town of Stettin, von Pohl's colleague, Dr. Hager, collated the details of 5,348 cancer deaths over a twenty-one-year span and found in each case that a subterranean water vein ran under the cancer patient's house. "Medical science has now a preventative measure which did not exist previously," noted von Pohl. "If one makes sure one's bed does not stand above a strong underground current and one tries not to work above these underground currents, one should not get cancer."

Two German physicians took von Pohl's data a couple of steps further in the 1940s, when they proposed an actual engineering scheme for the proposed telluric radiational currents. Manfred Curry, M.D., director of the Bioclimatic Research Institute in Ammersee, proposed the Curry Netting Screen, or Grid, which was a fine-mesh terrestrial grille extending around the planet. Curry's crisscross grid was oriented in two diagonally opposite directions—southwest by northeast, and northwest by southeast—in parallelogram sections about three and a half meters apart.

The second proposed radiational grid was developed by Ernst Hartmann, director of the Research Circle for Geobiology; according to Hartmann this grid, which runs diagonally to the Curry Net, is made of "standing walls of radiation." The Hartmann Grid is envisioned as a structure of radiations that rise vertically from the ground like invisible radioactive walls each nine inches wide; each

Hartmann grid rectangle measures about six feet, six inches by eight feet; like the Curry Net, its grid lines are electrically charged, alternately negative and positive. Frequently, where two rays or radioactive walls cross in the Hartmann grid, at a "Hartmann knot," this marks a geopathogenic zone of significance to human health.

The gridwork is magnetically oriented, while the space inside the invisible lines is a neutral zone, an unperturbed microclimate. "This network penetrates everywhere, whether over open ground or through dwellings," notes geobiologist Blanche Merz in her *Points of Cosmic Energy*. "According to Dr. Hartmann, the network forms a vast invisible whole, like a precisely woven net spread over the entire surface of the globe."

While the Hartmann Grid and Curry Net remain on the more speculative side of dowsing, the general concept of a regular patterning of telluric radiation lines has informed some important dowsing work. In 1972 Käthe Bachler, an Austrian mathematics teacher and dowser, was commissioned by the Pedagogical Institute in Salzburg to investigate the possible relationship of geopathic stress and school performance. Bachler tested 3,000 homes, interviewed 12,000 people in fifteen countries, and presented her findings in 1976 in a now widely distributed book (in Europe), *Experiences of a Dowser—Geobiological Influences on Man.*

Bachler found that 95% of slow learners had their beds at home situated above either water veins or Curry Net crossings, while the school desks of some children were positioned above "interference zones." In other words, Bachler was saying, somehow energetic emanations from the earth were directly interfering with the intelligence of schoolchildren—a fairly bold contention indeed. She identified ten certain physical indicators of geopathic stress and noted: "We should all relearn to pay more attention to the sensitivity of our body and let ourselves be guided by it."

But that's by no means the end of the mysterious trail of geobiological influences. According to continuing research by dowsers, geomancers, and Earth Mysteries investigators, these same subterranean water veins and radiational currents may in certain instances have salutary effects on human health and consciousness. Dowsers investigating various ancient megalithic sites in Europe discovered that these sites showed a proliferation of water veins, particularly under the high altars in old cathedrals and prominent standing stones in megalithic circles. Blanche Merz documented how a variety of prominent temples in India, Egypt, Tibet, and France were evidently meticulously designed to accommodate, even accentuate, the influence of the Hartmann grid intersections.

These discoveries threw the young field of geopathology into confusion. Hartmann and Curry had proposed invisible walls of radiation; the dowsers talked about underground water veins. Were they the same? Did the water veins carry a magnetic radiational charge? How could water veins be both injurious and beneficial at the same time?

Veteran British dowser Tom Graves in his *Needles of Stone Revisited* categorized the types of water veins and, using the *feng shui* terminology of Chinese geomancy, noted that "black" streams carry *sha,* or "demonic water in which the chi, or living energy, is converted to *sha,* stagnation, or 'noxious breath, stinking exhalation.'" Graves implied that the ancient Chinese geomancers had recognized the presence of injurious underground currents. Vermont dowser Sig Lonegren in his *Spiritual Dowsing* states that the presence of "primary water," which is a formation of underground water domes or blind springs from which radiate numerous water veins, is a prerequisite for a "power center or sacred enclosure" and is matched by a "yang energy line" (called energy ley or ley line) running above the ground.

Lonegren's empirical observation is that in some way the presence of water veins is crucial to the spiritual "success" or potency of sacred sites—stone circles and cathedrals, among others—which heighten and enhance human consciousness, even enact physical healing—Lourdes in France is a perfect example—yet is concurrently harmful when underneath beds. Lonegren's suggestion is that the specific site use, either sleeping (in beds) or consciousness expansion (at ancient sites), determines the health valency of these decidedly ambivalent subterranean currents.

Sarah Wooster, astrologer, dowser, and researcher, suggests a way out of this apparent Earth-energies paradox. "The lines of force at Stonehenge are fine for recharging your 'battery' or for meditation, but you wouldn't want to build your home there. It's a question of long-term exposure. If you spend fifteen minutes there in worship the effect is very different than if you sleep there every day."

But whatever the theoretical model used to explain the effects, practicing dowsers have ample empirical data testifying to the reality of such geopathogenic currents. Herbert Douglas, a retired lawyer and former trustee of the American Society of Dowsers in

Danville, Vermont, spent more than twenty-five years investigating the different effects of sleeping over water veins. He personally dowsed the bedrooms of at least 250 individuals, mostly in Bennington County in southwestern Vermont, and found as many as thirty to fifty line crossings of underground water. Based on his investigation of sixty cases of arthritis and nine cataracts, Douglas concluded: "In every single one of them I found dowsing reaction lines intersecting under the affected part of the body."

Douglas, like other old-time dowsers, is hesitant to develop a comprehensive model of causation, but that's the way dowsers are: practical, oriented to results, "down to earth." "It's not known precisely what is causing the effect although the consensus is that underground water seems a necessary element." The nebulous geopathic earth currents, many dowsers concede, must be seen in the larger context of influences from metallic ore and mineral deposits, geological faults and fractures, gravity and magnetic anomalies, radioactive hot spots, and the now pervasive human-made electromagnetic pollution.

Dowsing's success at practically and financially remunerative projects—locating wells, identifying ore and oil deposits—has gradually encouraged a few mainstream scientists to give it more credence. "We live in a region—the Earth's surface—of pronounced local electric field gradients, plus diurnal variations," observed Anthony Hopwood, considering the links among dowsing, ley lines, and electromagnetism in *New Scientist*. "The brain and neuromuscular system rely on tiny electrical signals, and it is hardly surprising that dowsing turns out to be a way of amplifying the instinctive response of this system to differences in electric fields."

Fortunately, the development in Germany of sophisticated instrumentation to detect biophysically subtle energies has prevented the young field of geopathology from relapsing into what its critics are eager to call "pseudoscience."

Quantifying the Geobiological Factor

Since von Pohl's day, individual research scientists have attempted to measure the suspected geopathic energies. Electrometer readings in the cellars underlying 7,000 "cancer beds" over dowsed water veins in Le Havre, France, in the 1930s showed an air ion concentration ten times above normal background levels.

In the 1970s, German scientist Jacob Stängle's scintillation counter registered a sharp increase in gamma radiation over underground water veins. Stängle resubstantiated von Pohl's original data from Vilsbiburg, after which he announced: "The principal objection against the existence of pathogenic stimulation zones, namely the inability to objectify them is no longer valid."

A recent development that further objectifies the presumed pathogenic stimulation zones comes from a German firm called Bio-Physics Mersmann with U.S. offices in Massachusetts. According to Ludger Mersmann, M.D., its director, the cause of geopathic stress is localized magnetic anomalies whose sharp field gradients upset delicate human physiological homeostasis. Mersmann carefully notes it isn't so much the presence of a subterranean magnetic field as unusual, sudden, local changes and quirks—anomalies—in the general field intensity.

To prove his hypothesis, Mersmann invented a geomagnetometer with data logger with which he can take precise, local magnetic field readings in a suspected geopathic zone such as a bedroom; his instrumentation generates a three-dimensional computer graphic showing the specificities of the disturbed magnetic field. "The geomagnetometer offers reproducible objective analysis in a scientific way of disturbed zones on site with the advantage of physical evidence," comments Mersmann. "Geopathic stress consists of several factors, maybe as many as twenty-five, but the main factor is a disturbed magnetic field. Here the natural homogeneous magnetic field meets with or turns into a nonhomogeneous field, resulting in a disturbed zone. These geomagnetic anomalies act upon the human organism as stimuli of a localized and chronic nature and, depending on the intensity and length of exposure, lead to impairment of health."

Mersmann's magnetic anomalies make more sense when contrasted with "normal" background geomagnetic field strength. The earth's natural magnetic field is measured at 0.5 gauss, or about 50,000 nanotesla (nT), which is actually an extremely weak field, several hundred times weaker than the field strength measurable between the two poles of a toy horseshoe magnet. Geomagnetic field strength varies slightly from zone to zone, and is subject to transient fluctuations, between the North and South poles, but not in correlation to the major features of geography and geology. Magnetic anomalies, or sudden field shifts, can range between 200 nT and 150,000 nT, says Mersmann.

As biometeorology informs us, widespread magnetic field shifts occur in connection with sunspot activity, but Mersmann is keying in on the tiny, minutely localized, sudden changes in field intensity. Typically in bedrooms over suspected geopathic stress areas, the gradient change from natural background to sudden anomaly is 10 to 20,000 nT.

Mersmann's precise magnetic field readings provide the necessary empirical, quantitative foundation to develop a scientific theory of geopathology. The starting point in Mersmann's model is the geological factor, by which he means some primary form of dislocation, fissure, or fault; the possibly noxious activity of water veins is a secondary factor, epiphenomenal to geological conditions. The geological factor produces a disturbance or anomaly in the local magnetic field, and this registers as a sharp, sudden, vertical fluctuation in an otherwise smooth, steady field.

The crucial factor for geopathogenic causation is the sudden change, either up or down, says Mersmann; the degree of geopathogenicity is directly related to the strength of the gradient change and the bodily site of geopathically induced illness seems to be exactly correlated with respect to the gradient change as well. "Some people live in fields of 30,000 nT while others have 50,000 nT, but this is not so important as the local gradient over the body lying in bed. This means different parts of the same body have different intensity lines and this disturbed zone, where the highest gradient is shown, is often the site of the cancer or illness."

Scientific data on the harmful effects of extremely weak magnetic fields on human health, which has been accumulating for two decades, supports Mersmann's hypothesis. As we noted above," the human body has composite and localized magnetic fields, as low as 1×10^{-9} gauss, or about one-billionth of Earth's magnetic field.

Studies in New York and Colorado show incontrovertible links between exposure to low-frequency, extremely weak electromagnetic fields—from high-voltage power lines, for example—and the onset of cancer, particularly childhood leukemia. "In addition to geopathic stress," notes Sarah Wooster in *Townsend Letter for Doctors*, "current research shows certain man-made electrical and/or electromagnetic fields to be another potentially serious health hazard adding further expanse to the definition of disturbed zones."

Biomedical research continues to deepen our understanding of possible internal effects from invisible fields. Helmut Ziehe, president of the International Institute for Baubiologie and Ecology in Clearwater, Florida, summarizes a dozen physiological changes that scientists have observed in humans occupying geopathic zones. These include in part: changes in electrocardiogram, pulse, blood sedimentation, pH, electrical cell polarity, and body immunological resistance parameters. According to Ziehe, a variety of subtle biophysical measurements—air ionization changes, increases in soil electrical conductivity, microseismic effects, intensification of radioactive and neutron radiation, anomalies in TV reception—are reliable indicators of geopathic "cancer points."

Overall the modern home presents us with an environment that is "a total mixture, a salad of electric waves," says Ziehe. The typical home has multiple injurious factors, from proximity to high-tension wires to toxic interior paint and 60 Hertz fluorescent tubes. "Behind an appliance there might be a wall, and that fridge is creating an electromagnetic field which goes right through the wall. Behind that wall you might have your bed, and you might sleep with your head right in the middle of that electromagnetic field. If somebody *knows* about these things, he won't do it, but the problem is people don't know."

The kind of precise biophysical data now accumulating makes the following conclusion by a leading German oncologist and geopathic researcher sound less fabulous. According to the late Hans Nieper, M.D., who operated a clinic at Silbersee Hospital in Hannover, Germany, and routinely advised patients to engage a water dowser to check their sleeping quarters for geopathogenicity, 75% of his multiple sclerosis patients "spend too much time in a geopathogenic zone." The MS patient should "avoid prolonged stays in such zones by all means since otherwise the electrical discharge of his cellular membrane potential will be reinforced," which, Nieper implies, worsens the illness.

"According to studies I have initiated, at least 92% of all the cancer patients I examined have remained for long periods—especially in respect to their sleeping places—in geopathogenic zones." Nieper further commented in a 1985 U.S. lecture: "This does not necessarily say that geopathogenic zones or their magnetic effect produces cancer, but rather it is the ultimate push button that then makes the thing happen."

The Ultimate Physiological Push Button

Other geopathologists have followed up Nieper's provocative statement regarding membrane potential discharge. Ludger Mersmann is one. Human biochemical reactions have an ultrasensitivity to magnetic fields and electron spin resonance changes, Mersmann explains. The sudden, dramatic magnetic field gradients he's observed over "geopathic beds" seem to upset this delicate homeostasis.

To explicate the correlations, Mersmann takes a foray into the technicalities of biochemistry. "Electrical cell membrane polarization, along with the intracellular electromagnetic linkages can be thrown into disarray with changes in spin oscillation and proton resonance of protein molecules and hydrogen bonds. This produces disturbances in the mesenchymal regulatory processes; it leads to hormone imbalances, pH shifts, autonomic nervous system malfunctions, and the eventual promotion of degenerative disease." Prolonged exposure to disturbed zones—residential exposure in particular—can produce blockages to healing and becoming well, even with holistic, natural medicines.

This is an important, though still underacknowledged, indicator of the negative activity of geopathic stress, says Mersmann. In an influential article in the British *Journal of Alternative and Complementary Medicine,* Anthony Scott-Morley of the Institute of Bioenergetic Medicine looked at how geopathic stress might block natural therapeutics. He proposed that habitual exposure to "geopathic disturbance" produced by "localized variations in the geomagnetic flux of the earth" might be a basic reason why natural therapies like acupuncture and homeopathy fail to cure definitively in some patients. He reasoned there must be other mitigating factors that compromised what was otherwise "excellent and appropriate therapy."

Scott-Morley reported that according to "experienced practitioners who are aware of these stresses," 30% to 50% of chronically sick patients exhibit some degree of geopathic stress. "A geopathic stress may be defined," wrote Scott-Morley, "as a geomagnetic disturbance which is geographically localized and which disrupts the homeostatic mechanisms of the sensitive patient. It does seem that geopathic stresses energetically weaken the body so that the patient may be more prone to disease-forming processes.

The geopathic stress is an energetic force which, in the sensitive patient, is sufficiently strong to overcome the natural regulation and equilibrium of the body energy." According to this model, then, when human physiological homeostasis is compromised by geopathic stress, various patterns of dysfunction and, potentially, degeneration set in.

The severe physiologically disruptive influence of geopathic stress was confirmed through another unusual manifestation. A report in *The American Dowser* in 1986 by the German engineer Robert Endrös and scientist Dr. Karl-Ernst Lotz linked unaccountable car accidents with geopathic stress zones.

Endrös and Lotz investigated 1,000 head-on collisions and found in every case they were within fifty to seventy meters of a geopathic stress zone with often several underground water streams. They conducted microwave radiation emission studies of human endocrine function within and outside these zones and concluded that somehow the geopathic locale immobilizes adrenaline, leading to sudden loss of acute vision necessary for fast reactions while driving a car, memory loss, and some decline in "vegetative-motor" function.

"This strong, recurring disturbance of the driver's endocrinal control system caused by successive underground water currents exhausts the hormone adrenaline, leaving a vulnerable driver," Endrös and Lotz concluded.

The Geopathic House:
Your Domestic Environment
May Be Harmful to Your Health

It's not only the presence of underground water and magnetic field anomalies and reversed cellular spin that constitute the full picture of geopathic stress. The building materials of the home itself may synergistically amplify the noxious influences of the naturally occurring geopathic zone underground.

This is the message from proponents of the German natural home movement called *Baubiologie* (meaning "biological architecture") which views humans, their clothing, and dwellings as a single living organism. These three living "skins" comprise a *Bauorganism*. If our home is a kind of bioarchitectural organism, this means we can have either a healthy or a sick home. According to Baubiologists, most of us have sick houses (*Krankheitsherd:* "sickness induc-ing dwelling")—our house itself may be injurious to health.

Baubiologie suggests that the "sick house syndrome" may result from an inappropriate combination of geopathic zone; unhealthy, toxic building materials (paints, plywood, artificial carpets, for example); and cumulative indoor electromagnetic pollution (*Elek-trosmog,* as the German Baubiologists call it). Houses with steel-reinforced concrete floors, says Helmut Ziehe, a leading proponent of Baubiologie in America, can distribute the geopathic radiation uniformly throughout the home in somewhat the same manner that the air-conditioning system distributed legionnaire's disease to conventioneers in Philadelphia some years ago.

"The 1990s will be an era of environmentalism as people become more aware of these contributing factors to disease," says another natural house advocate, Peter Sierck, a German-trained natur-opath who provides environmental testing for indoor pollutants in consultation with local physicians. "Is your home or workplace making you sick?" queries Sierck. He finds answers to this question through a combination of tests for the home and residents, relying on a German-innovated form of electroacupuncture called the Veg-atest—developed in 1978 by Dr. Helmut Schimmel as a method of electronic diagnosis and medication testing—that can specifically pinpoint geopathic stress in the human organism.

Schimmel's strategy, which he calls medication testing, is to ren-der acupoints measurable by instrumentation and to use them through a kind of kinesiological reflex method to determine a vari-ety of physiological effects. He found that the acupoints change their measurement readings when substances (such as allopathic or homeopathic medicines, vitamins, herbs, supplements) are intro-duced into the measurement circuit; this information has prescrip-tive value because the pathway can be used to gauge the potential efficacy of proposed remedies before they're taken.

Sierck and his M.D. colleagues cite a dossier of successful case studies in which conditions of asthma, sleeping disorders, and energy depletion, among many others, were resolved, after an initial diagno-sis revealed geopathic stress, by moving the bed. Despite its shocking simplicity, geopathy as a conceptual model remains controversial if not ignored. "There is not a lot of acceptance of the geopathic stress factor so far among American M.D.s," Sierck comments. Resistance is also lodged forcefully by real estate agents, who find geopathic revelations about their properties bad news at best. "They don't want to hear anything about this because by law if they know of any fault in a property they must report it to the prospective buyer."

The use of electroacupuncture diagnostic systems (also known as electrodermal screening) for identifying geopathic stress might become more widely known among M.D.s if the educational efforts of Walter Sturm, M.D., homeopath, and director of the Occidental Institute Research Foundation in Delta, British Columbia, come to fruition. Sturm's group is "an information bridge" for new developments in Germany—he considers German geopathic research about ten years ahead of anything happening in the U.S.—to the 600 M.D.s, acupuncturists, naturopaths, and chiropractors among his membership.

In Germany, about 50% of all physicians have some awareness of the geopathic factor, and among naturopaths, that number is about 70%, whereas in America, "It's still a rather unrecognized factor," says Sturm. As a practicing scientist-physician, Sturm knows that the new field is rife with hypotheses and intriguing theories, some of which may prove to be in error. A lot of the material published on geopathology by physicians in Germany is anecdotal rather than the rigorous result of double-blind scientific protocols, Sturm admits. "All we know is that whatever the nature of these lines, it is a great block to getting the patient well. We can very rapidly help these people by moving them out of their cancer houses."

In light of these findings we might do well to consider the possible importance of "geohygienic planning" in public health. After all, the notion of an intimate energetic relationship between planet and human isn't that recent. It's the basis of the ancient Chinese geomantic science called *feng shui,* itself a component of the comprehensive Chinese Taoist cosmophilosophical medical model. For millennia, *feng shui* has provided precise instructions on how to site one's house and bedroom favorably with respect to water veins and ambient environmental energies.

With this in mind, perhaps the statement by Ernst Hartmann, M.D., in his *Weather, Soil, Man* (1968) is not so completely insupportable. "The health and well-being of humans is intimately tied to the Earth on which they live and to its radiation. Once this is clearly understood, a door will be opened to a healthier, happier existence for everyone and diseases which threaten them like nightmares will disappear."

As a therapeutic prospect, certainly no physician will deny the desirability of geohygienic planning; as to how we accomplish this and by what means we assess its success, this will remain the stuff of scientific contention. Whatever the outcome, we can presume that geopathologist Gustav Freiherr von Pohl would no doubt be gratified that we're at least entertaining the question.

Environmental Illness: Equivalent Dysfunction in Self and Ecology

With Environmental Illness (EI), a multifactorial immunological malaise steadily gaining in incidence in America, we witness clear signs of the way dysfunction and disease are coincident in both the human and ecological environments, as if both poles of our world are equally, equivalently ill in a strange negative reciprocity. Here we have excellent, if grim, proof of the interconnectedness of human and outer environment. It has many names: Environmental Illness (EI), Total Allergy Syndrome, Twentieth-Century Disease, Chemically Induced Immune Dysregulation, Multiple Chemical Sensitivity.

The names may be multiple, but the message of EI is straightforward. Our total environment, inner and outer, is grievously ill. A steadily increasing number of Americans—one 1987 estimate by the National Academy of Sciences places it as high as 15%, and the numbers are predicted to steadily rise throughout the decade—can no longer live comfortably under the "normal" conditions of our postindustrial, high-tech world. Almost any substance can make them sick—the water, food, air, medicines, clothes, buildings, and just about any of the consumer products found in any supermarket, drugstore, hardware, or department store. In starkest terms, it's the twentieth century itself that's making people sick to death.

The prodigious technological expansion of the last 150 years has returned to us in the form of a ravaged, polluted outer environment and an allergic, cancerous, universally reactive inner environment. EI, as many holistic physicians struggling to discover treatments for this multifactorial disease attest, is a direct refutation of our national industrial profligacy. It's a direct rebuttal of our national way of life. And in the view of some observers, the beginning of survival is long past; it's now more a question of whether we can continue to survive. That 15% of Americans afflicted with EI may be only the environmentally sensitive front rank, the "wary canary" in the coal mine shaft, announcing bad fumes and probable danger. The symptom picture of EI is so diverse and its triggering agents so multitudinous that it challenges our conception of disease itself.

The Earth Day 1990 cover of the *New Yorker* expressed our plight with grim eloquence. It showed Atlas shouldering an Earth shrouded in black bands of pollution. Atlas didn't shrug, but he wore a gas mask. Many with EI must wear a gas mask and can't survive without a tank of pure oxygen in their room. But as environmentalists would say, where is the gas mask for Earth? The emergence of EI as a broad-spectrum malaise is a profound challenge for us to revise our understanding of self and environment. EI is a disease of the web of life itself, where both planet and people are environmentally ill.

The EI patient is, at worst, sensitive to nearly everything human-made in the modern world, to the whole twentieth-century technological environment of paints, plywood, carpeting, aerosols, electrical fields, natural gas—the list can be shockingly long. The EI patient suffers from more than sensitivity; it's a debilitating allergic reaction that often makes life in such environments unbearable. The EI patient experiences dysfunction at the immunological level. If anything, EI demonstrates the negative side of the indivisible interconnectedness of humans and the world, of inner and outer environments.

It is precisely on account of this interpermeation of self and world that Western allopathy is unable to comprehend the multifactoriality of EI or even, in many quarters, to acknowledge its existence as yet another immunological anomaly. With EI, there never has been a single candidate virus or bacteria or malfunctioning protein or gene implicated as the root cause.

Without a tangible, likely cause as a research focus, allopathic thinking tends to stall out, both in diagnosis and treatment. A multiaspected disease like EI simply does not compute according to allopathic rationality, so little in the way of therapies are devised. For the most part, if it hadn't been for the pioneering new specialty (within allopathy) of clinical ecology and its understanding of food- and substance-generated allergic sensitivities, EI would have remained largely immedicable, relegated to Western medicine's convenient pejorative category, psychosomatic.

But in the medical eyes of empiric physicians EI is an altogether different proposition: it makes sense and it can be treated. The core perception is that in EI the individual's immune function is severely compromised, leaving one overreactive to all manner of environmental toxins and stimulants, however benign they might be to other, non-EI patients. The diagnostic understanding and therapeutic strategies of empiric medicine in the face of EI illuminate many aspects of this interconnectedness of self and world that are otherwise obscured, ignored, or altogether unacknowledged in allopathy.

Yet despite the obvious physiological problems indicated by EI, the empiric insight shows us how inevitably there are antecedent, formative psychological, even spiritual issues, underlying even the most material kinds of physical dysfunctions. When we understand the true etiological pathways by which EI moves from subtle issues of identity and emotionality into immune system breakdown and universal sensitivity to environmental contaminants, we are witnessing how mind shapes matter and how illness is a material process of the psyche.

However, healing the EI patient alone is not enough, the empiric physicians caution us. Since EI is a disease interdependent and reciprocal with the outer environment, the ecological dimension of EI must be healed, too. EI is a disease with a large context—the composite environment of human and world. Unless both poles of this single environment are treated, EI will not be resolved. In the last several decades, numerous commentators, committees, even world convocations (most recently the Earth Summit in July 1992), have documented the environmental damages attributable to advanced Western culture and sought strategies to mobilize public and national action to halt the damage and begin programs of restoration.

Just as EI can't be truly, lastingly healed without some degree of environmental clean-up, effective environmental reform actually cannot happen until there is a change of attitude among individuals living in that environment. Again, EI unavoidably turns on the principle of *reciprocity,* that our inner immunological and outer ecological environments are really two aspects of the same single environment.

Environment, inner or outer, is created and regenerated fundamentally through consciousness, through a willed change of mind, attitude, and practice. For successful, enduring political and policy changes, we must make primary changes within ourselves as the foundation, knowing that the ecological crisis is the exterior aspect of an inner problem and can't be resolved without a spiritual rebirth of Western culture and its assumptions.

Our Destiny Is No Longer a Mystery

Speaking in his native Duwamish tongue to his tribal assembly in the Pacific Northwest in 1854, Chief Seattle considered the offer by the U.S. government to purchase his people's land. Chief Seattle, sensing the future, knew the role of Native Americans in North American history was at a moment of eclipse. "Every part of this Earth is sacred to my people," Chief Seattle said, in his now commemorated speech.

"We are part of the Earth and it is part of us. We know the white man does not understand our ways. One portion of land is the same to him as the next, for he is a stranger who comes in the night and takes from the land whatever he needs. This we know. The Earth does not belong to man; man belongs to the Earth. All things are connected like the blood which unites one family. Whatever befalls the Earth befalls the sons of the Earth. Man does not weave the web of life; he is merely a strand in it. Whatever he does to the web, he does to himself."

In closing, Chief Seattle contemplated the veiled future of the invading white man and the "special purpose" for which they were given dominion over the country and its native people. "That destiny is a mystery for us," he said. When the thicket and eagle, the swift pony and the hunt, were gone from the land, Chief Seattle added, it would mark "the end of living and the beginning of survival."

In the 1990s, America had reached that end of living and the beginning of survival and our destiny is no longer a mystery. Our destiny is spelled cancer, AIDS, heart disease, diabetes, alcoholism, lupus, Chronic Fatigue Syndrome, Alzheimer's—to enumerate only a few. Prominent and seemingly intractable among the new plagues is a clinical condition with symptoms that range across the board and against which conventional medicine has almost no treatments and would rather ignore.

While standard allopathic medicine shrugs its shoulders in the face of EI, holistic practitioners in a variety of complementary and adjunctive medical care fields all report high degrees of success in healing EI.

But there's a special condition. The fundamental condition for lasting human health is the inseparable need to clean up the Earth, to heal the planet of its environmental illness as well. EI can be "cured," but, as with AIDS and CFS, the price of treatment is high, not so much in dollars but in commitment to change. As any EI patient will report, it's nothing less than a profound and unilateral change in lifestyle.

"We are entering a period of consequences"

As Chief Seattle so presciently said, what humans do to the web of life, they do to themselves. "One thing we know: our God is also your God. The Earth is precious to Him. To harm the Earth is to heap contempt on its Creator." So, too, to heal the Earth is to offer praise to God's creation—humanity. The simple question is, Do we have the will to change? Chief Seattle's words were a prediction of EI. Our destiny is not a mystery anymore: we have to change our environment. When we clean up the Earth, we're cleaning up ourselves—that's the environmental web.

Our unearned carte blanche to change, upset, imbalance, and aberrate the planetary ecosystem, a subconsciously executed irresponsibility in which virtually all nations are now participating, has generated the extreme "immune deficiency" of our 4.5-billion-year-old host planet. It's an irresponsibility now widely recognized (but not acted upon) in the form of air, soil, and water pollution, ozone depletion, greenhouse gases, global warming, deforestation, acid rain, biodiversity extinction, overpopulation.

We know *about* these things—the knowledge capacity of the human intellect is prodigious—but as a culture evidently we do not *know* them, not directly—the wisdom capacity is, regrettably, not yet commensurate with our intellect—not deeply or passionately enough to act definitively to transform rampant abuse to mature cocreation.

We are still subconsciously guided by a dissociated ethics of action without consequences that institutionalizes and rationalizes our cultural alienation from nature. Our allopathic paradigm has schooled us in the unexamined dichotomy between self and environment—humanity *versus* nature—for centuries, producing the late-twentieth-century results of what Vice President Al Gore calls "the increasingly violent collision between human civilization and the natural world."

But of course: if Cartesian allopathy disallows free-ranging consciousness in the body and reifies the divorce of mind from body (which began as an opinion, not an observed fact), inevitably it will divorce us from the ecological web, making us intellectual antinatural orphans on a planet whose environmental riches are up for grabs.

Our actions, we hope, will have consequences that favor short-term exploitation, expediency, economic development, and "jobs"—the products of a "badly foreshortened" perspective, says Gore. Only an allopathic paradigm can so distort the truth of the situation by serving up the false dichotomy and torturous choice of jobs versus environment, people versus plants. It's a meretricious dialectic; we've been conned by the sophists who have locked up the true philosophers in a kind of paradigmatic Gulag.

The unexamined logic of alienated action seems consistent: If we are Western civilization, we seek unlimited riches from our material environment through continuous opportunistic development. And the inevitable though shocking consequence of our exploitative, soulless action is environmental collapse.

Environmental degradation is an epidemic of detachment, neglect, oblivion, inaction, dissimulation, distraction, and denial that has been intensifying for decades. It is a rapacious, shameless collusion of government, industry, and a disenfranchised citizenry. But we must admit we are willingly, if perversely, disenfranchised. There are no victims, no innocents; we are all culpable—presidents, prime ministers, politicians, CEOs chemists, farmers, individual consumers, *each of us*. Why did we sell the franchise rights on our democratic power? Victimization is an allopathic position, but not a category of real existence.

The allopathic paradigm would persuade us that our immune system is *invaded* by killer microbes and our political system *commandeered* by corporate interests, but this is wrong; we must own our passivity. We have all supported the environmental rip-off, explicitly or tacitly, with intention or unconsciously. We all make our monthly payments to the paradigm account. We are all on the hook, responsible; we all hold the buck. We are responsible for the environmental crisis because we construe environment as *separate* from our human self, as *out there*, as trees, plants, animals, birds, insects, the air, water, soil, clouds, mountains, the landscape.

At best, we are willing to acknowledge a relationship—and from this to develop a rationale for conserving, preserving, and protecting the environment as an asset—but not a fundamental coidentity as the world's mystical tradition has perennially suggested with revelatory pronouncements like *I am the world*. If each of us were to experience the world as *my body, my self, and I,* and know that this cognition is true, then we would have at once the necessary philosophical, paradigmatic rationale for a profound transfiguration of our environmental problems. We would have found our authentic position.

More than thirty years ago, Seyyed Hossein Nasr, an insightful Islamic scholar, interpreted the incipient global environmental crisis in its correct spiritual terms in his classic *Man and Nature.* The ecological crisis, Nasr wrote, is "only an externalization of an inner malaise and cannot be solved without a spiritual rebirth of Western man." In other words, just as humans are intrinsically connected ("wired") to the environment, so, in a negative mirror-image sense, our spiritual depredations are reflected in an environmental malaise.

As we see with AIDS survivors, what guarantees their remission is a total, unreserved self-transformation, a repositioning of their immunological environment through consciousness. So must it be with global ecology, a reorientation of our human participation in the planetary ecosystem, a remembering of our correct position. "It is still our hope that as the crisis created by man's forgetfulness of who he really is grows and that as the idols of his own making crumble one by one before his eyes," comments Nasr, "he will begin a true reform of himself which always means a spiritual rebirth and through his rebirth attain a new harmony with the world of nature around him."

To further this reborn harmony between humanity and nature, we need a deeper understanding of our multiple points of connection, of the ways in which our very organism embodies the activities of the outer environment.

References

Akasofu, Syun-Ichi, "The Dynamic Aurora," *Scientific American,* (May 1989).

—and Lanzerotti, Louis J., "The Earth's Magnetosphere," *Physics Today,* (December 1975).

Anderson, Craig A., "Temperature and Aggression: The Ubiquitous Effects of Heat on the Occurrence of Human Violence," *Psychological Bulletin,* Vol. 106, No. 1, (1989).

Archer, Victor E., "Geomagnetism, Cancer, Weather, and Cosmic Radiation," *Health Physics,* Vol. 34, (March 1978).

Arendt, Josephine, "The Pineal: A Gland that Measures Time?" *New Scientist*, (July 25, 1985).

Baker, Robin R., "A Sense of Magnetism," *New Scientist*, (September 18, 1980).

Barnston, A.G., "The Effect of Weather on Mood, Productivity, and Frequency of Emotional Crisis in a Temperate Continental Climate," *International Journal of Biometerology*, Vol. 32, No. 2, (1988).

Becker, Robert O., M.D., and Selden, Gary, *The Body Electric: Electromagnetism and the Foundation of Life*, William Morrow and Company, New York, 1985.

—*Cross Currents: The Perils of Electropollution, the Promise of Electromedicine*, Jeremy P. Tarcher, Inc., Los Angeles, 1990.

Bell, Iris R., M.D., *Clinical Ecology: A New Medical Approach to Environmental Illness*, Common Knowledge Press, Bolinas, 1982.

Best, Simon, "The Electropollution Effect," *Journal of Alternative and Complementary Medicine*, (May 1988).

—"What We Don't Know about Earth Radiation," *Journal of Alternative and Complementary Medicine*, (November 1988).

Bird, Christopher, "Dowsing and Geopathogenic Zones," *The American Dowser*, Vol. 27, No. 4, (Fall 1987).

—"Progress in Getting the Attention of the Medical Profession to Focus on the Study of Geopathogenic Zones and their Effect on Health," *The American Dowser*, Vol. 25, No. 4, (November 1985).

—*The Divining Hand—The Art of Searching for Water, Oil, Minerals, and Other Natural Resources or Anything Lost, Missing, or Badly Needed*, New Age Press, Black Mountain, 1979.

Blakeslee, Sandra, "Magnetic Crystals, Guides for Animals, Found in Humans," *The New York Times*, (May 12, 1992).

Brodeur, Paul, "Department of Amplification," *The New Yorker*, (November 19, 1990).

—"The Magnetic-Field Menace," *Macworld*, (July 1990).

—*Currents of Death: Power Lines, Computer Terminals, and the Attempt to Cover Up Their Threat to Your Health*, Simon and Schuster, New York, (1989).

Brodsky, Caroll M., "Multiple Chemical Sensitivities and Other 'Environmental Illness': A Psychiatrist's View," in *Occupational Medicine: Workers with Multiple Chemical Sensitivities, State of the Art Reviews,* Cullen, Mark, R., M.D., Editor, Vol. 2, No. 4, October-December 1987, Hanley and Belfus, Philadelphia.

Coates, Andrew, and Smith, Mark, "The Earth's Magnetic Field Yields Its Secrets," *New Scientist,* (December 12, 1985).

Coghill, Roger, *Electropollution: How to Protect Yourself Against It,* Thorsons Publishing Group, Wellingborough, 1990.

Cohen, David, "Magnetic Fields of the Human Body," *Physics Today,* (August 1975).

Cone, James E., M.D., and Hodgson, Michael J., M.D., "Occupational Medicine: Problem Buildings: Building-Associated Illness and the Sick Building Syndrome," *State of the Art Reviews,* Vol. 4, No. 4, October-December 1989, Hanley and Belfus, Philadelphia.

—and Harrison, Robert, and Reiter, Randy, "Patients with Multiple Chemical Sensitivities: Clinical Diagnostic Subsets Among an Occupational Health Clinic Population," in *Occupational Medicine: Workers with Multiple Chemical Sensitivities, State of the Art Reviews,* Cullen, Mark, R., M.D., editor, Vol. 2, No. 4, October-December 1987, Hanley and Belfus, Philadelphia.

Conoley, Gillian, "Living May be Hazardous to Your Health," *American Way,* (February 1980).

Cowley, Geoffrey, "An Electromagnetic Storm," *Time,* (July 10, 1989).

Cullen, Mark R., "Multiple Chemical Sensitivities: Summary and Directions for Future Investigators," in *Occupational Medicine: Workers with Multiple Chemical Sensitivities, State of the Art Reviews,* Cullen, Mark, R., M.D., editor, Vol. 2, No. 4, October-December 1987, Hanley and Belfus, Philadelphia.

—"The Worker with Multiple Chemical Sensitivities: An Overview," in *Occupational Medicine: Workers with Multiple Chemical Sensitivities, State of the Art Reviews,* Cullen, Mark, R., M.D., editor, Vol. 2, No. 4, October-December 1987, Hanley and Belfus, Philadelphia.

Czichos-Aust, Carolyn, "Dowsing, Part 1," *Environ,* No. 7, (1988).

Davidoff, Linda Lee, "Multiple Chemical Sensitivities (MCS)," *The Amicus Journal,* (Winter 1989).

Davis, Albert Ray, *Magnetism and Its Effects on the Living System,* Exposition Press, Smithtown, 1974.

DeMeo, James, Ph.D., "Response to Martin Gardner's Attack on Reich and Orgone Research in the Skeptical Inquirer," *Pulse of the Planet,* Vol.1, No. 1, (Spring 1989).

Dienstfrey, Harris, "Electromagnetic Man: An Interview with Caleb Gattegno on the Meridians and Acupuncture," *The Journal of Traditional Acupuncture,* Vol. X, No. 1, (Winter 1988-89).

Dubrov, Aleksandr Petrovich, *The Geomagnetic Field and Life,* Plenum Press, New York, 1978.

Endrös, Robert, and Lotz, Professor Karl-Ernst, "Unexplained Serious Car Accidents Involving Head-on Collisions and their Explanation by Geophysical and Biophysical Disturbances," *The American Dowser,* Vol. 26, No. 2, (May 1986).

Erlewine, Michael, "Dialogue: Michel Gauquelin, Michael Erlewine," *Astro-Talk, Bulletin for the Matrix User Group,* Vol. 6, No. 1, (January 1989).

Evans, John, *Mind, Body, and Electromagnetism,* Element Books, Shaftesbury, 1986.

Fox, Barry, "Electronic Smog Fouls the Ether," *New Scientist,* (April 7, 1988).

Galland, Leo, "Biochemical Abnormalities in Patients with Multiple Chemical Sensitivities," in *Occupational Medicine: Workers with Multiple Chemical Sensitivities, State of the Art Reviews,* Cullen, Mark, R., M.D., editor, Vol. 2, No. 4, October-December 1987, Hanley and Belfus, Philadelphia.

Games Ken, "The Earth's Magnetism—in Bricks," *New Scientist,* (June 11, 1981).

Gauquelin, Michel, *Cosmic Influences on Human Behavior,* Aurora Press, Santa Fe, 1985.

—*How Cosmic and Atmospheric Energies Influence Your Health,* Aurora Press, New York, 1984.

—*The Cosmic Clocks: From Astrology to a Modern Science,* Paladin/Granada, St. Albans, 1973.

Gilben, Susan, "TV Towers Breed Hot Spots," *Science Digest,* (November 1984).

Giovanelli, Ronald G., *Secrets of the Sun*, Cambridge University Press, Cambridge, 1984.

Gleick, James, *Chaos—Making a New Science*, Viking, New York, 1987.

Graves, Tom, *Needles of Stone Revisited*, Gothic Image Publications, Glastonbury, 1986.

Gribbin, John, "Geomagnetism and Climate," *New Scientist*, (February 5, 1981).

—"Magnetic Pointers to Stormy Weather," *New Scientist*, (December 25, 1986).

Hopwood, Anthony, "Dowsing, Ley Lines and the Electromagnetic Link," *New Scientist*, (December 20/27, 1979).

Joneja, Janice Vickerstaff, Ph.D., and Bielory, Leonard, M.D., *Understanding Allergy Sensitivity and Immunity: A Comprehensive Guide*, Rutgers University Press, Brunswick, 1990.

Kalkstein, Laurence S., and Davis, Robert E., "Weather and Human Mortality: An Evaluation of Demographic and Iterregional Responses in the United States," *Annals of the Association of American Geographers*, Vol. 79, No. 1, (1989).

Kissir, Susan, "Environmental Illness: When Everything Around You Makes You Sick," *Bestways*, (April 1990).

Kopp, J.A., "Healthier Living by Elimination of Soil Influences Detrimental to Health," *Effects of Harmful Radiations and Noxious Rays*, American Society of Dowsers, Danville, 1974.

Kopp, J.A., "The Present Status of Scientific Research on Soil Radiation," *Effects of Harmful Radiations and Noxious Rays*, American Society of Dowsers, Danville, 1974.

Kripke, Daniel F., "Photoperiodic Mechanisms for Depression and Its Treatment," *Biological Psychiatry 1981: Proceedings of the IIIrd World Congress of Biological Psychiatry*, edited by C. Perry, G. Struwe, and B. Jansson, Elsevier-North Holland Biomedical Press, New York, 1981.

Landscheidt, Theodor, *Sun-Earth-Man—A Mesh of Cosmic Oscillations*, Urania Trust, London, 1988.

Lanzerotti, Louis J., and Krimigis, Stamatios M., "Comparative Magnetospheres," *Physics Today*, (November 1985).

Laseter, John L., DeLeon, Ildefonso R., Rea, William J., and Butler, Joel R., "Chlorinated Hydrocarbon Pesticides in Environmentally Sensitive Patients," *Clinical Ecology*, Vol. II, No. 1, (Fall 1983).

Levin, Alan S., and Byers, Vera S., "Environmental Illness: A Disorer of Immune Regulation," in *Occupational Medicine: Workers with Multiple Chemical Sensitivities, State of the Art Reviews*, Cullen, Mark, R., M.D., editor, Vol. 2, No. 4, October-December 1987, Hanley and Belfus, Philadelphia.

Leviton, Richard, "Can The Earth's Stress Spots Make You Sick?" *East West*, (June 1989).

—"Current Affairs," *East West*, (May 1990).

—"How the Weather Affects Your Health," *East West*, (September 1989).

—"Environmental Illness—A Special Report," *Yoga Journal*, (November/December 1990).

Lewy, Alfred J., Kern, H.A., Rosenthal, N.E., and Wehr, T.A., "Bright Artificial Light Treatment of a Manic-Depressive Patient with a Seasonal Mood Cycle," *American Journal of Psychiatry*, Vol. 11, (November 1982).

Lonegren, Sig, *Spiritual Dowsing*, Gothic Image Publications, Glastonbury, 1986.

Loudon, Andrew, "A Gland for All Seasons," *New Scientist*, (July 25, 1985).

Maciocha, Edward, "Baubiologie, Germany's Surprising Natural-Home Movement," *East West*, (March 1987).

Maret, G., and Dransfeld, K., "Biomolecules and Polymers in High Steady Magnetic Fields," in *Strong and Ultrastrong Magnetic Fields and Their Applications*, F. Herbach, editor, Springer-Verlag, Berlin, 1985.

McAuliffe, Kathleen, "The Mind Fields," *OMNI*, (February 1985).

McLellan, Robert K., "Biological Interventions in the Treatment of Patients with Multiple Chemical Sensitivities," in *Occupational Medicine: Workers with Multiple Chemical Sensitivities, State of the Art Reviews*, Cullen, Mark, R., M.D., editor, Vol. 2, No. 4, October-December 1987, Hanley and Belfus, Philadelphia.

Merz, Blanche, *Points of Cosmic Energy*, C.W. Daniel Company, Saffron Walden, 1988.

Mooser, Stephen B., "The Epidemiology of Multiple Chemical Sensitivities (MCS)," in *Occupational Medicine: Workers with Multiple Chemical Sensitivities, State of the Art Reviews*, Cullen, Mark, R., M.D., editor, Vol. 2, No. 4, October-December 1987, Hanley and Belfus, Philadelphia.

Nasr, Seyyed Hossein, *Man and Nature—The Spiritual Crisis in Modern Man*, Unwin Paperbacks, London, (1968), 1990.

Nauss, D.W., "An Emptied Environment: Allergies Isolate Sufferers," *Dallas Times Herald*, (October 3, 1982).

Nero, Anthony V., Jr., "Controlling Indoor Air Pollution," *Scientific American*, Vol. 258, No. 5, (May 1988).

Noland, David, "Power Play," *Discover*, (December 1989).

Pan, Yaqin, Johnson, Alfred R., and Rea, William J., "Alipathic Hydrocarbon Solvents in Chemically Sensitive Patients," *Clinical Ecology*, Vol. V, No. 3, (1987).

Payne, Buryl, "The Global Meditation Project: Experimental Investigation of Human Effects on Sunspot Number and Geomagnetic Activity," *Interim Report*, Academy of Peace Research, Plymouth, November 1985.

—"The Power of Thought to Influence the Sun," *The Journal of Borderland Research*, (May-June 1989).

Pohl, Gustav Freiherr von, *Earth Currents—Causative Factor of Cancer and Other Diseases*, Frech-Verlag/GmbH and Co., Stuttgart, 1983.

Poore, Patricia, "Clinical Ecology: Medicine for the Chemical Sensitive?" *Garbage*, (April 1990).

Randolph, Theron G., M.D., and Moss, Ralph W, Ph.D., *An Alternative Approach to Allergies: The New Field of Clinical Ecology Unravels the Environmental Causes of Mental and Physical Ills*, Revised Edition, Perennial Library, Harper and Row, New York, 1989.

Rea, William J., M.D., "Chemical Hypersensitivity and the Allergic Response," *Ear, Nose, and Throat Journal*, Vol. 67, No. 1, (January 1988).

—and Mithcell, Monte J., B.A., "Chemical Sensitivity and the Environment," *Immunology and Allergy Practice*, (September/October 1982).

—and Johnson, Alfred R., D.O., "20th Century Illness," *Total Health*, (December 1986).

Richards, Bill, "New Study Strengthens Suspected Links Between Electromagnetism and Cancer," *The Wall Street Journal*, (July 16, 1987).

Rogers, Sherry A., M.D., *The E.I. Syndrome: An Rx for Environmental Illness*, Prestige Publishing, Syracuse, 1986.

—*Tired or Toxic: A Blueprint for Health*, Prestige Publishing, Syracuse, 1990

Ryan, Matthew, "Interview with James DeMeo, Ph.D.," *Wildfire*, Vol. 4, No. 2, (Jan/March 1989).

Schove, D.J., "Sunspot Cycles," *The Encyclopedia of Atmospheric Sciences and Astrogeology*, R.W. Fairbridge, editor, Dowden, Hutchinson and Ross, Stroudsburg, 1967.

Schoonmaker, David, "Are You Home Sick?" *Mother Earth News*, (March/April 1989).

Scott-Morley, Anthony, "Geopathic Stress: The Reason Why Therapies Fail?" *Journal of Alternative and Complementary Medicine*, (May 1985).

Siscoe, George L., "Solar-Terrestrial Influences on Weather and Climate," *Sunspot Cycles*, D. Justin Schove, editor, Benchmark Papers in Geology: 68, Hutchinson Ross Publishing Co., Stroudsburg, 1983.

Slesin, Louis, "People Are Antennas, Too: The Biology of the Electromagnetic Spectrum," *Whole Earth Review*, (Spring 1986).

Smith, Helen Mathews, "Ultimate Allergy to the 20th Century," *MD*, (July 1983).

Stovall, Trina, "Victims of the 20th Century," *Dallas Morning News*, Scene Magazine, (November 30, 1980).

Sutton, Christine, "A Magnetic Window Into Bodily Functions," *New Scientist*, (September 11, 1986).

—"A Magnetic Window into Bodily Functions," *New Scientist*, (September 11, 1986).

Terr, Abba I., "'Multiple Chemical Sensitivities': Immunologic Critique of Clinical Ecology Theories and Practice," in *Occupational Medicine: Workers with Multiple Chemical Sensitivities, State of the Art Reviews*, Cullen, Mark, R., M.D., editor, Vol. 2, No. 4, October-December 1987, Hanley and Belfus, Philadelphia.

Whybrow, Peter, M.D., and Bahr, Robert, *The Hibernation Response,* William Morrow and Company, New York, 1988.

Williamson, Tom, "A Sense of Direction for Dowsers?" *New Scientist,* (March 19, 1987).

—"Dowsing Achieves New Credence," *New Scientist,* (February 8, 1979).

Wisniewski, Zbigniew, "The Negative Influence of Water Veins, Part 1," *JBR,* (November-December 1987).

Wooster, Sarah M., "Geopathogenic Stress and Cancer," *Townsend Letter for Doctors,* (November 1988).

—"More New Concepts in Earth Mysteries, Earth Energies and Geomagnetism," *GN, Geocosmic News,* The National Council for Geocosmic Research Newsletter, Vol. 13, No.1, Fall 1988.

Ziehe, Helmut, "Interview in Acres U.S.A., Helmut Ziehe and Baubiologie," *The IBE Info-Sheets,* No. 3, (January 1989).

Chapter 4

The Holographic Human: Probable Locations of the Body

A Matrix of Connection for Complex Energy Systems

As humans, we are constantly engaged in reciprocal interaction with our environment, enmeshed in a perpetual energy exchange. Environmental energies of the Earth, atmosphere, and technology surround and permeate us every day. But now we need to deepen our inquiry to ask: how is the human organism connected to this web of environmental energies?

What is it about the human, in terms of anatomy, physiology, constitution, and consciousness, that makes this continual interaction possible, that provides the interface between the two poles of environment? In this chapter we explore an instructively new view of the human in terms of the holograph as an organizing principle and metaphor to help account for this interface.

The idea behind the holograph is that information about a large system is stored in equal and complete measure throughout that system; accurate information about the health and integrity of a human individuality is distributed, for example, in the eyes, the palms, ears, and feet. If you know the language, you can read out reams of information about the whole person from these miniaturized holographic systems within various body parts, regions, or systems.

Various empiric disciplines such as palmistry, reflexology, iridology, and acupuncture each document (and provide techniques for accessing) detailed holographic maps of the human as contained within apparent sections or parts of the whole body. A complete acupuncture system of meridians and treatment nodes has been described for the ears, the palms, and the solar plexus. From this perspective, the human body is a terrain of equivalent holographic maps, each offering a window into the human individuality.

But what about the larger system in this holographic topography? If we're dealing with a miniaturized acupuncture terrain in the feet, palms, ear, or solar plexus, any of these are subsets of the whole body acupuncture system—but of what larger system is this a holographic miniaturization? Acupuncture theory tells us that the human energy anatomy comprises "stems and branches" into the electromagnetic field of the earth and the solar system.

Here's where the holographic human stands revealed as a matrix of connection for complex planetary and extraterrestrial energy systems, as one holograph within an interdependent series of ever larger holographs. Hence the qualification in our chapter title on the apparent location of the human body. If the human totality represents the holographic presence (and distillation) of planetary and solar energies, we must say of the human body before us—mine, yours, our associates—that it is only *probably* located in this visible, tangible space. Other locations, according to the holographic metaphor, include the planetary environment, solar system, and cosmos.

Personality and Biography Written in a Palm Print

One evening, I sat in the offices of Ghanshyam Singh Birlaji, founder and director of the National Research Institute for Self-Understanding in Montreal. Birlaji—a slender, affable, passionately articulate man—holds an honorary Ph.D. in Jyotish from the All India Society of Occult Science in Delhi. For the last four decades, he has been studying the natal charts and palm prints of Western clients as a basis for life counseling.

Palmistry—the interpretive analysis of palm prints called *Samudrik Shastra*, "the science of human morphology," or chiromancy in the West—as the interpretation of the signs and lineaments of the body, particularly the palms, is one of Birlaji's specialties. In India, commercial astrologers must possess a university degree in *Jyotish*, usually an eight-year study program of the mathematical and astronomical principles and spiritual implications of the celestial bodies.

Palmistry in the West, is usually the target of pejorative dismissals by scientists. However, palm prints and horoscope in the hands of a competent reader like Birlaji can generate powerful information. I had never been to a palmist before and I knew nothing about the subject.

Ink prints of my palms lay on his desk. Birlaji held my palms like small blackboards on which he was inscribing squiggles and crescents with his pen as he made his remarks. This intricate network of lines across your palms represents a personalized signature engraved on your hand tissues by your nervous system. Palmistry in its purest form is "a set of investigative principles meant to reveal a human's own nature in his continual search for himself," said Birlaji. There is a consistent correlation between the way a person thinks and acts and palmar morphology, which makes palmistry potentially "a very useful tool to help a person understand herself better and to learn to rechannel his efforts." The implication here is that the palms are a map of a person's spiritual geography.

Most Westerners never suspect that palmistry can have such penetrative depth and interpretive finesse, that it can sketch a morphological gestalt from an unfamiliar client simply from deciphering flexion creases. "For each of these lines and mounts, we can compute fifty technical observations," Birlaji said. The palm, according to *Samudrik Shastra*, is a multilayered, intricately textured map of multiple factors, all converging into lines and mounts and offering descriptive, even predictive and therapeutic, applications.

The palm is a hologram, and as a holographic tool, palmistry is not unique. At least eighteen different holographic "body maps" or "somatic topologies" have been described. In each topology, complete information about the mind-body system is holographically encoded, in miniature, at one body locale, such as the eye, foot, hand, stomach, or ear. Could the concept of the holographic body, which is essentially a new mind-body paradigm in the West, have a tremendous positive effect on the future of Western medicine and noninvasive therapies or is it an interesting but ultimately unproductive mental exercise?

The Holographic Paradigm: Distributing Information

The holographic paradigm today enjoys increasing popularity and application as a versatile interpretive metaphor. It's become a highly serviceable way of conceptually framing a multidimensionally complex reality. It was originally founded on a technical development in optics. Back in 1947, Dennis Gabor discovered the mathematical principles for a new science of holography, a breakthrough that won him the 1971 Nobel Prize in physics, but it wasn't until the 1950s that laser optics would demonstrate the remarkable features of the hologram.

The hologram is a three dimensional photograph made with a laser. A wave field of light scattered by an object—an apple, for instance—is recorded on a glass plate as an interference pattern of intersecting waves. The plate, or hologram, is comprised of intersecting wave patterns much like ripples in a pond, except that they strike one, initially, as meaningless swirls and contours. According to the formulations of a nineteenth-century French scientist, Jean B. J. Fourier, wave forms could be converted into recognizable images—and the reverse, akin to how a TV converts electromagnetic frequencies into moving images—through a series of equations now known as "Fourier transforms" and understood by nonscientists as a language of wave forms.

Knowledge of Fourier transforms enabled Gabor to code images of objects into apparently blurred interference patterns—the hologram, which is basically a wave storage pattern. The virtual image (technically, an astral apparition) of the original apple is regenerated as a projection when either coherent light (laser) or ordinary light (in more recent developments) is focused on the holographic film. The sequence, then, is object to wave storage pattern (hologram) to virtual image reconstruction, in *reciprocal*, reversible relationship from wave pattern storage to object imaging and back again.

The hologram has several key features that make it immediately useful and penetrative as an extended metaphor, if not model, of reality. First, holograms have an enormous capacity for information storage in a minute space; something like ten billion bits of information are encoded in contiguous contour lines in one cubic centimeter of film. By the mathematics of Fourier transforms, the holographic interference pattern stores detailed information about the location and shape of the apple. "It is nature's way of storing information," noted Itzhak Bentov, the iconoclastic, independent scientist in his book *Stalking the Wild Pendulum.* "This kind of storage device is the most compact known in nature."

Second, the information is distributed throughout the system, such that if a hologram plate is shattered, a single fragment will reconstitute the original image in its entirety with only minor loss of depth-of-field and resolution. The same principle underlies the genetic code carried in our chromosomes, explains Bentov. "Each cell in our bodies carries all the information required to make an additional copy of our bodies." Third, by changing the angle at which the laser or ordinary light strikes the hologram, multiple images can be layered (or laminated) on the same surface, creating interpenetrating or overlapping visual and informational realities. In this manner, a prodigious amount of information can be encoded and stored in a comparatively minuscule surface area.

This is almost unavoidably necessary, because according to mathematician John von Neumann, in an average human lifetime the brain stores 2.8×10^{20} bits of information. As a technology, the hologram excels at encoding and decoding wave pattern frequencies—in multiplicity, if necessary—and acts like a lens to translate the frequency blur into coherent images. Again, it's the Fourier transforms that convert meaningless contour lines and irregular ripples into comprehensible information or images—in other words, they broker informational coherency.

Back in 1950, neurophysiologist Karl Lashley documented the remarkable degree to which intelligence in the brain is holographically stored, even when more than 90% of the brain is removed. Lashley was experimenting with rats, trying to find where in the rodent brain the memory function was located. First he taught the rats how to run a maze; then he systematically extracted portions of their cerebral tissue until only 10% remained. Lashley was astonished to note that the rats ran the maze as effectively with 10% of their brain as with 100%. The results convinced him that every individual cell of the cortex must store information of the whole brain while simultaneously performing its specific neural task.

The holographic paradigm was born when the neurophysiological research of Dr. Karl Pribram of Stanford and the theoretical physics of Dr. David Bohm of London's Birkbeck College were creatively fused in the mid-1970s. The theories of Pribram about brain function and of Bohm about the holographic universe were radical, very much against the grain of conventional scientific and physical models. Amply armed with clinical data, Pribram's always been one to shake the foundations of scientific thought in his field—"the Magellan of the brain," he was once called, "close at hand, if not a primary incendiary, at nearly all the major upheavals of prevailing thought about how the brain works," wrote Marilyn Ferguson in *Brain/Mind Bulletin* in 1977.

In 1966, Pribram sensed the emerging holographic technology and its implicit theory might prove metaphorically useful in explaining brain function. In 1971 he elaborated this "neural holographic process" in his landmark *Languages of the Brain*. The brain operates as a lens, Pribram proposed, performing Fourier transforms on the frequency data it receives from the outside world and converting it into meaningful images about the world. The frequency domain looks like a contour map gone wild. This is the chaotic blur of wave interference patterns that the brain then decodes according to an innate perceptual mathematics into useful information about the environment.

Another name for this frequency blur is the enfolded implicate order, says physicist David Bohm. Bohm rejected the randomness of the prevailing model of quantum mechanics and proposed instead a holographic universe, which he called the implicate order of "undivided wholeness," the primordial, primogenitive frequency domain that enfolds everything: time, space, past, present, future, all the opposites in creation. "In terms of the implicate order one may say that everything is enfolded into everything."

In the enfolded hologram of the universe, each part contains information about the "whole object," but not according to a point-to-point correspondence of object and recorded image, says Bohm. "That is to say, the form and structure of the entire object may be said to be *enfolded* within each region of the photographic record."

Our apparent world, said Bohm, is a holographic reconstitution—an unfolded, explicate order—of this antecedent, inclusive frequency realm. In the explicate order, "things are *unfolded* in the sense that each thing lies only in its own particular region of space (and time) and outside the regions belonging to other things." The dynamic relations between implicate/enfolded and explicate/unfolded Bohm called the "holomovement."

Bohm's new model of "holonomy" suggests a new, unsettling model of the electron, for example; it may not be a small discrete particle existing at a quantifiable space-time coordinate. "What is essential to this new model is that the electron is instead to be understood through a total set of enfolded ensembles, which are generally not localized in space. At any given moment, one of these may be unfolded and therefore localized, but in the next moment, this one enfolds to be replaced by the one that follows." Matter, in other words, and our "notion of continuity of existence," may keep jumping back and forth—holomoving—between an unexpressed, immaterial implicate state and an expressed, material, explicate state.

Now Pribram postulated that the brain stores and retrieves information, or memory, holographically, and not locally as most neuroscientists contend, and that it reconstructs images of the outside world through mathematical calculations performed in an intersynaptic frequency domain. "The essence of the holographic concept," Pribram wrote in *Languages of the Brain,* "is that images are reconstructed when representations in the form of distributed information systems are appropriately engaged. Holography in this frame of reference is conceived as an instantaneous analogue cross-correlation performed by matched filters. Many hitherto paradoxical findings regarding brain function in perception become understandable when the holographic analogy is taken seriously."

But by 1988, in an interview with *East West,* Pribram noted that it's no longer analogical but descriptive. It's a model of how the brain really works. Information, or memory, is distributed throughout the brain in patterns of nerve impulses that crisscross the cortex, says Pribram. The brain itself is a hologram. "It is thus the fact that the holographic domain is reciprocally related to the image/object domain that implies that mental operations (such as mathematics) reflect the basic order of the universe."

This basic order Bohm also calls the "implicate holographic." Pribram calls his latest perceptual model "quantum neurodynamics." At the neuroanatomical level, the holographic domain exists in the synaptic space between nerve dendrons. This dense and intricate feltwork of intersecting wavefronts and dendritic nerve endings Pribram calls the "holoscape." It's a kind of mathematically digitized spread function, a "processing domain" in which sense is made of holographically encoded information derived from the world, a little tendril of the implicate, enfolded order unfolding into the physical neuroanatomy of the human brain.

"Once you're in this frequency domain, all the facts of communication fit, but they don't make sense in the space-time domain. In the absence of space-time coordinates, the usual causality upon which most scientific explanation depends, must also be suspended." Instead, we must call on complementarities, synchronicities, and dualities as explanatory principles, adds Pribram.

Maybe the World Is a Splendidly Detailed Illusion

The theories of Pribram and Bohm have generated great interest in the application of holographic concepts to our understanding of consciousness and the universe. In a curious cycling of facts and theories, Gabor's technological breakthrough produced a potent metaphor that may be a relatively correct description of reality; yet another example of how technology unconsciously mirrors ontology, awaiting our conscious articulation of the connection.

Maybe the cosmos is a hologram, Bohm suggests; maybe what we take to be natural, automatic perception of a physical world is nothing more than the results of some neurological Fourier calculations in the brain, suggests Pribram.

Maybe reality is a "splendidly detailed illusion," the classic Hindu *maya*, suggests Michael Talbot in his synthesis of the paradigm, *The Holographic Universe*; maybe the world out there, our environment, is "a vast resonating symphony of wave forms, a 'frequency domain' that was transformed into the world as we know it only *after* it entered our senses." Or as Dr. John Battista, psychiatrist at the University of California at Davis, puts it: "Thus a new holographic model is being developed which emphasizes the interdependent, parallel, and simultaneous processing of events."

The implications of holographic modeling for humanistic psychologies, for example, is extensive and exciting. "Every aspect of the universe seems to be part of some larger, whole, grander being, and more comprehensive system," notes psychologist Ken Dychtwald. "Each particular aspect has the ability to be intimately knowledgeable about every other particular aspect within the master hologram."

In the holographic universe—or brain, or *body,* as we shall see—instantaneous cross-correlation and access is the hallmark. The holographic paradigm may vindicate many traditional, interpretive holisms—the butts of innumerable materialist sarcasms, such as palmistry, iridology, reflexology, and acupuncture, whose claims about an energetically interdependent mind-body system have never dovetailed comfortably—or rationally, mainstream scientists would like us to believe—with conventional Western medical and physical models.

But as Pribram remarks: "In the holographic domain, each organism represents in some manner the universe, and each portion of the universe represents in some manner the organisms within it."

So could it be that in each of these disciplines we may encounter a holographic microsystem, a body map, that encodes a full dossier of mind-body information?

The Mind at the End of the Palm

Palmistry, or chiromancy, has roots in the ancient Vedas of India from at least 4,500 years ago. It's an aspect of the astrologically coordinated science called *Hast Jyotish* ("that which radiates light"), says Ghanshyam Birlaji. "The hand is the most detailed, reliable, and accessible area of the human body for morphological analysis," he says. The multiple palmar features are a "throbbing" dermatological template for "the trend of thought, the impulses, the interplay of the five elements, and the changing sky of consciousness."

The science of *Samudrik Shastra* outlines a complete geography of the hand. In fact, palmistry is only an aspect of *Samudrik Shastra,* which correlates human shape, size, constitutional type, and body parts with psychological characteristics such as temperament, personality traits, and interests. Its conceptual system is vast and, for the West, controversial, because it correlates consciousness and energy patterns with physical morphology. That's challenging enough to our materialist beliefs, which do not allow such plasticity of matter and shaping by consciousness. But *Samudrik Shastra* takes its analysis yet further into the subtle realms by linking consciousness and palmar morphology with mental patterning, the unconscious, karma, astrology, and reincarnation, whose complex metaphysical drama is played out on the hands.

Let's consider the palmar terrain and its meaning. Our passive or inactive hand (the one we don't write with) reveals inherited traits, unconscious habits, experiential memory, and the unresolved residues of karma, says Birlaji. It embodies the "threshold image with which the present life was ushered in and contains the blueprint of one's destiny created by our own free will." The active hand represents our current trends—a progress report on the work-in-progress—in refining or abusing the inheritance. The palmar surface is further partitioned into ten districts called "mounts," which correspond to the planets; the twelve phalanges of the four fingers represent the constellations of the zodiac; while the thumb embodies the dynamic interplay of will, reason, and love.

The chiromantic interpretation encompasses a multidimensional spectrum of possible influences, from the past and present, all operative in an individual's life. These converging influences, in the philosophical vocabulary of India's ancient science, Ayurveda, include the three worlds (physical, astral, causal), the three primary energies (*sattvic,* uplifting; *rajasic,* activating; *tamasic,* enslaving), and the five elements (earth, air, fire, water, ether). "The rate of vibration, the depth of evolution, the height of one's highest generated consciousness are all visible in the hands," asserts Birlaji. "I see a completely different distinction of hands with a swami who has meditated for thirty years and a drug addict just released from the hospital."

What is particularly intriguing is that to an extent the palmar lines on both hands can change as we adjust our living, thinking, and feeling patterns—as the "trend of mental thought" changes, says Birlaji. Grooves may run deeper or smoother, broken lines may be mended, interference knots may dissolve. Both hands will give us irrefutable feedback on how we're conducting our life: The active hand will register changes in three to seven months while the inactive hand will adjust its interference wave pattern morphology in one to three years. More frequent fluctuations in mental attitude are registered by tiny horizontal lines in the "mental" district phalanges of the active hand.

According to palmistry, such interactive palmar imprinting is possible by virtue of the primacy of the mind, or consciousness, over matter, the body. *Samudrik Shastra* contends that it's the mental gestalt, our disposition in consciousness, that designs the palmar template in the first place—matter follows mind; the body takes its cues from consciousness.

"Thought energy constantly has a concrete effect on matter," explains Birlaji. "The hand analyst can decipher both the thought patterns and major karmic effects from the encoded somatic markers by reading the cellular structure and function as they manifest on a larger scale in the tissues. The organic condition of one's physical body is intimately associated with one's thoughts. Through the palm markings, we can trace our way back to these actual thought patterns, both conscious and, more importantly, unconscious, that gave rise to these physical effects."

Thus the whole body can be read if you know the morphological grammar. The final emphasis, says Birlaji, is always practical: the *prevention* of predicted, potential problems through more informed choices of action and living. "In its purest form, this discipline is meant as a tool for self-inquiry, facilitating informed choices in the use of one's free will, so that problematic situations, habits, and attitudes can be corrected or prevented." Or as Michael Talbot judiciously comments: "The lines and whorls in our palms may contain more about our whole self than we realize."

Energy Meridians Flowing through the Hands

The palm is host to another body map, though one less esoteric and easier to validate because it's part of a therapeutic practice. In 1971, Korean physician Tae Woo Yoo announced he had discovered a complete, though miniaturized, fourteen-meridian mini-acupuncture system in the hands. He mapped out 345 treatment points, bilaterally, on the hands, calling his new system *Koryo Sooji Chim.* Yoo mapped out the meridians and treatment points on both hands, then overlaid this with a hand map of all internal organs, from tongue to large intestine. The result was a graphic portrayal of the entire human body, acupoint energy systems, and material internal organs, holographically miniaturized within the hands.

In Yoo's somatotypic model, the middle finger represents the body's central axis. Acupuncture's Conception Vessel meridian runs down the inside palmar surface (in the body it vertically traverses the front), while the Governing Vessel (which vertically traverses the back of the body) streams down the knuckly back side of the hand. The left little finger represents the left leg, the index and ring fingers are the arms, and the right little finger represents the right leg. In general, meridians located on the back of the hands (nonpalmar side) correspond to posterior body meridians, while palm-side meridians reflect anterior body meridians.

In terms of our emerging holographic model of the body, what we have in *Koryo Sooji Chim* is basically a twice-compressed and miniaturized energy topology of the human body. Acupuncture, with its energy lines and acupoints, represents the first scale of miniaturization of the body's essential physiological, organic systems into a distributed energy topology; hand acupuncture represents a holographic condensation of that whole-body topology into a part of the body, the hands. Remarkably, acupuncture treatment on the hands alone can access body energy systems as effectively as whole-body treatment, a clinical fact that further corroborates the validity of the holographic premise.

The Zones of the Sole: Reflexing the Body Map on the Feet

"What we see on the feet is a mirror image of the human being itself, body and soul. We can use the feet like a map," explains Franz Wagner, Ph.D., of the Institute for Integrative Bodywork in Austria, writing in *Reflex Zone Massage*.

Wagner is referring to reflexology, or zone foot therapy, which appears to be another holographic map of the entire body imprinted on the feet and hands; it was first developed by an American physician in the early twentieth century. Reflexology lends itself to a striking visualization: the two feet can be imaginatively superimposed over the body or the internal geography of the body can be seen as miniaturized within the confines of the feet. Either way, it's a hologram. And the concept is validated therapeutically because when the body zones of the feet and hands are correctly manipulated, actual proprioceptive sensations are registered in the appropriate organs or muscles in the body at large.

The practice of foot massage for well-being and relief of symptoms apparently has ancient roots in India, China, and Egypt. In 1580, two European physicians published information on zone therapy, or indirect treatment, but in our time it was an ear, nose, and throat specialist named William Fitzgerald, working at St. Francis Hospital in Hartford, Connecticut, who outlined the zone therapy model in 1913. Fitzgerald, drawing on clinical observations with remote healing, divided the body into ten longitudinal zones, running like grid lines from head to hands and head to feet. His zone diagram portrays the human torso as if it were run vertically through a bread slicer. A particular zone is an energy-influence area that includes everything in that body zone from skull to toenails.

"Everything that happens in a specific zone of the body affects and is influenced by the organs of the body within that zone," postulated Wagner. "Disturbances in the flow of energy through these zones can be treated by massaging the feet." The feet and hands both contain a composite two-dimensional body map in which the reflex zones are sited according to anatomical realities. The body's right half is reflected in the right foot, while paired organs, such as kidneys, lungs, and ovaries, are shared between the feet. In the reflexive geography of the foot, the head, sinuses, and neck are reflected in the toes; the intestines, coccyx, and bladder live in the heel; and the principal organs are found in between.

Since Fitzgerald's pioneering studies eighty years ago, other reflexologists have refined and popularized the system. Kirlian photography apparently has shown that the energy field around the feet is "diminished" when there is an imbalance in the body area corresponding to the reflex area, suggests Nicola Hall in *Reflexology: A Patient's Guide*. Reflexologists postulate that the sedimentation of calcium crystal deposits in foot reflex areas, which they often notice in their foot massages, are possibly correlated with nerve endings and may indicate energy blockages in the body. Each foot has an estimated 7,200 nerve endings (effectively one-tenth of the 72,000 *nadis,* or subtle nerve endings in the entire body, as postulated by Hindu Tantric physiology), which have extensive interconnections through the spinal cord and brain with all body areas.

Contemporary reflexologists don't know how their system works, but some practitioners speculate about a possible overlay between foot zone areas and the twenty-eight acupoints from six acupuncture meridians that are known to pass through the feet. For reflexology, though, "the entire foot corresponds to the body whereas these acupoints represent the beginning or end of whole body lines." So it's two different though equally valid body maps coexisting in the same body space, which, as we learned above, exemplifies a basic information storage principle of holography.

The Little Human in the Ear

"Of all the remote acupuncture sites used to alleviate chronic pain, one of the most controversial areas is the acupuncture microsystem located on the external ear," states psychobiologist Dr. Terry Oleson, assistant clinical professor in the Pain Management Clinic at UCLA's School of Medicine in Los Angeles. "Auricular acupuncture has proven effective for the treatment of chronic pain, narcotic withdrawal, smoking, weight control, and hearing loss."

Specific acupoints for the relief of medical disorders were recognized on the ear at least 4,000 years ago in the *Yellow Emperor's Classic of Internal Medicine,* a key early Chinese acupuncture text, but it wasn't until the late 1950s that the Chinese published a "somatoypic ear map," as Oleson calls it, that charted a complete system on the ear, which was not simply the end points of full-body meridians. The funny thing is, a Frenchman found the ear acupoints first.

That French physician, Paul Nogier, is credited in the West at least with the diagramming of a complete acupuncture microsystem on both ears, a discovery he announced in 1957 in his *Treatise of Auriculotherapy.* Nogier also made an anatomical map of a miniature human, the classic homunculus of alchemical repute, superimposed on the ear; he envisioned this homunculus as an inverted human fetus. The head faces downward toward the lower lobule, the feet are at the ear's upper rim, and the body is situated in between. The little human in the ear, says Oleson, is best viewed as a person standing on his head, arched backward, with his back to his internal organs.

The homunculus in the ear is more than a peculiar revival of a medieval prescientific concept and it's more than an intriguing metaphor, too. It's another way of stating that in the ear is another hologram of the whole body. Somatotypic maps of the body have also been demonstrated in the brain. "Neuroanatomists have known for some time that there is an orderly representation of localized areas of the body at specific areas of the brain," explains Oleson. "Of all these brain areas, the homuncular arrangement of evoked neural responses in the thalamus most corresponds to the inverted fetus pattern represented upon the ear."

Research conducted by Oleson and his associates, reported in

1980, reached this conclusion: "Enhanced tenderness and increased electrical conductivity at localized areas of the auricle exhibited highly significant correspondence to areas of the body where subjects reported pain or some pathology." In a double-blind study, physicians conducting auricular diagnosis showed a 75.2% accuracy rate and could even pinpoint in which side of the body the problem resided. "These findings thus support the clinically derived hypothesis that there is a somatotypic map arranged on the external ear."

Oleson sees the same inverted-fetus motif of the ear reiterated in the body holographs of brain, hand, and feet. "In the brain the somatotype or homunculus is organized with the head parts lower than the body parts. It's always inverted. My theory for how it works is that there are nerves that connect to the ear from specific parts of the brain, which is organized like a holograph.

The ear holograph is, logically, connected to the brain holograph, which itself is connected to the whole body. The way we use the ear to affect the rest of the body is by working through the brain holograph." And this speculative master brain holograph is still a subset of the holographic *process* of the brain as it interfaces with the frequency domain of the outside world, as described by Pribram.

The Geography of the Eye: Another Body Map in the Iris

Iridology, or iris diagnosis, which postulates a body map in the lines of the iris, has, like palmistry, a long if poorly chronicled and somewhat abused European history. Ophthalmo-Somatic Analysis, as iridology is called in Germany, where much of its current research is conducted, was recognized by various luminaries like Hippocrates; instructors at the Medical School of Salerno, Italy; Philostratus; and the German scientist Phillipus Meyens, who in 1670 presented a systematic correlation of iris and body regions in his *Chiromatica Medica*. But it wasn't until the Hungarian physician Ignatz von Peczely formulated the topology of the iris signs and their correlations with organic disease in 1881 that iridology found itself on a formal, scientific footing.

"The eyes represent the end-weaving result of our genetic background," says Dr. Bernard Jensen, author of *Science and Practice of*

Iridology and a foremost iridology proponent. "Whatever genetic pattern our eyes take, that's what we have for our whole life." Iris topography is an early-warning system more capable of reflecting lifetime strengths or weaknesses ("risks," in iridology's illness-preventive vocabulary), than indicating current conditions. The morphological terrain of the eye, Jensen says, is imprinted prenatally, much as the inactive hand in palmistry presumably registers inherited tendencies.

For example, a competent iridologist can fulfill the predictive role of the observant doctor in a case in which a cancer is in its earliest, formative stages. That's because, as Farida Sharan says, founder of the British School of Iridology, and author of the textbook, *Iridology*, the eye encodes medically valuable, somatotypically holographic information. Anatomists say there are over 28,000 nerve fibers in the iris; for iridologists, says Sharan, this anatomical fact proves that information collected from all regions of the body is transmitted to the iris.

"The iris is a perfect microcosmic screen displaying symbolically the microcosmic realities of constitutional inherited strengths, weaknesses, pathways to disease, toxic accumulations, inflammatory and exudative conditions, personality, the emotional life, as well as revealing data on body systems and organs and their interrelated function." In short, the iris tells us, if we know how to decode its language, what's happening everywhere and anywhere within the body as a kind of "ecological iridology," says Sharan. "Iridology transforms the way we feel about our bodies. Our eyes radiate what we are at every moment."

The iris, say the iridologists, is an assessment map that registers genetically transmitted dispositions for health or debility, so for one skilled in its grammar, the iris may reveal "inherent quotients of energy" assigned to the various organs and body systems. The iridologist studies iris tissue, color, shape, structural patterns, pigment, signs, and minute changes, noting the iris' lovely bioarchitecture of "streams, flowers, and jewels," explains William Caradonna, a registered pharmacist and formerly vice president of the National Iridology Research Association (NIRA) in Laguna Beach, California.

"Each gland and organ has its place in the iris," Caradonna explains. "It's a slow-moving picture, a genetic map and lifetime x-ray. We can predict where a person is headed, what the risks are.

Then what we do with our environment and health makes us either live out or avoid these risks. We can work out a plan for preventive medicine, be it through nutrition, relaxation, or bodywork."

Paul Steutzer of the University of Munich, writing about iris constitutions, iridology, and the detection of precancerous conditions, notes: "The iris displays characteristic changes which allow the study of constitutional patterns, biochemical changes, and developing patterns of pathology long before overt symptoms emerge." Steutzer said that naturopaths have described twenty-three different iris constitutions and that the iris map is a holographic effect. "Since the single cell, through its DNA code, reflects the entire organism, larger cell conglomerates such as the ear, foot, and eye, can reflect the entire individual body as a type of homunculus, or miniature representation of the body, on some smaller organ or area.

"The character of the iris is unique in that disturbances in the coherence of the magnetic field surrounding the organs of the body become reflected in the stromal fibers of the iris tissue and also in the deposition of specific pigments."

Micro-acupuncture Holograms in the Body

The reflexology systems of foot, hand, and ear, the subacupuncture systems of hand and ear, and the iris maps of the eye all point toward a holographic model of the human body. Important information is distributed in multiple locations, even in the same location in overlapping storage patterns. For each body map a school, a dogma, and a therapy has arisen to negotiate the holograms found in ear, hand, foot, and eye, yet within their own provinces these disciplines maintain what remain separate, uncommunicating topologies. Might there be a unifying principle, a holographic body modem in effect that patches these different body maps together into some unified holographic topology?

Dr. Ralph Dale, teacher, author, and director of the Acupuncture Education Center in North Miami Beach, Florida, believes he has found one, based on data he's collected for more than two decades. The body functions according to a plan of micro-acupuncture systems, says Dale. In a provocative series of monographs, Dale has documented eighteen different micro-acupuncture holograms in the human body. "It is not only the ear but many, and perhaps all, parts of the body manifest a micro-acupuncture system whose reflexes are holographic reiterations of the gross anatomy," says Dale.

He describes micro-acupuncture systems—he prefers the term "somatic holograms"—from Japanese, Chinese, and German research all over the body: ear, foot, hand, abdomen, back, arm, leg, neck, scalp, face, nose, iris, tongue, wrist, temporal-sphenoidal line (cranium), head gravity line (cranium), anatomy impression area (cranium), and two in the teeth and gums. "The overwhelming evidence presented of the reiteration of the anatomy of the body in topological dynamics of these micro-acupuncture systems is a revelation that brings us closer to a theory of micro-acupuncture."

Dale mapped out the organ, systems, and glandular correspondences for each micro-acupuncture locale in the form of a homunculus, following Nogier's example of the inverted fetus in the ear. What he got was a kind of unified energy field map or somatic hologram of the entire human distributed like freckles across the body surface. The superimposition of the holographic human with its meridians and points provokes a stereo, holistic perception by the viewer. "The microsystems look like surrealistic ideas that couldn't possibly be true and of course are."

Dale worked out ten principles that he believes underlie micro-acupuncture topologies. There is a system in every part of the body. Every system is a holographic replica of the human anatomy. Each microsystem is intimately connected to the macrosystem. All systems potentially can be used both diagnostically and therapeutically. All micropoints are bidirectional patterns with relatively low electrical impedance. "Holographic integrity not only defines the energetics of our bodies, but expresses the reality of our universe and of each and every one of its parts."

Even more daring, Dale speculates that this holographic physiology might be found on the cellular level; after all, DNA is a kind of master hologram for the entire human, capable of reproducing—cloning, actually—our individuality. "If this is so, we would able to manipulate a single cell and balance the body's energies. The next step I hypothesize—and this is consistent with David Bohm's theories—is you can break the microsystem down such that every finger will have a complete micro-acupuncture system, all the way down to the cellular level."

Stems and Branches into the Cosmos

Today the Western medical establishment is gradually, grudgingly, accepting acupuncture as a viable, if unorthodox, discipline. Many of its claims have been empirically and clinically validated and its postulated Qi flows have been electrically quantified by specially developed instrumentation. So if acupuncture helps to explain, by way of context, the various somatic holograms we've been considering, especially reflexology and iridology, then it could potentially validate them as well. But here a larger question looms before us. If Dale's eighteen micro-acupuncture holograms relate holographically to the whole body macro-acupuncture system, what does this relate to? What is this a hologram of?

The macro-acupuncture system might have deeper, older roots in an antecedent "biological information signal system" that predates the human nervous system organization, suggests Stephen Birch, research director at the New England School of Acupuncture in Watertown, Massachusetts, and co-author of several technical, original works on acupuncture. In his forthcoming work, *Chasing the Dragon's Tail,* co-authored with the late Dr. Yoshio Manaka—during his lifetime Manaka was one of Japan's leading acupuncture theorists and director of the Oriental Medical Research Center at Kitazato Research Institute in Tokyo—Birch explores this possibility.

"Manaka has realized from his practice and observation where only tiny amounts of stimulation produce profound effects that there must be a signal system operating," says Birch. Here's how Manaka puts it himself in a recently translated paper: "There is a primitive signal and information system in our body which has embryological roots, but this is masked by the more advanced and complex control systems. Thus the original system is hard to find. This primitive system is able to detect and discriminate internal and external changes and plays a role in regulating the body by transmitting this information. This system serves as the *modus operandi* of acupuncture." Manaka's signal system is an interconnected system forming a functional structure that integrates the entire body. "This integrative structure operates under the holographic model," he said, "which means that the entire structure is reflected in each and every part."

Manaka substantiated this secret signal system in part through showing its sensitivity to color. Yellow, for example, associated in acupuncture with the earth element, was applied experimentally to the earth acupoint on various meridians. Manaka noticed changes in pulse and muscle tension at pain-pressure locations. He then postulated that the earth acupoints on all major meridians (one earth point per meridian) were "isophasal" (in the same wave pattern) to one another; similarly the meridian points for the other four elements were also isophasal throughout the meridian system.

Manaka derived the isophasal concept from his studies in mathematical topology as part of his effort to conceptualize body geometry. Such color stimulation in minute amounts, he contended, is certainly beneath the perceptual threshold of the nervous system, which means some other sensing system registered its energetic presence and set in motion a reaction, in this case, isophasal stimulation of the earth acupoints.

The theory of Five Elements, basic to acupuncture modeling, is the doorway into transpersonal energetics and possibly to the master hologram. Each of the twelve major meridians has an acupoint for each of the five elements, and each is in isophasal relation across the system; this gives us sixty elemental acupoints in all. If we use an analogy from computers, the earth acupoints are patched by modem to one another and can thus instantaneously communicate and interact through this isophasal or modemic connection. What may connect this body system with something transpersonal, with energy systems of the cosmos, is accounted for in Chinese medicine's theory of stems and branches.

Chinese medicine maintains that there are ten celestial stems (correlated with the five element acupoints on each meridian, each with a yin or yang quality) and twelve celestial branches (correlated with the twelve meridians) and that the five elements are in a periodic relationship with energy rhythms outside the body, in the Earth and solar system. This is our somatic wiring to the cosmos. Hourly, daily, monthly, and yearly cycles are mapped out for the periodic energy fluctuations in these stems and branches.

To make this vividly clear, let's consider the *Tzu* branch and its correspondences: *Chao Yang*/gall bladder meridian, 10-12 p.m., the month of November, the Chinese zodiacal animal, Rat; or the *Ch'en* branch, corresponding to the *Yang Ming*/stomach meridian, Dragon, March, 6-8 a.m. Among the stems, let's consider *Chia*:

this corresponds to the wood element, yang energy, and Jupiter; the *Wu* stem corresponds to the earth element, yang energy, and Saturn.

"The points that come open over the course of a ten-day repeating cycle are specifically the Five Element acupoints," says Birch. "What's happening in the body seems to be coming from a source outside the body and is probably related to the Earth's geomagnetic field. Its changes are being conditioned, meanwhile, by changes in the larger environment. Stem and branch theory is a way of rationalizing how changes in the larger cosmic environment manifest changes at the energetic level of the body. The use of stems and branches is a kind of holographic paradigm because they refer to huge and tiny time scale changes. At the energetic level the boundary of the skin simply doesn't exist."

Palpating the Big Open Mind on the Stomach

In *Hara Diagnosis: Reflections on the Sea,* Birch and co-author Kiiko Matsumoto describe the Japanese system of hara acupuncture based on one of the seven hirata zones (one of eighteen microsystems described by Dale). The hara (also called *tanden* or *chi hai*), situated just below the navel, is a major energy center, the bodily place of "moving chi between the kidneys." In Japan when people say *hara go ookii*—"big hara"—they indicate somebody who has an open mind. When someone is flushed with anger, they say *hara ga tatsu,* meaning "the hara stands up." Culturally, the Japanese have always placed great emphasis on hara, the abdominal region around the umbilicus, as have the Chinese, for whom it is "lower *dantien.*"

Hara is pivotal in the classical acupuncture of both cultures because the abdomen contains a primary energy map for the entire body. It's as if the mind were etched in acupoints around the belly button. Traditionally Chinese and Japanese acupuncturists have used palpation of the hara for diagnosis and often treatment. They considered it a technique of at least comparable merit to the more familiar wrist pulse diagnosis. Hara palpation, contend Birch and Matsumoto, is among "the most subtle and powerful diagnostic approaches" available for assessing predisease tendencies in the body. "We've speculated it corresponds to the gravitational center of the body and therefore to the total electric and magnetic field."

Classical acupuncture thinking says that the energies of Heaven, Man, and Earth interact to form the True Chi, one of whose main aspects is Source Chi, explains Birch. "It is in the Hara, the area of 'the Moving Chi between the Kidneys,' that all energies interact to create the basic or Source Chi of the body." According to the classic *Ling Shu* acupuncture text: "True Chi is the prenatal Chi from the parents, Chi of the breathing from Heaven and Chi of food and water from Earth, mixing together." The Hara was seen as the merging point of the various energies and the source of the True Chi, says Birch.

Birch further speculates that certain micro-acupuncture regions of the body, especially the abdomen, might be related to the chakras (literally, "spinning wheels"), or subtle energy/consciousness centers described by Indian Tantric physiology as situated alongside the spinal column. "Hara also has close proximity to the third chakra, the Manipura or solar plexus center, which we call lower *tan tien*. It acts as a very strong and specific organizing principle. Any change in the body field would manifest here first because it's a central processing point for field changes."

Indian Tantric concepts of the subtle body describe seven major and up to twenty-two minor chakra centers. While the seven principal chakras are arranged vertically with reference to the spine and the major endocrine glands, the minor centers are distributed throughout the body. There are chakras in the palms, soles of the feet, behind the knees, and clustered in the organic middle of the body, around the hara.

If Birch's speculations about hara diagnosis and the possible energetic linkages with the *Manipura* chakra are correct, then it's possible the reflexology models for hand and feet might be based in some manner on the energetics of the minor foot and hand chakras, acting as holographic affiliates for the whole-body somatic holograms, itself an affiliate of something cosmically grander.

The Energy Fields of Life and Their Celestial Antennae

Acupuncture theory thus recognizes that the human energy system, in its micro and macro expressions, is potentially a part of a larger energy web encompassing planet, solar system, and beyond. While Manaka's primitive signal system might predate and underlie the more developed central nervous system, the interconnected body system of connective tissue might be the physical interface for these holographic connections.

That's the contention of cell biologist James Oschman, instructor in the comprehensive studies program of the Rolf Institute and adviser to the New England School of Acupuncture. "Virtually all somatic therapies have examples of this kind of holographic interaction, where relationship of a part to the whole becomes apparent," comments Oschman. "Each approach articulates a possible mechanism by which parts of the whole may be interconnected by various types of energetic fields. The story that may be emerging is the same story Einstein was trying to articulate at the end of his life—namely, the equivalency of energies."

Oschman's thesis, which he drafted especially for the Rolf Institute—headquarters for a manipulative bodywork therapy called Structural Integration, or Rolfing, founded by Ida P. Rolf (1896-1979), a renowned Ph.D. biochemist-physiologist—is that connective tissue may form "an integrative electronic network allowing all parts of the organism to communicate with each other. The connective tissue is a continuous system extending into every nook and cranny of the body. As a candidate for a holographic fabric of the body, you don't have to look any further."

Connective tissue includes all the tendons, ligaments, fascial planes, all the organs and systems—even the cell, through its cytoskeleton, is "ensheathed" in connective tissue. Fascia, an intricate web of connective tissue coextensive with the entire body and its musculature, is paramount in the Rolfing model. Fascial tone and elasticity, say the Rolfers, are basic contributing factors in our overall bodily well-being. If one segment of this fascial web is "thickened" or disorganized, it can transmits strain throughout the body just the way a snag in a sweater noticeably distorts the overall weave.

Connective tissue is composed of insoluble collagen fibers, arranged in crystalline arrays, and embedded in a gel-like "ground substance." Connective tissue, says Oschman, is piezoelectric, an important clue to how it might broker the somatic hologram. To say it's piezoelectric means it generates electric fields when compressed or stretched. "It's as if the body were woven as a single fabric of piezoelectric collagen fibers," says Oschman. This weaving facilitates a continuous flow of information and energy through the "interconnected electronic fabric."

Oschman's electronic collagen body fabric is highly sensitive to larger energy fields surrounding the human. Harold Saxton Burr, probing this possibility at Yale University School of Medicine in the 1940s, called them "life fields," and his provocative observations have sparked further study ever since. In his *Blueprint for Immortality—The Electric Patterns of Life* (1972), Burr documented how all living organisms, from plants to humans, participate in the "ubiquitous field" with their "antennae to the universe" and are molded by "electrodynamic fields" that can be measured with standard volt meters. These fields of life, claimed Burr, are the basic blueprints for all organic life.

"Man is embedded in powerful fields from birth onwards," wrote Burr. "The universe is organized and maintained by energy fields that determine the position and movement of all particles of matter which are themselves condensations of the fields. Within our bodies molecules are arranged in intricate patterns that follow the lines of force of the various fields that influence them. The fields serve as a matrix or mold that preserves the configuration of the molecules comprising the body. The field maintains the pattern in the midst of a flux of components. This is the mechanism whose outcome is wholeness, organization, and continuity."

Since Burr's work, a small band of Western scientists has been gradually quantifying the presumed speculative existence of a subtle energy field about the human body. They are grudgingly admitting that just because you can't see it, doesn't mean it's not there. The groundbreaking but controversial research of Swedish radiologist Dr. Björn Nordenström at the Karolinska Institute on "biologically closed electric circuits" in the human body has shown that an innate positive electrical current that flows through the body may, when augmented, inhibit cancer-cell growth.

Nordenström, who first presented his work in a 1983 self-published textbook—*Biologically Closed Electric Circuits: Clinical, Experimental, and Theoretical Evidence for an Additional Circulatory System*—contends that the body has the equivalent of electric circuits and that this electrical activity may be the basis of the healing process. Studying the electrical properties of veins, arteries, capillaries, and blood in living animals, Nordenström discovered that the electrical resistance of the walls of the blood vessels was about 200 times that of the blood.

The body's electric circuits, part of the overall human "biological battery," are switched on (building up positively charged ions) by normal muscle use, injury, infection, or tumor. He reasoned that these vessels functioned as insulated cables, that the blood conducted electrical charge between cancer tumors (which had their own electric potential) and surrounding tissue, and that the capillary walls contained natural electrodes.

The body's electrical system Nordenström maintains, is as critical to human health as blood circulation; he further reasons that disturbances in this electrical circuitry might underlie the development of tumors. "If Nordenström is right, these circuits may explain many fundamental regulatory processes in the human body, and even the seemingly inexplicable therapeutic effects of acupuncture and of electromagnetic fields," notes Gary Taubes in *Discover*.

The organizing electrical and electromagnetic fields of life include Earth's electric, magnetic, and gravity fields, each of which itself encodes information about the larger celestial environment. The implication is that through the biological software of connective tissue, micro- and macro-acupuncture systems, the stems, branches and Five Element theory, the human body is a hologram of the energetic processes of the cosmos. We could, on this basis, hypothetically derive a weather forecast or predict sunspot activity or Mercury retrogrades from decoding the information lodged in our total-body hologram. Common sense provides a simple example of this majestic connectivity. Haven't we all heard some people say their big toe tells them when a storm is coming?

The Psychoenergetic Terrain: Mind and Body Meet in the Meridians

If the human body is a hologram of the energetic processes of the cosmos, what is the mechanism by which these energies work into the human being and our emotionality? According to at least two M.D. acupuncturists, one a psychiatrist, the other a physician, when you integrate the energetic principles of Chinese medicine with the psychological portraits of Western psychology, the result is a wonderfully illuminative model of the psychoenergetic unity of the human being.

Leon Hammer, M.D., of Saratoga Springs, New York, uses the twin eyes of Western psychiatry and Chinese acupuncture to create a cohesive, multidisciplinary diagnostic system, which he reports in *Dragon Rises, Red Bird Flies—Psychology and Chinese Medicine*. Drawing on thirty-nine years of psychiatry, with twenty-two years of Chinese medicine, Hammer links the energies of the Five Elements (water, metal, wood, fire, earth) with a Western model of psychological development.

Hammer sees in acupuncture the long-sought-after bridge between body and mind, a comprehensive clinical model that respects the presumed interrelations of psyche and soma. His hope is that the principles of Chinese acupuncture and Western psychology together might lay the rational foundations for a science of psychosomatics and a discipline of mind-body-spirit holism for Western medical practice.

Chinese medicine does not distinguish between a bodily and a psychoemotional function, explains Hammer. Both are expressions of chi, the vital, intangible life force. Chinese medicine recognizes the emotions as the Seven Internal Demons—anger, grief, fear, excessive joy, anxiety, worry, compassion. According to Chinese theory, these demons take expression simultaneously in the organ systems and emotional life of an individual and if unchecked or unresolved can lead to physical illness. "The disease process is *both* psychological and somatic at all stages," says Hammer.

Chinese medicine next correlates five of the demon emotions (specifically, joy, anger, worry, grief, fear) with its classical Five Element theory. This dynamic model describes the continuous energy transformations and recyclings among the elements of fire, earth, metal, water, and wood, that underlie material reality and its processes. The Five Elements, Hammer notes, are descriptions of psychoenergetic domains, a perception that enables Hammer to see Chinese medicine and Western psychology as "therapeutic partners." The Five Element system "provides the richest organization of correspondences between mind and body.

"By combining dynamic psychotherapy with Chinese medicine, we have an opportunity to embrace both approaches in a simultaneous and integrated fashion. I see the Five Elements as developmental stages in the evolution of a human being. My thesis here delineates an evolutionary approach to energetics reflecting developmental psychology."

Hammer aims to redefine the negative implications of the internal demons and cast them into a model of psychological development relevant for the Western psyche. Drawing on his psychoanalytical training and considerable experience in child psychiatry, Hammer realized that to promote health these basic energies must have a positive, natural function, and he began to see them developmentally. "As we grow and mature, each of these energies plays a role. But if they are not functional, that stage of life will be hurt, or if the stage of life has tremendous trauma, those energies will be affected."

Hammer has drawn on numerous case studies to integrate a Western psychological model of personality development into the psychoemotional domains of acupuncture. The result, constituting the bulk of his book, is a series of character configurations or portraits of personality disharmonies based on energy imbalances. As each organ-meridian system can have an excess or deficiency of Qi (and a predominance of either yin/passive or yang/active energy), these relative imbalances are also reflected in various personality types.

These energy-psychology pictures, Hammer cautions, are deliberately overdrawn and stereotyped, somewhat dramatic, possibly histrionic, examples of each energetic tendency. What's important, he stresses, is to see how they illustrate the potential, positive, and natural functioning of each meridian and organ energy and what a distortion or misdirection of these basic energies looks like in the context of human personality.

The Meridian Is the Hyphen in the Word "Psycho-Somatic"

Yves Requena, M.D., also uses the medical eyes of Western allopathy and the energetic eyes of Chinese medicine to describe character and constitutional tendencies in health and illness, which he summarizes in *Character and Health—The Relationship of Acupuncture and Psychology*. Like Hammer, Requena hopes this view will help legitimize the science of psychosomatics. "Acupuncture is simultaneously a basic and a highly differentiated model of psychosomatic expression," says Requena.

"Since the beginning of Chinese medicine, Chinese physicians have approached physiology and psychologic phenomena with the view that the two are not fundamentally different," Requena explains. "The meridians are the junction of mind and body. They influence each other. The meridian is the hyphen in the word psycho-somatic." In *Character and Health* Requena charts the psychosomatic laws of acupuncture and strives to present "a useful, consistent, and safe method for directing and prioritizing a self-directed program of health maintenance."

Like Hammer, Requena bases his model on the Five Element theory. He uses it to classify human psychosomatic behavior into an energetic anatomy of types and constitutions. Constitution, says Requena, means "the inherited vulnerability of one or more of the twelve organ-meridian systems of the body." This predominant predisposition—somatic, psychological, and potentially pathological—Requena calls a *terrain*. The terrain is a fundamental constitutional type and the energetic basis of character, explains Requena, and represents a basic tendency toward dysfunction or disease. "The notion of terrain is large, encompassing functional, organic, endocrinal, and characterological aspects."

Requena establishes his model of terrains and character types on the basis of what Chinese medicine calls the Six Energies. The twelve principle meridians and their element correlations are classified in groups of two to make six categories of paired meridians. Each pair connects the top and bottom of the body and in effect makes up a single meridian, which provides the acupuncturist trained in Requena's system with precise information about personality and physiological functioning.

For example, the *Tai Yang* pair comprises the Small Intestine (fire element) and Bladder (water element) meridians and corresponds with the climatic condition of coldness. The personality type is passionate; constitutionally, the person is vulnerable through the small intestine; physically, the *Tai Yang* type has a rigid bearing, a slender, noble posture, a tendency to stiff neck and dreads the extremes of heat and cold. Psychologically, the *Tai Yang* has a cold attitude, is distant and authoritative, has a faculty for learning and retention, a superior intelligence, shows emotional sensitivity, ambition, passion, single goal orientation, tends toward an austere lifestyle, can be stubborn, rebellious, and possessive, and expects a privileged relationship with the physician.

Consider a single Requennan character type—*Jue Yin*, Liver/Wood and Pericardium/Fire. The amount of precise medical correlations Requena can develop from this classification is impressive. "The pathology of *Jue Yin* is dominated by the physiology of the blood and liver, and this temperament is disposed to deficiency," Requena notes. He meticulously outlines the biological syndromes typically associated with an imbalance of liver chi: cardio-vascular, respiratory, urinary, gastroenterological, neurological, psychiatric, even problems in the ligaments and eyes.

It's on the basis of such comprehensive cross-correlations between Western organic anatomy and Oriental energy cycles that Requena can confidently conclude: "Acupuncture is a medical therapy that is rich in techniques to apprehend the most profound psychosomatic illness and mental dysfunction."

Searching for the Master Template

If the body maps give us the grammar for the holographic universe, what is the book its cosmically energetic words are written in? "At the basic level, the etheric body is the primary holographic template for the physical-cellular structure," contends Richard Gerber, M.D., in his *Vibrational Medicine,* a comprehensive synthesis of numerous subtle, energetic therapies into a larger model of "Einsteinian medicine."

According to Gerber, "There has been enough preliminary research with Kirlian photography to suggest the body really is holographic in nature. The holographic principle seems to be reflected at different levels of cellular physiology, structure, and function. Every cell in the body contains the information library required to create an entire new human being. Each piece contains the information of the whole body."

At the core of Gerber's vision for a new medicine is the realization that certain "energy-field patterns" within the body seem to precede the onset of illness. "We need to expand our database of information," he says, "combining the technological with the subjective, to get a fuller picture of what's happening in the human energy field." The true causes of disease, says Gerber, can only be apprehended by an Einsteinian medical perception.

Here the human is seen as a multitextured energy being whom vibrational medicine attempts to treat with energy compatible, complementary, and supportive with its own. "We are multidimensional beings of energy and light, whose physical body is but a single component of a larger dynamic system. The ultimate approach to healing will be to remove the abnormalities at the subtle energy level which led to the manifestation of illness in the first place. Vibrational healing methods work by rebalancing disturbances of structure and energy flow within the context of our multilevel inter-active energetic fields. This will be the greatest difference in approach between the traditional medicine of today and the spiritual-holistic medicine of the future."

Much of Gerber's contribution exists in his precise diagrams of "human multidimensional anatomy," a key component of which is the *etheric body* or aura. This usually invisible energy field, or sheath, described in Eastern, esoteric, and anthroposophic traditions and named after the fifth element—water, earth, air, fire, and ether—cocoons the physical form. In Gerber's model, the etheric body is the "primary holographic energy template" for the physical body. It carries "coded information for the spatial organization of the fetus as well as a roadmap for cellular repair."

The etheric body also contains the spatial roadmap for the organization of the mature physical form and it provides energizing nourishment necessary for both maintenance and regeneration. In vibrational medicine, says Gerber, the etheric body is the principal site of diagnosis and treatment because it is a key player in the origin and articulation of most illnesses. Disturbances in the etheric energy field, Gerber notes, precipitate dysfunctions, imbalances, and, eventually, degenerative processes in the physical.

The acupuncture meridian system, says Gerber, acts as an information transfer layout as well as a means of bringing in nutrient energy to the body. "It's the physical-etheric interface, between the etheric body, which is the holographic energy template, and the physical body. The two are mutually interdependent and co-stabilized. The etheric template is an informational pattern which precedes cellular structure. Many other higher energy systems feed into this and funnel down information."

Gerber diagrams the interfaces between subtle energy systems and physical, cellular structures in the body. He uses the analogy of a piano keyboard to illustrate what he calls the "human frequency spectrum." The various human energy fields of physical, etheric, astral, and mental each occupy an ascending octave on this frequency keyboard, explains Gerber; each is a faster-vibrating harmonic of its preceding neighbor, such that, for example, the "astral field" (the sheath of emotions, affects, and reactivity) vibrates faster and subtler than the "etheric field" (the energetic blueprint for the physical).

The human bioenergetic system is a multilayered interpenetrating organism of denser bodies (the physical) expanding out to subtler, finer bodies (astral and mental). Various energy systems—the acupoints and meridians of Chinese medicine, the chakra consciousness centers of Hindu esotericism, and the 72,000 nervelike *nadis* of Tantric physiology—are nested in this onion-skin fabric, and from this matrix they interact with the central and peripheral nervous system and the core physiological systems of the body. "The total balance and health of the human organism is a product of a balanced and coordinated functioning of both physical and higher dimensional regulatory systems," says Gerber.

The Palm at the End of the Mind

It all comes back to the palm again. Is it the signature of the master hologram for the holographic body? Wallace Stevens wrote gnomically in his "Of Mere Being": "The palm at the end of the mind/Beyond the last thought/ . . . The palm stands on the edge of space." Stevens was saying, it seemed to me, that the palm is the mysterious swinging door, the imprint of mind in this holographic universe between space and body.

The search for the nature and origin of the holographic body has led me out through my palm prints through cellular DNA, micro-acupuncture systems, numerous body maps and somatic topologies, electric fields of life, etheric templates, and out into the solar system and greater cosmos. The palm seems to represent a swinging door between holograms and the mind is the doorman. It's a very malleable world, Michael Talbot reminds us. "In a holographic universe there are no limits to the extent to which we can alter the fabric of reality."

The palm prints are the "subtle energetics of the divine nature," says Birlaji, drawing on the vocabulary of *Samudrik Shastra*. The flexion creases are the wave interference patterns of the frequency domain or enfolded implicate order imprinted on the palmar surfaces, we might say, drawing alternatively on the technical language of Pribram and Bohm. Further, the holographically encoded information we carry around with us in the palms may be useful not only for disease prediction and prevention, but also for our individual development and spiritual evolution. Whatever vocabulary we employ, it's clear that the micro-acupuncture somatic holograms considered here exemplify the cardinal features of the holographic paradigm.

Information is distributed throughout the system, from the microcellular to the macrobiological domains—holographic theory tells us this. Homunculi flourish like spring dandelions throughout the body. The information is encoded in wave interference patterns in the form of reflex zones, iris topologies, palm prints, auricular meridians, all requiring precise decoding according to a kind of new Fourier somatomathematics into meaningful, interactive images of the whole.

Any piece of the integrated electronic fabric will regenerate the original image, which means that the nose map and scalp map and foot map will each equally project back the original composite human image with its morphological terrain contoured with meridians. Overlapping, multilayered body maps are not at all contradictory or mutually exclusive, but represent the holographic versatility to store immense amounts of information in virtually the same space.

That's why the palm contains the equally valid maps of hand acupuncture, reflexology, palmistry, plus a minor chakra. And because the holograms encode information from Bohm's enfolded implicate order or Pribram's frequency domain or Talbot's holographic universe, all of which are outside our conventional spacetime, causal framework, readouts can encompass information from the deep genetic past, the unconscious, the present, and the predictive, probable future.

The final implication, not yet conceptualized by somatic holographers, is that the human body, composed of myriad smaller holographic projections, is itself in its entirety, an enfolded implicate frequency domain, a cosmic hologram awaiting our astonished illumination. The mystics always caution us, things are not what they seem. The holographic paradigm provides palmistry's more esoteric and controversial claims a context for validation.

According to *Samudrik Shastra*, the accumulated karmic tendencies of thousands of lifetimes accruing to one soul are encoded in the dermal signature of the inactive hand. As I contemplate my left palm, I realize with a sudden mental lurch that if I accept this outrageous hypothesis, the significance of my palms held now before me would be suddenly, tremendously transformed. Before me, as it would be for anyone engaging in this riveting consideration, would be the *holoprint*, as we might call it, of a 10,000-lifetime-old human individuality.

Here we would have the cumulative organic signature of that master hologram, the palm at the end of the mind, which, upon contemplation, would reciprocally reveal to us the mind at the end of the palm. In the holoprint of the palms we could behold the master library and multidimensional gestalt, a "paradigm of Buddha consciousness" requiring only the mathematical, intuitive decoding to regenerate the original enfolded implicate coherency—the original object. If we could do this perceptual transformation, what would it reveal? We next turn to Rudolf Steiner's anthroposophy for a possible answer.

The Human Is a Mirror Image of the Spiritual World

One of anthroposophy's immediate assets for us is that it postulates an expanded model of the human constitution that takes into account the holographic human. Anthroposophy's extended human anatomical model gives us the clues we're seeking for an authentic relationship between bodily based consciousness and the outer environment.

The theoretical structure underlying anthroposophy is exceptionally complex and detailed, both in scientific precision and spiritual depth. For those habituated to a conventional perceptual framework, it can seem arcane, even baffling, and it certainly requires hard study and long contemplation to master. Yet the sweetness of the philosophical fruits obtainable by making the effort is considerable.

Never opposed to rationalism, Steiner wanted to enrich its information and conceptual base with the results of empirical research. In the case of medicine, he wanted to extend allopathy's scientific, deductive method beyond the physical, bodily domain and leaven it with spiritual (clairvoyant) insight. That was his intention, in fact, with the whole range of human knowledge—agriculture, music, poetry, speech, education, history, philosophy, and cosmology.

Self-knowledge is knowledge of the world and world knowledge is knowledge of the self, Steiner never tired of telling his associates. Investigation in one realm (self-inquiry) reciprocally illuminates its complementary domain (the world); we find the world in the self and discover the self in the world because the two realms are basically mirror opposites. Steiner indicated ways to extend science's rigorously obtained observations of the physical world into the sub-tler human realms of the etheric, astral, and Ego sheaths of the human, planet, and cosmos.

Behind anthroposophy's apparent esotericism lies a complete model of the world, a kind of bio-organic cosmology, encompass-ing human, plant, animal, mineral realms, the stars and planets, and myriad spiritual beings and intelligences—with everything in its proper place. The human is not an isolated, material being, but belongs to and comprises the whole universe, declared Steiner. The human organism is the "sense-perceptible" reflection of something spiritual and supersensible.

There is far more to the human being than meets the average, nonclairvoyant eye. There is "an invisible man [human] within us," composed of the mutually interpenetrating etheric, astral, and Ego spiritual bodies that leave their formative imprint on the physical organism. This fundamental observation, which Steiner termed the fourfold image of the human, illustrates how the natural world, the environment, is subsumed in the human being, how it lives within the human—as the human. Before we illuminate this concept, we need to appreciate how Steiner envisioned the human being in our cosmic context.

According to Steiner, the kingdoms of plants, animals, minerals, and the starry cosmos are all constituents, in concentrated, micro-cosmic form, of the living, organic, independent human being. In other words, the cosmic, planetary, and natural environments all find their place within the living human and reciprocally, the human organism is the condensed microcosmic expression of the cosmos. There is a core identity at the basis of the human, natural, planetary, and cosmic worlds—of all expressions of environment.

The human is the cosmos in microcosm and the cosmos is the human in macrocosm; hence the astonishing isomorphism of human, world, and universe. "Man as he stands on Earth is indeed a shrunken universe," said Steiner. "Man is the world. We weave mankind out of the cosmos. We have within us shadow-images of the great world, and all the members of our constitution—the physical, etheric, and astral bodies and the I—are worlds for divine beings. Man is so complex because he is truly a mirror image of the spiritual world. He begins to feel as though he were intergrown with the entire cosmic structure in spite of the fact that he feels himself in his complete independence."

The whole cosmos took part in the formation of the human physical body; we can behold the presence and intelligence of the cosmos through the life of our internal organs. "One finds the entire spiritual organization of the macrocosm spiritually within one's own organs."

Each of our bodily organs—heart, liver, spleen, kidney, lungs—is produced, shaped, and maintained by cosmic forces, by the powers and potencies of the planets of our solar system and the stars of the galaxy. The Sun contributes and energetically maintains the heart; Saturn underlies the spleen, Mercury the lungs, Jupiter the liver, Venus the kidneys, Mars the gall bladder, and the Moon supports the brain and reproductive organs. Thus any perturbations in the magnetic fields of Sun, Moon, or planets, however slight, will be registered in the human etheric biofield and physical organism.

It's a bold, perhaps preposterous, proposition at first acquaintance, but when contemplating the contemporary man or woman Steiner evokes the archetypal human, the first created human, and its cosmic formative elements. Everyone since, including us today, has been patterned, with minor variations, according to this primal human template. "Behold Cosmic Man through human organology," declared Steiner in what's become a famous dictum of environmental equivalency.

Through his own considerable clairvoyant research, Steiner understood that when we die—it is axiomatic in Steiner's view that human consciousness survives the dissolution of the physical body—among the peculiar experiences we're likely to have is the perception of the cosmos as the extended, diffused, organological body of the human. If our human organs are made from cosmic forces, then these organs, or their formative, prematerial energies, must be present in some form in the cosmos.

When we're dead, the cosmos is our residency, so it's logical to expect an encounter with our organs in another form. Disincarnate, it's as if we see our insides spread out before us in the vast reaches of cosmic space, in the preorganic, prematerial form of the stars and planets of the galaxy. Behold human organology in the elements of the cosmos, we might say, reversing Steiner's declaration. Every aspect of our physical organism seems spread out boundlessly into cosmic infinity, more like forces than discrete organs.

After all, this macrocosmic view of the human is implicit, if widely disbelieved, in astrology, which describes the psychophysiological mechanics of this relationship. Astrology tells us that the signs of the zodiac influence or "rule" different parts of the body: the constellation Taurus rules the neck; Leo rules the heart, Cancer the breast, Pisces the feet. Medieval astrologers, in fact, customarily depicted the human being as spangled with the signs and zoomorphic images of the zodiac, with the bull at the neck, the lion at the heart, the fish at the feet. It's a dramatic, highly suggestive image of what the esoteric tradition calls the "microcosmic human," that the human being is a miniature flesh-and-blood version of the cosmos. That's also the perception behind the famous Hermetic dictum, *As Above, So Below.*

Somehow the composition, both organic and psychological, of the human is a small, compact version of the energetic reality of the stars and planets of the cosmos; the human is the cosmic environment in living miniature. Steiner contended that the origin of each of our principal internal organs is a cosmic body: behind the heart stands the Sun; behind the neck there dwells Taurus.

Each of the zodiac's twelve houses contributes a single aspect of the human being. Taurus, for example, not only rules the neck, it contributes—creates—the neck, throat, larynx, faculty of speech, and the potential for clairaudience. It's more accurate to say the human neck *is* the constellation Taurus and that we wear the Taurean stars like a jeweled necklace. Similarly, Leo in conjunction with the Sun, contributes the heart, illumined feelings, the warmth of selfhood; again, while astrology says Leo rules the heart, it might be more precise to say, Leo *is* the heart. The constellation known as Leo lives *as* the human heart. As Steiner puts it, "The heart can only be formed from the Sun when the Sun has within it the forces of the constellation of Leo."

In this disincarnate moment, we see what our true form is, our supersensible self, Steiner explains; beholding it objectively, we see it's something like a majestic, dynamic picture. "The cosmic germ of man's physical body is experienced in pre-earthly existence as a cosmos. The forces streaming from this archetypal picture have the same effect as a radiant body. This cosmic picture of Man shines spiritually, as the luminous picture of his own form. He feels his soul nature spread out far across this cosmos." It feels as if the entire universe is our inner being; where we once had an organic pulsating heart, liver, and stomach, now we behold "the spirit-seed of the human physical body as a universe of vast magnitude."

This cosmos is actually our future physical body expanded to a universe. Reciprocally, in the time between death in one life and subsequent rebirth in the next—reincarnation is another fundamental metaphysical tenet of Steiner's anthroposophy—this immense cosmic human seed begins to contract and condense, until it finally appears as our incarnate, microcosmic physical organism. All this suggests a question: if the physically incarnate human is a microcosmic expression of the cosmos, what really is the cosmos?

The Human Is a Living Picture
of the Universe

In a sense all of anthroposophy is the complex answer to this fundamental inquiry. Throughout his career Steiner sought to answer this question in different ways. One of his most evocative answers was to suggest that the human being is a picture of the living spirit comprising all the spiritual beings in the universe. The outer form of the human represents a living picture of the working-together of all the hierarchies of the spiritual world, Steiner explained.

By hierarchies, he meant what traditional esotericism calls the families of higher angels; Steiner's angelology is more precise than most and ranks the hierarchies according to function, cognitive range, and serial appearance in the Creation. What's important here is to appreciate that, if Steiner is correct, the full range of hierarchical spiritual intelligences has legitimate, lawful residency within the human being, as organs, processes, and strata of consciousness.

For example, the Aborigines of Australia see themselves as humans living *within* the projected thoughts of the gods; our world is the Dreaming of the Ancestors and "the interiority of the gods is our external reality." In a similar manner, Steiner asserted that as humans we are "souls embedded in cosmic thought, links in the thought-logic of the cosmos." When the angels think, their thinking is so powerful, it thinks humans into existence; humans are the materialized thoughts of the hierarchies.

An "intelligible" picture of humankind, says Steiner, shows us the ranks of the spiritual hierarchies, their deeds and thoughts, with humanity as its dynamic product. "Our whole world-system is the consolidated clairvoyance of the Gods, of the higher Hierarchies.

Thus when we look at the human being with supersensible knowledge, behind every part of him we see a world of spiritual cosmic beings."

The Cosmic Composition of the Human Being

Now, it's reasonable to ask if the summation of the hierarchies constitutes some microcosmic condensed expression of something even larger. "The entire Cosmos first appeared as a gigantic Being in the Saturn sphere and the whole man is seen as a gigantic cosmic Being appearing as the sum total, as the inner-organic, cooperative activity of generations of Gods," wrote Steiner. With variations, this is a fairly common theme in different cosmogonies.

In Qabala, this being that is the size of the cosmos is called Adam Kadmon and is the macrocosmic expression of Man, the primal first human before biology or gender. In the Gnostic tradition, 365 angels contributed to the creation of the first Adam of Light. For this to make sense, we need to review Steiner's model of cosmogony, his theory of how the world was created. A fundamental tenet of Steiner's anthroposophical model is that the human and cosmos evolved together, that in the human we find all the concentration of all the forces and intelligences of the cosmos, and that in the environment, the natural world, we find the differentiated mirroring of these cosmic/human forces.

To understand the evolution and elaboration of the human being, we must simultaneously appreciate how the cosmos came into being, because they are two complementary poles of the same process.

Steiner's cosmogony is radically different, often disturbingly so, from the orthodox astrophysical view of the origin of the solar system. But as Fred Wolf, a physicist himself, suggests, much of what modern science upholds as physical fact and "proven" theory is often nothing more than an interesting explanatory myth of only probable truth. So maybe the standard astrophysical story of cosmic creation is as outlandish as Steiner's, which has the epistemological advantage of being based on rigorous clairvoyant, empirical investigation.

Steiner places our planet Earth within a sevenfold developmental sequence in which our solar system is seen as one cosmic body. Humankind appeared and evolved within this solar context, as did each of the nine celestial families of the three "angelic" hierarchies. In other words, the creation, elaboration, and progression of the solar system, humanity, and the spiritual hierarchies were synchronous, coincidental events, a situation that augurs well for a close working relationship across environmental dimensions.

The first stage of cosmic evolution Steiner calls Old Saturn, a gaseous, amorphous milieu in which the mineral, warm essence of the human physical body was first created. Here *Saturn* refers not to the individual planet but to a quality or condition of the cosmos as a single emergent being—the Saturn condition. Next came Old Sun, an airy, swirling environment in which the human etheric body was created. Again, when Steiner uses the term *Sun,* he doesn't mean our Sun, but a cosmos-wide condition called Old Sun. Also, at each successive stage, different families of spiritual beings within the hierarchies were active and made their own evolutionary advances. On the Old Moon, dominated by water, the astral body was incorporated into the emerging human.

The fourth stage is called Earth. This marked the materialization and mineralization of the solar system of which our planet Earth was one microcosmic aspect among many, including the discrete planets such as Saturn, satellites such as the Moon, and the super-bright Sun. In the Earth phase of cosmic evolution, physical matter appeared, things became visible, and a nascent, evolving humanity was given the Ego, or I-consciousness, the unique patrimony of the creator gods. Cosmic evolution doesn't stop at the Earth stage, however. There are three more planetary stages (or cosmic conditions) the world is yet to pass through before the triune evolution of humanity, solar system, and hierarchy is completed: Jupiter, Venus, and Vulcan.

Now let's insert the elements of the complete human being into this cosmogonic model. According to Steiner, the physical body incorporates the mineral sphere and the element of earth. The human physical body corresponds to a primordial, primogenitive Old Saturn stage of the cosmos. The germ of the human physical body was actually the first phase in the creation of the human, characterized as a kind of gaseous warmth, although in terms of visible, tangible manifestation it was the last and most recent.

Next came the etheric body. What had been the appearance of life on Old Saturn has now become actual life on Old Sun. On the Old Sun the "human mineral" from Old Saturn was animated, made alive. Old Sun adds *life* to the human mineral in the form of the etheric body, the animated life of wisdom. During the Old Sun period the Kyriotetes, or Spirits of Wisdom, members of the Second Hierarchy, imparted the ether body to evolving humanity, later, the Exousiai or Elohim, Spirits of Form, would also contribute to this life body. The Kyriotetes' substance itself is ether, "mobile, power-filled wisdom, or life," so the human etheric body is an emanation of the Wisdom Spirits. Steiner likens the Old Sun human to a plant: it's phototropic and sentient, but not self-aware. As the Kyriotetes pour the ether or life body into the human, the Sun itself, previously dark, begins to radiate. Life begins. Signs of inner activity appear in the germinal human.

In the Old Moon stage, the human astral body was formed; this is the basis for soul life, emotions, desires, affects. In the Earth phase, the individual I, or the possibility for self-aware, independent selfhood, was imparted to the evolving human being, now incarnate in physical, mineralized, living, animate matter—the biological human form. During the Earth stage, the etheric body keeps the human in contact with the cosmos and is the seat of activity for another member of the Second Hierarchy, the Exousiai, or Elohim, the Spirits of Form.

On Earth, the etheric body is an image of the cosmos, of the entire starry heavens, filled with its activities, sounds, and intelligences. For the most part, we aren't aware of the prodigious, swirling activity in our etheric body, but sometimes at the moment of falling asleep, we can catch a glimpse and it's as if we are watching a fabulous, multidimensional movie made from all the forgotten scenes of our life.

The Geomythics of Environment: Aboriginal Dreamtime and World Making

Steiner's anthroposophic cosmology gives us a macrocosmic model for our human connectivity with the larger environment. For more instruction on the microcosmic, practical grounding of this view, we turn to one of the world's oldest surviving native cultures, the Australian Aborigines. For them, human identity and the landscape have always been equivalent.

The matrix we seek, according to tribal beliefs and shamanic practices, is the dreamtime (*alcheringa*), that fecund, eternal, creative moment of world making in which all living things in the environment—people, animals, birds, insects, trees, fishes, waterholes, mountains, and thus the environment itself—were generated on the first day by these primordial, primogenitive ancestors. The landscape is compounded of the "dreamings" of the ancestors. They left manifold clues to their acts, Aboriginal traditions tell us: a totemic, mythopoeic landscape, beaded with totem emergence places and threaded with song lines, animated traces of the ancestors' great deeds; this animistic terrain provided the basic elements for a ritualized Aboriginal geomancy.

When the dreamtime (before time began) epoch ended, explains Australian storyteller Johanna Lambert, "the energy and vibrational patterns from the exploits of the great Ancestors congealed the initially limitless space into the topography and forms that we now experience as the material aspect of the universe." The land, its features, and energy qualities, represent the imprint of dreamtime dreamings, Lambert says.

The Aboriginal song lines and ritual totem centers represent significations of the cosmogony of the dreaming ancestors in the landscape. The original creation myths thus live in the landscape as animistic presences and mnemonics; the Aboriginal landscape is geomythically alive. Further, the Aboriginal culture shows us how environment is made by *geomythopoeisis,* which means "the living myth creates and lives as the Earth landscape."

Earth's surface is a "ledger of cosmology," as each dreamtime story has its geomythic nexus in the sacred landscape. Our world is the dreaming of the ancestors, the living expression of their creative thoughts, say the Aborigines; more formally put, this means the interiority of the gods is our external reality. The landscape is thus inherently sacred and deeply, irrefutably meaningful.

Song Lines for the Eternal Ones of the Dream

We don't normally regard agriculture as a disastrous innovation in human evolution, but one day in Tasmania an Aboriginal elder named Uncle Bul made it strikingly clear to researcher Robert Lawlor just how profound an effect the decline of the old hunter-gatherer lifestyle and the advent of agriculture exacted on the Western psyche.

The crux of the problem, the old man told Lawlor, is that through agriculture "white men have lost their dreaming." That's a loss of major significance, because according to the Australian Aborigines, when "white men"—or any people, themselves included—lose their dreaming, they've lost the crucial nexus that weaves together Heaven and Earth, women and men, nature and humanity, and makes long-term cultural survival and true prosperity possible.

During trance vision, Uncle Bul sees a "web of intersecting threads" on which scenes of the physical world, dreams, and prophetic visions are hung like cinematic beads—an aspect of the original dreaming that created our world, in other words. "But inner fears break that glimpse of an invisible webwork, leaving only a world of isolated things"—and inner fear *is* the psychological state of most of Western humankind. "Some of the young Aboriginal men today talk and act very smart, but they no longer have the vision, 'cause they have the same fear inside as white fellas," continued the elder. They can't feed themselves off the land like Uncle Bul, who knows the whereabouts of all the roots and berries. "Anyone who does not know how to find food and feed himself is always frightened inside like a little child who has lost his mother and with that fear the vision of the spirit world departs."

What more indigenous people can there be than the Australian Aborigines, whose Latinate name itself means "the very first, from the beginning, of the source" and whose myths establish them as the oldest surviving culture on the planet? Anthropologists credit them with a 60,000-year history, but according to Aboriginal elders, their race is much older. "We have been here since the time *before* Time began. We have come directly out of the Dreamtime of the great Creative Ancestors. We have lived and kept the earth as it was on the First Day."

That's a contention hard to substantiate and a state of mind almost impossible to conceive, yet the archaic consciousness of the First Day Aborigines may hold "a recollection of our origins, a guiding code, a potency, and a seed for the rebirth of Western culture in which land and spirituality are inseparable," says Robert Lawlor. Lawlor is an American author who has lived in the wilderness of Tasmania (one of Australia's seven states) for seventeen years, studying firsthand the ancient lifeways of these First Day custodians. Lawlor writes with passion and lucidity about their redemptively pristine world-view in his book, *Voices of the First Day: Awakening in the Aboriginal Dreamtime.*

As Lawlor understands the Aboriginal world-view, those immaculate first days on Earth didn't include agriculture, either as animal husbandry or tilled crops. That wasn't because those ancient forebears didn't know about agriculture; the lack of any form of agriculture in Aboriginal Australia, even today, explains Lawlor, was a conscious choice. The Aborigines chose against agriculture because it profoundly contradicts the tenets of dreamtime law, the basis of their society.

"The activities and religion of agriculture began the externalization of human attention, which turned away from the dreaming toward the physical manipulation of the material world," explains Lawlor. "With the adoption of agriculture, populations became increasingly geographically fixed, their survival dependent on regional fertility and weather patterns. The earth was seen as something to be cleared, exploited, and managed at will. Agriculture first encouraged then required a structured moral polarity to replace the deep empathic participation of the hunter-gatherers as the foundation of religious sensibility."

The Aborigines say no to agriculture because it severs their profound participation in the dreamtime—and that's the pith of their existence. If there's one word from Aboriginal culture that's already marched into Western culture it's *dreamtime* or the dreaming, what the Pintupi tribes call *tjukurrtjana,* and others calls *alcheringa*—"the eternal ones of the dream." The material, living, perceivable world, called *yuti,* comes from the formative dreaming, which is a fluid, creative state of astral lucidity. It's "the absolute ground of being or the fundamental universal continuum from which all differentiation arises," explains Lawlor.

"In Aboriginal cosmology, the universal manifesting field is consciousness, which simply externalizes or dreams the world of thoughts, forms, and matter." In the beginning was the dreaming and the entire world was created by the ancestors during this timeless epoch of *tjukurrtjana,* say the Aborigines. The ancestors traveled across the barren, inanimate vastness of Australia hunting, skirmishing, making camp, fighting, loving, creating, "and in so doing they shaped a featureless field into a topographical landscape." Their dreams and adventures created the witchetty grubs, emus, kookaburras, wallabies, wombats, kangaroos, lizards, snakes, wattle, banksia, and humans of that primordial world.

The Ancestors Dreamed
the World into Being

"Everything was created from the same source—the dreamings and doings of the great Ancestors," says Lawlor. The phenomenal world appears as the "external objectification" of the dream visions of the Ancestors; all life forms are differentiated aspects of the original dream of Light. The transcendent world of *tjukurrtjana* is accessed again through the Wombat Dreaming, the Honey Ant Dreaming, through the dream memories eternally inscribed in the Aboriginal landscape. Song is the link, but song to the Aborigines means creative mantric sound.

The great ancestral beings were "vast, unbounded, intangible vibratory bodies" who spoke their dreams of the plants and animals by "naming" their specific vibratory pattern—making the Word flesh, as we say in the Christian West. "They created by drawing vibratory energy out of themselves and stabilizing this energy and by specifying or naming—the inner name is the potency of the form or creature," explains Lawlor. Thus as the Aborigines see themselves as humans living *within* the projected thoughts of the gods, our world is the dreaming of the ancestors and "the interiority of the gods is our external reality."

During the dreamtime the physically animate world was sung, or named, into existence—so if you want to remember these profoundly creative names, look to the landscape, listen to the *song lines* that maintain the mythopoeic connection between the ancestral Heaven and the human Earth. The Aboriginal song lines represent the primordial cosmogony of the dreaming ancestors written intricately like a musical score in the landscape. The terrain is geomythically charged, it remembers the Creation, so to disturb the topography in any way "is to obscure the meaning and history of humanity and reality."

Earth's surface is a "ledger of cosmology," as each dreamtime story is designated and remembered by the place where it occurs—by the dreaming tracks called song lines. The primordial creative act of geomythopoesis continues in and *as* the landscape; for the Aborigine, the landscape comprises the primogenitive living myth. "Everything in the natural world is a symbolic footprint of the metaphysical beings whose actions created our world. As with a seed, the potency of an earthly location is wedded to the memory of its origin. The Aborigines called this potency the dreaming of a place, and this dreaming constitutes the sacredness of the earth."

The ancients sang their way all over the world, British nomad-journalist Bruce Chatwin was told during his Outback peripatetry to learn the secrets of the Aboriginal landscape. "They sang the rivers and ranges, salt-pans and sand dunes," Chatwin writes in his *The Songlines*. "They hunted, ate, made love, danced, killed: wherever their tracks led they left a trail of music. They wrapped the whole world in a web of song." Each of the antediluvian ancestors, while singing their way across the landscape, "left a trail of 'life-cells' or 'spirit-children' along the line of his footprints"—a kind of "musical sperm."

Each ancestor's song covered the ground in "an unbroken chain of couplets," says Chatwin, each couplet marking the double foot-falls of the wandering ancestor, "each formed from the names he 'threw out' while walking," each comprising another segment of the dreaming track. Each tribe's ritual and cyclical responsibility is to maintain, if not regenerate, its ancestral song line, reiterating the tribal song cycle "in the correct sequence" as part of their dream journey across the symbolic landscape.

This is their conception and practice of communal ecology, environmentalism at the metaphysical level. Failure to do this or mistakes in singing could "uncreate the Creation." The seasonal Dream Journey is itself "a hagiographic history of the people's origins" along a "totemic landscape saturated with significations," notes Australian poet James Cowan, in his *Mysteries of the Dreaming*. The Aboriginal landscape, says Cowan is "fully humanized," because the land they traverse is a part of themselves. "The Dream Journey on the ritual level is a way of renewing contact with themselves, since they and the land are inseparable."

Spirituality and Landscape Breathe Together

That's why the Aborigines insist on maintaining the Earth as they found it on the First Day, in its original perfection. That's because the First Day is the epiphany of the Golden Age only vaguely recollected in Western myths. The landscape itself bears the direct imprint of the creative acts and meanings of the world-creators and thus is the impression of the Golden Age itself. "The

Earth to the Aborigines is the memory, a symbolic language, of the entire metaphysical dimension, its forms, processes, and thoughts. You don't disturb this imprint because it's like destroying the memory of the race."

Hence for the Aborigines landscape and spirituality are indissolubly bound and every moment is a revelation of the First Day. "This initial moment was thought to be the most vigorous and most potent," comments Lawlor. "The First Day was symbolic of the capacity of the world, humanity, and the cosmos to perpetually renew itself."

Aboriginal ritual—in fact, all of Aboriginal culture—is a perpetual reiteration of the dreamtime Creation. In their unfailing adherence to this mythic dimension, the Aborigines maintain their tribal sections of these journeying pathways that crisscross the entire Australian continent "as a symbol and memory of the primordial Dreaming, of the invisible, metaphysical prototype" bearing its voices and seeds.

So seamless is the Aboriginal dreamtime cosmogony that geomancy and animism are inseparable. In the West we're slowly growing acquainted with the ancient science of the energetic landscape called geomancy; meanwhile our anthropologists still regard animism—the notion that nature is permeated with individualized spirits or conscious intelligence—as primitive and outmoded. But in the Aboriginal experience, the landscape still bears the mythopoeic energy of the First Day and if they listen they'll hear the original songs of the plant and animal species—their dreaming.

That's why, for the Aborigine, place, or *ngurra*, is the basis of personal identity. *Ngurra* means "country, camp, or place," a landscape feature formed through the metaphysical activities of the mythic ancestors as they dreamed the world into being. To the Aborigines place is thus inseparable from meaning, from the original activities that gave it form, notes Lawlor. The landscape is inherently sacred and meaningful and a part of each tribal member. "The question of identity, of *who* I am, is resolved in the Aboriginal consciousness by knowing the full implications of *where* I am."

The Aboriginal forms her personal identity from a knowledge of her place of birth, by studying the landscape's mythopoeic pedigree. "The first thing that happens after an Aboriginal birth is that a small hollow is dug in the earth and the infant is placed in it," explains Lawlor. "That place marks her indissolvable relationship with the landscape for the rest of her life. She has certain responsibilities to perform with respect to that hollow because that's the beginning of her identity and the center of her country. It's a personalized *axis mundi* in a completely mythologized landscape, the exact point in the geomythic terrain where she connects to the Heavens." Each location is mythically alive—with its unique energy pattern, its precise sound, and with the dreamtime totem signature of a single plant or animal species.

Let's say one's place of birth is a site of Opossum Dreaming. This means some of the preformative energy that contributes to the spirit of that species emanated from this part of the landscape, says Lawlor. As part of your initiatic training, you revisit this site with your precision tool of natural magical science, the *didjeridoo* (a long hollow flutelike musical instrument) and re-create the vibratory essence or sound signature of Opossum Dreaming. Then through a process of synesthesia—in which your five senses intermingle and fuse and you hear colors and see sounds—"that sound of the *didjeridoo* allows you to enter into the essence of the place and the sound appears to you as the animal totem."

Opossum Dreaming Is but Another Aspect of Yourself

You recognize the Opossum Dreaming as yet another aspect of yourself because in the dreamtime, animal and human characteristics were originally combined in the proto-ancestral personalities. Each animal species represented a subjective emotional state of the gods. Only in the manifestation stage of *yuti* were animals and humans distinguished, says Lawlor. "At the completion of the Dreaming, the Ancestors disappeared into the earth as potencies and, at the same time, permanently separated their human and animal powers. Humanity's internal psychological states and emotions are externally symbolized in the behaviors and bodily forms of animals."

Through sharing the Opossum Dreaming as your geomantic totem, you automatically enter into kinship relation with all your brothers and sisters of this same species. One clan is descended from the kangaroo-man ancestor of the dreaming, for example, which means all clan members have special responsibilities to the kangaroo, its stories, ceremonies, and multiple kangaroo dreaming sites in the land. "The spirit of the species is believed to flow from the spirit world into the physical world at a particular site. This spirit of the species actually *possesses* the region, not the clan that represents it." Aboriginal society is thereby woven together in a web of geomancy, animism, totemism, and initiatory experience—from birth.

So as a newly initiated Aborigine, you inhabit your destined node in the web of song lines that weave the sacred landscape. The Aborigine recognizes this landscape as an extension of his body. "As they travel and expand their cultural knowledge, memory and the spatial world expand together as an extension of self. The songlines that criss-cross the landscape flow as his own veins and arteries. Like the human body, the country is considered nonsegmentable. Internalized mythic knowledge and its topographical image, painted on their bodies in initiations, are the only graphic maps of their countryside the Aborigines possess." From the dreamtime, then, comes the profound nexus of geomancy, animism, kinship, ritual, and spirituality.

Lawlor isn't the first modern commentator to serve up Aboriginal sexuality to Western intellectual culture. Back in the early decades of this century, when Sigmund Freud argued that subconscious sexuality underpinned much of Western psyche and culture, Freudian enthusiasts like Geza Roheim in *The Gates of the Dream* and *Australian Totemism* rushed to interpret Aboriginal culture as the classic example of a well-preserved infantile sexuality, as an antecedent phase of European civilization.

But what was a pejorative for Roheim has now, some seventy years later, grown worthy of emulation, suggests Lawlor. How remote, after all, are these Aboriginal views from the leading-edge thoughts and speculations of our own time? Aren't the morphogenetic fields of biologist Rupert Sheldrake just another form of the polymorphous dreaming of the ancestors?

The extravagant popularity of Findhorn and its nature spirit communications put animism back on the Western cultural map in the 1970s as a metaphysically legitimate concern. The planetary event called Harmonic Convergence in 1987 catapulted the forgotten science of geomancy and its catalogue of sacred landscape sites into widespread public awareness. The interwoven philosophies of deep ecology, ecofeminism, and engaged Buddhism uniformly advocate extending personal identity to include the plant and animal world in a new identity called the Ecological Self.

The spirit of Aboriginal culture provides eyes through which we may view, as if from the outside, our deteriorated and purulent condition." Our reacquaintance with the Aboriginal dreamtime, that "pure process of consciousness and image of wholeness," may "free us to dream the dreams of the next cycle in which humanity is reintegrated with the earth and the beauty and spirit of the natural world," says Lawlor.

Standing Up for Gaia: The Deep Ecological World without Boundary

A little of the impulse linking self and environment implicit in Steiner's anthroposophy and the Aboriginal dreamtime is beginning to show up in mainstream Western science and culture. This is most notable in the Gaia Hypothesis, the perception of our planet as a self-organized, homeostatic unity, as a single geophysiological entity of presumed sentience comprised of myriad interdependent life forms.

In the late 1970s, British atmospheric scientist James Lovelock pinned the ancient Greek nom de plume for our planet—Gaia, a titular name for the Goddess of Earth—on his grand systems model of planetary life. Lovelock encouraged us to radically expand our perceptual horizons: don't think in terms of local landscape or bioregion, think of the entire planet as a single, integral environment, whose planetary life subsumes all other forms of Earthly life.

Enthusiasts ever since have extrapolated Lovelock's cogent metaphor somewhat beyond his original intentions, investing the Gaian unity with sentience, purpose, even divinity, using it as the foundation for a planetary ethics. Hence the Gaian ethos. Our indivisible environment, the Gaian ethos tells us, is the planet in its totality. Perhaps this was how the Greeks originally perceived the planet, as a "Her" with planetary integrity and a legitimate role in the solar system.

The Gaian ethic provides the metaphorical and philosophical rationale for a host of complementary ecological views that redefine our human relationship with our planetary environment. These Gaian extensions include deep ecology, engaged Buddhism, ecofeminism, and a polyglot borrowing from native peoples' shamanism; all of these are often categorized as components of a new ecophilosophy.

In terms of what Lovelock calls "planetary medicine," these newer expressions of a Gaian ethos come closer to embodying what on a planetary scale approximates the values of empiric, holistic medicine, certainly when compared to the allopathically inspired attitudes and practices of mainstream environmentalism, not to mention our culture's standard (and irresponsible) industrial approach to the environment.

The fertile alliance of ecophilosophy with Buddhist spirituality have birthed a planet-encompassing ethos called DharmaGaia, in which the spiritual practice of an individual is conducted in the context, and on behalf of, the whole planet. A Buddhist needn't break stride to acknowledge that the Buddha Mind is as big as the planet—and bigger. The nexus of feminism and the Gaian perspective has generated a potent form of ecofriendly "green" political activism in the form of ecofeminism, bioregionalism, watershed politics, and the transnational Greens political movement. Concurrently, interest in the American new age community has sprung up in the wisdom traditions and shamanic experiences of native peoples on this continent and elsewhere; many are probing these lineages for insight in formulating a profounder, Gaian relationship with the world environment.

In this wide-ranging search through the planetary archives for new, sustainable Earth-based spiritualities and ecofriendly consumer habits, many have intuited that behind the biological complexities and interdependent relationships of ecology stands another dimension—the geomantic.

Geomancy—meaning "divination of Gaia"—is an old word recently dusted off for reuse to describe an unfamiliar realm of energy and subtle configuration lying behind or invisibly within the apparent ecological terrain. Traditionally in the medieval and Renaissance period, the term denoted a system of divination in which marks and configurations on the ground signified future predictions; today geomancy has taken on more of an energy and Earth mysteries connotation.

Lovelock's Geophysiology and the Planetary Physician

In the 1970s, atmospheric scientist James Lovelock formulated the outlines of his now famous Gaia Hypothesis, which has been widely debated, repudiated, extolled, and metaphorically extended ever since. Not insensitive to poetic nuance, Lovelock christened his integral planetary ecosystem, *Gaia,* a potent metaphor that's been richly elaborated ever since.

Strictly speaking, enthusiasts have expanded the Gaia metaphor somewhat beyond the rigorous physiological context Lovelock originally had in mind. For Lovelock, Gaia isn't alive, purposeful, or a Goddess; Gaia is a homeostatic physiological system the size of a planet that continually self-regulates its temperature and chemistry despite perturbations, which are often human-made.

Our Earth, postulated Lovelock on the basis of his worldwide atmospheric and climatological research, is a unified, self-regulating, living organism. The remarkable consistency of an unstable atmosphere at a constant composition over billions of years necessarily indicated some kind of automatic regulating agency and control system—"the presence of the invisible hand of life"—in favor of life, Lovelock reasoned.

For Lovelock, the evolution of biological species and their material environment is so tightly coupled that together they comprise a single, indivisible living organism. Earth's minerals, plants, animals, oceans, atmosphere—all are components of one large self-sustaining organism. Homeostasis of the oceans, climate, atmosphere, and planetary crust (the environment) is maintained by "active feedback processes operated automatically and unconsciously" by the resident biota (life). Lovelock christened this planetary regulator *Gaia,* after the ancient Greek concept of an Earth goddess.

It was NASA's startling photographs in the late 1960s of our blue-white planet that initially birthed the Gaia Hypothesis in his thinking, says Lovelock. That riveting astronautical view of our home planet as a whole entity inspired Lovelock with an unconventional "top-down approach to Earth and life science, the approach that physiologists use for living systems." A physiological model for understanding the Earth had actually been suggested in 1785 by James Hutton, the father of modern geology, when he lectured before the Royal Society of Edinburgh, Scotland. "I consider the Earth to be a super-organism," Hutton declared, "and that its proper study should be by physiology."

But that was the eighteenth century, when scientists were comfortable with a total systems model like physiology. Mainstream science in our day is still dominated by that "apartheid of Victorian biology and geology," a late-nineteenth-century conceptual remnant that divides the world into incommunicable geological and biological models, says Lovelock. Scientific specialists abound, each with his separate, proprietary turf, each with her expertise of minutiae, but almost nobody dares to take the holistic generalist's view—except Lovelock. With that characteristic flair of the English nonconformist, Lovelock would have none of this "disastrously fragmented science" and set out to remold scientific vision on a Gaian scale.

Lovelock first introduced his planetary perspective on biology, humanity, and evolution in 1979 with *Gaia: A New Look at Life on Earth*. Here he outraged scientists but rallied many others outside science, probably because his Gaian vision was on the edge of everyone's intuition. Lovelock's "detached, extra-terrestrial view" of Earth as a homeostatic organism evolving over time, even though what he self-effacingly called a "rough pencil sketch" at first, has catalyzed public discussion ever since.

As Lovelock formulates his Gaia model, unity and synthesis are key. A single evolutionary science can properly describe the history of planet Earth because the evolution of species and their environment "are tightly coupled together as a single and inseparable process." The Earth's atmosphere, oceans, climate, and crust are regulated at a "comfortable" state for life by the combined behavior of all living residential organisms. This homeostasis, says Lovelock, is maintained by continual active feedback happening automatically and "unconsciously" in the planetary biota.

In his second book, nearly ten years later, *The Ages of Gaia*, Lovelock presented a "testable model" for Gaia as a living organism and answered the technical objections raised by his critics in the preceding decade. He traced the evolution of Earth from the earliest epoch (the Archean, the time of our biological godparents, the cyanobacteria) into modern times and the ubiquitous ecological crisis. Lovelock reperceives the particularities of the environmental crisis—acid rain, ozone depletion, the carbon dioxide-greenhouse effect-climate loop, nuclear radiation—according to enlarged Gaian parameters. These are "perturbations," says Lovelock, that "momentarily" stress Gaia into achieving a new planetary homeostasis.

In *Healing Gaia*, Lovelock takes the stance of a geophysiologist. He's a planet doctor who gives us the "top down view of the Earth" according to the systems science of living organisms. The result is a highly valuable work, persuasively reasoned, amply documented, and handsomely produced; it's a physician's desk reference and treatment primer on a Gaian scale. With an allopath's classic bedside manner, Lovelock sagely explains the intricacies of Gaian anatomy, planetary biochemistry, circulation, climate regulation, symptomatology—typified by exfoliation, acid indigestion, an ozonemia, and greenhouse fever—and treatment options, as the family of man huddles in deep concern around a global ecosystem in great distress.

If Gaia is the organic regulator, how does She do it? To answer this Lovelock forwards the "old-fashioned transdisciplinary" approach of geophysiology, a bold revisioning that sees geological and biological processes as interdependent, automatic phases of a single, evolving planetary system, the superorganism called Gaia. "With geophysiology, a single evolutionary science, a theory of the living Earth, describes the history of the whole planet. We have to model the global system on the basis that we're dealing with a responsive physiological system, not just an inert, dead planet that happens to have life on it, which is the standard model most scientists use."

The Essential Theoretical Basis for Practicing Planetary Medicine

Geophysiology, then, is about the blood and nerves and sinews and health of our planet, metaphorically speaking. It's the foundation text for any study of planetary medicine. For Lovelock, it's the crucial whole systems science that takes a top-down look at the whole Earth. "Geophysiology offers a different view and a different set of priorities for global environmental problems," explains Lovelock.

With this, Lovelock established the "essential theoretical basis" for the profession of planetary medicine. "We need, as well as science, an empirical approach like medicine for our environmental ills." As the first in what he hopes will be a new breed of planet doctors, Lovelock diagnoses complex, intractable environmental problems—acid rain, ozone depletion, nuclear radiation, methane pollution, greenhouse gases—as health crises and "perturbations" in the homeostatic life of a four-billion-year-old living planet.

"There is nothing to stop us from going through a routine examination of the temperature charts and the biochemical analyses of the body fluids of Gaia's planetary biology," Lovelock says. "With any class of environmental problem, such as tropical rain forest clearance, we look at the whole system, try to envisage what it would do in a state of health, then compare that with what's happening to it now. We look for physical signs of damage, the way a physician does. We measure temperature, pulse rate, and come to empirical conclusions, rather than exact scientific answers. These conclusions suggest remedies, treatments, or at least palliations. We can take action in advance of hard and fast scientific conclusions and expensive models based on these issues. Inevitably there will be mistakes, but the net effect will be beneficial."

In Lovelock's Gaian diagnostics, "ozonemia is the dermatologist's dilemma." The fear of skin cancer, the apparent medical consequence of ozone depletion, led at first to a "global hypochondria" and the panicky ozone wars that sought to reduce the level of ultraviolet exposure to zero. This was a humanist but not a Gaian analysis, based on inadequate atmospheric modeling, and thus "one of the truly great scientific myths of the century," contends Lovelock.

Ultraviolet radiation is part of our natural environment and has been there as long as life itself, states Lovelock, and it's not really the point anyway. Ozone depletion is "a warning of other more serious surprises yet to come"—the "carbon dioxide fever" and the climate-threatening greenhouse effect, for example. Ozonemia is one aspect of a complex interdependent Gaian web of rain forest clearance, chemicalized agriculture, methane gas pollution, acid rain, and desertification. These are all dangerous "geocidal acts," warns Lovelock, perturbations that could precipitate a planetary "shudder" and a sudden Gaian shift to a new, possibly posthuman, homeostasis.

Lovelock's geophysiology gives him both the tool for diagnosis and the means for prescription. Overall, the planetary outlook isn't that bleak, actually—that is, from Gaia's point of view. "Nothing we do will wipe out the system. I don't have to be optimistic for Gaia. She's looked after herself for so long, She won't be worried by us."

Mother Earth will eventually always correct imbalances, says Lovelock, but it might mean a shift in the type and nature of her living biota, including humankind. Gaia, metaphorically speaking, is neither a doting, tolerant mother, nor a fragile, delicate damsel, suggests Lovelock. "She is stern and tough, always keeping the world warm and comfortable for those who obey the rules, but ruthless in her destruction of those who transgress." If not ruthless, perhaps startlingly efficient in her methods, such as using a volcanic eruption to cool down the planet.

So when Gaia recovers from her present interglacial warm period, her planetary fever, She may do so with an apocalyptic shudder. Left to herself, Gaia would be relaxing into another normal, comfortable ice age, explains Lovelock. "She may be unable to relax because we've been busy removing her skin and using it as farmland and adding a vast blanket of greenhouse gases to the already feverish patient. In these circumstances Gaia is much more likely to shudder and move over to a new stable state fit for a different and more amenable biota."

How amenable a biota is humankind, anyway? "We are a responsive species and therefore one that will pull back from geocide in time," emphasizes Lovelock. His concern is that the human response might be "iatrogenic, with consequences more severe than those of the poison." Lovelock is optimistic, but he's really not a humanist. He doesn't categorically put the human interests first in this "very democratic planetary community," the superorganism called Gaia.

This is no tenure for anyone, any species, on this planet. Humankind may represent Gaia learning to think consciously, but this becomes a dangerous assumption if it promotes arrogance. If we seriously foul our nest and treat our planet badly, we can be voted out and destroy ourselves, warns Lovelock. Meanwhile, he's taken on the vacant position of "shop steward" and "speaker of the house" for the other Earth household "partners in Gaia, the bacteria and the less attractive forms of life."

More than steward, Lovelock sees himself as an Earth trustee, which entails accountability to future generations. "I see the world as a living organism of which we are a part—not the owner, nor the tenant, not even a passenger on that obsolete metaphor 'spaceship Earth.'" When we think geophysiologically, when we understand our intimate place in the superorganic life of Gaia, we will profoundly reconsider our present habits of exploitation. We'll see with a shock that our contemporary frenzy of agriculture and forestry is global ecocide. "Would we mine our livers for nutrients? Would we raze our hair and plant our scalps with tomatoes?" Probably not, but we might plant some trees, adds Lovelock. Gaian homeostasis begins with the local activity of individual organisms, says Lovelock—and that includes the responsive human.

Understanding the Gaian model instills an awareness of "the significance of the individual organism," Lovelock stresses. "It is always from the action of individuals that powerful local, regional, and global systems evolve. It's up to us to act personally in a way that is constructive," advises Lovelock. "Living with Gaia is a personal responsibility and each of us will develop a personal solution to the problem," suggests Lovelock. "It gives you a gloating feeling of righteousness, that you're on the side of the angels," concludes Lovelock with a twinkly grin.

That's the kind of planetary medicine a lot of Westerners could start administering to a feverish Gaia today. "Thinking of the Earth as alive makes it seem, on happy days, in the right places, as if the whole planet were celebrating a sacred ceremony."

An Act of Ecological "Self-Realization"

This sacred ceremony may also represent an act of global self-awareness. We turn to Norway, where an ecophilosophy called deep ecology provides another link in the Gaian ethos. Deep ecology got its formal start in Norway about twenty years ago, when Arne Naess, a philosophy professor now in his eighties at the University of Oslo—"the most influential Scandinavian philosopher of this century," declares Australian deep ecologist Warwick Fox—coined the term and outlined its protocols in a landmark 1972 paper.

"The deepness of normative and descriptive premises questioned characterizes the movement," said Naess. "The issue of deep ecology is to ask deeper questions. We ask, which society, which education, which form of religion, is beneficial for all life on the planet as a whole. What we need today is a tremendous expansion of ecological thinking in what I call ecosophy, or a shift from science to earth wisdom." Naess credits the beginnings of the international deep ecology movement to the 1962 publication of Rachel Carson's *Silent Spring*, which "insisted that everything, not just politics, would have to be changed."

Naess is not an ecologist waxing philosophical, but a truly philosophical mind using the traditional tools of this discipline to reformulate our human relationship with the natural world. Ecology is a limited science that employs scientific methods; philosophy is a "forum of debate on fundamentals"; but ecosophy, argues Naess, is "a philosophy of ecological harmony or equilibrium" that includes "*both* norms, rules, postulates, value priority announcements *and* hypotheses concerning the state of affairs in our universe." The deep ecology movement, says Naess, is "rich in philosophical implications" as it aims for "wisdom rather than science or information."

Naess' ecosophical model has three tenets. The first is ecocentrism, which refers to adopting an ecology-centered or Earth-centrist approach to our interactions with the environment rather than the standard anthropocentric, or human-centrist approach. Ecocentrism considers the nonhuman world to be valuable "in and of itself," said Naess, to possess "intrinsic value" and "a right to live and flourish" irrespective of any utilitarian values affixed by humankind. His second premise is that we must ask deeper, more penetrating questions about the realities of our human-to-nature relationship, looking for root causes of the multiple, interdependent ecological crises rather than focusing on symptoms.

"The term *deep* is supposed to suggest explication of fundamental presuppositions of valuation as well as of facts and hypotheses," explains Naess. Third, we can usefully expand our parameters of individual identity, to identify more widely and deeply with the world in an act of ecological "Self-realization." The opposite of a widened self, or the failure to expand self-identification to include the environment, is alienation, a root cause of the ecological crisis.

This expanded sense of self spontaneously motivates us to defend the environment and the integrity of the world, says Naess. "Considering the accelerating rate of irreversible ecological destruction worldwide, I find it acceptable to continue fighting ecological unsustainability. Long-range local, district, regional, national, and global ecological sustainability is the criterion of ecologically responsible policies as a whole."

"Not until I discovered the writings of Arne Naess did I find a label for my feelings," comments deep ecologist Bill Devall, an author, academic, activist from northern California who, like others, was moved to a deeper consideration of what Naess calls the "ultimate norms": biocentric equality, core democracy in the biosphere, maximal Self-realization in mixed communities as an approach to being in the world. Naess' ultimate "norms and tendencies," the bedrock tenets of his ecosophy as a philosophical ecology, "express a value priority system" not derived from ecology by logic or induction.

"Ecological knowledge and the lifestyle of the ecological field-worker have *suggested, inspired, and fortified* the perspectives of the Deep Ecology movement," says Naess. The consideration of ultimate norms, the foundation of deep ecology, is a largely interior task, what Gary Snyder once called "the real work," Devall points out.

First to be questioned is the size of one's self. Naess contends one's sense of self-identity—the bodily and psychological parameters of individual selfness—should, properly, encompass a forest or a watershed, perhaps an entire bioregion: "a mixed community of humans, bears, sheep, wolves, trees, and mountains." The California poet Robinson Jeffers called this "falling in love outwards," and it's a profound experience—"an affective conversion experience," says Devall—that can lead to a deeper, ecologically widened, more empathic, *transpersonal* self.

That's why Australian deep ecologist Warwick Fox calls Naess' third tenet "transpersonal ecology," because "it clearly points to the realization of a sense of self that extends beyond (or that is *trans-*) any narrowly delimited biographical or egoic sense of self. Broadening and deepening our identification—or our sense of felt commonality—with the world around us leads us from a relatively narrow, atomistic, isolated, or particle-like sense of self to a wide, expansive, participatory, or field-like one."

This sense of one's body extending into the landscape is the deep identification California poet Gary Snyder had in mind with his term "reinhabitation." For Bill Devall and a growing worldwide community of ecologists, philosophers, feminists, Buddhists, artists, Greenpeace-type activists, and native peoples, it's taking the form of a grass-roots coalition in defense of nature.

The broad movement is generally called "deep ecology" to distinguish it from "shallow environmentalism." Devall notes that the deep, long-range ecology movement extends the principle of interrelatedness into every aspect of our daily lives. The experience of deep identification with nature, says Devall, inevitably initiates a painful awareness of what ecologist Aldo Leopold once called "the wounds of the world."

But this kind of compassion-generating insight must precede activism and brings with it a constant, deep questioning of social norms. "Before changing paradigms or political ideologies or social institutions, we must change the way we experience life," suggests Devall.

Deep ecology offers instruction at both ends of the pole, for both penetrating introspection and appropriate activism, while its rich vocabulary—bioregionalism, ecocentrism, biocentric egalitarianism, ecological self, ultimate norms, maturity—reflects its far-ranging, philosophically radical concerns. Deep ecology "is a hope-filled, affirmative approach to being in the world in the sense of getting back to our roots," notes Devall. "Bearing witness to our emotional wounds, our alienation from the rest of nature, we can move into healing relationships with a watershed, with our bioregion, with Gaia.

"Supporters of deep ecology do not engage in political activism to advance the ego, to gain power for the sake of power over other persons, but to advance and affirm the myriad of beings, the integrity of our broad and deep self." We are best positioned to help the world when our selves are "very broad and deep," when compassion toward all beings and insight into the web of nature well forth out of our own suffering, adds Devall. The deep ecologist necessarily takes a courageous stance as "gentle ecowarrior" or "bodhisattva warrior," helping as much as one can, "as much as we have energy to bear witness to on this earth."

"I am part of the rain forest protecting myself"

Deep ecologist John Seed, founder of the Rainforest Information Center in New South Wales, Australia, and an international activist, evokes the ambiance of this ecological self-expansion. "'I am protecting the rain forest' develops into 'I am part of the rain forest protecting myself. I am that part of the rain forest recently emerged into thinking.' The thousands of years of (imagined) separation are over and we begin to recall our true nature."

When the definition of human self encompasses plants, animals, and mountains within sight, the minimal Self dilates into maximal Self, says Devall. That's because, according to deep ecology, truly, Self *is* bioregion or, unilaterally, the ecological web. "*Self* realization means not only humans but all other beings are free at last, liberated from the social jail, the constrictions of the dominant mindset. Whales are free again to follow their own destiny." When one thinks like a mountain, says John Seed, who facilitates this transformative experience in his Council of All Beings group rituals, "one thinks also like the black bear, so that honey dribbles down your fur as you catch the bus to work." At this level of identification, *Self* means organic wholeness, the whole natural world—environment—in allegiance to the maxim, "No one is saved until we are all saved."

Seed's Council of All Beings deep ecology initiations are an attempt to shift humans from the center stage of anthropocentrism to a humbler biocentric position of "nothing special," what Aldo Leopold called being "a plain member of the biotic community." Deep ecology refuses to validate the prevailing cultural assumption that "humans are the center of the universe, the source of all value, the crown of creation," says Seed. The world is not a pyramid topped by humanity but rather an extensive web "of which we are one strand interconnected with all the other strands."

Forests are not a resource for human economic gain, but the matrix out of which humans and all other life forms grew over a span of one hundred million years, argues Seed. Human intelligence, which we prize so highly, "is just a tiny subset of the intelligence of this rainforest, which gave birth to it, and an even tinier subset of the intelligence of Gaia herself, the integrated, functioning living being which is our planet."

Although human intelligence, etiologically, is a tiny subset of Gaian intelligence, suggests Seed, the deep ecology perspective allows us to experience "our *actual self* stretching back over these vast periods of time," so that when a person says "I" this encompasses a "much vaster reality." Converting to an ecosophical view isn't something for us to entertain in our leisure, either, urges Seed. We need "a total revolution in human consciousness"—today, if possible. "The only thing that will save us, it seems, is an almost instantaneous awakening within human beings as to where our true self-interest lies—something that will be so enlightening that all our present religious and cultural conflicts will just fade into a kind of mist."

When we start cultivating this widened ecological self, the "metaphysical chasm" between the values of the dominant worldview and deep ecology becomes evident, explains Devall. The prevailing attitude about individual human self and environment is Newtonian, fragmented, mechanistic, utilitarian, based on human dominance over all species and resource management of the environment. Nature is "humanized" into a marketable commodity and all crisis solutions are technological—behavioral aspects of what George Sessions, another key figure in the American deep ecology movement, calls "the anthropocentric detour."

Putting "Humanity First!" during the last two millennia and increasingly since the Industrial Revolution, says Sessions, has been a costly, mistaken detour from ecocentric "Earth First!" priorities, which, if it continues unchecked, "will lead inexorably, perhaps with the best of intentions, to an accelerating decline of the earth and all its inhabitants."

In contrast, deep ecology emphasizes harmony with nature, biospecies equality, the principles of diversity and symbiosis, complexity in contrast to complication, simple material needs, frugality, recycling, appropriate low-energy technologies, bioregional identity, local autonomy and decentralization, and the primacy of the quality of life over standard of living. "Naess challenged people to begin *thinking* in a dialogue process," notes Devall. "Deep ecology *combines* the day-to-day problems of environment, including human health problems, with the global, cultural, psychological, long-range problems."

Deep ecology fosters what Naess calls a gestalt form of perception that sees wholes, not fragments. Naess terms this "the rejection of the man-in-the-environment image in favor of the relational total field image. Organisms are knots in the biospherical net or field of intrinsic relations. This deeper stream addresses questions which draw us to major realignment in our self and in our thinking and calls us to long-range solutions from an ecological perspective." They give us new tools for repositioning our environment.

References

Allen, Michael D., and Wolf, Harri, "A Comparison of Applied Kinesiological and Applied Iridological Findings," *Iridology Review, Journal of the National Iridology Research Association,* Vol. 1, No. 2, (Autumn 1987).

Allen, Paula Gunn, "The Woman I love is a Planet; The Planet I love is a Tree," in *Reweaving the World: The Emergence of Ecofeminism,* edited by Irene Diamond and Gloria Feman Orenstein, Sierra Club Books, San Francisco, 1990.

—*Grandmothers of the Light: A Medicine Woman's Sourcebook,* Beacon Press, Boston, 1991.

Bates, Betsy, "Eye Abnormality May be Heart Disease Indicator," *Los*

Angeles Herald Examiner, (November 19, 1987).

Battista, John R., "The Holographic Model, Holistic Paradigm, Information Theory and Consciousness," in *The Holographic Paradigm and Other Paradoxes: Exploring the Leading Edge of Science,* edited by Ken Wilber, New Science Library, Shambhala, Boston, 1982.

Bayly, Doreen E., *Reflexology Today: The Stimulation of the Body's Healing Forces Through Foot Massage,* Thorsons Publishers, Rochester, 1987.

Begley, Sharon, Wright, Lynda, Church, Vernon, and Hager, Mary, "Mapping the Brain," *Newsweek,* (April 20, 1992).

Becker, Robert O., M.D., and Selden, Gary, *The Body Eelectric: Electromagnetism and the Foundation of Life,* William Morrow and Company, New York, 1985.

—*Cross Currents: The Perils of Electropollution, the Promise of Electromedicine,* Jeremy P. Tarcher, Inc., Los Angeles, 1990.

Bentov, Itzhak, *Stalking the Wild Pendulum—On the Mechanics of Consciousness,* Destiny Books, Rochester, 1988.

Birlaji, Ghanshyam Singh, *Systematic Palmistry—An Introduction to Palmistry,* National Research Institute for Self-Understanding, Westmount, Quebec, 1983.

Bohm, David, *Wholeness and the Implicate Order,* Ark Paperbacks, Routledge and Kegan Paul, London, 1980.

Borelli, Peter, "The Ecophilosophers," *The Amicus Journal,* (Spring 1988).

Bradford, George, *How Deep is Deep Ecology?* Times Change Press, Ojai, 1989.

Briggs, John, and Peat, David F., "Interview with David Bohm," *OMNI,* (January 1987).

Burr, Harold Saxton, *Blueprint for Immortality—The Electric Patterns of Life,* C.W. Daniel Company, Saffron Walden, 1972.

Byers, Dwight C., *Better Health With Foot Reflexology,* Ingham Publishing, Saint Petersburg, 1983.

Chatwin, Bruce, *The Songlines,* Picador/Pan Books, London, 1987.

Cowan, James, *Mysteries of the Dreaming: The Spiritual Life of Australian Aborigines,* Prism/Unity, Bridport, 1989.

Dale, Ralph Alan, Ph.D., *The Micro-Acupuncture Systems, Books I-IV,* Dialectic Press, Surfside, 1978.

Devall, Bill, "Political Activism in a Time of War," *ReVision,* Vol. 13, No. 3, (Winter 1991).

—*Simple in Means, Rich in Ends—Practicing Deep Ecology,* Peregrine Smith Books, Salt Lake City, 1988.

—and Sessions, George, *Deep Ecology: Living as if Nature Mattered,* Peregrine Smith Books, Salt Lake City, 1985.

Dowie, Mark, "The New Face of Environmentalism," *World Policy Journal,* (Winter 1991/92).

Dychtwald, Ken, "Reflections on the Holographic Paradigm," in *The Holographic Paradigm and Other Paradoxes: Exploring the Leading Edge of Science,* edited by Ken Wilber, New Science Library, Shambhala, Boston, 1982.

Fox, Warwick, "Self and World: A Transpersonal Ecological Approach," *ReVision,* Vol. 13, No. 3, (Winter 1991).

—*Toward a Transpersonal Ecology: Developing New Foundations for Environmentalism,* Shambhala, Boston, 1990.

Gerber, Richard, M.D., *Vibrational Medicine: New Choices for Healing Ourselves,* Bear and Company, Santa Fe, 1988.

Goosmann-Legger, Astrid I., *Zone Therapy Using Foot Massage,* C.W. Daniel Company, Saffron Walden, 1986.

Hall, Nicola M., *Reflexology: A Patient's Guide,* Thorsons Publishing Group, Wellingborough, 1986.

Grove, Richard H., "Origins of Western Environmentalism," *Scientific American,* (July 1992).

Hameroff, Stuart Roy, "Ch'i: A Neural Hologram? Microtubules, Bioholography, and Acupuncture," *American Journal of Chinese Medicine,* Vol. 2, No. 2, (1974).

Hiss, Tony, *The Experience of Place,* Alfred A. Knopf, New York, 1990.

Ingham, Eunice D., *The Original Works of Eunice D. Ingham,* Ingham Publishing, Saint Petersburg, 1984.

Johnson, Denny, *What the Eye Reveals, Book One: An Introduction to the Rayid Method of Iris Interpretation,* Rayid Publications, Goleta, 1984.

Kelley, Kevin W., *The Home Planet*, Addison-Wesley Publishing Company, Reading, 1988.

Kraft, Kenneth, "Engaged Buddhism: An Introduction," in *The Path of Compassion: Writings on Socially Engaged Buddhism*, edited by Fred Eppsteiner, Parallax Press, Berkeley, 1988.

Kriege, Theodor, *Fundamental Basis of Irisdiagnosis*, L.N. Fowler and Company, Romford, 1986.

Lambert, Johanna, *Wise Women of the Dreamtime: Aboriginal Tales of the Ancestral Powers.* Inner Traditions International, Rochester, VT, 1993.

Lawlor, Robert, "Voices of the First Day—Awakening in the Aboriginal Dreamtime," *Inner Traditions,* Rochester, 1991.

Leviton, Richard, "How the Body Programs the Brain," *East West,* (August 1988).

—"Mind/Belly Theory," *East West,* (February 1990).

—"The Holographic Body," *East West,* (August 1988).

—"Tuning in to Vibrational Medicine," *East West,* (October 1988).

—"Vibrational Medicine," *Yoga Journal,* (March/April 1989).

—"Healing With Nature's Energy," *East West,* (June 1986).

—"Voices from the Dreamtime," *Yoga Journal,* (September/ October 1992).

—"The Father of Gaia," *East West,* (November/December 1991).

—"The Island Within," *Yoga Journal,* (January/February 1992).

—"Gaian Spirituality," *Yoga Journal,* (May/June 1992).

—"Home Sweet Home—A Blue and White Jewel," *East West,* (February 1989).

—"On the Wild Side, Notes from off the Trail," *East West,* (March 1991).

—"World Without End," *East West,* (August 1989).

Lovelock, James, "Gaia: The World as Living Organism," *New Scientist,* (December 18, 1986).

—"Geophysiology," *The Gaia Magazine,* No. 3, (1991).

—"I Speak for the Earth," *Resurgence,* No. 129, (July/August 1988).

—"Stand Up For Gaia," *Resurgence,* No. 132, (January/February 1989).

—"The First Leslie Cooper Memorial Lecture Given at Plymouth on 10 April 1989," *Journal of the Marine Biology Association,* Vol. 69, (1989).

—*Healing Gaia: Practical Medicine for the Planet,* Harmony Books, 1991.

—*The Ages of Gaia: A Biography of Our Living Earth,* W.W. Norton and Company, New York, 1988.

—"On the Brink," *The Gaia Magazine,* No. 1, (1990).

—and Epton, Sidney, "The Quest for Gaia," *New Scientist,* (February 6, 1975).

MacRobert Alan M., "Reality Shopping: A Consumer's Guide to New Age Hokum," *Whole Earth Review,* (Fall 1986).

Macy, Joanna, "What's So Good About Feeling Bad?" interview by Jonathan Adolph and Peggy Taylor, *New Age Journal,* (January/February 1991).

Manaka, Yoshio, M.D., Itaya, Kazuko, C.A., "Acupuncture as Intervention in the Biological Information System," edited by Stephen Birch, unpublished manuscript, 1988.

Matsumoto, Kiiko, and Birch, Stephen, *Five Elements and Ten Stems: Nan Ching Theory, Diagnosis and Practice,* Paradigm Publications, Brookline, 1983.

—*Hara Diagnosis: Reflections on the Sea,* Paradigm Publications, Brookline, 1988.

Meyer, Michael, "The Way the Whorls Turn," *Newsweek,* (February 13, 1989).

Morris, David, "The Four Stages of Environmentalism," *Utne Reader,* (March/April 1992).

Naess, Arne, "Identification as a Source of Deep Ecological Attitudes," in *Deep Ecology,* Tobias, Michael, editor, Avant Books, San Diego, 1985.

—"Politics and the Ecological Crisis: An Introductory Note," *ReVision,* Vol. 13, No. 3, (Winter 1991).

Neher, Andrew, *The Psychology of Transcendence*, Prentice-Hall, Englewood Cliffs, 1980.

Nelson, Richard, *The Island Within*, North Point Press, San Francisco, 1989.

Oleson, Terrence D., Ph.D., and Kroening, Richard J., M.D., "A Comparison of Chinese and Nogier Auricular Acupuncture Points," *American Journal of Acupuncture*, Vol. 11, No. 3, (July-September 1983).

—and Bresler, David E., "An Experimental Evaluation of Auricular Diagnosis: The Somatotypic Mapping of Musculoskeletal Pain at Ear Acupuncture Points," *Pain*, Vol. 8, (1980).

Oschman, James L., Ph.D., "Structure and Properties of Ground Substances," *American Zoologist*, Vol. 24, No. 1, (1984).

—*The Connective Tissue and Myofascial Systems*, The Rolf Institute, Boulder, 1987.

Pearce, Fred, "Gaia: A Revolution Comes of Age," *New Scientist*, (March 17, 1988).

Porritt, Jonathon, "Seeing Green: How We Can Create a More Satisfying Society," *Utne Reader*, (November/December 1989).

Pribram, Karl H., "What the Fuss is All About," in *The Holographic Paradigm and Other Paradoxes: Exploring the Leading Edge of Science*, edited by Ken Wilber, New Science Library, Shambhala, Boston, 1982.

—*Languages of the Brain: Experimental Paradoxes and Principles in Neuropsychology*, Prentice-Hall, Englewood Cliffs, 1971.

Roth, M., and Wolf, H., "An Introduction to Applied Iridology," *Iridology Review, Journal of the National Iridology Research Association*, Vol. 1, No. 1, (Spring 1987).

Scheller, Melanie, "Do the Eyes Have It?" *Medical SelfCare*, (July-August 1987).

Seed, John, "Rainforest Man," interview in *Timeless Visions, Healing Voices*, edited by Stephan Bodian, The Crossing Press, Freedom, 1991.

Sessions, George, "Ecocentrism and the Anthropocentric Doctor," *ReVision*, Vol. 13, No. 3, (Winter 1991).

—"The Deep Ecology Movement: A Review," *Environmental Review*, (Summer 1987).

Sharan Farida, M.D., *Iridology: A Complete Guide to Diagnosing Through the Iris and to Related Forms of Treatment*, Thorsons Publishing Group, Wellingborough, 1989.

Simon, Allie, Worthen, David M., M.D., Mitas, Lt. John A., "An Evaluation of Iridology," *Journal of the American Medical Association*, Vol. 242, No. 13, (September 28, 1979).

Snyder, Gary, "Buddhism and the Possibilities of a Planetary Culture," in *The Path of Compassion: Writings on Socially Engaged Buddhism*, edited by Fred Eppsteiner, Parallax Press, Berkeley, 1988.

—*The Practice of the Wild*, North Point Press, San Francisco, 1990.

Spretnak, Charlene, "Ecofeminism: Our Roots and Flowering," in *Reweaving the World: The Emergence of Ecofeminism*, edited by Irene Diamond and Gloria Feman Orenstein, Sierra Club Books, San Francisco, 1990.

—"Gaian Spirituality," *Woman of Power*, No. 20, (Spring 1991).

—*States of Grace: The Recovery of Meaning in the Postmodern Age*, HarperSanFrancisco, San Francisco, 1991.

Steiner, Rudolf, *Anthroposophical Spiritual Science and Medical Therapy: Second Medical Course*, Mercury Press, Spring Valley, 1991.

—*At the Gates of Spiritual Science*, Rudolf Steiner Press, London, 1970.

—*Cosmosophy, Vol. 1*, Anthroposophic Press, Spring Valley, 1985.

—*True and False Paths in Spiritual Investigation*, Rudolf Steiner Press, London, 1927.

—*Man as a Picture of the Living Spirit*, Rudolf Steiner Press, London, 1972.

—*Planetary Spheres and Their Influence on Man's Life on Earth and in Spiritual Worlds*, Rudolf Steiner Press, London, 1982.

—*Man's Being, His Destiny, and World-Evolution*, Anthroposophic Press, Spring Valley, 1984.

—*An Outline of Occult Science*, Anthroposophic Press, Spring Valley, NY, 1972.

—*The Spiritual Hierarchies and Their Reflection in the Physical World*, Anthroposophic Press, Spring Valley, NY, 1970.

—*True and False Paths in Spiritual Investigation*, Rudolf Steiner Press, London, 1985.

—*Human and Cosmic Thought*, Rudolf Steiner Press, London, 1961.

—*Man and the World of Stars*, Anthroposophic Press, New York, 1963.

—*Philosophy, Cosmology and Religion*, Anthroposophic Press, Spring Valley, New York, 1984.

—*Supersensible Man*, Anthroposophical Publishing Company, London, 1961

Stuetzer, Paul Howard, "Iris Constitutions: Iridology and the Detection of Pre-Cancerous Conditions," *Iridology Review, Journal of the National Iridology Research Association*, Vol. 1, No. 1, (Spring 1987).

Talbot, Michael, "The Universe as Hologram: Does Objective Reality Exist, or is the Universe a Phantasm?" *Village Voice*, (September 22, 1987).

—*The Holographic Universe*, HarperCollins Publishers, New York, 1991.

Taubes, Gary, "An Electrifying Possibility," *Discover*, (April 1986).

Thompson, William Irwin, editor, *Gaia 2, Emergence: The New Science of Becoming*, Lindisfarne Press, 1991.

Wagner, Franz, Ph.D., *Reflex Zone Massage: Handbook of Therapy and Self-Help*, Thorsons Publishing Group, Wellingborough, 1987.

Wexu, Mario, D.Ac., *The Ear: Gateway to Balancing the Body*, Aurora Press, New York, 1975.

Wolf, Harri, and Vahjen, James, *Instructional Iris Analysis*, Case Studies, National Iridology Research Association, Santa Fe, 1979.

Zoeteman, Kees, *Gaiasophy: An Approach to Ecology*, Lindisfarne Press, Hudson, NY, 1991.

CHAPTER 5

Mysteries of the Body:
Remaking Our Inner Environment

Participating in the Life of the Body

Through our considerations of environmental energies and the holographic human, it should be clear by now that as human organisms we are intimately, intrinsically embedded in the environmental web of life. Energies from the external environment have a measurable physical and psychological impact on the human organism, and the theory of holography provides a vivid metaphor for extending our understanding of how the multifaceted human organism participates in the web of environmental, planetary, even cosmic energies. According to the theory of the holograph and its extension to the human organism, at many levels intricate models of order and connection, from cosmic to physiological, keep us embedded in a multishelled environment.

So this is the mechanism of connection and relatedness and describes our relationship to an "outer" environment, but how do we fare in relation to our "inner" environment? We are "wired" to the outer environment via multiple holographic systems of order within the human organism; this connection focuses our relation-ship with the environment outwardly. Does the same connection work inwardly? Does consciousness have any efficacy *in* here, with-in the human organism? Is this inner environment in any way mutable in response to will, desire, or acts of consciousness? Is it more than allopathy's "stupid meat machine"?

This chapter answers, resoundingly, *yes,* and will provide numer-ous convincing examples in support of this conclusion. Our rela-tionship with ourselves, with our own organism, if this doesn't sound solipsistic, can be participatory and cocreative. We just have to be willing to expand our sense of what's possible and of what self-identity authentically consists.

Empiric medicine documents several phenomena—placebo response, psychoneuroimmunology (PNI), spontaneous remission, multiple personality disorders, the survival of consciousness in coma—that demonstrate vividly how mind can profoundly alter the bodily environment when applied with at least marginal awareness. Imagine what range of malleability is possible with focused con-sciousness, the bolder empirical spokesmen urge us.

Making Pleasure-Inducing Drugs in Your Head

In 1986, Los Angeles psychotherapist Evelyn Silvers, Ph.D., hit upon a stunning way to help drug addicts kick their habit. She showed them how to make the drugs in their heads—or at least experience their effects. Already a decade earlier, Silvers had used a combination of authoritative suggestion and guided visualization to help patients produce apparent "brain drugs"—neurotransmit-ters associated with specific emotional states—that produced the same calming, numbing, or consciousness-altering effects as their accustomed heroin, alcohol, cocaine, or tranquilizers.

Silvers told her clients that their brain's "inner pharmacy" could generate the drugs to treat any situation, such as the most unre-lenting pain. Silvers instructed each patient to imagine building up a large supply of the neurotransmitter endorphin (a known internal painkiller or natural opiate) in his or her brain, then to mentally inject the endorphins into the bloodstream.

Everyone, including Silvers, found the results impressive: chronic, immedicable pain radically improved or disappeared; the clients felt *as if* they were experiencing the actual drugs. Afterward many of her patients, practicing the "brain drug" technique on their own, were able to wean themselves off their habitual painkillers. Then in 1986, buoyed by these successes, Silvers decided to try out her methods on a group of entrenched drug addicts, with histories of four to forty years of addiction to heroin, Valium, alcohol, or cocaine.

This was a desperate, hardened group indeed, most of whom had long since abandoned career, family, and productive living for a downward-turning spiral of addiction, physical pain, guilt, and ineffectual drug fixes. Silvers taught them the brain pharmacy technique, but, elaborating a little, told her group that not only can the brain generate its own painkillers, but it can biochemically replicate the effect of any street drug. She won the addicts' trust when she explained that in her view the brains of addicted people are deficient in certain normally innate neurotransmitters that produce the normative conditions of feeling happy, in control, calm, and balanced. Chronic addiction, Silvers told them, is a desperate form of self-medication not in principle unlike the use of insulin to shore up an underactive pancreas.

Silvers wasn't trying to justify the lifestyle of drug addiction, but to biochemically rationalize the strong addictive cravings that held them all in bondage, and to show them a way out. She reasoned, just a little in advance of medical findings, that in so far as our brains have the necessary receptor sites to bind to the neuroactive chemicals present in the street drugs, this must mean that addictive substances are in some way equivalent in composition and purpose to neurochemicals made "in house," like external replacements for internal deficiencies. If true, then learning how to generate these brain drugs on demand could dissolve the addictive cravings for "outside" drugs and revolutionize the whole approach to drug addiction therapy.

Silvers instructed her clients to mentally build up a large store of their favorite drug, then, on her signal, to release the "drug" throughout their system. The simulated drug fix was so strong Silvers had to wait twenty minutes for the group to gain enough coherency to discuss their experiences. You now have learned how be in control of the drug, Silvers advised her astonished group. "I find this a superb example of how awareness can heal," notes Deepak Chopra, M.D., who reports Silver's results in his *Unconditional Life.*

"Once a plausible tool was offered, the mind allowed itself to break out of an old boundary."

The brain is a neutral agent with no will of its own, says Chopra; it can maintain or abandon an addiction depending on how it is directed. "The brain cannot free itself; it needs instruction from the mind." The brilliance of Silver's methodology, says Chopra, is that it credits the mind-body connection with the ability to accomplish whatever it chooses, acknowledging a therapeutic carte blanche in which the brain is "the mind's infinitely resourceful servant, able to carry out what it was told to do. When Silvers offered these addicts a drugless fix, they discovered on the spot that addiction was not a prison but an illusion."

If we make our own reality, then we can make it better, says Chopra. Chopra's concern is not just our physical or psychoemotional health; he wants to provoke healing in the metaphysical foundations of our existence. He wants to heal our "hurt awareness." Reality for most of us is a highly subjective, personalized field of experience, comments Chopra. The forces that shape our personal reality are unconscious beliefs, attitudes, perceptions, the boundaries of subjective conditioning—what the ancient Indian sages called "mistakes of the intellect."

We suppose, mistakenly, that the world is solid, material, static, and formidable, yet the rishis assure us it's really a mirage of molecules, a mask of maya, and a "layer of trick effects." If reality is malleable, who's in charge? The self, answers Chopra, the "potentiality of untold possibilities" and the field of pure awareness at the heart of atoms, molecules, human bodies, and galaxies. If he's right, then obviously our health is entirely negotiable.

Better health means better metaphysics, he implies, guiding us progressively through the conditioned personality to the silent, witnessing ground of being behind it all. Chopra's thesis of unconditional life is really about preventive holistic medicine at the ontological level of being. So with great slyness, like a magician performing before our disarmed skepticism, Chopra constructs the philosophical rationale for meditation and transcendental experience. There is no cure from the outside anyway, Chopra warns us. Ill health arises from the field of subjective conditioning and personal reality, and only a resolute, courageous turning inward will set in motion the innate healing forces. And don't wait until you're dying to finally address this, adds Chopra. "Disease is no way to solve the core issues of life. People have to be trans-formed *before* the crisis."

That's the ideal of course, but it's better to be transformed some-time than never. Silvers' casefile of her work with clients suffering from drug and alcohol addiction, rheumatoid arthritis, cancer, and AIDS, yields numerous other surprising examples along the same lines. There was a family from Chicago, she relates, in which a woman, whose husband and son were both M.D.s, had terminal cancer, or so her oncologists told her. They had exhausted all the therapeutic options but nothing had produced a cure or even remis-sion. The last oncologist they consulted, admitting he couldn't pro-vide any useful therapy at this point and that she would quite likely die in a few weeks, advised her husband and son, in private, to make her last days wonderful, perhaps with a vacation. They did this, but added one factor that made all the difference, says Silvers.

They didn't tell her the oncologist's negative prognosis. "Instead, they gave her hope and good reason to be joyous. They said she was in remission and that the doctor had said she was going to live a long and healthy life."

They fêted her to a lovely vacation and she lived another fifteen years, restored by the medicine of hope. The patient made mirac-ulous use of the "illusory" good news, turning a compassionate fib into a medical reality. "Her mind obviously relaxed, the tension flushed out of her body, the fear and feelings of hopelessness were gone, so her neurochemistry was able to work at its normal level to activate the immune system," notes Silvers. "Someone was merely told she could relax because she was fine. The body's healing sys-tem took over and she was helped."

Biology Is Dramatically Mutable through Acts of Consciousness

That's basically a placebo response, comments Silvers, in which you get medical effects without the apparent involvement of any drug substance. The only drug was, technically, misleading infor-mation not medically appropriate (but certainly humanistically) for the situation. A change in attitude, a shift in emphasis, and sud-denly a terminal, immedicable condition goes into remission.

It's all in the mind, as skeptical M.D.s used to say of presumed hypochondriacs whose mental disposition would somehow precipitate the illusion of bodily discomfort. The doctors "knew" the patients were always faking it. But what physicians once dismissed scornfully as spurious, psychosomatic illness, may actually hold the key to unlocking the mystery of how illness and healing are generated by the mind.

The placebo response—ridiculed by allopaths as a clinical nuisance, as the therapeutically digressive power of suggestibility, and the ultimate pejorative for a biochemically ineffectual drug—may be the mind-body mechanism that completely repositions our understanding of the healing response and therapeutic efficacy. "The placebo should not be a pejorative term," says Silvers. "There are therapeutic placebo interventions that are successfully applied. Not understanding all of the underlying mechanisms does not imply a placebo response is a nonactive treatment process. If one thinks of placebo of being worthless medication, it's a narrow concept of what placebo is or is capable of doing."

Reinterpreting the allopathically maligned placebo response puts us merely at the threshold of a vast field of unexploited mind-body-mediated therapeutic effects. If the placebo effect—you give a fake drug and it works as well as the real one because doctor and patient expect it to—actually veils the innate healing response of the human organism, activated purposefully by the mind, which is commissioned by our positive attitudes to begin healing, then a great deal more is possible. If the placebo inadvertently awakens the healing power of expectant belief, then if this force were to be marshaled directly and purposefully, quite likely nothing could stand in its way. It would convince us, at last, that mind and consciousness do in fact shape matter, that biological environment is in fact wildly mutable according to our beliefs.

In this chapter, then, we'll visit the placebo response, then consider what scientists now regard as the probable biochemical underpinnings of placebo activity, a rapidly growing discipline called psychoneuroimmunology (PNI), which maps mind-body, molecular, and immunological communication networks and shows how the nervous system (the mind) "talks" to the immune system (the healing response). Next, we'll investigate the intriguing psychological anomaly of multiple personalities in which different resident personalities completely reorganize bodily physiology, again illustrating how biology takes its cues from the mind.

Perhaps this is a fundamental principle of biology itself. Close on the heels of personality multiples we'll chart the mysteries of the coma and the possible survival of consciousness beyond its material, biological context, the body. What do these seemingly disparate fields have in common? They all indicate that environment—whether it's microbiological, physiological, or psychological—is dramatically mutable through acts of consciousness and that at its core the molecular self-identity of our human mind-body may be continually form-changing according to how we think about ourselves.

Placebo Response—The Therapy of Expectant Belief

As Evelyn Silvers indicated, placebo in allopathic circles generally has a negative connotation. The word "placebo," which is Latin, meaning "I shall please," first entered the English language in the twelfth century as a church colloquialism for a vespers service for the deceased; later in Chaucer's day, it suggested a degree of "supine sycophancy"; still later, it meant "flattery" and "flatterer," then by the seventeenth century, it meant a soothing courtesy; in 1787 Quincy's *Lexicon* described placebo as a "commonplace method of medicine," then in the 1811 edition of *Hooper's Medical Dictionary*, placebo was defined as "any medicine adapted more to please than benefit the patient."

In the 1930s, three scientists at Cornell University developed the now standard protocol of the double-blind controlled experiment for drug evaluations—"the gold standard of medical research." Here the pure placebo (a therapeutically worthless, inactive, neutral substance made to physically resemble the drug) was administered in trials alongside the active pharmaceutical to yield presumably objective data on the actions of the drug. If the active drug produces more results than the placebo, that must mean it works, so the doctors reasoned. Neither physician nor patient were informed which substance was the new drug and which the placebo so that their "innate enthusiasm" and expectation would not distort its pharmacological activities.

Thus the placebo became mandatory as a control in evaluative trials, but unethical in medical practice because after all it is deliberately deceptive and manipulative. It would be charlatanry to give a patient a fake, dummy pill, a mere placebo. For allopathic doctors it was almost unconscionable to prescribe a physiochemically

inactive drug—a placebo—to a patient requiring true pharmaco-
logically potent medicine. The "benevolent deception" exemplified
by placebos, wrote Sissela Bok in *Scientific American* almost twenty
years ago, "represents an inroad on informed consent, damages the
institution of medicine, and contributes to the erosion of confidence in medical personnel."

The last thing allopathic physicians want a patient to believe is
that a physiochemically inert substance—"a mere placebo"—could
have *real* therapeutic benefits, other than mentally suggested but
fundamentally spurious, discountable results. That's counter to the
materialist paradigm of medicine itself—only physical substances
(drugs) can produce physical effects (remission of symptoms plus
side effects).

These days most doctors and researchers consider the placebo
effect—apparent therapeutic results from the suggestibility and
expectancy of the patient, often fostered by the physician—as a
nuisance variable, an artifact that muddies up research, "noise in
the system" that contaminates therapy and obscures objective
pharmacological results. Scientists want to see the unimpeded,
specific physical actions of a new drug, not artifacts produced by
an overly suggestible mind.

Unspecific, mind-produced effects, or the placebo response, are
invalid in drug trials and must be screened out; that's why scientists
exalt the double-blind approach.. But as Leonard White, Bernard
Tursky, and Gary Schwartz, editors of *Placebo—Theory, Research,
and Mechanisms,* note, "This methodological refinement guided by
a narrowly conceived orientation tacitly recognizes placebo effects
as a clinical reality, but dismisses them from further consideration."

In the mainstream of medical thinking, then, placebo is an
exclusionary classification, the category for all nondrug-produced
results. "For many doctors, the practice of placebo medicine has an
unsavory scent about it," notes Andrew Weil, M.D., a natural medicines proponent and author of *Health and Healing.* "It seems to
involve deception and trickery and so is not clearly distinguishable
from quackery." Trickery and deception, for an allopath, means the
willful administration of a physiochemically inactive drug merely to
please the patient.

AIDS added another adjective to the placebo pejoratives: cruelty. In the 1980s, when AIDS activists pressured drug companies
and the FDA to accelerate drug development, testing, and

approval, the use of placebo became equated with inhumane medical care (and, in some cases, was eliminated from the drug trial protocols), or cruelty, because in the life-and-death intensity of AIDS, for an HIV-positive patient to use a fake, inactive drug instead of something powerful like AZT or pentamidine could mean the difference between survival and death.

"Murder by placebo," cried AIDS activists when NIH sought 3,200 HIV-infected adults for double-blind control studies with AZT in which one-third of the participants would receive a placebo drug. Project Inform, a national AIDS information group, charged that NIH's Protocol 019 amounted to the outright sacrifice of 1,000 individuals for whom not getting AZT might cost them their lives. Biologist Mathilde Krim of the American Foundation for AIDS Research underscored the dark side of placebos in drug trials when she said: "If you have any evidence that it has an effect, you don't have a right to give a placebo."

Reinterpreting the "Mere" Placebo Effect

But perhaps we've completely misunderstood the meaning of placebo. Baffling, contradictory clinical and empiric data may soon turn the negative positioning of the "mere placebo effect" on its head. The case for a reinterpretation of placebo has been building for three decades, ever since H. K. Beecher published a paradigmatically distressing paper 1961 called "Surgery as Placebo," in *The Journal of the American Medical Association (JAMA)*, not a magazine known to tolerate procedural heresy. Here he recounted the history and implications of the surgical treatment for angina pectoris (heart pain from constricted vascular blood vessels) that had been prevalent in the U.S. throughout the 1950s.

It turns out that sham surgery produced the same results as internal mammary arterial ligation, then the standard surgical procedure. In an experiment, surgeons told some of their patients they would undergo the standard operation, whereas in fact all the doctors did was to open and close their chests, never tying off the artery. In other words, they did intentional placebo surgery. The quality of the results with patients receiving "placebogenic relief" was dramatic and sustained, comparable to standard surgical results, and sometimes better; they had increased exercise tolerance, required less nitroglycerin, and showed a more vigorous electrocardiogram.

In a 1959 study, both objective and subjective criteria revealed placebo heart surgery to be as effective as actual arterial ligation; in fact, 43% of patients receiving sham, placebo surgery reported a sense of improvement compared to only 32% who actually had been ligated. "This history has a sobering moral," notes Adolf Grünbaum, Ph.D., philosopher at the University of Pittsburgh. It might implicate other common surgical procedures as similarly placebogenic. "It bears further monitoring to what extent the positive results from coronary artery bypass surgery are placebogenic."

The 1950s generated another classic placebo case study, this one involving a patient with advanced lymphosarcoma. When the patient was put on an experimental drug called Krebiozon, his enthusiasm for the probable therapeutic outcome (remission) was so extreme that, according to his physician, "the tumor masses had melted like snowballs on a hot stove, and in only a few days, they were half their original size." The injections were continued until the patient experienced full remission and was released from the hospital to resume a productive, healthy life. Then two months later, when newspaper reports announced that Krebiozon was ineffectual, the patient, learning of this, spontaneously relapsed and his lymphosarcoma returned.

His doctors, wishing to save him and at the same time to test the possible regenerative capabilities of the mind, devised a single-blind study: they told him a new version of Krebiozon had been developed that overcame the limitations of the earlier form. With the patient's expectations aroused to a "fevered pitch," the doctors gave him a saline water injection.

"Recovery from his second near terminal state was even more dramatic than the first. Tumor masses melted, chest fluid vanished, he became ambulatory, and even went back to flying again," noted Bruno Klopfer, who summarized the case in 1957. He remained this way for another two months, until the AMA announced that nationwide tests had definitively shown Krebiozon to be a "worthless drug" for cancer treatment. On learning this, the patient was devastated and was readmitted to the hospital, where, having lost his faith in his Krebiozon-mediated cure, he died in two days—in effect, according to his expectations. If Krebiozon was worthless, his remission was illusory, and therefore, logically he had to die, which he did.

The Krebiozon debacle argues powerfully for the viability of the placebo response, even if in this example it was out of control, playing the patient's physiology like a puppet. What saved this patient evidently was his expectant, ardent *belief* in the efficacy of Krebiozon, not the drug itself. The paradox is keen: when the doctors told him Krebiozon worked, it did and he went into remission; when they told him it was worthless and couldn't work, it didn't and he relapsed. Perhaps the drug itself had nothing to do with his remissions and relapses; maybe it was a smokescreen for his own powerful faith in medicine.

Another classic example illustrates the placebogenic power of healer belief. According to Robert Ornstein, Ph.D., of Stanford University, and David Sobel, M.D., of Kaiser Permanente Hospital in San Jose, California, writing in *The Healing Brain,* a doctor was treating an asthma patient who had difficulty keeping his bronchial tubes dilated. Fortunately, the physician knew of a brand-new bronchial drug and ordered it immediately from the drug company. Within minutes of application, the asthma patient was breathing freely. Intrigued with the instantaneous results, the doctor gave the patient an inert placebo instead (but didn't tell him) to measure the range of effects of this new bronchial drug. Shortly the patient complained that the drug wasn't working as well any longer and his breathing was getting difficult again.

This convinced the physician that the real bronchial drug was most impressive and he contacted the pharmaceutical company for more information. Then came the shocker. They told him they had accidentally sent him a placebo sample. It was the physician's ardent belief that this new drug was genuine and effective that turned a placebo into an active medication.

"The patient responded in both cases to the *doctor's* differing expectations of the treatment," says Sobel. "The doctor communicated to the patient in very subtle ways, perhaps tone of voice, facial expressions, or word choice, whether he thought the treatment would be efficacious or not." For Sobel the story highlights the untapped power of placebos. "The placebo makes a statement that we have within us a certain self-regulatory mechanism, a self-healing mechanism, which can be mobilized given proper situational and environmental cues."

Most doctors, less bold than Sobel, don't want to admit it, but the anomaly of the placebogenic effect may be far more widespread and therapeutically important than they think; but we have to invert the phenomena and comprehend its positive message about the healing process and the powers of mind. As Beecher commented: "Many 'effective drugs' have power only a little greater than that of placebo. To separate out even fairly great true effects above those of placebo is manifestly difficult to impossible on the basis of clinical impression. Many a drug has been extolled on the basis of clinical impression when the only power it had was that of a placebo."

It will surprise many to learn that the prescription of antibiotics for virus-produced sore throats, which comprise the vast majority, and their therapeutic result, is a placebo response. Antibiotics work against bacterial infections, but are ineffective against viruses; this hasn't prevented antibiotics from becoming a "very popular form of allopathic treatment" for sore throats, notes Andrew Weil.

In his own practice, Weil has observed numerous case histories of patients with viral sore throats who experienced rapid cures within two days of beginning antibiotics; but he's fully aware that it's not the physical antibiotic that's effecting the cure. "It can do so only by eliciting a placebo response, and the prevalence of such cures indicates the extent of real faith in the power of antibiotics on the part of both doctors and patients. Antibiotics are real drugs with intrinsic effects; however, those effects are irrelevant to the course of a viral infection."

What is relevant is the expectant belief that the antibiotic will work; here the "intrinsic pharmacological activity of the substance"—the sine qua non of allopathic magic-bullet drug therapy—is, ironically, the true sugar pill. That's why Weil calls them "active placebos," physiochemically active drugs (or procedures) that cannot medically be effective in a particular context yet produce placebo effects. For Weil, all medical treatments are active placebos, and the newer ones work the best, at least for a while. "One should use a new remedy as much as possible while it still has the power to heal," remarked Sir William Osler of Johns Hopkins University perhaps a century ago.

As public belief in a new drug fades, so evaporates the bright halo surrounding its direct actions and so dwindles its potential to work as an active placebo, adds Weil. Take Darvon, for example. Introduced in 1957 as a powerful nonaddictive painkiller midway in strength between aspirin and morphine, Darvon (a synthetic opiate, propoxyphene) flourished until the 1970s, when drug addicts began abusing it, doctors questioned whether it in fact reduced pain as competently as the earlier analgesics, and patients reported less pain relief from using it. "Doctors tend not to see the diminishing placebo returns as a change but rather to think the drug was not very good from the start and longer experience has made its limitations clear," says Weil.

Placebo—The Benign Lie That Heals

In a comprehensive review article on placebo and the art of medicine, Canadian naturopath Peter Bennett, N.D., notes the astonishing range of placebo-mediated physical effects, incontestable proof of "the lie that heals," as allopaths put it.

According to the medical literature, documented symptoms and side effects of the placebo response include, in part, anorexia, diarrhea, epigastric pain, headache, palpitation, pupillary dilation, rash, depression, anger, and drowsiness. Conditions that have been clinically shown to respond favorably to the administration of placebos include angina, arthritis, diabetes, gastric ulcers, hay fever, hypertension, pain, rhinitis, tremor, common cold, asthma, PMS, and many others. A. K. Shapiro, writing in the *American Journal of Psychotherapy* in 1959, commended the placebo effect: "Placebos can have profound effects on organic illness, including incurable malignancies."

Studies in the mid-1980s indicated that placebo used as an active analgesic for pain was 56% as effective as injections of actual morphine; another study proved that placebo was 54% as effective as aspirin for headache relief. According to a *JAMA* article by Beecher in 1955, fifteen studies, involving 1,082 patients, indicated that placebos have an average effectiveness of 35.2%—"a degree not widely recognized." A study reviewing placebo analgesia from 1959 to 1974 showed that 36% of 908 pain patients experienced more than 50% pain relief from placebos. A 1976 study of 288 cancer patients at Carnegie Mellon University indicated that 112 (39%) claimed 50% or greater pain relief from placebo medications.

A 1934 study involving 105 patients with warts revealed that of those treated with the standard drug, sulpharsphenamine, 52.5% achieved remission, while those treated with a dose of distilled colored water, or placebo, had 47.6% remission. An earlier study from 1927 indicated that one physician cured 44% to 88% of warts (depending on type) in patients by the power of suggestion alone.

More recently, results from a 1993 study of nearly 7,000 patients receiving five different placebo-based treatments led Alan H. Roberts, psychologist at the Scripps Clinic and Research Foundation in La Jolla, California, to conclude that, for mild medical problems, the placebo effect will produce positive outcomes in about two-thirds of patients, which is twice as high as normally expected.

Sometimes brand-name recognition (though false) on a placebo product heightens its effect. A British study of women with headaches found that 40% who took an unbranded placebo aspirin reported considerable pain relief, 50% felt better with branded placebos, 56% with unbranded aspirin, and 60% with branded aspirin. Evidently it was the packaging and expectation associated with the branded aspirin, not its active ingredients, that made the difference.

More recently, a researcher at the University of California Medical Center in San Francisco demonstrated that a placebo is as effective as 6 to 8 milligrams of morphine, a standard dosage. The investigator administered naloxone (a drug that blocks the analgesic effects of endorphins and opiates) to patients already under placebo medication for relief of pain; just as it would for morphine, the naloxone blocked the pain-relieving effects of the placebos. "We've always known that placebos can be potent painkillers," commented Jon Levine, the study's researcher, "but until now it was assumed that their action was psychological. Now we know placebos have direct physical effects on the chemistry of the brain."

What is even more remarkable, placebos produce "nocebo effects," the same kinds of unpleasant or injurious side effects normally associated with the physical drug. For example, placebo aspirin produces nocebo effects of ulcer-like pain. One double-blind study revealed that 30% of patients involved with placebo medication (in place of oral contraceptives) had 17% more headaches, 14% increased menstrual pain, and 8% increased nervousness and irritability. In another study involving a placebo vaccine for colds, 7% of patients receiving the "inactive" medication had such strong effects they needed additional medication. Of cancer patients who were told they were receiving a potent new strain of chemotherapy, but who actually got a placebo, 31% of them lost their hair just as they would have had the chemotherapy been chemically real.

Remarkably, placebos mimic active drugs, producing the same toxic reactions; they replicate the pattern of drug responses of the active drug, such as time-effect curves, cumulative effect, and carryover effects; they even produce drug dependency equivalent to the kind patients often develop with tranquilizers or narcotics. Women who took placebo contraceptives experienced an astonishing range of physical symptoms, including lumbar pain, headache, dysmenorrhea, nausea, acne, blurred vision, and palpitations.

In his 1955 study, Beecher documented thirty-five different toxic side effects from placebos, culled from fifteen different studies. Placebos can produce adverse reactions in asthma patients equivalent to the ingestion of allergenic substances. When forty asthmatics were told they were inhaling an allergenic substance (it was a placebo made of salt water), nineteen, or almost 50%, experienced bronchial obstruction, and twelve of the nineteen developed wheezing and full-blown asthma symptoms. In a corollary study, the same researchers noted that fifteen of twenty-nine asthmatic patients experienced bronchospasm after inhaling a placebo solution they thought contained allergenic materials.

"What is this thing that directs a cure in 30-50% of patients without doing anything?" queries Bennett. "I see this great hole in the doctor-patient relationship. This is the healing response by another name. It's an amazing idea that medicine tries to rule out the underlying movement of the body to heal as an unreasonable variable. The bottom line tool of all great physicians is knowing how to access the inner resources, or the placebo response, of the patient. Health practitioners need to be equipped with a better understanding of placebo therapeutics." In Bennett's view, it's not the "lie that heals" that is at play in placebogenic results, but rather the catalytic field between patient and doctor, "the relationship between the patient and doctor which stimulates a natural self-healing mechanism via psychologic, symbolic, and biologic intervention."

For Michael Murphy, co-founder of the Esalen Institute and author of *The Future of the Body*, a study of evolutionary possibilities for human nature, the placebo response is evidence of human transformative capacity. Placebogenic effects highlight the underappreciated fact that humans "possess largely untapped capacities to balance and restore their own functioning" and to "mobilize latent transformative powers—for either sickness or health—without external devices. Expectant faith, in short, stimulates healing behavior, along with positive imagery and mood." Consciousness marshaled for a cause has efficacy in the life of the body.

Laughter and the Chemistry of Healing

Physician, heal thyself, or as the late Norman Cousins, M.D., put it, physicians must help patients find the doctor within. Cousins put the placebo response on the medical map in 1979 with his best-selling account in *Anatomy of an Illness* of his unexpected recovery from ankylosing spondylitis.

The disease—deterioration of connective tissue in the spine, first diagnosed in Cousins in 1964—should have killed him according to allopathic statistical prediction, but Cousins had other plans. "I have learned never to underestimate the capacity of the human mind and body to regenerate—even when the prospects seem most wretched," said Cousins, who cured himself with ascorbic acid, the Marx Brothers, and the "chemistry of the will to live."

Not interested in the verdict of his pessimistic physicians—they gave him one chance in 500—Cousins refused to subscribe to the requisite fear of decline and death his disease warranted and embarked on "a mammoth venture in self-administered placebos." Cousins, who would survive his illness by twenty-seven years, self-prescribed the Marx Brothers—and anything funny, books, movies, jokes—for the laughs: "I made the joyous discovery that ten minutes of genuine belly laughter had an anesthetic effect and would give me at least two hours of pain-free sleep." The placebo, Cousins observed, is not a pill but a process that translates the will to survive into a physical reality, demonstrating "the capacity of the human body to transform hope into tangible and essential biochemical change."

No longer a "dummy drug," the placebo is "an authentic therapeutic agent" pointing medical science, if they will pick up the cue, "straight in the direction of something akin to a revolution" in the theory and practice of medicine. According to Cousins, our "healing system" is how the body mobilizes its resources to decommission disease, but it's our "belief system" that activates the healing system. Allopathic drugs may be powerful, but the activated will to live, a positive, faithful attitude in the possibilities for recovery, and the *vis medicatrix naturae,* "the healing power of nature" and "the biology of hope," may be even stronger, suggested Cousins. And the placebo is free: it comes with life, with being human. "The placebo is the doctor who resides within," and the superior physician is the one who inspires and empowers that inner doctor to heal the organism. "The placebo, then, is an emissary between the will to live and the body."

But the emissary itself is expendable, a mere intermediary to catch our attention. "If we can liberate ourselves from tangibles, we can connect hope and the will to live directly to the ability of the body to meet great threats and challenges." That, says Cousins, is the great, unfulfilled challenge of the placebo response: it's a doorway into unlimited self-healing. As placebo researcher Frederick Evans, Ph.D., of Rutgers Medical School, comments, maybe we need to reposition how we regard placebo. "The placebo effect should be considered as a potent therapeutic intervention in its own right, rather than merely a nuisance variable." Evans advocates that physicians understand placebo as if it were a legitimate, active pharmacological agent worthy of independent investigation. In this way, doctors might pick up that placebogenic cue Cousins alluded to and get on with the conceptual revolution in store for them.

Despite the allopathic insistence on isolating the specific pharmacological activity of drugs in its evaluative trials, in effect rigorously quarantining any influence from patient belief or physician enthusiasm, this may be a fool's quest. Belief and enthusiasm may be the vital force that enables drugs to work at all; certainly that's true in about 35% of the cases, as Beecher revealed years ago. The medical anomaly continuously posed by placebo statistics may force doctors to revise their model of pharmacological agentry and put themselves back into it—to reconsider the entire context in which medication is administered. Why should they want to screen out the doctor's benevolent influence?

Perhaps it's time to reemphasize the therapeutic value of an avuncular bedside manner. That revision will require a more radical change in valuation of the double-blind protocol, which allopaths contend "absolutely screens out the contaminating influence of belief," Weil says.

A Non-drug with Specific Intent

The concept of "specific agentry" reigns supreme in allopathic pharmacology, but this may be a major theoretical fallacy. "A drug no more effective than a placebo is, like a placebo, no drug at all," explained Berton Roueché in the *New Yorker* back in 1960, unknowingly summarizing the conceptual contortions into which placebogenic success had tied allopathic thinking. In an earlier day, the placebo response was a way of indicating the therapeutic efficacy of the physician's presence, his touch, his concern, his healing words—the contaminating, "iatroplacebogenic" influence of the doctor's bedside manner and his belief that the patient would get better. As Francis Peabody once remarked in a now famous dictum: "The secret of the care of the patient is in caring for the patient."

The history of medicine, Weil contends, is actually the history of the placebo response, in which, quite frequently, ineffective remedies, founded on faulty knowledge, produced cures—as they still do. It's the chronicle of how strong belief heals, set against an allopathic insistence to regard the mind as an imaginary organ with no business in the body. One 1974 estimate suggested that 35% to 45% of all prescriptions are for substances that cannot have the intended effect for which they were prescribed; that means, if they work, it's pure placebo. In one study, 59% of the drugs recommended for colds (antibiotics, penicillin, and sulfonamides) were technically incapable of producing any beneficial results against the viral infection. The most active treatments have "the brightest placebo halos," says Weil, because they have been invested by patients and physicians alike—and the whole of medical orthodoxy—with enormous expectant belief in their efficacy.

That's why Weil calls much of contemporary allopathic medicine active placebo response; the fact that the doctor is doing something, giving you a pill, making an injection, performing a surgery, means help is on the way and recovery is around the corner. If you believe in allopathy, it will probably work that much better for you. Placebo analgesia and other demonstrably molecular effects "hint at what incredible potential may exist within human psychological abilities," comments T. D. Borkovec, Ph.D., of Pennsylvania State University. "The possibility that what one believes to be true may actually influence what does become true is nothing short of spectacular in its implications." Perhaps it's spectacular for physicians, but surely not for physicists, for whom a quantum, indeterminate universe that responds to intent has been the norm for decades, as we learned in our visit with shamanic physicist Fred Alan Wolf.

Intent is the environment-remaking energy of belief, the placebo response in full flower. These spectacular implications should be put to immediate constructive use in medical practice, argue psychologists Sherman Ross and L. W. Buckalew. Most doctors still regard the placebo response as an embarrassment, as something that detracts from their power, authority, and expertise, so fixated are they on specific physical agentry. "We would suggest that, to the contrary, recognition and appreciation of the 'powerful placebo' can add appreciably to the efficacy of any indicated therapeutic treatment." And it might help heal the estranged doctor-patient relationship, too, suggests Howard Shapiro, medical professor at Yale University, and author of *Doctors, Patients, and Placebos*. "Placebos can help physicians regain confidence in the symbolic reality of medicine and help restore the bond between themselves and their patients."

So it's time to turn the placebo response around, remove its negative valuation, and appreciate it for what it demonstrates about mobilized self-healing. Doctors should rule the placebo response *in* and try to find more ways, more frequently, to elicit the healing response rather than always relying on powerful physical drugs, says Weil. Implicit in allopathy's insistence on powerful, fast-acting drugs, surgery, and risky, expensive, biochemical, mechanical interventions is a deep distrust and "profound lack of faith" in the body's innate self-healing capabilities, says Weil. "It is more an arrogant disregard of the wholeness and holiness of the human body."

Physicians should tell patients from the start that they will *cure themselves* through learning techniques to control their bodily responses, just the way Silvers showed her drug addicts how to simulate the narcotic effects in their minds. That's because the agentry that's truly at play in the placebo response—this "agent of infinite range," said Roueché; "one of the oldest and most broadly effective medical remedies known," said Morton Hunt in *Longevity*—is the awesome, unexploited mind-mediated, psychosomatic mechanism of self-healing, the innate homeostatic healing response of the life force. Or, as Peter Bennett says, "Belief is relief."

The placebo response, mediated by faith and expectation, mobilizes the patient's "healing power of expectant belief." Placebogenic medicine is the therapy of strong intention—faith healing in a sense. "I claim here that the nocebo and placebo phenomena comprise a whole in which the culturally fostered expectations of persons (causally) effect what is expected," states Robert Hahn, psychologist at the University of Washington in Seattle. "Simply put, belief sickens; belief kills; belief heals."

What is the placebo response? By some remarkable mechanism, strong belief changes the outcome of material, biochemical

processes. The placebo response is therapeutic change precipitated by a patient's "own intentional actions," formulated as an
expression of faith in a therapeutic procedure, notes William Plotkin
of the Durango Pain Management Clinic in Durango, Colorado. In
Plotkin's view, placebo effects are a "subclass of self-healing" in
which patients are always the "immediate therapeutic agents";
placebo responses are strongest with persons who are "highly moti-
vated to improve" and who have a developed understanding of
their own "behavioral eligibilities."

The creative, active use of the implicit principle of placebo
response—the belief that I am eligible for healing, that my biochemical behavior is changeable according to my intent—and our
latent self-healing skills is a "competence-mobilizing procedure,"
says Plotkin, that enhances "our *sense* of competence, autonomy,
and self-control." The fact of positive, therapeutic placebo responses poses a challenge for the modern healing arts to develop methods for "freeing persons to exercise their self-healing competencies"
and for taking charge of the remarkable pathways by which strong
belief is transformed into biological results.

In the last two decades the biochemical mechanism underlying
the placebo response has gained a name: it's called psychoneuroimmunology (PNI), and it's showing us how the mind talks to the
cells, and what is even more important, that they listen.

PNI—Awakening the
Self-Healing Competency

The language of this conversation between mind and molecules
is based on neurotransmitters, "informational substances" including hormones, neuropeptides, growth factors, and lymphokines,
communication molecules that keep the lines open between brain
and body. Scientists estimate there are perhaps 100 to 200 different neurotransmitters, or information molecules, that are coded for
intercellular communication in this fluid interface, forming what
researchers Candace Pert and Michael Ruff, then at the National
Institute of Mental Health (NIMH), called a "neuropeptide and
psychosomatic network" founded on a vocabulary of biochemicals.

Neuropeptides, or "brain hormones," are short chains of amino
acids that regulate the key human activities and sensations: sleep,
hunger, sex, stress, emotions, and pain; prominent examples

include norepinephrine, glutamate, cortisol, serotonin, ACTH, and dopamine. Pert and Ruff found that certain white blood cells had receptor sites ("molecular antennae") tuned specifically to receive biochemical messages from the brain, conveyed by these neurotransmitters.

One of the first and most important neurotransmitters to be discovered by Pert in 1973 was endogenous morphine, or endorphin, a family of natural, painkilling opiates. The endorphin discovery led Pert, Ruff, and other researchers to a gradual appreciation of the human brain as a prodigious manufacturer and consumer of physiochemically active drugs. It also provided a probable explanation for the mechanisms of three mysterious (for allopaths) forms of analgesia, including acupuncture, electrical brain stimulation, and the placebo effect because clinical evidence suggested that the placebo response worked by stimulating endorphin release.

"The brain is just a little box with emotions packed into it," quipped Pert, arguing that neuropeptides and their cell receptors constitute a biochemistry of emotions or molecular atlas of affective states. "And we're starting to understand that emotions have biochemical correlates. We know the molecular structure of pleasure."

The brain-body connection may have even deeper, more intimate wiring, according to a new discovery that classifies ATP—adenosine triphosphate, a ubiquitous molecule involved in energy transactions and found inside nearly every living cell in the biological world—as a neurotransmitter. The discovery was made by Dr. Geoffrey Burnstock of University College, London, in 1970, but none of his colleagues believed him; it took him twenty-two years to convince them he was right. Not only does ATP provide the energy that makes biological life possible, but it also transmits messages outside the cells between the brain and intestines, heart, lung, reproductive organs, bladder, and immune system.

It also took Burnstock considerable effort to persuade them of the validity of his second hypothesis, that nerve cells release multiple neurotransmitters. Burnstock's current research question is to find out why all the major cells of the immune system have receptors for ATP. "This may help us understand how the immune system and brain interact," he notes.

For years, popular and scientific literature has been rich with anecdotal confirmation of this vast communication network that

PHYSICIAN

enables the brain to talk to the estimated 100 trillion cells comprising the human body. Close relationships, familial, and community support—"the ties that bind"—evidently have positive
immunological affects. A study of thirty elderly men and women
living in a retirement home showed enhanced immune competence
(higher levels of NK, or "natural killer," cells and antibodies) as a
result of being visited three times weekly for a month by loved
ones. A study conducted at the University of New Mexico School
of Medicine showed that among 256 healthy elderly people, those
who enjoyed confiding relationships had demonstrably more vigorous immune function, lower serum cholesterol and uric acid levels.

The sense of control that comes with accurate medical information
also enhances immune competency. A British study revealed that
women undergoing a gynecological operation who read a booklet on
dealing with preoperative fear and postoperative symptoms fared
much better than women in a control group provided with minimal
information. The informed women recovered faster, experienced less
fear, anxiety, pain, and lower heart rates and blood pressure. A Stanford University study revealed the link between emotional conflict
and the onset and elaboration of rheumatoid arthritis. Emotional factors such as loneliness, stress, isolation, worry, dissatisfaction, lack of
control, poor coping ability, and "giving up," have been linked with
immune suppression and the onset of disease. A longitudinal study of
280 men and women who interpreted setbacks according to a pessimistic frame of mind, had significantly lower immune function, as
measured by T-lymphocytes and NK cells.

On the other hand, when Harvard psychologists showed students
a film designed to instill feelings of love and caring, they noted
increases in salivary IgA, an antibody that provides protection
against colds and upper-respiratory infections. A study of college
students by psychologists at Carnegie Mellon University showed
that optimism promotes health and is a reliable predictor of physical well-being. Norman Cousins demonstrated how ten minutes of
laughter can increase endorphin and enkephalin levels in the brain.

Similar examples along these lines are copious and could fill a
book, which they did in Blair Justice's valuable compilation and
commentary, *Who Gets Sick*. Justice, a psychologist at the University of Texas Health Science Center in Houston, documents how
responsive the body is to our thoughts. "Because thoughts themselves are electrochemical events, capable of initiating physical

effects, this response is not only real but also powerful." As one NIMH neuroscientist (quoted by Justice) declared: "Talk therapy changes chemistry. It's perhaps the profoundest way to change it."

Mastering the technique of cognitive reappraisal and mobilizing the faith to heal, says Justice, are keys to facilitating the self-healing response. Our body is the best druggist, and we may access its psychobiological pharmacy through a variety of placebogenic strategies, from love, positive thoughts, optimism, laughter, visualization, creative imagery, encouraging the brain to write the neurochemical prescription for health. Our thinking styles and learning experiences can change cell structures within the central nervous system, says Justice, a fact we can put creatively to use. "The fact that both drugs and cognitive therapy can help many people who are depressed affirms the two-way influence of biology and behavior—which includes the internal behavior of our minds as well as the external behavior of our bodies."

Or as David Sobel and Robert Ornstein put it, beliefs, endorphins, and the intrinsic pain-relief system are all aspects of the pharmacy within.

The diverse field of mind-body interactions has a general umbrella term—psychoneuroimmunology, or PNI—first coined in 1981 by one of its leading researchers, Dr. Robert Ader of the University of Rochester School of Medicine. Of course a great deal has been catalogued under Ader's PNI rubric that, like James Lovelock and his neo-Gaian advocates, strictly speaking, Ader might not have intended. Ader was running Pavlovian-conditioning and immunological experiments with rats to test the hypothesis that the central nervous system could directly influence immunological activity. Ader trained his rats to depress their immune system in response to the stimulus of drinking saccharine-sweetened water.

First, he gave them the sweet water followed by an injection of cyclophosphamide (an immune suppressant), until the rats learned the conditioning; then he gave them the sweet water alone and noticed the same immunodeficient results, indicating that for these conditioned rats, a taste of sweet water was equivalent to an injection of cyclophosphamide. His results showed that mental association, even in rodents, could depress immune activity. By extension, this suggestibility in humans Ader termed the "psychosocial factor," including the effects on health of personal relationships, environment, behavior, attitudes, thoughts, stress.

"It was an elegantly simple experiment that demonstrated a clear connection between the behavior conditioning and immune changes," note Locke and Colligan. For Ader, who announced his results (after replicating them many times) in *Science,* it marked his moving into a new dimension of medical discovery, that scientifically uncharted realm where mind, nervous system, and immune function interconnect. "It would appear that, to a greater or lesser extent, all pathologic processes are subject to the influence of psychosocial interventions of one kind or another," Ader commented.

"Your unconscious mind may be smarter than you"

For the most part, these powerful psychosocial interventions, whether originating in the doctor or patient, tend to be unacknowledged, subliminal, even unconsciously undertaken. As Brendan O'Regan, staff researcher for the Institute of Noetic Sciences in Sausalito, California, notes in his *Investigations* monograph on placebos, "One of the missing elements in contemporary placebo research clearly is attention to the role of the unconscious mind in mediating placebo effects."

The surprising placebo statistics—efficacy ranging from 35% to 56%—may be due to unconscious interventions alone; were the mind to be fully, consciously engaged in the placebo process, these numbers would probably be a lot higher. The major cognitive and executive systems involved in the placebo response, suggests O'Regan—"the real, ongoing dynamic structure of mental processes"—are probably beyond the ken of ordinary awareness and involve "a large proportion of unconscious activity."

"Your unconscious mind may be smarter than you," says *New York Times* science writer Daniel Goleman in an article about the "ordinarily invisible, building blocks of irrational opinion, prejudice, and neurosis." Recent studies indicate the cognitive unconscious, formerly regarded by most cognitive scientists as simple-minded, may instead be extremely intelligent, says Goleman. This cognitively smart unconscious might be the competent agent behind the mystery and wonder of spontaneous remissions.

While placebos and spontaneous remissions demonstrate the human capacity for dramatic psychosomatic change and our inherent, underutilized powers of self-regulation, they are largely the results of unattended mental functioning and not the product of the "conscious cultivation of particular capacities," explains Michael Murphy. "This is the case because we typically develop extraordinary attributes through activities that involve self-awareness, whereas a placebo's effectiveness generally depends upon its subject's *lack of awareness*."

Spontaneous remission is the sudden, inexplicable, total recovery from presumed incurable, immedicable, hopeless conditions, without any apparent medical intervention. As with placebos, the popular literature is copious with anecdotal examples; even the staid *Cancer* and the *New England Journal of Medicine*, perhaps grudgingly, occasionally run articles on these unpredictable medical flukes and aberrations, as they tend to regard them. In 1966 two surgeons at the University of Illinois College of Medicine published their analysis of the scientific literature in which they found 176 legitimate reports of spontaneous remission in most forms of cancer.

In 1976, Eric Peper and Ken Pelletier identified 400 cases of spontaneous remission from cancer; when biofeedback pioneers Elmer and Alyce Green examined the pre-remission circumstances of these patients, they noted the only common factor present was a change of attitude in favor of hope and positive attitude. A 1984 report published by Stanford University researchers found that 23% of 83 patients with non-Hodgkin's lymphomas experienced a spontaneous remission lasting from four months to six years. In 1992, the Institute of Noetic Sciences (INS) published its annotated bibliography of about 1,000 cases of spontaneous remission from the past forty years (about 3,000 medical articles in 860 different journals published in twenty languages) involving a broad range of diseases from cancer to warts, heart ailments to tuberculosis.

"We have found cases of remission from almost every kind of illness, not just cancer," says O'Regan, and "we have many cases of remission with no medical intervention at all." These comprise one-fifth of the cases O'Regan found. Allopathic physicians have their estimates—one spontaneous remission out of 750,000 lung cancer cases between 1950 and 1974; one cancer case out of 80,000; or, according to a 1985 estimate, one out of 20,000 diagnosed cancer cases—but since most doctors disbelieve in the phenomena and may discount or ignore many more cases, the incidence is probably much higher.

There's a more significant reason for the low incidence or minimal evidence of spontaneous remissions, as Stephen Hall usefully highlights. It takes some time for an "incurable" case to go into spontaneous remission; the habit of modern allopathy is to treat immediately as soon as the diagnosis is made—hit them aggressively with chemotherapy, antibiotics, radiation, or surgery as soon as possible. After the 1950s "whatever clues spontaneous remission might have suggested got swamped in the wave of drugs," notes Hall.

A recent landmark study indicates that the occurrence of spontaneous remission (SR)—namely, the disappearance of a disease without medical treatment or treatment considered adequate—may be far more widespread than most people thought. Brendan O'Regan and Carlyle Hirshberg of the Institute of Noetic Science published a massive annotated bibliography in 1993 drawing on the world's largest database of medically reported cases of SR: specifically, 3,500 references from 800 journals in twenty languages and across the spectrum of diseases. "Remission is potentially an extremely rich area of research that can allow us to see important, little-known psycho-biological processes in action in a way that may provide important clues to understanding the self-regulating processes in the body," they wrote.

For Brendan O'Regan, former INS project director, people who have experienced a spontaneous remission represent a medical goldmine that must be studied. "These are nature's successes, nature's success against cancer." All cases of spontaneous remission, but especially those that involved no allopathic medical intervention, says O'Regan, "give us the strongest evidence that there is an extraordinary self-repair system lying dormant within us." A handful of physicians share O'Regan's sentiments, regarding spontaneous remissions as "'whispers of nature,' infrequent but tantalizing clues about the ways the human body can rally itself to fend off mortal disease," says Hall.

Allopathic physicians tend to react with unlimited disbelief and incredulity when supposedly terminal patients fail to abide by the statistical certainty of their mortality, such as Harold Whitely, a lung cancer patient who refused to die twenty-five years after his doctor's grim prognosis. It was as if he had cheated fate. "Why is this man not dead?" queried his doctor. "He's really the only lung cancer patient that's been going for, well, forever. I'm still looking for someone to tell me why. This wasn't supposed to happen."

In this case, summarized by Stephen Hall in *Health* magazine, Whitely first went to his doctor in 1966, when he was fifty-five, complaining of breathing difficulties and an enlarged lymph node above his collarbone. The lab biopsy indicated oaT-cell carcinoma, a rapidly proliferating form of lung cancer that "is like a death certificate," said his doctor, who estimated Whitely would survive one to two more years at best. Ironically, Whitely didn't get the full picture and understood only that he had a tumor, but not a mortal one; he left without receiving any treatment. Whitely returned to his doctor five years later with no signs of lung cancer, according to radiology exams; the tumor mass had disappeared. Somehow the "laboratory of his ingenious self-healing cells" had produced a cure, says Hall.

It's intriguing to speculate what might underlie the biology of spontaneous remission in this startling case from the work of Arnold Mindell, Ph.D., formulator of dreambody process work. A little boy with an incurable brain tumor was brought to Mindell by his parents. Two brain surgeries had failed to arrest the tumor's progression. How do you experience your tumor, Mindell asked the child—how does it hurt? "It hurts like a hammer," the boy replied. When Mindell asked him to repeat his remark, the boy struck his knee when he said "hammer." He kept pounding his knee until Mindell knew he understood its dreambody message. "After a minute or two, he looked at me a bit sheepishly and said the 'hammer' told him to get to work, watch less television, and do his homework."

Psychologically, the tumor embodied a conflict of discipline versus leisure being waged in the boy, so he and Mindell worked out an inner peace treaty in which he would watch some television then do all his homework. The child's health improved radically and soon his tumor disappeared according to x-ray analysis. What reversed the process of destruction and produced the remission? Awareness, says Mindell.

"Up until the moment when the conflict became conscious, he had been living in a psychologically closed system that was trying to balance itself." The normal, lazy boy was struggling with an industrious, disciplined boy; the irresolution of their conflict hammered away at the boy, producing the tumor. "The two were killing each other, and there was no one 'home' to mediate their conflict."

Yogic Vigilance in the Face of a Body That Listens

One important way to keep your symptoms from continually returning is to be yogically vigilant in your thinking, says Michael Talbot, author of *The Holographic Universe*. Don't keep sending your body the wrong messages, because it's always listening and has ears everywhere. "The body is a hologram with consciousness and mentality distributed throughout the system. We are an ocean of mentalities; we are legion, full of voices. We must be careful what we say to the multiple voices of our body. Our body listens to everything we think and feel. It takes our wishes literally, so we must be vigilant."

In the course of trying to heal his spleen through creative imagery, Talbot waxed impatient and scolded his spleen for underachievement. Shortly after, a psychic told Talbot his spleen was very upset and confused. "Never, never get angry at your body or your internal organs," she advised a chastened Talbot. "Your spleen became ill because it thought it was doing what you wanted. That was because you were unconsciously giving it the wrong directions. Only send it positive messages."

In Talbot's view illness is clearly self-created, but the creation usually happens below the threshold of ordinary consciousness. "Science shows us we have all these life-threatening viruses in our body all the time, but they don't strike, they remain latent. What seems to activate them are our propensities and belief systems. The level at which we decide to become ill is deeply unconscious, a deep-level of programming." And watch out for self-organizing thoughts, he adds.

Unconscious illness programs can develop into self-organized, autonomous disease entities, warns Talbot. Our negative thoughts can organize themselves and take on a biological life of their own. It's the creative power of mind used negatively. Self-organizing negative thoughts can empower disease conditions indefinitely. "Your bodymind can resemble Amazonian animal life with a jungle of denizens, each with its own agenda." Years ago while in Tibet, the Buddhist scholar and adventurer Alexandra David-Neel projected the thought-form of a monk so powerfully that all her companions saw "him." The trouble was, he wouldn't go away, says Talbot. It took her as much focused psychic energy to dissolve the apparition as she had expended in his creation.

But we can also project positive outcomes, positive self-organized thoughts of health, says Talbot, who does this regularly. He often programs his immune system to get stronger rather than wilt in the face of a potential cold infection. "I always make affirmations. I'm going to *build resistance* to this cold or hay fever. I don't buy into limitations. We're like babies at the controls of a 747 jumbo jet. We have vast power before us but we don't know how to work the switches. This is how we relate to our health. We need vigilance in the face of all the mental chatter. We mustn't pollute our bodies with negative thinking. We have extraordinary healing abilities, the vast distributed intelligence of body and mind." Even if the mind resembles the House of Representatives in full debate.

The clinical data of multiple personality disorders is incontrovertible evidence that illness is largely a drama of the psyche played out in biology, suggests Talbot, who cites several provocative case studies in his book. An acute medical condition possessed by one personality suddenly vanishes when another personality takes over—all within the same physical body. All but one of the multiple selves of a man were acutely allergic to orange juice, breaking out in severe rash after consumption.

But if the "host" switched to his nonallergic subpersonality, the rash instantly disappeared and he could drink orange juice with no negative reaction. Another multiple was stung by a wasp, which caused his eye to swell shut. He was in great pain, so his psychiatrist undertook some ingenious first aid. He induced an "anesthetic personality" within the multiple's repertoire to take charge; the man's pain and swelling disappeared. Other studies scientifically document the mutability of diabetes, epilepsy, even tumors, depending on the disposition of the dominant subpersonality.

Multiple-personality phenomena such as these clearly indicate an intimate relationship between psychological state and physiology. If allergies or diabetes can be turned on or off according to the resident personality, the startling implication is that these medical disabilities somehow serve the agenda of that subpersonality, and at some level are entirely optional, like preferred furnishings.

It suggests that in a queer way illness might be a movable prop for a host personality. It places the meaning of illness squarely in our laps as a self-generated event. "If the psyche of an individual with multiple personality disorder is a kind of multiple image hologram," concludes Talbot, "it appears that the body is one as well, and can switch from one biological state to another as rapidly as the flutter of a deck of cards. This suggests that somewhere in our psyches we all have the ability to control these things."

The Exceptional Patient—
Key to the Miracle of Healing

Equally as remarkable as patients who experience spontaneous remission are individuals who persevere against all medical odds in recovering from supposedly incurable diseases and restoring their health. Retired Yale surgeon Bernie Siegel, M.D., calls such individuals exceptional, and has chronicled their stories in two exceedingly popular books, *Love, Medicine, and Miracles* (1986), and *Peace, Love, and Healing* (1989). You should never say a disease is 100% fatal, Siegel admonished his audience at an AIDS conference in Washington, D.C., a few years ago. "I'm interested in paths of possibility, not probability. You can't tell the future from looking at a lab report."

The fact that people survive terminal illnesses is by now amply documented—Siegel referred to 4,000 published articles—but what's missing is the psychological biography of these survivors, these exceptional patients. It's not a miraculous spontaneous remission, says Siegel who habitually asks patients why they healed, but the hard-earned results of a determination to prevail over the illness. "The answer I hear over and over is, 'When I learned I was going to die, I finally started living. I began doing what I really wanted to do. And the by-product was that I got better.'"

How does he typify the exceptional patient who wins a cure against medical expectation? "Ultimately the individual who learns to be the *crazy, unique, refreshing,* exceptional patient is more likely to be the one who achieves a *cure.*" For Siegel, this is empirical evidence that the mind and body communicate with each other, forming an intelligent unit; the immune system responds both to "live" and "die" scenarios as projected by the mind. In fact, it responds most favorably to "unconditional love," hope, and will, the most powerful immune-enhancers known, contends Siegel. "You have a lot of control over your own body—and you can create a healing environment. The idea is to turn on your body's intelligence, to help it heal itself."

Siegel's immense popularity and the persuasiveness of his work has inspired a new genre of self-help and recovery biography literature. "I refuse to become a cancer patient," exclaims one of ten exceptional patients profiled in Wendy Williams's *The Power Within.* Each of Williams's subjects exemplifies hope and courage. "I am a human being—who also has cancer." The cancers they have are grim indeed—glioblastoma, lung, breast, ovarian, leukemia, brain—but their unconventional feisty determination to refute the biological negativity of their cancer is inspiring. Their stories are about affirmative choice—"how a person decides to live *after* the cancer diagnosis."

Williams takes an informal Studs Terkel approach to this folk history of life and death issues played out on the field of cancer. She lets the ten individuals tell their stories in their own colloquial way, but brackets their narratives with the uninspired prognoses of the M.D.s, pronouncements usually expressed in "weeks expected to live" and professional allegiance to actuarial tables. "Life is not controlled by statistics," retorts Williams. "Life is a pact made between an individual being and the spiritual forces of the universe." Healing cancer, as *The Power Within* suggests, seems to be a renegotiation of that pact; as fortification for that task, this book provides light and digestible nourishment.

In his collection of recovery biographies, *Making Miracles,* practicing psychologist Mark Roud, Ed.D., also plays Studs Terkel to eleven officially incurable "extraordinary patients" whose self-willed "spontaneous remissions" restored their lives and health on a new key while astounding the medical experts. Roud invites each to relate their story of medically predicted death and unexpected "miraculous" recovery, then supplements their autobiographies with a professional analysis. One woman recovered from a metastasized lung cancer; one man cured his fifth round of lymphatic cancer; one man cured his meningeal carcinomatosis; another was a twenty-year wheelchair paraplegic who eventually walked.

What is the secret of these "experts at exceptional survival?" Diet, emotions, attitude, will, faith, unconditional love are all involved, but healing is individual, says Roud. It's founded on "the ill person's self-understanding. Their experience has demonstrated that each individual must discover for himself or herself what is life-giving." All this makes Roud's almost anthropological inquiry into the intimacies of health a salutary addition to the growing literature of self-healing.

So when we adopt the kind of self-healing attitudes highlighted by Siegel, Williams, and Roud, we're standing on the threshold of what Ayurvedic physician Deepak Chopra, M.D., calls quantum healing, the mind-borne realm of infinite choice in which environment may be remade according to our expectations. Ayurveda, the ancient medical philosophy of India, cures the reality of the patient first, explains Chopra, one of the system's foremost advocates in the U.S. Ayurveda is both a medicine and a mystery knowledge, a therapeutic praxis and a philosophy of awakening, "a system for curing delusions, for stripping away the convincing quality of disease and letting a healthier reality take its place."

Ayurveda seeks to lead the patient away from the apparent reality of his symptoms and the seemingly convincing perception that being sick is his dominant reality, into the quantum realm where anything is possible depending on our intent. Ayurvedic techniques, which include meditation, "lead the mind to a 'free zone' that is not touched by disease," says Chopra, who reminds all his clients that illness scenarios are ultimately self-created, mental ideas that convince us at the cellular level, as the following case study indicates.

A middle-aged radiologist consulted Chopra after receiving a diagnosis of leukemia from another specialist at a leading cancer institute. He decided to postpone the experimental drug protocols they had recommended; he came to Chopra to find out how to produce a spontaneous remission. Right away, Chopra perceived that the radiologist's medical obsession with statistics and their presumed import was undermining his chances; his client's sense of hope was hobbled by the absence of any cases of spontaneous remission from his kind of leukemia in the scientific literature.

Why don't you tell yourself you have some other form of cancer in which the hopes for remission are brighter, suggested Chopra, handing him his first straw. Later, he suggested the radiologist defer blood tests because bad results would depress his spirits and immune system and make it harder to keep living as if he were healing; then Chopra recommended not calling it "cancer" at all, but rather a mysterious, unnamed "chronic disease."

"So far, I have done nothing for this man except change the label on his disease, but from that he changed his whole appraisal," remarks Chopra in *Quantum Healing*. With his condition repositioned, the man was ready to begin Ayurvedic treatment at Chopra's clinic. "Now we have a chance to witness the birth of a cure."

The Quantum Blueprint for Healing

In Chopra's view, placebo response, spontaneous remission, exceptional patients, and repositioning disease concepts are all aspects of the fluidity and freedom of the quantum approach to healing. The body is a quantum field whose blueprint for health or illness is always subject to revision, explains Chopra. It's the "observer effect" of quantum physics played out in biology: how you look at it and what you're looking for determine what you see. We are thoughts that have learned to create a physical body, says Chopra, a quantum field in which we can justifiably assert that the brain and the immune system *are* each other and that a neuropeptide "moves with thought, serving as a point of transformation."

The placebo response, spontaneous remission, even faith healing, give us our first vivid insights into the mechanism of creation whereby material reality (biological change) comes into existence, Chopra comments. Specific biochemicals and neurotransmitters become the bodily mediators of our focused attention in a field of all possibilities.

The new physics disallows the classical bifurcation of reality into field and matter, says Chopra. "The field, which is consciousness, is the only reality—pure potentiality, which is our own awareness, the pure potential for information states. Thoughts are quantum events in the field of energy, impulses of energy and information." The field is without limitations and it's only our conceptual restrictions—Chopra calls these, variously, cultural indoctrinations, consensus reality, reality maps, the superstition of materialism, and the "hypnosis of social conditioning"—that can rein in our ability to regenerate biology.

The war in the mind-body system, the fear born of duality itself, and the mistake of the intellect that refuses to believe everything (both sickness and healing) is happening inside the mind-body unity—here we have the chief cause of all illness, contends Chopra.

"As we experience our own spiritual essence, our intentions can be triggers for bodily transformation. In Ayurveda we see the body as a network of intelligence and pranic energy, as a bundle of consciousness, a function of our level of awareness. Consciousness conceives, governs, constructs, and becomes physical matter through converting impulses of energy and information into material events." Through inner stillness and meditation, says Chopra, awareness reveals itself to us as the maker of reality, as unconditional life. "If you knew how to control the creation of impulses of intelligence, you would be able not only to grow new dendrites but anything else."

Chopra's pronouncement about nerve cell regeneration may not be so unachievably idealistic, according to recent work at the University of Calgary Faculty of Medicine. There two neurobiologists in 1992, treating nerve tissue from mice in vitro with a powerful stimulatory protein called epidermal growth factor, discovered that some of the stem cells (15 of 1,000) bloomed into connective glial cells and neurons. Scientists had always believed that the mammalian brain, unlike the liver, skin, stomach lining, and immune system, was incapable of regenerating nerve cells; the results of this study could overturn that assumption completely, and introduce new therapeutic options for neurodegenerative diseases like Parkinson's, Alzheimer's, and Huntington's.

"Just because the brain doesn't repair itself normally, doesn't mean it can't repair itself," said Dr. Samuel Weiss, one of the study's two investigators.

Multiple Identities Bloom in the Human Psyche

The baffling phenomenon of multiple personality disorders (MPD) also highlights the astonishing plasticity of the mind-body. MPD is a truly discomfiting fact for our scientific paradigm to embrace; some call it the "UFO of psychiatry," for others it's "mind in many pieces."

In MPD numerous apparently separate and autonomous selves (subpersonalities or fragments) cyclically occupy self-referential prominence in the psyche of an individual. The average number of multiple selves per psyche is placed at eight to thirteen, but it can be far higher: among famous, clinically evaluated or popularly reported cases, Sybil had 16; Eve had 22; Billy Milligan had 24; Cassandra had 180; Truddi Chase, the contemporary subject of the mass-market bestseller, *When Rabbit Howls,* had 92. In addition to the observable shifts in personality among multiples within one individual, even more startling are the effects on physiological, neurological, and immunological variables.

Studies conducted by NIH on MPD individuals have shown

dramatic shifts in brain activity, cerebral blood flow, and hemispheric dominance, as measured by EEGs (electroencephalograms), as the subpersonalities switch dominance; further, there are striking differences in allergic reactivity; and some female multiples have three menstrual cycles per month. Each subpersonality has a separate name, age, memories, abilities, handwriting, gender, IQ, racial and ethnic background, even foreign-language fluency.

The changes that a subpersonality, during its moment of dominance, produces on the biology of the individual are awesome. The degree of change argues strongly for the view that human biology acts according to a script written by the personality, and that our organic well-being is a psychological drama played out in matter. It also raises fundamental questions about the solidity, permanence, and authority of the individual self: non-MPD people take it for granted but is it a fiction?

Frequently a pronounced medical condition, such as diabetes or allergenicity, will temporarily vanish as subpersonalities change their "shift" within the individual. One study showed that all but one of a patient's multiples were allergic to orange juice; when the subject drank orange juice, his skin broke out in a prolific rash unless this single nonallergenic subpersonality was in charge, in which case there was no dermatological reaction. An individual may show physiological symptoms of diabetes, epilepsy, or hypertension, but when a nonepileptic, nondiabetic, or nonhypertensive personality switches into dominance, these symptoms disappear, as if retracted by the previous personality as so much biological baggage. Warts, scars, and skin rashes similarly come and go with subpersonality dominance.

Multiples evidence great differences in sensitivity to pain. In a classic example, a Yale psychiatrist was treating a multiple who arrived one day with an eye swollen shut from a wasp sting; he was in severe pain and couldn't wait even one hour to see an ophthalmologist. The psychiatrist, remembering that one of this patient's subpersonalities was an "anesthetic" self who never felt pain, invoked this self to assume control of the patient's body for the next hour and impart its analgesic effects. Within a couple of hours, the pain and swelling had disappeared and the ophthalmologist's services weren't required; the anesthetic personality had transformed the individual's physiology by the mere assumptions of its presence.

Subpersonalities can mitigate the effects of alcohol, instantly sobering up an intoxicated individual. They respond to drugs differently: one personality requires five milligrams of a tranquilizer while another fails to respond to even 100 milligrams; and if one personality is a child, and takes an adult's amount of medication, it can produce the effects of drug overdose—all this in the same body. Differences have been documented in handedness, visual acuity, optical needs, eye color, shape and curvature of the eyes, optical refraction, color blindness, facial expression, accent, vocabulary, body language, phobias, voice pattern (according to spectral analysis of their "voiceprints"), and speed and frequency of healing.

These multiple perspectives are cogent evidence for the many-chambered self, comment Judith Hooper and Dick Teresi in *The 3-Pound Universe*. The "often astonishing gifts of their satellite personae" consistently observed in MPDs, "make a strange showcase for the untapped potentials inside every brain."

The facts of MPD, comments Michael Talbot, who reviews some of the field's rich literature in *The Holographic Universe*, "offer further evidence of just how much our psychological states can affect the body's biology. This suggests that somewhere in our psyches we *all* have the ability to control these things." For Talbot, the MPD facts illustrate the holographic nature of the human mind-body. "If the psyche of an individual with MPD is a kind of multiple image hologram, it appears that the body is one as well, and can switch from one biological state to another as rapidly as the flutter of a deck of cards."

Recent studies on the probable psychogenesis of MPD (85% of people with MPD are women) indicate that 97% have a childhood history of trauma, incest, beating, torture, or abuse, suggesting that the qualities of dissociation, hypnotic trance, and fragmented multiplicity arose as a defense and coping mechanism, a "psychophysical athleticism" and "fluidity of childhood" carried into adult life, as Michael Murphy phrases it. NIMH researcher Frank Putnam noted a correlation between the huge changes in mood, cognitive style, and configurations of hormonal, neuronal, and muscular reactivity in MPD individuals with the two facts that children can switch emotions rapidly and flexibly according to circumstances and that MPD tends to originate in terrible abuses received during childhood.

Recent child physiological and developmental studies suggest a picture of natural, fluidic multiplicity in self-identity in two ways.

First, apparently a child's brain contains hundreds of times more nerve endings than an adult's, thereby making the child highly impressionable to experiences and more open to learning. "Thus, instead of small seedlings needing time and proper input to grow, children's' minds actually resemble more closely luxuriant bushes whose branching cells are 'pruned back' over the course of development," explains Susan C. Roberts in an MPD survey article in *Common Boundary*.

Second, apparently children do not have a continuous self-consciousness and sense of stable observing self, Roberts reports; rather, they "move through a progression of different states," such as a "crying state," a "bright and shiny state," and so forth. It's only through attainment of adulthood that this natural, prolific multiplicity of identity congeals into a consistent observing self, "an overarching construct that yokes all the still-discrete states together." That's the norm; severe childhood trauma can shatter the standard developmental sequence into dozens of self-identity fragments, generating an MPD individual.

In this sense, MPD distorts the innate psychomutability of young children into a contortion of self and biology as adults. MPD indicates a remarkable human skill—the plasticity of the mind-body and of self-referential focus—shown in negative, distorted relief, a perverse, unintegrated form of extraordinary functioning, says Murphy. "Like certain religious adepts, multiples alter their flesh and consciousness through highly focused intention, hypnosis-like trance, and the retention of childlike mutability, though they do so in a dissociated and psychologically destructive manner."

Murphy cites the research of psychiatrist Eugene Bliss, who hypnotized MPD patients to find out how they switched personalities. One explained her "perfected method of self-alteration" to him as follows: "She lies down, but can do it sitting up, concentrates very hard, clears her mind, blocks everything out, and then wishes for (another identity), but she isn't aware of what she is doing."

That's the key of course: it's an *unconscious* strategy. For MPDs it's the survival skill of protean polymorphous personality, but for more psychologically integrated individuals, the mechanisms of MPD might indicate ways to access unexploited but extraordinary healing and creative powers. As Deepak Chopra insightfully queries, the implications of MPD, spontaneous remission, and placebo response may hearken to the same quantum mutability of the mind-body: "Is there any difference between my patient making her angina disappear and a multiple personality doing the same thing?"

Mysteries of the Coma:
Time-Out with the Dreambody

Taking its place alongside the placebo response, PNI, and multiple personality disorders, and the startling implications these pose about the efficacy of consciousness independent of and interdependent with its material context, the body, is the coma and its mysteries. In Western medical thinking, coma is the dead end of conscious life, the reduction of the human self to an inert vegetable existence of bare sentience.

But maybe something else is happening during the apparent "lights out" experience of coma. The materialist-reductionist model may collapse in the face of evidence suggesting the survival and activity of consciousness beyond the viability of the physical body, as demonstrated by the "dreambody" life of comatose people.

Anecdotal and word-of-mouth stories about unusual experiences in coma have been appearing in the public press for years. Allopathic scientists may dismiss them as circumstantial but not substantive, but some of them are plainly riveting. Consider Mary Kay Blakely, who offered *Redbook* readers a firsthand revelation of her own coma experience at age thirty-six. She was working as a freelance journalist when a combination of influenza, flu, emotional confusion, and diabetes sent her into a coma. Like any well-trained news reporter, Blakely took good notes—in this case, from inside her coma. Her *Redbook* piece, later expanded into a book *(Wake Me When It's Over),* claims to be a first-person narrative of her experience of the coma.

Contact with close, supportive friends helped a great deal, says Blakely. Her partner was with her most of the time during the hospital ordeal. "When Larry spoke or touched me, I heard and felt him but couldn't speak or touch in return. My body was like a broken transmitter, able to receive but not send any messages." Then Blakely's sister arrived, with whom she was a childhood bosom buddy, and this began to make the difference. "In my dream I'd heard people talk about me, around me, over me, but until Gina arrived, no one had spoken directly to me. Gina brought faith. Her belief in my survival was absolute."

In the end Blakely was "completely rewired by nine days of hallucinations." She finally woke up "into an atmosphere of unconditional love, as an adult, knowing that my family and friends had forgiven me and passionately wanted me back, however contentious and difficult. I re-entered the world, shaken but whole. The personal responsibility I'd abandoned became my own again."

For Blakely, the coma experience had been meaningful, even transformative; it had not been a lacuna of consciousness in her life, an empty space, dead time. That's exactly the kind of startling testimonial of the inner psychological journey of the comatose that would be appreciated by Jungian coma therapist Arnold Mindell, whose dreambody views we have briefly explored earlier. Possibly the only difference is that he usually conducts his psychoanalytic counseling *inside* the patient's coma, understanding coma to be a process of consciousness conducted by the dreambody, or self, to achieve a goal. If Mindell's observations are credited, it could push us right to the edge of our understanding of the coma experience— and on through into something else entirely.

The coma is like an extended dream state, an inner process trying to unfold to deepen our self-knowledge, a dream that has seized the body, claims Mindell in *Coma: Key to Awakening*. A certified Jungian analyst from Zurich, Switzerland, and now director of the Process Work Center in Portland, Oregon, in recent years Mindell and his colleague-wife, Amy, have traveled extensively, teaching and training students in his unique somatic practice called process-oriented psychology. First off, Mindell questions the belief that comas are unconscious, inaccessible states. "There are powerful, dramatic, and meaningful events trying to unfold themselves in comatose states," says Mindell. One such event is the innate drive for self-knowledge.

"Except for those with severe structural brain damage, all the comatose people I have seen have awakened and verbally communicated powerful experiences." Coma, says Mindell, can be part of the psychological maturing process. "Comatose people are wakeful human beings going through one more meaningful step in their process of individuation. Over the last fifteen years the people I've worked with around the world who have remained in coma for long periods of time are people who are trying to work on themselves to seek something internally. The coma is one of the best ways of doing this. The coma allows you to be quiet, internal, to focus on things inside. There's no internal dividing line with your inner experiences between coma, dreaming, Near-Death Experiences, even occasional psychotic episodes."

Doorway into an Awareness of Life beyond the Body

If in some way the comatose patient actually makes constructive use of his down time once he's in coma, what kind of psychological factor propels one into this kind of traumatic leave-taking from conventional life in the first place? "If there was nobody around with whom they could communicate about their problems," says Mindell. "It's an act of metaphysical desperation and a relationship signal. It says the man needs to experience and work through a dreamlike state because there's nobody around with whom he can do it. These are not just people who are physically handicapped; they are potentially creative people with whole lifetime stories happening to them."

This understanding then translates into coma prevention, says Mindell. If we approach the noncomatose with an attitude of wanting a deeper relation, wanting to find out more about one another, in ordinary states of consciousness, the tendencies to slip into coma will be reduced. Mindell reports experiences of entering the room of a comatose patient who suddenly awakens to tell him of a deep dream state or stories from outer space. "As soon as we leave, she will go back into coma, or she will re-create that coma to protect herself against the kind of treatment she gets from other people. If the nurse comes in, just to clean her back or roll her over, she reproduces the coma, but as soon as we're there, the person awakens."

Mindell assures me the remarkable alarm clock effect he has isn't related to any celebrity status as a coma therapist he may have with patients. Typically he and Amy enter a room unintroduced. What the patient hears is a caring voice willing to engage in a dialog. This is the beginning of Mindell's process-oriented work. It treats the coma as a dreaming process trying to unfold and express itself through the body for the purposes of self-understanding. Mindell takes a phenomenological approach to the whole matter.

"The governing idea behind my work is a mixture of scientific realism, phenomenological respect for individual experiences, and the suspicion that everything that happens contains the seeds of our totality," says Mindell. "I work with the client's perception. I take what they are saying as facts unto themselves, as a description of their experience. I've learned to follow people and facts and realities as closely as possible. A phenomenological approach accepts the comatose state as it is described and allows the signals descriptive of this state to unfold into a process."

The signals are what Mindell calls "minimal body cues"—coughs, eye rolls, tongue clicks, facial grimaces, finger twitches, changes in breathing. It may strike many as a fabulous concept, but Mindell claims these minute physical reflexes are consciously intended and can be the therapist's thread into the dream state, where the comatose patient is trying to conduct business. The dreaming process (or dreambody) is reflected through the physical body in these minimal movements, says Mindell. "They are a thread into the psyche to find a way to connect to the deepest part of the human being where she feels creative and is co-creating her dream world."

Mindell's clinical anecdotes vividly make his point. He once worked with a man dying of stomach cancer. After a major operation, the patient pointed to his stomach, grinned and said, "It's still growing." He flexed his delicate stomach up and down to illustrate. "It gets bigger and bigger all the time!" he croaked. Mindell asked him what would happen next. The man suddenly realized he had dreamed the previous night of an explosion in his body. "That was the first time I realized the man had been dreaming his healing as it was trying to happen physically," says Mindell. "Paradoxically, his cancer was an attempt to heal him. This was a man who never exploded. He kept everything inside, all his thoughts and feelings."

In *Coma,* Mindell graphically relates the use of process-oriented psychotherapy with a coma patient named Peter. One day Peter had a troubling cough accompanied by facial grimaces. Mindell imitated the cough but exaggerated the facial expressions. Soon the cough disappeared and Peter, though still, paradoxically, in some degree of coma, begin to sing, then talk. Meanwhile, his body was swollen with water from kidney failure. Mindell considered the significance of this and said, "Why didn't I think of this before? The inner spirit has a rough time in such a small bottle!"

Mindell encouraged Peter to uncork the bottle at his throat and let the spirit out of the bottle. "Then Peter began to shout just for the sake of shouting. We screamed and shouted together for a long time. Apparently it was this spirit in the bottle making rattling noises through bronchial pneumonia and blowing up the body through kidney failure. If somebody tells me he experiences himself as a spirit locked into a bottle, that's a picture of a state trying to unfold, like a picture trying to become real."

In Mindell's view, coma therapy is just a highly refined method of communication. "We're singing their song so they feel supported. Not only do we want to get inside the coma, but we want to get the comatose dreamer to believe in what's happening. In coma you have some of the deepest issues you've never worked on. Why live? Why not just die? What's my life all about? These deep questions become experiences, and by tapping into these experiences, the keys to life unravel."

The coma experience, Mindell stresses, is a very special dream trying to deepen our understanding. "In this blackest hole of life, the processes that have been waiting inside of us our whole lives seek completion and realization. The sooner people believe in their trance and coma states, the more readily they are resolved. So we encourage them to remember. That's the way out for them. The experiences themselves are the road out of the coma."

Mindell doesn't rest his case without making one last point. Maybe coma isn't "this dark hole of life" as most M.D.s contend, says Mindell. Might this medical-psychiatric cul-de-sac called coma be a major opening into a broader field of consciousness? "Oh my God and how!" says Mindell. Rather than the dead end of conscious life, coma may turn out to be, in Mindell's words, the key to awakening. "Coma and all these physical symptoms, all the dreadful pathological things that happen to us—they could all be a doorway. The stronger the symptom, the more powerful the enlightenment. Such cases lead me to the idea that awareness can also be located outside of the physical body."

A Father's Love—Life inside His Son's Coma

The astonishing lucidity Mindell teases out of the comatose dreambody for others gifted with clairvoyant sight is a personally corroborable reality. Consider the experience of Mike Booth, an English father whose teenage son, Aaron, spent several years in deep coma after sustaining a brutal head injury. "The initial prediction was that with such massive bleeding in the brain coupled with brain stem injury, Aaron would be lucky if he was ever anything more than a vegetable," admits Booth. A parent's nightmare had crashed into his life. Maybe it was the traditional British stiff upper lip, but once he got his bearings, Booth took a much more plucky view of his son's future than the somber physician's report would justify.

"I was shocked when I got to the hospital and saw Aaron on the life-support system and realized the gravity of the situation. It took me a week before I was able to overcome the shock enough to be able to really tune into what had happened, to get beyond the appearance of things." When he got beyond the dismaying medical appearance of things, Booth was with his son every step of the way. He never lost sight of Aaron during the two years of his coma. He talked to him, counseled him, admonished him, even went to the zoo with him. As Booth recounts his experience, he went right inside the coma and stood beside Aaron as he went through an intense inner psychological process. "The coma doesn't look the same from the inside," says Booth.

Booth has a gift many grieving fathers might wish to have, too. He's clairvoyant. He could see what Aaron was doing as a spiritual being outside his brain-damaged body. He understood Aaron's intention in precipitating the coma. He realized the coma was more than a medical issue alone. What Booth reports is of course highly controversial and probably won't change the minds of too many M.D.s overnight, but it might encourage some parents who don't want to be daunted by what appears to be an unmitigated disaster. "I've always had the conviction Aaron would be able to maintain himself and fulfill his function in this world ever since the accident happened. I saw directly that Aaron was involved in an initiatory process in his coma on the other side of life. I saw he had been taken out of his present situation for the purposes of going through an initiation within a culture that doesn't provide that for children entering adulthood."

What Booth has to say about his son's experience of coma puts it in the same paradigm-shifting category as deep dream and trance states, patient reports of awareness during anesthesia, and Near-Death Experiences (NDEs). All of these by now are widely reported—and widely debated. Traditionally coma is regarded by both physicians and patients as the black hole of consciousness, a dark, empty land at the end of the body from which few return to tell any tales. Physicians struggle to perfect their emergency life-support procedures yet often remain as helpless in the face of this physiological impasse as the coma patients themselves. For many, coma is a one-way street. So maybe a second opinion on coma is in order.

Booth's story poses a provocative question. Can consciousness somehow be present and active in coma even though the brain and body are barely functioning? Should we treat the comatose differently? As the kind of remarkable inner experiences people in coma might be having come to light, this could radically shift our understanding not only of what is coma, but the nature of personality, awareness, the dream life, and the survival of consciousness outside the body. Coma, in this view, wouldn't be a total absence of consciousness, only an altered state of perhaps heightened awareness, somehow independent of the physical body. Coma research like this could open up a mind-wobbling possibility that standard medical textbooks never dreamed possible.

Why was Aaron undergoing an initiation through the coma experience? I asked Booth. "In other cultures in the past, when a child got to the point of puberty, he was taken out of the tribe and given various keys to help him enter manhood at a spiritual level. Our Western culture no longer has that facility. So Aaron's being elected this particular method of coma to go through to an initiatory process." What is the initiation all about?

"We could talk about the grey-robed guys standing around Aaron, talking to him about various metaphysical things, but the experience has to do with educating him in his feelings," says Booth. "He's learning how one feels differently as a child than as an adult, how we shut down when we have to grow up. He's learning about the difference in the quality of the feelings that happen when we begin to shut down. The process Aaron's involved in is how to remain open and yet still grow to the point of understanding that he has to function in the world."

The inner psychological need for this kind of initiation at puberty alone was not enough to propel the young curly-headed Aaron into the grassy bank. A decade ago Booth separated amicably from Aaron's mother, with whom Aaron spends the bulk of his time. Family breakups, increasingly common in the West, can have deep-seated repercussions in the children, Booth reasons. His analysis of the kind of repercussion it had on Aaron is both rigorous and startling. "What's happened for me is I've seen the consequences of the dissolution of the nuclear family, what happens to the psyches of the individual concerned in this family when it disperses. So these two factors—the soul purpose, for which he's been prepared in this life, linked with his personality function in relation to his mother—precipitated the coma."

Booth's clairvoyance may have produced insight into his son's traumatic experience, but it also posed an excruciating moral dilemma. As a father, how much should he intervene in Aaron's process? It became a constant tug in his mind—wanting his son back, wanting to heal him, yet knowing Aaron must complete his process in freedom—explains Booth.

"The emotional part is always concerned. This is the concern of the genetic father, to do with love and caring at a human level. I would really like my son back as he was and not have him be going through all this stuff. The other side is my position as a healer. If I heal him, help him out of the coma, but do nothing to understand why he's in this situation, then I deny him the experience that his soul has selected. It's like a healer helping a blind woman get off a train—when she's actually trying to get on."

For many months it was unclear whether Aaron was getting on or off the train of his life, whether he would live or die. (The story has a relatively happy ending: Aaron eventually returned and slowly regained possession of his body and faculties.) "I could very easily at various points in the last two years have helped Aaron to come back, except he may very well have been, at that point, wishing to get on and leave. It has to be his responsibility for his life and body—not anybody else's, not even his father's."

Despite the constant temptation to intervene and bring his son back from the nether world, Booth kept his ground as a compassionate observer. In a paradoxical way, he simply continued his role, if in another guise, as the father of a teenager. "At various points I was in direct mind-to-mind contact with Aaron. At some points I saw he wasn't associated with his body enough even to worry about it. Once I found him at the local zoo looking at the animals. He wasn't even aware he didn't have his body with him, that it was being maintained in a distressing state in the hospital. He was quite happy to be looking at the animals. 'Maybe you've noticed you don't feel some of the things you felt before,' I said to my disincarnate son, trying to get Aaron to realize he'd left his body behind. 'Maybe there might be a reason for that.'"

Another time Booth lay in the bathtub at the home of Aaron's mother. Aaron walked into the bathroom—through the closed door. The dialogue was most unusual, yet shows a father's exacting respect for Aaron's individuality and spiritual freedom. "What are you doing in here while I'm having a bath?" inquired Booth. "I didn't realize you were in here," replied Aaron. "But you didn't even open the door," continued Booth. "I didn't think I needed to," said Aaron. "Well, doesn't that seem wrong to you?" asked Booth. "Maybe I'm asleep," admitted Aaron. "Maybe you ought to reflect on that a little," concluded Booth, returning to his suds, his privacy restored.

The Conscious Imagination of a Healthy Environment

The dominant theme in our consideration of placebo response, PNI, spontaneous remission, multiple personality disorder, and coma has been the prevalence of relatively unconscious and latent but extraordinary restorative, self-healing human capacities that are somehow suddenly mobilized to produce healing.

Might not these latent transformative abilities in which mind clearly shapes and directs biological matter be brought into conscious control? Doesn't the spontaneous though unconsciously directed mutability of psychological and physiological environment imply that the vastly potent mind might consciously re-create environment? "We live only part of the life we are given," notes Michael Murphy. "I firmly believe that all of us can realize at least some of the extraordinary possibilities described here."

As with the phenomena we've already surveyed, the literature of conscious use of the mind to alter biology is richly anecdotal. In her *Imagery in Healing,* Jeanne Achterberg, research director at the University of Texas Health Science Center in Dallas, presents the case of a minister at a Los Angeles metaphysical church. One day he told his congregation that in the mid-1970s, when consulting an oral surgeon for advice on a persistent mouth sore, he was informed that the lesion was a malignant tumor; the surgeon recommended excision of the lesion along with a large portion of his jaw. The minister wasn't enthusiastic about this prospect, which might render him unable to speak, so he took a meditation retreat along the Oregon coast. He devoted his meditations toward the healing of his mouth tissues, visualizing them returning to normal health. His second biopsy, made a few weeks after his return home, indicated complete remission of the tumor.

Achterberg also recounts the directed self-healing experience of the well-known paranormal investigator Stanley Krippner, Ph.D. Earlier in his life, Krippner had abdominal surgery, but the incision wouldn't heal and drained copiously, so his doctors suspected graver internal complications. Krippner consulted an intuitive friend who received the impression that something was amiss with four stitches. Krippner actively imaged these misplaced, irritating stitches as passing out through the drainage tubes, which they did two days later, after which the incision promptly healed.

"I am always touched by such stories," comments Achterberg, because they represent "conscious efforts to use the imagination," for some, "the most difficult mental work" they had ever undertaken. "More than any research, they support the very special abilities of human beings to heal themselves when nothing else can."

When appreciated in complement with corroborative clinical research, the anecdotally reported validation of these very special human abilities is even further justified. Back in 1963 J. V. Basmajian published evidence in *Science,* not a journal known to fool around with mentally directed healing, indicating that humans could learn voluntary control over individual cells, specifically, a single nerve fiber in a bundle of nerve fibers. The prolific research and clinical results of biofeedback innovators Elmer and Alyce Green in the 1960s at the Menninger Foundation extended the scientific appreciation of human control ("psychophysiologic self-regulation") over normally autonomic functions. "Recent research has established that it is also possible to influence such autonomic processes intentionally, volitionally, by directing physiological changes via one's focus of attention," notes Elmer Green in *Beyond Biofeedback.*

We can do this, says Green, through a form of autogenic training: "The idea is to *visualize, imagine,* and *feel* that the change is happening, and then just *let it happen.* Do not interfere with the body's tendency to cooperate." It's as if the body needs a cue or indication, supplied by conscious, focused intention, and then a little time and space to respond by producing the "consciously programmed sensation." The Green's contribution was to demonstrate how, through using instrumented biofeedback as a somatic teaching device, conscious control and psychosomatic self-regulation could be extended over "normally unconscious and involuntary body processes."

Intriguing research conducted in the early 1980s at Michigan State University by John Schneider and C. Wayne Smith demonstrated the responsivity of the human immune system to active, focused imagery procedures. Their findings, comments Achterberg, who summarizes their work, "suggest that the imagination, in and of itself, without years and years of meditation training, and without biofeedback, can control certain functions of the neutrophils." A neutrophil is one of several granules (along with eosinophils and basophils—collectively called granulocytes) present in phagocytic cells of the immune system, which are involved in the digestion (phagocysis) of foreign materials.

Eight men and eight women were selected for this study on the basis of general good health and a willingness to believe it possible they might learn to control their own immunological function. Blood samples were taken, personality inventories assessed, slides of neutrophils were shown, relaxation and imagery methods were demonstrated.

The group was asked to spend twenty minutes visualizing the activity of neutrophils within their own immune system, to imagine them acting as free-ranging garbage collectors that gathered biological toxins and removed them from the body. Afterward their white blood cell count was compared with values obtained before the exercise; all sixteen subjects showed a drop in white blood cell count from 8,200 to 6,400, with an average neutrophil depletion of 60%. Insofar as the students had actively visualized neutrophils removing toxic materials from the blood, it was reasonable, if not encouraging, to see a drop in their count after the exercise. The visualization, after all, was highly specific to neutrophils.

Researchers also noted that there was a big drop in neutrophil adherence to cell walls; although the students had been asked to visualize the neutrophils as adhering to cell walls, apparently these were flushed out of the system, and uninstructed, nonadhering neutrophils remained. But when the participants imaged the neutrophils as adhering during the imagery procedure, the count doubled, rising from 28% to 56%.

According to Achterberg, these experiments were repeated in Schneider's lab and elsewhere with even tighter controls and with the same results, persuasively ruling out chance expectations. "Imagery appears to have a direct impact on the function of the neutrophils, at least for those who believe it will."

The relationship between belief and will and their combined power to affect, even reform, the environment when focused through effective imagery will assume greater importance as the book proceeds. What's needed next is to identify the meeting place between inner and outer environments, what I will call the etheric interface. Not only a meeting place, the etheric interface will prove to be a prime theater for the effective operation of consciousness in contacting, informing, and reforming the environment.

References

Achterberg, Jeanne, *Imagery in Healing—Shamanism and Modern Medicine*, New Science Library/Shambhala, Boston, 1985.

Angier, Natalie, "New Nerve Tissue Generated from the Brain Cells of Mice," *The New York Times*, (March 27, 1992).

Beecher, H.K., "The Powerful Placebo," *The Journal of the American Medical Association*, Vol. 159, (1955).

Bennett, Peter, N.D., "Placebo and the Art of Medicine," in *A Textbook of Natural Medicine*, edited by Joseph E. Pizzorno, N.D., and Michael T. Murray, N.D., John Bastyr College Publications, Seattle, 1988.

Blakeslee, Sandra, "Finding a New Messenger for the Brain's Signals to the Body," *The New York Times*, (August 11, 1992).

Blakely, Mary Kay, "Halfway to Heaven!" *Redbook*, (July 1989).

—*Wake Me When It's Over—A Journey to the Edge and Back*, Times Books, New York, 1989.

Bodian, Stephan, "Field of Dreams, An Interview with Arnold Mindell," *Yoga Journal*, (March/April 1990).

Bok, Sissela, "The Ethics of Giving Placebos," *Scientific American*, Vol. 231, No. 5, (November 1974).

Borkovec, T.D., "Placebo: Defining the Unknown," in *Placebo—Theory, Research, and Mechanisms*, edited by White, Leonard, Tursky, Bernard, and Schwartz, Gary E., The Guildford Press, New York, 1985.

Browning, Frank, "Murder by Placebo?" *Hippocrates*, (July/August 1989).

Chase, The Troops for Truddi, *When Rabbit Howls*, Jove Books, New York, 1987.

Chopra, Deepak, M.D., *Quantum Healing: Exploring the Frontiers of Mind/Body Medicine*, Bantam Books, New York, 1989.

—*Unconditional Life: Mastering the Forces that Shape Personal Reality*, Bantam Books, New York, 1991.

Cousins, Norman, *Anatomy of an Illness as Perceived by the Patient: Reflections on Healing and Regeneration*, Bantam Books, New York, 1981.

Dow, Mary Louise, with Wagenheim, Jeff, "Encounters with a Medicine Man," *New Age Journal*, (July/August 1992).

Dreher, Henry, "Are You Immune-Competent?" *Natural Health*, (January/February 1992).

Evans, Frederick J., "Expectancy, Therapeutic Instructions, and the Placebo Response," in *Placebo—Theory, Research, and Mechanisms*, edited by White, Leonard, Tursky, Bernard, and Schwartz, Gary E., The Guildford Press, New York, 1985.

Goleman, Daniel, "Your Unconscious Mind May be Smarter Than You," *The New York Times*, (June 23, 1992).

—"Placebo Effect is Shown to be Twice as Powerful as Expected," *The New York Times*, (August 17, 1993).

Green, Elmer and Alyce, *Beyond Biofeedback*, Knoll Publishing, Ft. Wayne, 1977.

Grünbaum, Adolf, "Explication and Implications of the Placebo Concept," in *Placebo—Theory, Research, and Mechanisms*, edited by White, Leonard, Tursky, Bernard, and Schwartz, Gary E., The Guildford Press, New York, 1985.

Hahn, Robert A., "A Sociocultural Model of Illness and Healing," in *Placebo—Theory, Research, and Mechanisms*, edited by White, Leonard, Tursky, Bernard, and Schwartz, Gary E., The Guildford Press, New York, 1985.

Hall, Stephen S., "A Molecular Code Links Emotions, Mind and Health," *Smithsonian*, (July 1988).

—"Cheating Fate," *Health*, (April 1992).

Hiller, Stephanie, "A New Answer to Cancer," *Yoga Journal*, (September/October 1993).

Hooper, Judith, and Teresi, Dick, *The 3-Pound Universe*, Jeremy P. Tarcher, Los Angeles, 1986.

Hunt, Morton, "Faith, Hope & Placebos," *Longevity*, (May 1991).

Hurley, Thomas J., III, "Placebo Effects: Unmapped Territory of Mind/Body Interactions," *Investigations*, Institute of Noetic Sciences, Vol. 2, No. 1, (1985).

Johnsen, Thomas C., "Christian Scientists and the Medical Profession: A Historical Perspective," *Medical Heritage*, (January/February 1986).

Justice, Blair, Ph.D., *Who Gets Sick—How Beliefs, Moods, and Thoughts Affect Your Health*, Jeremy P. Tarcher, Los Angeles, 1988.

Keyes, Daniel, *The Minds of Billy Milligan*, Random House, New York, 1981.

Kline, David, "The Power of Placebo," *Hippocrates*, (May/June 1988).

Klopfer, Bruno, "Psychological Variables in Human Cancer," *Journal of Prospective Techniques*, Vol. 31, (1957).

Leviton, Richard, "Mysteries of the Coma," *East West*, (September 1990).

Locke, Steven, M.D., and Colligan, Douglas, *The Healer Within—The New Medicine of Mind and Body*, New American Library, New York, 1986.

Mindell, Arnold, Ph.D., *The Leader as Martial Artist: Techniques and Strategies for Resolving Conflict and Creating Community*, HarperSanFrancisco, San Francisco, 1992

—*Coma—Key to Awakening*, Shambhala Publications, Boston, 1989.

Murphy, Michael, *The Future of the Body: Explorations into the Further Evolution of Human Nature*, Jeremy P. Tarcher, Los Angeles, 1992.

O'Regan, Brendan, "Multiple Personality—Mirrors of a New Model of Mind?" *Investigations*, A Bulletin of the Institute of Noetic Sciences, Vol. 1, No.3/4, (1985).

—"Placebo—The Hidden Asset in Healing," *Investigations*, Institute of Noetic Sciences, Vol. 2, No. 1, (1985).

—"Psychoneuroimmunology: The Birth of a New Field," *Investigations*, A Bulletin of the Institute of Noetic Sciences, Vol. 1, No. 2, (1983).

—"Healing Remission and Miracle Cures," *Noetic Sciences Collection, 1980-1990—Ten Years of Consciousness Research*, Institute of Noetic Sciences, Sausalito, (1991).

—and Carlyle Hirshberg. *Spontaneous Remission: An Annotated Bibliography.* Institute of Noetic Sciences, Sausalito, CA, 1993.

Ornstein, Robert, and Sobel, David, *The Healing Brain: Breakthrough Discoveries About How the Brain Keeps Us Healthy,* Simon and Schuster, New York, 1987.

Parsons, H.M., "What Happened at Hawthorne?" *Science,* Vol. 183, (March 1974).

Peel, Robert, *Health and Medicine in the Christian Science Tradition,* The Crossroad Publishing Co., New York, 1988.

—*Spiritual Healing in a Scientific Age,* Harper & Row, San Francisco, 1987.

Plotkin, William B., "A Psychological Approach to Placebo: The Role of Faith in Therapy and Treatment," in *Placebo—Theory, Research, and Mechanisms,* edited by White, Leonard, Tursky, Bernard, and Schwartz, Gary E., The Guildford Press, New York, 1985.

Resnick, Susan Kushner, "The Benefits of Suggestion During Surgery," *Natural Health,* (May/June 1992).

Roberts, Susan C., "Multiple Realities, How MPD is Shaking up Our Notions of the Self, the Body, and Even the Origins of Evil," *Common Boundary,* (May/June 1992).

Ross, Sherman, and Buckalew, L.W., "Placebo Agentry: Assessment of Drug and Placebo Effects," in *Placebo—Theory, Research, and Mechanisms,* edited by White, Leonard, Tursky, Bernard, and Schwartz, Gary E., The Guildford Press, New York, 1985.

Roud, Paul C., M.D., *Making Miracles—An Exploration into the Dynamics of Self-Healing,* Warner Books, New York, 1990.

Roueché, Berton, "Annals of Medicine—Placebo," *The New Yorker,* (October 15, 1960).

Schreiber, Flora Rheta, *Sybil,* Henry Regnery Company, Chicago, 1973.

Schwartz, Tony, "Doctor Love—Bernie Siegel and his Controversial Theories of Self-Healing," *New York,* (June 12, 1989).

Sliker, Gretchen, *Multiple Mind—Healing the Split in Psyche and World,* Shambhala, Boston, 1992.

Talbot, Michael, *The Holographic Universe,* HarperCollins, New York, 1991.

Weil, Andrew, M.D., "Stimulating the Placebo Response," *Natural Health,* (July/August 1992).

—*Health and Healing: Understanding Conventional and Alternative Medicine,* Houghton Mifflin Co., Boston, 1983.

White, Leonard, Tursky, Bernard, and Schwartz, Gary E., "Placebo in Perspective," in *Placebo—Theory, Research, and Mechanisms,* edited by White, Leonard, Tursky, Bernard, and Schwartz, Gary E., The Guildford Press, New York, 1985.

Williams, Wendy, *The Power Within: True Stories of Exceptional Patients Who Fought Back with Hope,* Harper & Row, New York, 1990.

CHAPTER **6**

Etheric Interfaces: Common Ground for Body and World

We now shift into the third phase of the argument of *Physician*—the unity of self and environment. Once the unity is established, healing of the environment, both immunological and ecological, can begin. This chapter examines some of the notable healing interfaces, or places of connection, between the human and the environment, starting with the field of music therapy.

Musical Healing: Bridging Immunology and Ecology

Central to the healing effect of music is a clay statue. According to Hafiz, the fourteenth-century Sufi poet, in the beginning God made a clay statue as an image of divinity and asked the human soul to enter it. But the soul refused, regarding this forced incarnation as an imprisonment; after all, the soul was used to flying freely about the celestial world, unbound and unlimited. So God requested the angels to play their music and this brought the soul such ecstasy that in order to better comprehend this music of life, it willingly entered the clay body—the human form.

But angelic music was more than God's lure, as Hafiz comments: "People say that the soul, on hearing that song, entered the body; but in reality the soul itself was the song."

Not only is the human soul musical in essence but so is the world, from stars to atoms, quarks to planets, the mystics and scientists tell us. Everything is vibration, or, as the ancient Hindus called it, *Nada Brahma*. The world is sound; all of creation, even emptiness, is vibratory sound. God, or Brahma, the primordial creator and power in the cosmos, is a current of sound, and "the inner consciousness of man and of all living things," says musicologist Joachim-Ernst Berendt. "One singularity, the primal sound of being: Being itself"—that's Nada Brahma.

The sages tell us that the primordial sound of *AUM* is a semi-audible high-pitched electrical vibration that manifests at ten levels, including, as the Chinese said, the *hum* of the dragon, the *growl* of the tiger, referring to rarified qualities of the environment. Nor are the audible and visible worlds too far apart. After all, only forty octaves separate sound from light, or the electromagnetic spectrum, in the vibratory continuum of reality; and the electromagnetic spectrum itself encompasses seventy vibratory octaves.

Much of reality is hearable, potentially. The rose, upon blossoming, has an audible sound, according to photoacoustic spectroscopy, that is like the drone of an organ. A single cornstalk has a demonstrable sound; atoms have individual resonating sounds that collectively form chords, or molecules; the atom is a tiny musical note and even a stone is frozen music.

All of nature exists as a vast oscillatory spectrum. "It is the song of life *par excellence,* an immense choir, millions and billions of sounds that fuse into a grand polyphony, a harmony beyond human imagination," says Berendt in his book, *The World Is Sound, Nada Brahma.*

According to scientists at Yale University, the six visible planets, including Earth, have distinct sounds, based on their magnetospheric waves, and their spectrum spans eight octaves. Mercury has a quicky, busy, chirping, quicksilvery sound, astrophysicists tell us, while Saturn is a slow, dreamy melody, and the Sun is a great musical instrument comprising eighty different overtones. Johannes Kepler, the seventeenth-century German astronomer, anticipated all this when he plotted the harmonical structure of the solar system; around 1619, he discovered that the planets' elliptical orbits produce sonic oscillations in a geometrically orderly scale based on whole-number ratios. Then in 1773, Johann Bode formulated Bode's Law, which mathematically shows how the planets form a chain of musical octaves; each planet's orbital speed is a sound signature of its cosmic pitch, said Bode.

An earlier researcher of cosmic music named Pythagoras had christened this effect the Harmony, or Music, of the Spheres. "Study the monochord," advised the Greek polymath, referring to his famous example of a single stretched and vibrating string, which he likened to the cosmos, "and you will know the secrets of the universe." The ratios of the musical intervals, mathematically demonstrated by Pythagoras' monochord, demonstrated a universal law of harmony, descriptive of planetary motions, the laws of music, and inner soul life.

There is *so much* to hear: the human ear can distinguish 1,378 different tones within the vibratory range of 16 Hz and 25,000 Hz (Hertz, meaning cycles per second). Philosophical musicologists like Hans Kayser argue that the world is better, more deeply, understood through hearing, not viewing, which is why he called his 1946 work on harmonics, *Akroasis,* from the Greek word for "hearing." Kepler's harmonic proportions are spiritual realities that are part of us, said Kayser. "There are powers above and shapes written in the sky which sound in your own soul, which concern you most vitally, and which belong to the Godhead as much as do you in your innermost self."

The Sound Shapes of Matter

Not only does musical sound animate matter, but it may well form it, too. That sound shapes matter and imparts structure was unarguably demonstrated by Swiss scientist Hans Jenny in the 1960s. Using electronic sound oscillators and sophisticated photographic equipment, Jenny documented the reality of wave phenomena underlying matter (a new field he called cymatics) by filming the instantaneous shaping effects of tones, music, and vocal sound on various substances (sand, iron filings, lycopodium powder, water, mercury) spread on a metal plate.

Jenny meticulously catalogued the symmetrical, geometrically perfect structures and elegant sound mandalas that resulted from directing hundreds of different frequency and rhythmic combinations, from single tones and intervals to complex musical harmonies, through the plate. As the sounds increased in frequency, so did the complexity of the figures generated.

Jenny's astonishing images resemble the geometric yantras of Tantric iconography as much as they do the formation of continents, or the intricate vasculature of a liver cell. In his experiments, the inorganic matter on the metal plate kept its structure as long as the specific formative sound continued; for Jenny, this indicated that organic structures in nature, including the tissues and organs of the human body, are upheld by specific longstanding frequencies. "If biological rhythms operate as generative factors at the interval-like frequencies appropriate to them, then harmonic patterns must be necessarily forthcoming," he wrote in 1974. Cymatics, as a vibratory model of reality, was also the key to a musical therapeutics, Jenny realized.

This suggestion was picked up in the 1970s by English osteopath Dr. Peter Guy Manners who developed his unique Cymatic Instrument as a means of delivering therapeutic sound to the human body in the range of 60 Hz to 30,000 Hz through a handheld skin-contact applicator. Disease, in Manner's cymatic model, is a harmonic imbalance, the result of an unfavorable deviation in the body's fundamental vibration, which itself is the summation of numerous interdependent organ, tissue, and molecular vibrations. Jenny's work had proved that sound has a formative effect on every atom, cell, molecule, and organ; this means the human body is a great and complex sound resonator comprised of many octaves of biological systems potentially in harmonious, musical relationship.

Biological forms are a nested hierarchy of harmonics, of multilayered frequencies. Our body is filled with implicit biological music, the rhythmicity of our organic life, breathing, and nerve conductivity. Health is maintained through regulating the harmonics of the body, said Manners; when the individual harmonics of the heart, liver, spleen, bones, and muscles vibrate in harmony, we are in harmonic pulse and healthy. "But if any part loses its tune or goes out of phase, then we are in trouble"—until we reproduce those necessary harmonic signals through the Cymatic applicator to reestablish an organ's innate sound. Manners, and a handful of other cymatic therapists, has worked successfully with conditions such as bone fractures, arthritis, muscle strain, whiplash, slipped discs, fibrositis, paralysis, and rheumatism, but after twenty years, he considers the field to be still in its infancy.

Cymatic therapy may be still in its early days, but the field of musical therapy—healing with music, voice, and sound—is among the oldest and most holistic of medical approaches. Novalis, the eighteenth-century German mystical poet, formulated its potential clearly: "Every sickness is a musical problem. The healing, therefore, is a musical resolution. The shorter the resolution, the greater the musical talent of the doctor." Again, much earlier, back in the sixth century B.C., that preeminent musical doctor, Pythagoras, had understood the therapeutic qualities of music.

The practical thrust of his science of celestial harmonics was to show his students how to retune their inner life and bodily health through musical laws. Pythagoras, credited today as the founder of music therapy, sang calming melodies to his disciples, based on the principle that melody and rhythm, which originate in cosmic laws, cannot fail to restore the human soul, or emotions, to concord and harmony.

According to his biographer, Iamblichus of Chalcis (250-325 A.D.), Pythagoras tempered, even transformed, the passions, from rage to sorrow, of his students with appropriate melodies applied as salutary medicines. In the evenings, with his lyre and voice, he liberated his disciples from the "perturbations and tumults" of the day, purified their intellectual power, rendered their sleep quiet "and their dreams pleasing and prophetic." In the morning, he freed them "from nocturnal heaviness, relaxation, and torpor, through certain peculiar songs and modulations." Pythagoras, Iamblichus said, held that music "contributes greatly" to health, and is capable of producing, if used in an appropriate manner, "the most beneficial correction of human manners and lives."

The search for the beneficial use of music in that appropriate manner has occupied music healers ever since. It's not surprising that about sixty years ago the prominent psychics Edgar Cayce and Alice Bailey both announced that music would be foremost among therapeutics of the future. The field of music therapy gradually arose in the West with the maturing of the twentieth century, such that today music therapists, composers, performers, and educators of diverse traditions apply Pythagorean principles of music, voice, sound, and universal harmonics to affect human healing, from physical complaints and emotional disturbances to spiritual awakening.

Music can make profound differences in the treatment of autism, dyslexia, Alzheimer's, and depression; reduce anxiety and stress during medical interventions; palliate trauma and chronic pain; generate deep states of relaxation and brain wave entrainment; stimulate inner visionary experience and provoke psychological integration; provide a stairway into spiritual insight and illumination; and help the dying gain repose through a sacramental form of musical midwifery.

Composing Self-Health
with the Body's Sound Physician

In June 1990, Pat Moffitt Cook's physician diagnosed a pelvic mass and recommended immediate surgery for a presumed cancer. "Instantly my wholeness was threatened," comments Cook, then thirty-four, a musician, composer, and multicultural music scholar. Cook's doctor assured her she could not heal herself, that only surgery could remedy this obvious pathology; when she enlisted his support in an experimental program of holistic, alternative healing, including music, he politely fired Cook as a patient.

"From the beginning, I had to find my own way," Cook reflects. "Music became the crucial healing element in my journey. I decided to compose my own health." What better way to put to use her wealth of musical knowledge and fifteen years of study than in this directly personal context. It would be a two-year initiation—a "vibratory transition based on greater understanding and inner knowing"—into the therapeutic realities of music.

Cook supported her healing process with several prominent music-oriented approaches, including toning (free-range vocalization focused on body areas), Guided Imagery and Music (music-assisted psychotherapy involving active imaging), and the Tomatis Method (retraining the ear through listening to frequency-filtered music—all are three discussed below). She thought about music a lot: "A musical composition is a perfect model for understanding wholeness."

The elements of melody, rhythm, harmony, instrumentation, and voice weave a mood picture over time, which is a lot like the human soul, leading us to breakthrough, release, and completion. Cook became acutely aware of inner-body sounds; she used her voice like a musical scalpel, penetrating and dissolving crystallized energy and emotional patterns. "Music-supported healing brings a person inside; we start rearranging the way we think, feel, and interact with the world," says Cook.

When she finally had surgery, she had the anesthesiologist play prechosen music during her operation and recovery. The mass on her ovary wasn't cancer, but endometriosis; not fatal, but problematic enough to provoke her musical odyssey, a gift that when unwrapped, revealed the miracle within music. Her illness had been a test of her belief in the healing powers of music, its powers to heal the psyche through self-understanding and deep insight.

That she still needed surgery didn't mean she hadn't experienced healing through music, Cook insists; she had seen vividly all the ways music can deepen, enrich, and clarify her life. The illness had been in effect a prod to put her music work in full gear. "These trainings, realizations, and therapies were, and still are, themes in composing health. I had woven in as major themes what would help me recognize and achieve a sense of wholeness."

The Living Energies of Color: Healing with the Hues of the Soul

In color and light therapy, we encounter another healing modality in which the healing agent—the *physis*cian, the wielder of *physis*—is a natural energy component of the human being. We are made of sound and light, music and color.

Even within the eclectic field of complementary medicine, color therapy is still a cutting-edge modality, not yet widely practiced or understood. Color healers most commonly use tinted screens, chromatic cards, projected lights, visualizations, and liquid color applied to the body, and advertising designers use colors to subliminally manipulate viewers. The latter is called Aura Soma and was developed in England in the 1980s; its founders liken their system to looking through "God's shop window."

The shop window is a chromatic display of more than 100 "Balance" bottles, colored body oils that tune in to and balance the human aura. Each dual-toned bottle is an emulsified balance of essential oils and aroma essences on top, water-based herb extracts on the bottom, in hues of yellow over red, pink over turquoise, green over gold.

Aura Soma, claim its originators, pharmacist-chiropodist Vicky Wall, cranial osteopath Margaret Cockbain, and former mandala artist Mike Booth, is "a non-intrusive soul therapy," a kind of spiritual restorative based on the living energies of color. What you're most likely to see when through "God's shop window"—Vicky Wall's favorite term for Aura Soma's "brilliant jewels" in bottles, which she first formulated in late 1983—is the "higher dimensions of being, the higher part of yourself, and your personal color code."

For Aura Soma, a unique system in which the color selections are both diagnostic and therapeutic, the responsibility for healing falls predominantly on the client. Through the Balance selection, the client self-diagnoses and self-prescribes, drawing the appropriate remedies from the shop window, because the selection *is* the therapy.

The sensitive practitioner is on hand mainly for interpretation, to clarify "all the qualities, gifts, and obstacles that lie inside a person's shop," says Booth. This clarification can be a remarkably insightful, intimate, even formidable self-perspective from an outsider whom you wouldn't think could know such personal things about you. Your inner self is an open secret spoken through your color choices, says Booth. You just need to understand the language, to know what colors *mean*. The language of an Aura Soma interpretation ranges the gamut of personal health as it's expressed in physical, emotional, and spiritual issues. Booth explains: "The color bottles access your inner, essential parts, showing what you need for the full development of your potential. *You* pull out the remedies that are most relevant for you at this time."

Aura Soma's headquarters in Tetford, Lincolnshire, in the north of England, is called Dev Aura. Dev Aura was Vicky Wall's poetic statement to the future about "the promise" of color therapy. *Dev* means divine or deva, the little elemental spirits that assist nature and the plant kingdom of planet Earth—metaphorically speaking, *plant-net* Earth, the net or web of etheric plant energies says Booth. "These little beings, or devas, are part of the plant network, and when those plants network, then the devas cooperate for the benefit of the whole Earth." When that happens, everything comes into harmony. But there's still a missing link.

That missing link is the human kingdom. "Between the angelic kingdom, which is the *aura*, the whole of the light body that surrounds the Earth, and the world of the *devas*, is Man. We call our house Dev Aura because it brings humans in to make the interface between the devas and the aura, comprised of the beings of light, the angels, and the whole of the light body that surrounds Earth. And at that interface between the three kingdoms, of dev, aura, and humans, we have the living, radiant energies of color—the *aura soma*."

"The aura is the map of the soul"

We are bodies made of living color and energetic radiance, say color therapists like Mike Booth. "We are Hue-man beings, beings of a hue, so it's time we showed our true colors," Booth explains. Showing our "hue-man" colors, so to speak, is a revelation of *Aura Soma* itself—"the light of our being made manifest in living energies," says Vicky Wall. As aura is the light (as in *Aurora,* the Greek goddess of morning light, which is to say the rainbow spectrum of colors) and soma is the energetic body of being, so Aura Soma is "the mirror of the soul," says Wall. "The personal aura is the soul essence of the human being."

Wall speaks of the chromatic light of being, the human aura, with the authority of experience. Wall was gifted with the second sight since childhood, a clairvoyance that revealed an individual's auric secrets or majesty, as she related in her therapist's memoir, *The Miracle of Colour Healing.* "Words, clothing, appearance, all were of no importance; nothing could distract me from the true person within. I was fully aware of their emotions, their thinking."

With this literal in-sight, Wall held the diagnostic key to health and illness, because disturbed, inharmonious auras always presage physical illness. "It is essential that the aura be known and treated first. This is nearly always the root cause of sickness which, physically, mentally, and spiritually, is the outward manifestation of inner auric disturbance. Not only does the Balance system act as a barometer of physical and emotional conditions, it is informative of past, present, and future events. It provides knowledge of the true self which, once revealed and understood, can be healed."

The aura, then, is the map of the true personality, the mirror of the soul in a state either of health or disturbance, says Wall. The renowned sleeping prophet and medical clairvoyant Edgar Cayce corroborated Wall's contentions years earlier in his booklet *Auras,* published in 1945. "I do not remember a time when the human beings I encountered did not register on my retina with blues and greens and reds gently pouring from their heads and shoulders. I do not even think of people except in connection with their aura, the weathervane of the soul."

David Tansley, the late radionics pioneer and a distinguished British therapeutic contemporary of Wall's, also testified to the primacy of the aura. All life forms—human, animal, plants, even minerals—radiate "a surrounding field of energy" into the environment, Tansley explained in *The Raiment of Light*. "Color is a form of vibratory energy. To clairvoyant sight the human aura is alive with glowing ethereal emanations and coruscations of color. These flares and flickerings of color reflect our emotions and give form to our thoughts."

With sensitive practitioners like Wall and Booth, Aura Soma charted the territory of the human aura with precision. Their results, Booth claims, are in accord with the ancient model of the Indian Vedas and represent an intriguing description of what we might call the energetic, radiant hue-man. The human being is part of a universal wavelength that includes all life forms in nature. Everything is light vibrating at particular frequencies described as the electromagnetic spectrum, explains Booth. That includes the human and our multiple bodies arrayed subtly in dovetailing envelopes around our physical form like delicate eggshells of light.

The first layer of the auric field is the electromagnetic field, an electrical corona discharging very close to the skin, which has been measured by modern devices like Kirlian electrophotography. Next comes the etheric body, the formative field of life forces that maintain the physical, and comprising the dualistic world of emotions, either positive or negative. The astral body, the subtlest of the human electromagnetic shells, is "a unified field within all of us, relating to the world of the higher dream body, the higher emotions, the inspirations within the being," says Booth. These three membranes of light enclose the aura and the "chakras."

The subject of chakras, or the seven vital energy centers arranged vertically around the spine in accordance with the endocrine glands, is itself an entire complex science of psychic cartography, Booth notes. Everybody talks about chakras these days, but what can we accurately say about them? As the old Vedic texts explained, the chakras, or spinning color wheels, are like mini power centers energizing distinct color regions in the body. "The ancient Vedas determined that various areas of the human body related to specific wavelengths, such as the sacrum with red, the stomach with yellow, the throat with blue, the heart with green, the brow with indigo. They called these color areas chakras, which means that within a particular body region there is a vibration, a spin, a particular wavelength that is also a colored light."

Aura Soma extended the classical Vedic model of a color-coded human anatomy with epicenters in the individual chakras. Wall postulated a human body wrapped in distinct color bands from red to violet, feet to head, intermeshing at the borders. Whole areas of the torso, not just the vortices of chakra centers, vibrate at a particular color frequency. Red, the slowest human vibratory band and normally associated with the root chakra, envelops the body from the feet to the sacrum, said Wall; and green, the mid-spectrum hue of harmony, is the predominant color band of the entire upper chest cavity, from sternum to collarbone.

The chakras are "the very core of the aura," observes Vicky Wall, the rarefied region in which Aura Soma's work begins. The auroral flickerings of the chakras are the barometer of our inner life. So the aura comprises this modulating rainbow of chakras, but within this there is still the "aura soul core, the true aura." This soul essence has a particular color and is a distilled reflection of our potential, our gifts, our life purpose and lesson—for example, the blue/blue of peaceful communication of my first bottle. "To ensure that the energies flow in harmony, that the complete being of mind, body, and spirit, is 'in tune,' each chakra should be fully open and in balance," Wall contends. "By feeding back the appropriate color, whose wavelength is the key to the chakra needing help, the weakened wavelength is reinforced. This sets in motion the regenerative and healing processes within the body cells themselves."

Not only does Aura Soma's Balance match the color resonance of essential oils, herb extracts, and aroma essences with the human auric color bands, but it imparts the living energies of three kingdoms to midwife its color healing. Aura Soma brings the wavelengths of color, herbs, and gems within the same band of color vibration into the same area of the body, thereby blending their resonant wavelengths, says Booth. The red Balance blends, for example, include the energetic essences of red gems like ruby and garnet, along with the red flowering plants, so it's red energy from three different realms. "The three kingdoms of mineral, plant, and human are united within the same color vibration to bring about the healing response."

Validated by a Century of Color Healing Research

Aura Soma may be the most comprehensive of contemporary color therapies, but it takes its place in the context of more than a hundred years of Western research and innovation in the color-provoked healing response. "The medicine of the future is light," comments Jacob Liberman, O.D., Ph.D., in his excellent study, *Light: Medicine of the Future*. "We are healing ourselves with that which is our essence. Not only is light responsible for the emergence of all life, but life literally is light. Life is truly color-full! Light must be embraced as potentially one of the most powerful disease-prevention tools at our disposal."

Although the ancient Egyptians and Greeks recognized the Sun as the original healer and established color healing temples like Thebes and Heliopolis, says Liberman, it wasn't until the 1870s that Western physicians, predominantly in America, started to probe the therapeutic benefits of life-giving color.

Animal and human bodies are living energy systems kept in balance by the Sun, declared General Augustus Pleasanton in 1876. He reported that blue light, either from the sun or artificially derived, effectively stimulated the glands, nervous system, and secretive organs of animals and people. In 1877 a prominent physician named Seth Pancoast discovered that sunlight filtered through panes of blue or red glass relaxed or accelerated the human nervous system. In the next year Dr. Edwin Babbitt, in *Principles of Light and Color*, described his Chromo Disk, a device that projected light through filtered disks onto the body, and his Chromo Lens, a method of passing solar potentized water through color filters to produce "solar color tinctures."

The preliminary color work of Pleasanton, Pancoast, and Babbitt was largely ignored by professional colleagues, but in 1908 the scientific world took a major step forward in justifying the efficacy of color therapy. Dr. Walter Kilner, a practicing physician at London's St. Thomas' Hospital, developed a photographic process called the Kilner Screen that made the human aura relatively visible, thereby offering doctors a remarkable diagnostic potential.

The aura is triple layered, transiently disfigured in infections, but permanently distorted in pathological conditions, Kilner reported in *The Human Aura*. With the Kilner Screen a physician could now see aspects of the human auric field, a perception that formerly had been available only to medical clairvoyants. Kilner's revolutionary work was refined in the 1930s by Cambridge biologist Oscar Bagnall, who developed an improved screen. Like Kilner he observed light rays extending outward from the inner human aura through an outer pale-blue auric haze and into the environment.

The human raiment of light received further clarification

through the recent work of John C. Pierrakos, a practicing clair-voyant M.D. Pierrakos described the "thrilling phenomenon" of the cloudlike auric envelopes and their precise chromatic pulsa-tions relative to body metabolism, breathing rates, emotional states, humidity, and air ionization. Pierrakos, like Kilner, postulat-ed that the aura sprang from a "longitudinal core of energy" in the physical body, possibly connected with the central nervous system, that radiates outward through the skin to activate the immediate atmosphere and form the triple aura.

The practical, diagnostic correlations of the subtle human anato-my with medicine were advanced in 1967 by neuropsychiatrist Shafica Karagulla when she investigated the applications of clair-voyance for aura diagnosis. Karagulla worked with a team of sensi-tives, matching their psychic perceptions of internal organs, auric colors, and the functional integrity of the chakras with known phys-ical pathologies. For Karagulla's sensitives the healthy etheric body was a matrix of light frequencies penetrating the body like a "sparkling web of light beams"; the etheric webs of unhealthy peo-ple, however, showed gaps, holes, and a texture like scar tissue.

The chakras were "spiral cones of whirling energy," reported Karagulla in *Breakthrough to Creativity*. Breaks or disturbances in these spiral cones indicate an imbalance in the function of the physical body in that area, Karagulla explained. "If any of these major vortices show a dullness or irregularity or 'leak' in this cen-tral point or core, we look for some serious pathology in the phys-ical body in the area."

While scientists and clairvoyants continued to substantiate the human aura as an index for physical well-being, other researchers probed the versatility of color for practical healing. One of the most persistent of these innovators was Dinshah Ghadiali, who developed his Spectro-Chrome Tonation system of "attuned color waves" in the 1920s. Color healing evidently was an inflammatory topic earlier in this century, because Gha-diali spent more than forty years embroiled in a running battle over his system with the kingpins of U.S. medical authority—the American Medical Association, the Food and Drug Administra-tion, even the U.S. Post Office—who strenuously opposed dis-tribution of his color projectors.

Ghadiali knew that every chemical element in an excited state gave off light and absorbed energy from light. This cycling activity formed a set of colored bands called spectral emission lines. Ghadiali correlated the primary color emission for each element with its known physiological function in the human body, contending that chemical elements were linked with specific color waves and that colors represented chemical potencies of subtler vibrations. Ghadiali reasoned that if this same major color were used therapeutically on the body, it would enhance that element's activity.

In Ghadiali's model, color's radiant energy restored balance at the body's energetic, not physiological, level. Through the tonation process, Ghadiali used a set of twelve precisely adjusted color filters enclosed in a projector that shone light directly onto body regions mapped according to chemical element, physiology, and color band.

Maybe colored light projected through the eyes was the key to balance. That was the supposition of another American scientist, Dr. Harry Riley Spitler, both an M.D. and optometrist, who introduced his new ocular light therapy, called syntonics, in 1927. Spitler discovered that alterations in light received through the eyes was the "master key" to the brain's major control centers and through this, body function, behavior, and physiology. Spitler's syntonics system used thirty-one different color filter combinations, adjusted to each individual's nature, to balance and integrate the nervous system, and his College of Syntonic Optometry, which he founded in 1933, is still operating today.

Meanwhile in London, Dr. E. C. Iredell, a surgeon at Guy's Hospital in the 1930s, treated postoperative cancer patients with encouraging results with the Focal Machine, his own color instrument. Green was the color most generally used, producing in patients a "cool, pleasant, and soothing" sensation like flowing water. In the 1960s, Dr, Max Lüscher, a Swiss physician, developed a seventy-three-color-panel test model that correlated color preference with psychology, glandular balance, and psychic stress in individual clients. The Lüscher Color Test, which takes eight minutes, reveals valuable diagnostic information for physician and psychotherapist alike.

While therapists like Babbitt, Ghadiali, Spitler, and Iredell were seeking new color instrumentation, other scientists investigated color's healing efficacy in controlled laboratory studies, further substantiating its therapeutic claims. In 1958 Robert Gerard documented the psychophysiological effects in the autonomic nervous system and visual cortex of viewing colored (blue, red, and white) lights. Gerard noted that red increased the viewer's blood pressure, respiration, and anxiety levels, while blue enhanced the relaxation response. In the same year Dr. Harry Wohlfarth documented how specific colors affected respiration, pulse rate, mood, and blood pressure; these increased maximally under yellow, orange, and red, but decreased maximally under black, blue, and green.

Biologists in the 1970s, including Nobel Prize winner Albert Szent-Gyorgyi, began documenting the dramatic effects of color on biological activity. Reports came out that specific colors increased the rate of enzymatic reactions and could stimulate specific enzymes to be up to 500% more effective. In 1975 Richard Wurtman, M.D., reported in *Scientific American* that each year 25,000 premature U.S. infants were successfully treated with blue light in maternity wards for neonatal jaundice. In 1982 Sharon McDonald, M.D., reported that in a clinical study of sixty middle-aged women with rheumatoid arthritis treated for fifteen minutes with blue light "significant" pain relief was experienced by the majority of her subjects.

In 1990, John Anderson, M.D., reported that for 72% of patients suffering severe migraine headaches exposure to blinking red lights through eye goggles eliminated the condition within one hour. Pink may be the ultimate tranquilizer and the best antiriot device around. In the 1980s U.S. prison authorities learned that the tranquilizing effects of "bubble gum pink" arc lights or pink rooms rapidly reduced aggressive, hostile behavior; in fact, muscle-strength reduction occurred within 2.7 seconds. Pink's remarkable sedating, muscle-relaxing effect has been extended successfully into geriatric, adolescent, and family therapy practices.

"Even the color-blind are tranquilized by pink rooms," explains Alexander Schauss, clinical psychologist and director of the Institute for Biosocial Research in Tacoma, Washington, who first documented the effects of "being in the pink."

Gradually contemporary science has quantified the old folk wisdom that expressed its understanding of the intimacy of color, human health, and subtle anatomy in cliches like "seeing red," "feeling blue," "in the pink," "green with jealousy," and "black with rage." "These all relate to actual changes which take place in the colors of our own electromagnetic field due to changes in our emotions," explains color healer Mary Anderson in her concise review, *Colour*

Therapy. Standard methods of color treatment are eclectic and highly innovative, but all proceed from this basic understanding.

In the late 1970s, American optometrist Jacob Liberman began investigating syntonic light therapy, wanting to experience for himself how using different portions of visible light—different colors, in effect—therapeutically projected *through* the eyes could successfully treat various bodily conditions. Liberman developed a way to use specifically chosen colors to precipitate and clarify deep-set emotional problems which, he found, were in effect color-coded in the psyche. "One of my most important clinical discoveries was that the colors to which people were unreceptive correlated almost 100% of the time with the portions of their bodies where they housed stress, developed disease, or had injured themselves," says Liberman.

For example, a patient who felt consistently uncomfortable in the presence of blue often had a history of chronic sore throats, dental problems, difficulties with verbal expression, and tonsillectomy, all of which correlates quite tangibly, Liberman contends, with the throat chakra energy center whose "soul color" is universally regarded as blue. Liberman further noted that when a patient with throat problems had resolved the issues triggered by treatment with blue, "then looking at these colors, which was originally uncomfortable, actually stimulated feelings of joy and euphoria."

The body is light dependent, a living photocell, explains Liberman. He found that rather than treating overt organic disease, it's more important to look at what's underneath. It's not the imbalance in the nervous or endocrine system at fault, but different unresolved states of mind underlying those physical manifestations that affect the overall receptivity of the organism. "When we contain our energy, it produces a solidification in the body, like light slowed down, becoming solid matter. If we don't express emotions they 'solidify' in the body like tiny biocrystals. The energy stagnates in the body when it should be open like a flowing river. Light is one therapeutic key opening all the doors."

Life Force Healing:
Homeopathy's *Similia Similibus Curentur*

We turn our attention now to study a single representative empiric modality at work—homeopathy—highlighting its rationale, strategies, and outcomes. In homeopathy, we witness the collegiality of healing, between physician and client, medicine and patient, and between client and illness process; synergistically, these forces heal the self's environment. Homeopathy has flourished as a legitimate, self-contained, and therapeutically successful medical system for nearly 200 years, ever since the German physician Samuel Hahnemann formulated its principles and developed its pharmacopoeia.

A system of therapeutics implies a theory of disease and a coherent model of the human in health and illness, and so we find this fully articulated in homeopathy. Homeopathy's meticulous attention to the integrity (and symptomatology) of the individual as the seat of a multifactorial illness process reveals volumes of insights about our energy, even spiritual foundations. Should we embrace the homeopathic medical revelation, it could profoundly reorient our understanding of, literally, the human environment, from molecular immunology to psychological identity—comprehensive health, in other words.

As such, homeopathy indicates a rational basis for a reordering of Western medicine according to empirically demonstrated principles, both gross and subtle, material and intangible, constituting health.

Case Study: Making Her Life Livable Again

At forty-six, Kay Barton's life had become almost unlivable. She had systemic lupus erythematosus, an autoimmune disease in which the body's immune system attacks its own tissue. The symptoms usually include fever, anemia, skin rashes, arthritis, kidney dysfunction, low white blood cell count, and, in Barton's case, which her physician diagnosed as moderately severe, she had recurrent pericarditis, or inflammation of the outer lining of the heart. This kind of searing pain, said Barton, felt like "a big hunk of metal in my chest, the way a heart attack must feel."

Her medical history was formidable, too. At twenty-three, she became paralyzed from the waist down in a car accident, but after eighteen months of physical therapy and life in a body brace, she regained her mobility. At forty-four, she reinjured her traumatized back, was hospitalized and disabled, and had been unemployed since. She had high blood pressure and felt exhausted, depressed, apathetic, despairing, and had a tremendous fear of death.

Her physical viability was maintained primarily by a downwardly spiraling carousel of high-technology drugs. She took prednisone (60 milligrams daily, at the high end of dosage for autoimmune diseases), an anti-inflammatory, antibiotics, drugs for blood pressure, heart stabilization, pain, and sleep problems—eight medications in all. She hadn't been able to drop her prednisone dosage below 20 milligrams daily without dangerous flareups, and these could happen even in the higher, 30- to 60-milligrams-daily range. Kay Barton's life, it seemed, was falling disastrously apart. Nor did modern medicine offer her any hope of patching it together.

"The normal prognosis for lupus is that it's of unknown cause and has no cure," comments Stephen King, N.D., a naturopathic physician specializing in homeopathy, who treated Barton for four years. "The disease, if the patient is lucky, will remit. Barton was told by her allopathic doctors she'd have to stay on prednisone the rest of her life."

Excavating the Layers of Illness

Negotiating Barton's case was like "peeling off the layers of an onion, a kind of medical archeology, and at each new level, there was an increase in her vitality," says King. In August 1984, after taking Barton's entire symptom picture, King prescribed a daily homeopathic microdose of *Cactus grandiflorus* (night-blooming cereus). His plan was to gradually wean her off chemical drugs, since an immediate withdrawal from prednisone, says King, could have precipitated a dangerous attack of pericarditis. In homeopathic provings, *Cactus grandiflorus* produces symptoms like pericarditis plus heart palpitations and depression. "The remedy is matched to the total symptom pattern. You could bring in another lupus case and I would prescribe a different remedy."

Over the next five months, King and a consulting rheumatologist managed the reduction of Barton's drugs as she made "steady progress." She had more energy, her depression abated, she lost ten pounds, dropped her dependency on six drugs, had no further lupus symptoms, and returned to work part time. Her prednisone was reduced to every other day without producing flareups. Then Barton's symptom pattern shifted to the next layer. "At this point a lot of anger and bitterness came up in her," says King. "This was old resentment and frustration toward her family—feelings that had been underlying the apathy and exhaustion and which may originally have contributed to her lupus through stress and a weakening of her immune system."

So in February 1985 King took Barton off *Cactus* and prescribed *nux vomica* (poison nut) once daily. *Nux vomica,* which contains strychnine, produces irritability, nervous cramping sensations, and is suitable for people with an anxious, hot temperament. She showed steady progress again, and within four months started working full time. By May 1986, only twenty months after beginning her homeopathic treatment, Barton went off prednisone completely, something her M.D.s had never envisioned possible. Barton was unquestionably better, says King, but there would be two more stages to her recovery.

In July 1987, when she was only on blood pressure medication, Barton had a recurrence of her old back pain. When driving, she experienced an unbearable phobia about car accidents; she also reported an anomalous energy slump at 6 p.m. every day. The "drug picture" that most matched these symptoms, King discovered, was *Hypericum perforatum* (St. John's Wort).

The immediate result of taking *Hypericum* as the sole remedy was a predictable, transient intensification of her back pain, which soon passed, as did her energy slump and phobia, and Barton passed into the fourth layer of wellness. She became sad and wept frequently, experiencing great remorse about her recent anger toward her mother, who was in a nursing home. King prescribed *Natrum muriacticum* (potentized table salt) for her grief, and within a short time, Barton announced she had been "freed from her prison." Her gloom had been transmuted into a newfound caring and creativity. "She went through this last level of grief and came out the other side, much more optimal in her health and freedom," observes King.

Thus after four years of diligent homeopathic care, King and Barton have dramatically overturned allopathy's grim foreclosure on Barton's future. At the end of 1988, Barton was completely off seven drugs, taking only small amounts of blood pressure medication. "She has progressed considerably," says King. "She's well and happy, able to work full time, and lives in a normal manner."

Since homeopathy was formulated almost 200 years ago by German physician, pharmacist, and medical iconoclast Samuel Hahnemann (1755-1843), its disciplined, highly trained, holistic practitioners have achieved similarly impressive cures of acute and chronic disease, from nineteenth-century cholera epidemics to late-twentieth-century immunological dysfunction, where allopathy, relying on nineteenth-century bloodletting or twentieth-century antibiotics, has often foundered.

Hahnemann's "Provings": Physician as Researcher

In the early years of his long medical career in eighteenth-century Germany, Hahnemann grew increasingly disillusioned and discontent with medicine's prevailing doctrines and retired from active practice for fourteen years, from 1782 to 1796, to search for a fundamentally new approach to medicine. Although he had taken his medical degree only a few years earlier, in 1779 at the University of Erlangen, he was already an astute, critical physician. Medicine at the time was dominated by the views of the German "Natural Philosophers" and the orthodox codifications of Cullen and Brown. Bloodletting and the administration of strong, compound prescriptions (eight to ten drugs) were widely practiced, but Hahnemann vigorously opposed both. With so many medicines applied simultaneously in strong doses, how could the physician tell which one, if any, was efficacious?

Hahnemann was a rationalist, gifted with an independent mind, notes Karl Koenig, M.D. "He is up in arms against all the theoretical nonsense of his time and accuses his fellow physicians of their inability to help and to heal." So Hahnemann lived quietly for fourteen years with his wife as a medical recluse and scholar, translating texts, conducting independent research, and reformulating his approach to therapeutics, seeking that "new principle for ascertaining the curative powers of drugs."

Hahnemann, said Johann Wolfgang von Goethe, his contemporary, a few years later, is "that rare combination of philosophy and learning, whose system must eventually bring about the ruin of the ordinary receipt-crammed heads, but is still little accepted by practitioners, and rather shunned than investigated."

Hahnemann was convinced that physicians of his day did not understand how drugs worked, how they effected cures, or why they didn't. He reasoned that the only way to understand the action of a medicine was to observe all the reactions and symptoms—including mental and emotional—it produces in a healthy individual; this method of empirical testing and observation Hahnemann called "proving" (from the German *Pruefung*, meaning "test" or "trial"). In the course of translating Cullen's *Materia Medica*, one of the standard medical texts of the day (Cullen was a renowned physician, founder of the Glasgow School of Medicine), and reflecting on a passage about Peruvian cinchona bark (quinine) in 1790, Hahnemann had an idea. He wanted to disprove Cullen's contention that cinchona bark was effective against intermittent fever because its astringency tonified the stomach.

To make his case, Hahnemann experimented on himself to find the secret of cinchona's efficacy, taking "four drams" twice daily. As soon as he discontinued taking the bark, the symptoms disappeared. His disputatious method was daring and practical, and would set the tone for homeopathy's future. His empirical results were startlingly clear: cinchona produced in him all the symptoms normally associated with intermittent fever. The deeper meaning of the results was that one fever could cure another by virtue of the similarity between both. "Peruvian bark, which is used as a remedy for intermittent fever, acts because it can produce symptoms similar to those of intermittent fever in healthy people," he wrote.

From this firsthand data Hahnemann could evolve his now classic "Law of Similars," which held that as physicians we may wisely imitate nature, which sometimes cures a chronic disease by "superadding another," by employing a medicine that can produce a very similar "artificial" disease—*similia similibus curentur,* "like cures like." As he explained in a foundation essay in 1796 ("An Attempt Concerning a New Principle for Discovering the Healing Forces in Remedies"): "By choosing a remedy for a given natural disease that is capable of producing a very similar artificial disease, we shall be able to cure the most obstinate disease. In order to cure gently, quickly, unfailingly, and permanently, select for every case of disease a medicine capable of calling forth an effect similar to that which it is intended to cure."

With the revolutionary principle of "like cures like" in hand, Hahnemann knew he had to make therapeutics practical by developing a reliable, empirically tested *materia medica*. The only way he could accomplish this formidable project was through direct provings of individual medicinal substances on *healthy* subjects—on himself. "Nothing then remains but to test the medicines we wish to investigate on the human body itself," Hahnemann declared boldly. On his own, or with the assistance of family members, students, and close colleagues, Hahnemann "proved" ninety-nine substances, presenting the detailed symptomatic reports of "changes, symptoms, and signs" for each remedy in his *Fragmenta de Viribus Medicamentorum Positivis* (1805) and *Materia Medica Pura* (1811-21).

He started with herbs and metals (mercury and arsenic) because these formed the basis of most allopathic drugs of his time; later he extended his "provings" to include herbs recommended from European folk medicine. He even tested known poisons on himself in "solution, dilution, and small administration," demonstrating that presumed injurious substances like belladonna, strychnine, aconite, viper poison, and various spider and snake venoms could have curative power.

By the end of the nineteenth century, Hahnemann's homeopathic followers would have proved a total of 600 substances; by the 1990s, that number, comprising the homeopathic pharmacopoeia, had grown to about 2,000. "The provings of these substances yield groups of symptoms which define precisely how the healthy organism reacts to the specific stimulus represented by each substance," explains medical historian Harris Coulter. And that precise catalogue of symptom groups forms the rational, empirical basis for how each substance may be most effectively used in treatment.

Why the Organism Responds to "Similar Suffering"

To his contemporaries, of course, it seemed that Hahnemann was intent on poisoning himself to develop his "true" *materia medica*. "The best will always be those that the healthy, unprejudiced, conscientious, sensitive physician undertakes on *himself*," he wrote in his *Organon of the Rational Art of Healing*, his major homeopathic testament, first published in 1810, and expanded many times afterward during his life. "This so natural, so absolutely necessary, so uniquely valid proving of the pure, characteristic action of medicines,"—in this way did Hahnemann extol the virtues of empirical research for a rational basis of a new medicine he called homoeopathy, from the Greek, *homoios* ("similar") and *pathos* ("suffering").

Hahnemann positioned homeopathy clearly against the prevailing trend of "enantiopathy" (or allopathy, from the Greek, *allos* "other" and *pathos* "suffering"), in which a symptom complex is treated by a substance *opposite* in effect, producing the opposite symptoms. Allopathy's enantiopathic practices, founded on the oppositional principle of *contraria contraris,* produced effects, particularly with respect to chronic diseases, that were at best "temporary" and "palliative," said Hahnemann, and he urged his colleagues to "abandon this method."

For example, let's consider the homeopathic and enantiopathic treatment of constipation. The enantiopath would prescribe a laxative of strong, repeated dosage to produce diarrhea, whereas the homeopath would give a substance that produces constipation in a healthy individual, such as opium, in a highly dilute, single dose. In this simple example we see revealed the profound chasm, both conceptual and therapeutic, between allopathy and homeopathy.

According to Hahnemann's Law of Similars, a substance that is symptomatic or toxic for a healthy person can be therapeutic and healing for a diseased person when taken in infinitesimal, highly dilute doses. Ipecac root, for example, taken in botanical quantities, produces nausea and vomiting, yet when taken in homeopathic dilution, often cures nausea in dyspeptic patients.

Dynamis—Life Force and the Disease Process

The fundamental differences in therapeutic approach between homeopathy and allopathy arise from their positioning of the etiology, process, and resolution of disease, from their scale of observation of the human being in sickness and health. Hahnemann was a vitalist, contending that disease represents a dynamic, originally immaterial disturbance arising in a human individual and manifesting in a pattern of symptoms, both organic and psychoemotional.

As a vitalist, Hahnemann was part of a centuries' old ad hoc attempt to evolve a cure based on the life force and the inherent dynamis of nature; he joined the company of such medical pariahs as the alchemists, Gnostics, animists, and other naturalist-magicians. When Hahnemann said dynamic, he meant the "spirit-like" *dynamis,* the vital life force that literally animates (breathes life into) the human organism. Hahnemann's *dynamis* is equivalent to the older Greek concept of *physis,* the Chinese medical conceptualizations of *Qi,* and the Western metaphysical *etheric.*

The *dynamis,* said Hahnemann in his *Organon,* is a life-giving, regulatory, instinctively feeling, fundamental energy, it's what distinguishes a dead corpse from a living human. "In the healthy condition of man, the spiritual vital force, the *dynamis* that animates the material body, rules with unbounded sway, and retains all the parts of the organism in admirable, harmonious, vital operation . . . so that our indwelling, reason-gifted mind can fully employ this living, healthy instrument for the higher purpose of existence."

The vital force, although it animates the human body, is not in itself directly experienceable, only its effects and qualities. According to James Tyler Kent, M.D., (1849-1916), one of America's most distinguished nineteenth-century homeopathic physicians, included among its qualities: a constructive, formative intelligence that operates the body's organismic economy, keeping it "continuously constructed"; it dominates the body it controls, yet it's changeable, adaptable with respect to the environment, keeping the human body "in a state of order, in the cold or in the heat, in the wet and damp, and under all circumstances."

These formulations are in accordance with classical empiric descriptions of the *physis*. The *physis* (or *Natura*) is the innate healing power of the whole organism; this inherent force for cure is spontaneous and reactive, quickly summoned into action to respond to environmental energies, be they disruptive or supportive. Even though the *physis* is a kind of generic energy informing all human organisms, it is highly individualized with each person. That is why illness and disease—symptomatology—can be virtually infinitely varied, as each body expresses its unique dynamic pattern.

According to empirical thought, the *physis* should guide the physician, should be the doctor's mentor; or, as Harris Coulter writes, "The physician's practice must imitate that of the *physis*." The physician's role is to aid the *physis* in achieving a cure because, as an ancient Greek medical text *(Epidemics)* said: "The *physies* are the physicians of disease." As such, the *physis* is self-acting: "Though the *physis* is unschooled and uninstructed, she does what is proper [to affect healing]," said the *Epidemics*. When symptoms arise, the empirical physician regards these positively as signs of the struggle of the *physis* against the morbific influence.

"Now, if the *physis* does everything for the preservation of living creatures," wrote Galen in the second century A.D., "this too is reasonable, that she should be the first to heal diseases." Fourteen centuries later, Paracelsus, another central figure in the empirical tradition, reiterated Galen's observation: "Then our own nature is itself our physician, which is to say, it has in itself what it needs."

Thus, if the *dynamis* (Hahnemann's renaming of the *physis*) maintains health, then aberrations and derangements of the *dynamis* must precipitate illness, Hahnemann reasoned. In this way, it is the "morbidly affected vital force alone that produces diseases." The symptom picture, or composite pattern of "morbid phenomena" reveal all the internal changes under way in the individual, "that is to say, the whole morbid derangement of the internal dynamis; in a word, they reveal the whole disease."

Hahnemann, like many homeopaths after him, was cognizant of the organic pathologies participating in illness, but he never accorded them the same etiological primacy as the allopaths; to him, they were epiphenomenal, secondary characteristics in the work of the *physis* to rebalance the organism. "Homeopaths have always felt that pathological data are basically speculative and changeable, and for that reason are not a reliable basis for therapy," says Coulter. "Symptoms, however, are unchanging." And, frankly, neither Hahnemann, nor most of his homeopathic successors, contend that microbiological agents or pathologies are the causes of illness, but rather symptoms (or products) on an already initiated *physis*cal process.

"The conviction that disease is caused by bacteria is probably one of our greatest illusions," notes George Vithoulkas, probably the twentieth century's most renowned homeopathic scholars. Microbial etiology, the bedrock upon which the whole edifice of allopathic theory sits, says Vithoulkas, is a wrong assumption. "Today more than ever, mental shock is recognized as the sole exciting cause of a series of diseases." Or as the nineteenth-century American homeopath James Tyler Kent said: "The bacteria are results of the disease. The microscopical little fellows are not the disease cause, but they come after. They are the outcome of the disease . . . but the cause is much more subtle than anything that can be shown by a microscope."

Diseases correspond to a human's affections, said Kent, and should be understood as the outward expression of our affective interior. "The internal state of man is prior to that which surrounds him; therefore, environment is not cause; it is only, as it were, a sounding board; it only reacts upon and reflects the internal."

Homeopaths prefer talking in terms of susceptibility and predisposition to disease than in terms of causes. What allopathy customarily construes as causes, as disease agents, as prime etiological factors, are, according to homeopathic thinking and observation, secondary *results* of something antecedent—Vithoulkas' "mental shock" or Kent's "much more subtle" event—that precipitates a pattern of symptoms.

Symptoms, pain, and pathologies are sense-perceptible signs of an immaterial adjustment in the *dynamis* well under way; we say "adjustment," because the *dynamis* is inherently homeostatic, always seeking to resolve its temporary "untunement" and restore balance within itself, with a little help from the "wise physician" and his homeopathic pharmacopoeia.

"By giving a remedy which resembles the disease the instinctive vital force is compelled to increase its vital energy until it becomes stronger than the disease, which, in turn, is vanquished," wrote Hahnemann.

Generational Taints Are Like Seeds for Illness within the Organism

Yet it was when, in the late 1820s, he contemplated the observed fact that for some of his patients cures were only temporary, that Hahnemann hit upon his profound concept of *miasms.* By miasm, he meant a common denominator, a chronic, underlying, even inherited disease pattern or predisposition upon which other illnesses and symptom pictures might arise. We might think of the miasm as a specific form, stamp, or distortion given to the individual *physis,* affecting its expression in the organism. The miasm is a far more subtle theory of the continuity of energy patterns across generations than the materialistic model of genetics so favored by allopathy.

There are three fundamental miasms (from the Greek, meaning "taint, contamination") that underlie all chronic diseases and are transmitted from generation to generation in a form of what we might today call metagenetics, said Hahnemann: psora, syphilis, and sycosis. These are influences that can engraft predispositions to illness upon the human constitution, overpower the life force, and get transmitted across the generations. "Unable to extinguish them without assistance, the vital force is powerless to prevent their growth or its own gradual deterioration, resulting in the final destruction of the organism."

Of these miasms, psora, characterized by skin eruptions (from the Greek *psora,* meaning "itch"), the oldest and most fundamental of the three, accounts for seven-eighths of all chronic disease, Hahnemann speculated. "The psoric miasm is the most ancient, most universal, most destructive, and yet most misapprehended miasm, which for many thousands of years has disfigured and tortured mankind," he wrote in 1827. The second and third miasms, syphilis and sycosis (from the Greek *syco,* meaning "fig," hence figwort disease, i.e., gonorrhea), are both associated with venereal diseases, which, Hahnemann speculated, were once, in historical times, as rampant as the plague, affecting nearly everyone, leaving a "taint" that was carried down through the generations.

Implicit in miasmic theory is the idea that "there exist *layers of predisposition* which underlie the waxing and waning of temporary ailments," writes George Vithoulkas. "These must be taken into account in treatment intending to be completely curative." These layers of "predisposing weakness" exist in a definite and rational sequence and must be peeled off in order through careful homeopathic prescribing.

Hahnemann's concept of miasms is complex but profound, presupposing the evolution of the disease process over time and across humanity; yet it has also a symbolic, descriptive sense in terms of categorizing diseases in terms of their depth of residency or penetration within the human organism. The psoric miasm works through the skin, the outermost layer of the human organism; the syphilitic involves the internal organs, producing cankers and sores as evidences of discharge; whereas the sycotic miasm is set still deeper, in the mind, producing mental symptoms.

"The degree of chronic weakness of the defense mechanism is a direct result of the intensity of the miasmatic influences," explains Vithoulkas. But he adds that the newer tuberculosis miasm, postulated by Kent, is a combination of the psoric and syphilitic miasms; the practical result of this complex combination of miasms is the perception that in any individual there are "layers of predisposition," miasmatic strata that underlie the "waxing and waning of temporary ailments," and which must be systemically peeled off, layer by layer, in the course of treatment.

"Each layer is always the result of the underlying ones, and there is a definite sequence to the presenting layers," says Vithoulkas. "To peel off each miasmatic layer in succession, even assuming that correct prescriptions are made each time, can take many years of painstaking and patient effort."

The profound concept of miasms is amplified and in effect explained by Hering's Law of Cure, named in honor of its promulgator, Constantine Hering, M.D., (1800-1880), a major post-Hahnemannian homeopathic thinker. A major conceptual contribution to homeopathic understanding came from this German émigré who settled in Philadelphia in 1852 and was later known as the father of homeopathy in America. Hering formulated three principles of homeopathic healing, building on Hahnemann's foundation; his formulations were prodigiously documented as his *Guiding Symptoms of Our Materia Medica* takes up ten volumes of 500 pages each.

Hering's Law of Cure states that healing begins in the deepest part of the body and moves outward to the extremities, and begins in the emotional-mental layers and moves outward into the physical. In terms of miasms, Hering was proposing that illness moves from the most deeply entrenched miasms, which tend to be the syphilitic and sycotic, then, in the process of resolution (cure), move out to the skin, the psora, the oldest miasm. Skin eruptions and diseases in this light are regarded as highly favorable signs of progress in resolving the disease picture, indicating the passage of the aberration from the interior to the exterior.

Hering also said that healing flows from the upper trunk (e.g., arthritic neck pain) to the lower parts (e.g., finger joints), and that it progresses in reverse chronological order of the original appearance of symptoms; patients therefore often reexperience symptoms from old conditions in the course of healing. Hering's postulations, read in reverse, describe the process of disease taking hold of the person, and are thus doubly valuable. In other words, as a disease shifts from an acute to a chronic stage, the symptoms shift from the extremities to the interior, from the lower trunk to the upper, and from the peripheral organs to the vital ones.

According to Hering's Law "mental illness" is a comprehensible extrapolation from a continuum of effects, an extreme form of a general morbific process set in one of the body's most vital organs, the brain. "Only such patients remain well and are really cured who have been rid of their symptoms in the reverse order of their development," Hering noted. Illness and recovery have a natural process, an innate therapeutic logic that must be respected and aided by the physician to facilitate healing.

Disease Is Appropriate
to the Individual Constitution

Homeopathy does not palliate symptoms, allopathy does, and in this distinction we behold the fundamental schism in therapeutic thinking between these two approaches to illness. As Richard Grossinger notes in his insightful commentary on homeopathic practice in *Planet Medicine:* "Homeopathy is based on the responsiveness of the defense mechanism rather than on the intercession of the physician. Temporary relief is always given to the organism only at the expense of an ultimate return to full health."

The allopath strives to curtail, suppress, or remove the symptoms, regarding success here as tantamount to cure, but for a homeopath, this is a dangerous practice based on a mistaken understanding of the illness process. Allopathy, in following this course of action, achieves at best a "superficial palliation," says Grossinger, that drives the disease deeper into the constitution, "because its mode of expression is cut off each time." Diseases never go away; they simply retreat into deeper layers of the human being.

Here Grossinger highlights one of homeopathy's remarkable perspectives, namely, that disease is appropriate, meaningful, teleologic, and necessary for the health of the human. Disease is appropriate because the illness matches the organism's basic susceptibility; it's tailor-made at a molecular level. When the disease manifests itself through pathologies, it is announcing an antecedent disturbance on what Hahnemann called the "dynamic plane," and what we might today refer to as the subtle bodies, principally, the etheric and astral bodies.

The presenting symptoms and pathologies, says homeopathy, represent the organism's "extraordinarily refined response" to a vibrational distortion within. "The disease is a property of the constitution itself and lies beneath any concrete manifestation, beneath any separation into mental and physical," explains Grossinger.

Everything potentially reflects it and all symptoms—a wart, a nightmare, sensitivity to cold, diarrhea, weeping—are equally valid and revelatory, he adds, highlighting the holographic principle at work. Further, the body is unilaterally intelligent and economical, wasting no energy on superfluous, digressive symptoms. "It would not be able to produce these idiosyncrasies unless it meant them (i.e., unless something inward spoke in terms of them)," says Grossinger.

In its style of straightword symptomatic communication, the expressivity of the dynamis illustrates the principles of Arnold Mindell's dreambody process, which acknowledges the egalitarianism of all mind-body signals. If this is true, if we have a holographic, dreambody, polysymptomatic expressivity, as homeopathy asserts, the last thing we should do is palliate it with suppressive medicines, which is the allopathic response, because we can thereby actually do great damage to our health.

Allopathic drugs, founded on biochemical contraries, not homeopathic similars, inevitably superimpose on the constitution a new drug disease that must be counteracted, says George Vithoulkas. If the allopathic medicine suppresses the peripheral symptoms, it drives the disturbance deeper into the organism, forces the dynamis defense mechanism to establish a new state of equilibrium at a deeper organic level, and weakens the "vibration rate" of the organism. "Consequently, if the drug is powerful enough, or if drug therapy is continued long enough, the organism may jump to a deeper level in its susceptibility to disease."

You might palliate the stomach ulcer but precipitate a violent irritability and paranoia because you've pushed the process deeper into the organism. Through vaccinations you may gain protection from certain infections, but at the expense of having lost enough useful susceptibility on superficial levels to produce a symptomatic reaction, says Vithoulkas.

In other words, you may be immune to the flu, but you'll get cancer instead. Disease, says homeopathy, is not alien to us, but a necessary elaborative and refining process of our organic being. If we cut off the disease's mode of expression, which uses the body tissue as a medium, this drives it ever deeper into our organism in search of a venue for expression. The symptoms and pathologies indicate the response of our organism, "a system-wide recognition of the existence of disease within itself," Grossinger explains, "and a synchronous attempt to allow the disease to express and vent itself with the least damage to the vital organs."

The key point is that palliation only *seems* to preempt the disease; but if you preempt the disease, disturbing its organic process, you only shortchange your health and postpone the moment of true resolution. You will eventually pay the price in terms of reduced health. Allopathic palliation is superficial and insubstantial; "it drugs the organs without strengthening their response," says

Grossinger, producing chronic, aggravating side effects. Ultimately, homeopathy tells us, we must experience and process the message of the disease; it's unavoidable and the longer we postpone it by continually pushing it further into the interior, the more biologically traumatic it will be when we begin unwinding it through homeopathic remedies. It's not a pleasant prospect, but a real one, to say that in undertaking a course of homeopathic treatment things may get worse before they get better.

Hering's Law of Cure states that old suppressed pathologies will return and be expressed organically in the reverse order as current ailments are resolved. In light of this, the apparent recurrence of old symptoms is a positive sign. In effect, we must reexperience all the layers of the disease through superficial flareups and recurrences of symptoms until the "disease core" has been unwound, expressed, and transmuted. That's what Hering's Law of Cure and Hahnemann's miasmatic stratification imply on a practical level.

"Homeopathy is nonpalliative by principle," says Grossinger. "It often requires suffering. It proposes only an unwinding of the disease by a passage through the elements that make it up in time and space. Homeopathy is a creative use of disease to bring about human transformation and, ultimately, health; allopathy is a means of antidoting the dangerous and reactive disease process, and, at worst, limiting human potential to what can be achieved in a drugged condition."

The logical extension of the homeopathic argument is startling: allopathic suppressive therapies may be unilaterally "sanctioned malpractice," suggests Grossinger.

Case Taking—The Chorus of Symptoms Reveals the Remedy

Acknowledging the potential miasmatic complexity of the disease picture, Hahnemann emphasized the homeopathic interview, on taking the complete case of each patient. This of course is one of homeopathy's hallmarks, the basis for the individualizing of therapy.

Hahnemann knew the "wise physician" must collect all the facts from the patient, all the details—organic, proprioceptive, emotional, psychological, spiritual, family medical history—to form an exact impression of the symptom picture, and with this symptomatic gestalt match it precisely against a specific remedy picture in the homeopathic repertory of remedies. Hahnemann urged his students to ferret out "the most striking, singular, uncommon, and peculiar signs and symptoms," knowing that often the idiosyncratic revealed the entire case.

At a certain level, the diseased patient and the remedy are equivalent, notes British homeopath L. R. Twentyman, so that we can intelligently speak of the *Sulphur* disease or the *Lycopodium* patient: "We learn to speak of a patient as the remedy which is called for by his totality of symptoms." All diseases are afflictions of the whole organism, Hahnemann said; there are no diseases, only sick people, and no "external malady" can arise, persist, or worsen, without the "cooperation" and "instrumentality" of the whole organism nor without the "consent of the whole of the rest of health, and without the participation of the rest of the living whole (of the vital force that pervades all the other sensitive and irritable parts of the organism)."

The homeopath, while taking the patient's case, must pay attention to the smallest, most seemingly insignificant details, and thereby exercise "faithfulness in recording the disease picture," Hahnemann urged his students. It's a perceptually formidable task.

"In practice, homeopathic diagnosis falls somewhere between an on-the-spot encyclopedic research project and an instantaneous comprehension of a unity," notes Grossinger. The kind of qualitative personal method of medical history taking Hahnemann insisted on runs counter to the abstract quantitative approach so favored by allopaths who tend to view patients as so many units in a diagnostic assembly line. There is no generic prescription in homeopathy, such as an aspirin for a headache or antibiotics for an infection; similar symptoms usually arise out of a completely different dynamic totality and must be treated with a unique, individual repertorization.

Homeopathic case taking calls for time, intellectual labor, and a "very fine and subtle observation of the patient's symptoms," all of which are out of step with the "socio-economic determinants" of modern allopathy, notes Harris Coulter.

The examining homeopath must weigh carefully the particular conditions of the patient's daily activities, living and sleeping habits, diet, domestic situation, dreams, thoughts, attitudes, irritations, mannerisms, appearance, style of dress and speech, family medical background, previous use of medicines and drugs. Each patient is a new, unique, open case; there are no pat formulas for the homeopath, only accurate, empirical perceptions, the knowledge that symptoms are gestures of the disease process.

"The physician must presume the true picture of every epidemic to be new and unknown and must thoroughly examine it," advised Hahnemann. In sharp contrast to allopathy's brief, imprecise, diagnostic sketches, as prevalent today as in Hahnemann's time, the homeopath's immersion in a patient's totality, in her full symptomatic presence and whole image, is crucial for the "individualizing examination of a case of disease."

The fundamental difference between allopathic and homeopathic case taking, comments Karl Koenig, is that for the latter "the chorus of symptoms indicates a remedy, but for the former it describes a disease." The allopath seeks to identify and name the disease, then find a substance to counteract it (*contraria contraris*), whereas the homeopath isn't interested in the disease, but uses the symptoms to identify the remedy (which, were he healthy, would actually produce the condition) that will encourage the patient's innate life force to vanquish the disease state (*similia similibus curentur*). Hahnemann wasn't interested in this Hippocratic "natural historian" approach to disease classification; that kind of "tabulated and ordered survey" is the proper work for scholars, not healers. "But for the physician as a practitioner of the art of medicine it would be of no value whatsoever."

Hahnemann disregarded the disease and affected organ altogether, says Koenig. As Richard Grossinger pithily remarks, whereas an allopath, looking directly at a diseased organ or a corpse, sees the active pathology, for the homeopath "these are only the hit-and-run effects of an assailant that has long since fled." Hippocrates sought the disease, extrapolating from nature its morbific influences on the human, but Hahnemann reversed this, taking the empiric path from the human back to nature, in search of the remedy. "He did not clearly realize that he had actually reversed the Hippocratic path," says Koenig.

Hippocrates, who died in 355 B.C., walked away from the silent mystery tradition, which had provided initiation into the mysteries and relationships between humankind, nature, and the cosmos, and out into the bright light of the awakening power of human thinking, Koenig explains. But at that time, the nascent penetrativeness of human thought wasn't sufficient to plumb the relationship between the human and the divine, and this understanding gradually disappeared. It would remain so for 2,160 years (a full astrological cycle, incidentally) until 1805 when Hahnemann published an essay, "Aesculapius in the Balance."

Here Hahnemann praised Hippocrates as having been remarkably close to the "discovery of the science of medicine"; although Hippocrates was unsurpassed in the faculty of "pure observation," he was "destitute" in the knowledge of medicines and their application, said Hahnemann. The line of generations since him only "degenerated and wandered more or less from the indicated path," and the art of the "pure observation of disease" was abandoned—until Hahnemann, argues Koenig.

Hahnemann fulfilled what Hippocrates had begun: the new art of healing. "He divined the new path of medicine: back to the mysteries."

The Mystery of the Microdose— Less Is Much More

Once the remedy has been identified, then it's a question of matching the remedy's potency with the demands of the patient's situation. One of the more puzzling facts of homeopathic therapeutics is that the strongest potencies are actually those preparations that are the most dilute, what an allopathic chemist would call the weakest, that contain, technically, no quantifiable physical trace whatsoever of the original substance. In fact, the higher the potency, or dilution, the more "etheric," literally immaterial, and powerful the remedy.

In developing his repertory of "provings," Hahnemann discovered a way in which a substance that in its gross, botanical form might become curative in its subtle, potentized form as a remedy. He called this chemical translation process, based on serial dilutions and succussion (vigorous shaking), "dynamization" or "potentization." The result, he announced in 1799, is the infinitesimal microdose.

"By means of this ever-increasing dynamization, the material ultimately refines and transforms itself completely into a spiritualized remedial force," said Hahnemann. By means of its special procedure, homeopathy "develops the inner, spirit-like medicinal powers of crude substance to a degree hitherto unheard of and makes all of the exceedingly, even immeasurably, penetrating, active, and effective." Through this "remarkable transformation,"

Hahnemann explained in his *Organon,* the homeopathic preparation of remedies develops the latent, sleeping dynamic powers, previously imperceptible, in substances (in his time, largely plants). "The crucial observation," comments Vithoulkas, "was that the more the substance is succussed and diluted, the greater the therapeutic effect while simultaneously nullifying the toxic effect."

Homeopathic medicines are prepared from a variety of sources today following Hahnemann's original indications. In his time, he insisted that homeopaths prepare and dispense their own remedies, bypassing the allopathic apothecaries, whom he judged unfit to appreciate the complexity and precision of the homeopathic repertory. Remedies from plants, which comprise about 80% of remedy substances, include, for example, *Bryonia* (wild hops), *Calendula officinalis* (marigolds), and *Rhus toxicodendron* (poison ivy). Among fish, animal, and reptile sources, there are *Apis melliflica* (honey bee), *Sepia* (the inky fluid from cuttlefish), and *Lachesis* (bushamaster snake venom). The repertory also includes remedies made from potentized minerals such as *Natrum muriaticum* (sodium chloride), *Silicea* (salica), and *Argentum nitricum* (nitrate of silver).

Beyond the Measurable Chemical Limits of the Paradigm

A homeopathic dilution of 12C (which is quite a low dose) technically no longer has any molecular trace of the original substance because at this point it exceeds what chemists regard as their equivalent of the speed of light, the boundaries of material presence: Avogadro's number. Amadeo Avogadro was an influential chemist and contemporary of Hahnemann who postulated that the number of molecules in one mole of any substance is 6.0253×10^{23}. Practically, this means that any dilution beyond 12C cannot possibly contain even a single molecule of the original substance. Chemists and doctors of his day adopted Avogadro's number as a constant, a limit to the possible therapeutic efficacy of a material substance, reasoning that if it wasn't molecularly present, it couldn't possibly be active. Hahnemann's blithe transgression of this presumed inalterable limit "seems to violate our usual understanding of physics and chemistry," notes Vithoulkas.

This assumption of a material limit to possible therapeutic efficacy in a drug substance would form the bedrock of the allopathic rejection of the pharmaceutical impossibility of homeopathy and its ultramolecular dose—an attitude that remains firmly in place.

It won't help materialist allopaths in their attempts to rationalize the mysterious efficacy of homeopathic remedies to learn that the remedies may be prepared radionically without any involvement of the original botanical, mineral, or animal substance. Innovations in this century by Ruth Drown, Malcolm Rae, and David Tansley culminated in the development of the Mark II Potency Stimulator, a radionics device, which now enables homeopaths in England and Australia to prepare their remedies in minutes. At least 2,000 "magnetically energized geometric patterns" for the standard remedies were ascertained then printed on small cards; these are inserted into the radionics device, which projects their vibrational signature into a vial of water or sugar pills, which then transmit the charge to the human organism when the drops or pills are consumed.

It gets even more subtle. In the 1980s, Stephen Kane, an English inventor, developed a radionics device that obviates the geomagnetic cards; instead, the remedy signatures are programmed into a crystal, which the homeopath accesses by calling up the appropriate signature on a small computer console. According to homeopathic practitioners, the therapeutic results obtained from radionics or standard succussion-dilution are identical.

And it gets even more subtle. Accomplished psychics trained in the homeopathic repertory can send homeopathic remedies telepathically to patients, or to themselves, as needed. According to one such practitioner, if you want to give someone *Arnica montana* for relief of acute fear or trauma symptoms, you visualize the plant itself (not the potentized remedy) and project this thought form upon another visualization of the patient. Here the delivery of the prescription is, literally, in the practitioner's head: both the remedy and the patient. The dosage strength is determined by how long the person is exposed to the visualization of the arnica plant, in a manner akin to f-stops in photography that regulate light exposure.

Homeopathy pushes the paradigm of physical matter and causality beyond the level comprehensible by most people. The fact that it works helps a lot in dealing with this uncomfortable paradox that it is exceedingly difficult to define the mode of operation of a modality that produces healing. In the case of classical homeopathy, there is no physical trace of the original substance; only an energy imprint held in water. In radionic homeopathy, there is no water and there never was a physical substance involved; only a geometric abstraction of the energy field of the particular plant. In psychic homeopathy, there is a return to the original plant substance but in its etheric thought-based form, as projected by the practitioner.

After all, what is a homeopathic remedy? Homeopathic medicines, suggests Grossinger, are "parallels, vibrations, spiritual entities, intelligences, messages, qualities of substances, not quantities."

The Allopathic Paradigm Collapses in *Nature*

In mid-1988, the homeopathic community measured its own progress and saw its belief system in striking perspective as scientists pondered the "unbelievable, supernatural, extraordinary" results of a clinical study from Paris. Scientists in Italy, Israel, Canada, and France jointly conducted laboratory studies using a microdose of an antibody (a homeopathic dilution, essentially) to see if it would cause a reaction among certain white blood cells called basophils. Their independently obtained results—they were replicated in seventy experiments and clearly indicated that microdoses were effective—were coordinated through the lab of immunologist Jacques Benveniste of the University of Paris.

The scientific paper that the researchers prepared passed through considerable peer review before it was published in *Nature,* Britain's premier scientific journal, on June 30, 1988. *Nature's* editors, however, were so skeptical of the experiment's conclusions—that a microdose containing no molecular traces of a substance could be biologically active—that they published an unprecedented "editorial reservation"—"When to believe the unbelievable"—to chaperone the article into the materialist belief system of its readers. The implication, if tacitly couched, was that *Nature* didn't believe in the validity of the research. "We are certain these results must be wrong, but we have been unable to disprove them," one editor confided to *The New York Times.*

"The essence of the result," said *Nature,* "is that an aqueous solution of an antibody retains its ability to evoke a biological response even when diluted to such an extent that there is negligible chance of there being a single molecule in the sample." Welcome to the mysteries, the homeopaths said to themselves, acknowledging the paradigm-shattering fact of the infinitesimal dose, a belief-system time bomb primed by Hahnemann almost 200 years ago.

The provocative results were obtained in six labs in four countries by reputable scientists—that, even *Nature* would have to grant, is proper scientific procedure. Hahnemann's demonstrated fact of the therapeutic efficacy of the infinitesimal dose was always an alarming contradiction to the rigorous materialist reductionist model underlying allopathy; it refused to fit into the marvelous edifice of theory and hypothesis erected over centuries.

Orthodox scientists have always balked at the suggestion that a substance can have a biological effect when it is so highly dilute as to not technically be materially there. Scientists have assumed since the time of Avogadro, Hahnemann's contemporary, that when a substance is diluted 24 times by a 10:1 ratio, no molecules are any longer present. What so alarmed *Nature* was that the researchers used a substance diluted 120 times at a 10:1 ratio and it appeared to produce action. "There is no physical basis for such an activity," stated *Nature* in desperation. "There is no objective explanation for these observations." There is, as any homeopath will tell you; it's just that to make the case you have to abandon the predominant Cartesian, materialist, mechanistic, rationalist, allopathic view of the world that has so entranced the West for centuries.

Nature spoke for most scientists when it noted Benveniste's results "strike at the root of two centuries of observation and rationalization of physical phenomena." Mainstream *physical*-oriented scientists didn't like the idea that "an unexpected observation requires a substantial part of our intellectual heritage should be thrown away." It's much easier to throw away the experiment—especially if you have the power to squelch or discredit paradigm-exploding results—so with astonishing celerity the medical-scientific establishment responded to the paradigm assault with antibiotic vehemence. The July 28, 1988, issue of *Nature* published a retraction of Benveniste's article.

In *Nature's* opinion, the homeopathic heresy was halted by the fresh look their investigative "team of experts" focused on Benveniste's data. "The phenomenon described is not reproducible in the ordinary meaning of the word," they stated, adding that the microdose hypothesis is "a delusion" that is "as unnecessary as it is fanciful." The fact that for two hundred years homeopathy had achieved remarkable cures for diseases that have stumped the allopaths had no bearing on the theoretical impossibility of their pharmacy.

However, as much as *Nature* may have self-righteously railed about the unscientific nature of Benveniste's protocols, its own style of investigation was decidedly spurious. In their visit to Benveniste's lab in Paris, *Nature* editor John Maddox was accompanied by the magician-debunker James "The Amazing" Randi, his assistant, and Walter Stewart (neither an M.D. nor a scientist) from the U.S. National Institutes of Health. Hardly a highly credentialed team to staff an inquisition. The "scientific" investigative team observed seven replications of Benveniste's experiments, then declared the whole business chimerical.

Evidently, the *Nature* team had no patience for one of the more provocative speculations Benveniste presented at the end of his original article. He proposed that as none of the original molecules were measurably present, yet the dilution still produced effects, perhaps the molecular information had been imprinted somehow on the water, which then retained the memory or signature. The concepts of memory, signature, resonance, and template of course are central to the homeopathic model of the intangible efficacy of the microdose.

In making his speculations, Benveniste was edging his way into perilous waters indeed. Surely he sensed the contiguity of a heretical domain because after he dropped his suggestion for a new "metamolecular biology" he let the subject go—for the moment. In 1991, when his new work was published in the journal of the French Academy of Sciences, thus signaling to the world his continuing interest in the "heresy," *New Scientist* was moved to reconsider the "'Ghost Molecules' Theory Back from the Dead."

In Benveniste's new experiments with homeopathic microdoses of an antibody, he found that 39% of the experiments had a noticeable effect on white blood cells. "If proven, this would shatter the laws of chemistry and vindicate homeopaths who say that extremely dilute drugs can have a physical effect," noted *New Scientist*'s David Concar. Not surprisingly, Benveniste's research report was turned down by *Nature* and *Science*, whose scientific materialist edifice stands to lose a great deal when Benveniste's clinical trials are finally vindicated.

From a therapeutic point of view, whether Benveniste ever convinces the allopathic skeptics or not is inconsequential; it's indisputable that homeopathy *works;* the fact that scientists can't prove *how* is basically their epistemological problem.

Water's Memory and Other Paradoxes of Physical Matter

But a crucial, irrepressible question had been raised, no matter what *Nature's* magicians thought they had successfully debunked. Can water remember? Can the ghosts of molecules produce biological effects? Can water retain a phantom imprint of a substance it once contained? If true, the discovery would radically shift science's adamant materialist fixation and presumption of linear causality into the fluid dynamics of energy interactions and interdependencies.

The *Nature* community would not have been quite so alarmed, notes energy cartographer Richard Gerber, M.D., had they been less intellectually provincial and more current with the emerging Western scientific literature that was bringing energy back into matter in medical thinking. In 1979, for example, Dr. Bernard Grad of Montreal's McGill University showed that barley seeds exposed to water treated by a psychic healer sprouted more often, achieved greater height, and had higher chlorophyll content than those grown in a regular saline solution. In 1985, sophisticated instruments measured increases in the magnetic field emanations of healer's hands during the healing act. Further, Grad found that psychic energizing actually had shifted the atomic bond angle of water—certainly a quantifiable change along the lines M.D.s and Ph.D.s. love to see.

Certainly water can remember, Gerber would say. It's been proven, too. Homeopathic remedies are "subtle energy medicines which contain the energetic frequency or 'vibrational signature' of the plant," Gerber postulates. "What Hahnemann may actually have been doing is empirically matching the frequency of the plant extract with the frequency of the illness."

In terms of a vibrational paradigm, Hahnemann's Law of Similars, Gerber suggests, was an ingenious method of energetic frequency matching. Disease and health conditions may have vibrational orbits like electrons, such that transitions between modes could be provoked by slight energy shifts. "Homeopathic remedies are able to deliver that needed quantum of subtle energy to the human system through a type of resonance induction."

Gerber may be highlighting a profound interdependency when he links the energetic nature of the plant with the illness in a kind of frequency isomorphism. According to British homeopath Ralph Twentyman, when Hahnemann grasped the disease as an entity through its deeds and appearances in the symptoms, he was at the threshold of a profound understanding. For Hahnemann, says Twentyman, "the 'idea' which unites all symptoms into a unity is really the same idea which in a changed metamorphosis comes to expression in the remedy—the plant, for instance, as it grows in nature."

The "image-idea" of the remedy, the penetrative homeopath comprehends, is the same as the "unifying idea" of the disease or symptom picture. That's why the homeopath speaks more than metaphorically, but truly, when she describes a client as "a *Lycopodium.*"

In this light, *Nature's* posture of paradigmatic insult "to a substantial part of our intellectual heritage" from Benveniste's experiments is understandable. Acceptance of Benveniste's data commits allopathic materialists to paradigm-death under the blade of their own "Cartesian guillotine," as British anthroposophist Owen Barfield eloquently puts it. "The Newtonian model of medicine does not account for, nor believe in, these other energetic systems," says Gerber. "It's much easier to deny the efficacy of vibrational medicines like homeopathy than to extend an outdated model of understanding to incorporate higher energetic phenomena. The Einsteinian model of matter as an energy field gives us a framework in which we may realistically view and comprehend these subtle energy systems."

Cultivating a More Mobile Way of Medical Thinking

One would prefer to persuade rather than force allopathic conservatives into an appreciation of how it might be possible for post-Avogadro substances to be biologically active. British anthroposophic scientist George Adams proposed a new way to understand the mystery of potentization in terms of the "peripheral forces" of nature.

After all, in terms of the "rough and ready common sense and prevailing scientific notions" it is strange indeed to accept Hahnemann's outrageous statement that through potentization (which means in effect the removal through successive dilutions of all molecular traces of the original substance) the plant, animal, or mineral substance brings forth its "medicinal virtue" in a therapeutically enhanced form. "Thus our dilutions represent a truly wonderful unveiling, nay more, a calling-to-life of the medicinal and healing spirit of the substance," wrote Hahnemann. As Werner Junge notes, "A natural scientific establishment of homeopathy presupposes the inclusion of other dimensions besides the ones considered by modern physicists."

In an effort to rationalize the enigma posed by Hahnemann's potentization, we need "a more mobile thinking," says Adams, writing in the *British Homeopathic Journal*. He proposes that what is unveiled during potentization are the "ethereal formative forces," which in their essence are peripheral forces that move in from the vast omnidirectional expanse of the cosmic periphery toward the living center of humans, plants, and animals, and are active in that context without being bound to matter. These etheric peripheral forces, explains Adams, are the means by which the "purely spiritual essences to which the specific virtues of living things are due" are brought into matter. They exist in contrast to "centrist forces," expressed in terms of quantity and weight, the apparent virtues of solid matter.

So, if matter is maintained and fructified by "ethereal, peripheral forces of life, working in toward the earth from the surrounding heavens," this can explain how a potentized substance might be more effective than a molecularly gross one. If the substance is the bearer of "ethereal virtues" or formative forces derived from the cosmic periphery, says Adams, then its effect will be enhanced, not by concentration but by expansion.

In other words, when a materially gross substance is potentized beyond Avogadro's limit, the innate etheric formative, peripheral forces latent within it are "unveiled" and made available in their natural energetic milieu, what Hahnemann called the dynamic plane and Rudolf Steiner called the etheric world. Here it might be useful to fold our understanding of *dynamis, Qi,* and *physis* into the concept of etheric and assume that in these four words we are referring to an identical function (or location) of subtle energy.

The higher the potency of a remedy, which is to say, the more ethericized the substance becomes, the stronger the formative force and thus the more therapeutically powerful its effect, says Adams. In short, the etheric pattern is stronger than the physical substance.

Thinking and the Life of the Etheric Body

Rudolf Steiner vividly described the generally unrecognized nature of the etheric body. It is crucial to human health, illness, healing, and for our environmental relations. We've encountered the etheric body numerous times in the context of empiric, holistic therapeutics (where it is often, imprecisely, called the energy field surrounding the organism), but now we must work to comprehend its significance, because this is central to what follows in the remainder of the book.

The etheric body (sometimes called the "body of formative forces") is a kind of unconscious, active plantlike being within us; in fact, the etheric body represents the plant kingdom and the element of water in the human organism. "Basically, it is what implants actual life into us. It fills us with life. It is what contains the forces of growth and also those of nourishment," says Steiner. The etheric body is what individualizes the *physis*, giving it our unique soul imprint and bearing this as an active memory or formative force.

The etheric body is composed of the formative life forces engaged in the processes of growth and repair; they maintain the body's structural and organizational plan and overcome entropic tendencies. The etheric body is made of "streaming movements," said Steiner, that maintain the form and condition of all our internal organs; the heart, for example, is maintained by an "etheric heart," underlying the physical brain is an "etheric brain." The etheric body is understood to be materially insubstantial, an energetic copy of the physical form enfolding it like a thin robe of light: "a living, interpenetrating flow," said Steiner; "a supersensible entity active in all living beings," said German anthroposophic scientist Hermann Poppelbaum.

This etheric body, anthroposophy contends, contains a complete blueprint of all our organic life processes, including nourishment, growth, and reproduction, of the physical body. You might say it bears an imprint of a kind of spiritual DNA, a map of our organic destiny. That's why anthroposophists speak of the etheric body as bearing the "life organization" of the human. The intimate working relationship (and energy equivalency) of the human etheric body with the plant kingdom makes it easier to understand why the majority of the holistic pharmacopoeia, from herbalism to homeopathy, is botanical in origin.

In distinguishing physical from etheric energies, the anthroposophic scientist Ehrenfried Pfeiffer notes that chromosomes and genes, for example, are carriers, not originators, of the fundamental human pattern. To attribute organic effects to genetic inheritance, in other words, is tautological. The original pattern is "an inherent, immaterial activity," the organizing etheric force field which is "the creative force which acts out of cosmic order and wisdom in order to create and maintain life." Physical energies are executive while etheric forces are creative, says Pfeiffer. In other words, the etheric directs the physical.

The essence of the human etheric body is similar to the energy of the plant world: lush, passive, willowy, delicate, vital, vibrant, totally responsive to sunlight. If you take all the botanical species of nature—something like 270,000 varieties—and condense their essence into one form and wrap this around the human, that will give you at least a metaphorical idea of what anthroposophy means when it says the etheric body incorporates the entire plant kingdom. "Anthroposophical science of the spirit," notes Christof Lindenau, a German anthroposophical writer, "shows that each human being bears a portion of the etheric world individualized within himself."

The etheric body is rhythmic, harmonious, cyclic, moving in time, marked by "mobility, movement, formative activity in rhythmic or musical sequence, in fact, the quality of time," Steiner said. During sleep, the lively streaming activity of the etheric body is particularly evident as "a kind of humming and singing, a changing murmur . . . resounding music . . . at the same time radiant with light."

Paying no heed to the philosophical proprieties of the prevailing Cartesian mind-versus-body model, Steiner declared that thinking is an activity of the etheric body. The seat of thinking is not our brain but our etheric sheath, Steiner said. The etheric body is actually "the bearer of our whole intellect" because the "ordinary thought-forces of man are the refined forces of growth and differentiation." The etheric body represents "a picture world, which is also a world of weaving thoughts." This picture-world is the "true form of the etheric body" and as "picture-etheric body" it is also the body of "formative forces," Steiner said.

In other words, the etheric body bears not only the "life organization," but the "thought organization" for the human, whose structure "corresponds completely to that found to underlie the life organization," points out Lindenau. Thinking and growing are somehow twin expressions of the same energy. This also means that errors in thinking, at the etheric level, account for illnesses in the physical; conversely, when you establish correct etheric think-ing (or picture-thoughts), you are able to effect healing and disease reversal in the physical.

Whereas the etheric life organization organizes physical processes such as breathing, warming, digestion, secretion, and sustenance, the etheric thought organization organizes their etheric counter-parts such as perception, memory, distinguishing, questioning, and grasping totalities. It's the same energy, simply deployed in two dif-ferent spheres by the human etheric body. In fact, as Poppelbaum points out, there is a "dialectic of morphogenesis" and a "morphology of thought forms."

This means the shape and pattern of differentiation by which the plant unfolds and functions is similar in kind to how we think, thereby accounting for "the remarkable correspondence between the formative processes of the body and the processes of thought," says Poppelbaum. For example, the development of left-right symmetry in plants corresponds to the symmetrical structure of logic; the loss and regeneration of plant organs (leaves, roots) cor-responds to how we forget then reconstruct a "train" of thought. "These parallels exist because both morphogenesis and thinking have a common basis in the etheric body."

A Theophany Weaving Pictures in the Etheric Body

The implications here are remarkable. Steiner links thoughts, pic-ture-images, the Sun, formative life forces, and the plant kingdom all in one etheric energy sheath. We think with the same forces with which we grow and heal; this is why, as empirical medicine tells us, errors in thinking (how we picture our self-image, for example) can generate physical illness. Further, Steiner noted that whatever evolves in time is connected with the etheric body; the etheric body is a time repository for memories of incarnate existence.

We witness the truth of this observation in the commonly report-ed Near-Death Experiences (NDE), in which a person in a life-threatening situation or a moment of near mortality sees his entire life flash before him in a powerfully vivid tableau.

In fact, according to Steiner, this was an aspect of the baptism in the ancient mystery initiation. Candidates were deliberately almost drowned by their mentors to provoke a temporary loosening of the etheric from the physical so as to afford them a glimpse of their etheric thought pictures. Such a glimpse into their energy biography was also an introduction to their destiny or, as other traditions know it, "karma." This lifetime tableau, says Steiner—"the great memory-tableau of [one's] past life in the form of a vast picture"—is stored in the human etheric body and is spooled out spontaneously at the moment of death like a personalized videocassette biography. Glimpses are also accorded during dreams: "When we go to sleep at night, all our thought pictures and memories actually remain in the etheric body," said Steiner.

In the early decades of the twentieth century, Steiner predicted that as the century grew, at first a small number, then larger numbers, of people would begin having this glimpse of the etheric body spontaneously. Eventually a "natural etheric clairvoyance" would become a new part of the standard human organism. "People everywhere will gradually begin actually to see, although only in shadowy outline and in its first elements, what we call man's etheric body." This new faculty will enable humans to see in their environment aspects of the etheric world that previously had been entirely closed off to them, Steiner said. The etheric will come into view as "at least a shadowy picture" as humans become able to "perceive the connection between deeper happenings in the etheric world."

So when we wish to find the seat of thinking, of intellectual activity, we turn to the etheric body, not the physical brain. Thinking is nothing less than the etheric body's natural activity. The etheric is a thought organism with a life and force of its own, and that life consists of pictorial imagining and living pictures, "this self-imagining world formed out of the universal thought-weaving of the cosmos."

It is the human etheric body and its microcosmic world of flowing, weaving thoughts that bears our whole intellect. Thought isn't so much words, sentences, or concepts, but interlinking, living pictures—"forms of thoughts, of *flowing thoughts* . . . everywhere thought . . . the thought-processes of the Universe individualized." Normally, all of this remains in what we call the subconscious; for even the initiated, a clear perception of the etheric body in its time-life as a weaving, flowing picture tableau, is not easily had. After death, things change, and we are able to perceive its true form for a short time.

Whose flowing, weaving thoughts are these that comprise the human etheric body? In providing an answer to this question,

Steiner inducts us into the spiritual world, opening a profound vista of supraphysical influences and agencies. The human organism is not an accident of nature, but a theophany of spiritual intelligences. The human etheric is formed by a powerful "Imagination driven outward" by the Exousiai or Elohim of the Second Hierarchy of cosmic spiritual intelligences, Steiner said. As "Gods," the Elohim's thoughts literally inform us.

Their world-making pedigree is actually well-known to Western culture, although under a different name; the Christian Bible mistranslates (or oversimplifies) "Elohim" from the Hebrew as "God" or "Jehovah." The Elohim reveals itself through its activities, which are prolific, weaving imaginations. This weaving of picture-thoughts, which knits the human etheric body, is the expression or signature of the spiritual world itself.

The cosmic picture world is the true form of the etheric body, and this picture-etheric body is the seat of the vital, formative forces that shape and maintain the human physical form.

The Archetypal Relations between Plant and Man

The implication here is that not only are health, illness, and healing centered in the etheric body, but also the visionary capacity, the ability to receive supersensible impressions from the spiritual worlds. We also see how if consciousness inhabits or visits the etheric body in a wakeful state, insofar as the etheric body is the legislator of energy and structure, for the physical body, this is a crucial point of access for using consciousness to effect the bodily environment.

The popularity and alleged therapeutic success of "creative visualizations" suggests that many people have similarly made this discovery and are relying on the etheric body and its weaving, pictorial imaginations as a place of high therapeutic efficacy.

The crucial life forces that shape and permeate the outward physical body, facilitating growth, health, and nutrition, are at the same time united with the etheric picture-thought weaving. During sleep the etheric body is inwardly mobile, the site of continual lively activity: the Music of the Spheres, a flooding stream of warmth, a phosphorescent glow—"a reflection of the whole universe shines into the etheric body of man, the whole starry heavens are in the etheric body."

All of these qualities, Steiner said, are an "outer revelation, the external clothing, the revelation, the glory of mighty cosmic beings," the Exousiai. The activity of these exalted Sun-beings, their flowing and mutual influencing, itself forms the human etheric organism. Thus we can say it is the living thought-pictures of the cosmos, working through the activities of the Second Hierarchy, that generate the human intellect and thinking, and shape and maintain the physical human body. Our physical body is made of etheric thoughts.

This means that learning to think *alively*—to enliven our thinking—is to seize hold of the same etheric forces that are the formative energies shaping and maintaining our physical organism. It's the same energy, simply deployed in two different spheres by the human etheric body. In one direction, this energy maintains our physical life; in another, it is the matrix for our thinking. The crucial life forces that shape and permeate the physical body, facilitating growth, health, and nutrition, are at the same time united with the etheric picture-thought weaving activities of thinking.

Enlivened thinking, or a perception animate with living imaginations and life-filled pictures, trades in the same currency as our etheric life forces. This is precisely the means by which an empirical therapy effects healing. In other words, thinking and healing are inseparably connected; potentially, we think with healing energy because both thinking (in the alive, weaving-picture sense) and healing are activities of the etheric domain. This also means that our physical body is made of (or from) etheric thoughts. The etheric body is the key, then, to both diagnosis (the perception of the energy imbalance underlying the pathology) and treatment (the rebalancing of etheric life forces through natural remedies).

As such, the etheric body is the foundation for the efficacy of natural human-centered medicines because it is the intelligent energy matrix antecedent to and thus formative for the physical body.

That's why the etheric body is the great healer, the repository of restorative energies. In a sense, the Ego, in drafting the blueprints for a given physical incarnation, selects from a multitude of plants those it will use to weave the individual human etheric body. *Equisetum* (horsetail), for example, is, in its essential nature, correlated with the human kidneys and astral body and as such provides an archetype for kidney processes—the *idea* of the kidney process expressed as the living plant *equisetum*. It's as if with kidney problems, we lack the formative life force idea of *equisetum;* through the application of the appropriate remedy (in this case, a certain potency of *equisetum),* we thereby restore what is properly an innate constituent of the human organism.

The life force—call it homeopathy's *dynamis,* acupuncture's *Qi,* or the Greek doctor's *physis*—is thus the "idea" of the plant. By extension, human etheric vitality is the same as the totality of the plant kingdom, as the whole botanical archetype, or idea. This is why anthroposophical physicians talk about "the archetypal relations between plant and man." It is part of the unity of human self and physical world that is at the basis of Pandora's covenant.

References

Adams, George, "Potentization and the Peripheral Forces of Nature," *British Homeopathic Journal,* Vol. 78, No. 2, (April 1989).

Amber, Reuben, *Color Therapy,* Aurora Press, Santa Fe, 1983.

Anderson, Mary, *Colour Therapy: The Application of Colour for Healing, Diagnosis, and Well-Being,* The Aquarian Press/Thorsons Publishing Group,Wellingborough, 1990.

Beardsley, Timothy M., "Now You See It . . . " *Scientific American,* (September 1988).

Begley, Sharon, "Can Water 'Remember'? Homeopathy Finds Scientific Support," *Newsweek,* (July 25, 1988).

Berendt, Joachim-Ernst. *The World is Sound, Nada Brahma. Music and the Landscape of Consciousness.* Destiny Books, Rochester, Vermont, 1987.

Birren, Faber, *Color Psychology and Color Therapy,* The Citadel Press/Lyle Stuart, Secaucus, New Jersey, 1979.

Browne, Malcolm W., "Impossible Idea Published on Purpose," *The New York Times,* (June 30, 1988).

Brusatin, Manlio, *A History of Colors,* Shambhala Publications, Boston, 1991.

Carpenter, Mary, "Homeopathic Chic," *Health,* (March 1989).

Concar, David, "'Ghost Molecules' Theory Back from the Dead," *New Scientist,* (16 March 1991).

Cook, Pat Moffitt, "Composing Self-Health," in *Music and Miracles,* Compiled by Don Campbell, Quest Books, Wheaton, 1992.

Coulter, Harris L., *Homoeopathic Medicine*, Formur, St. Louis, 1972.

—*Homoeopathic Science and Modern Medicine: The Physics of Healing with Microdoses*, North Atlantic Books, Berkeley, 1981.

—*Divided Legacy, A History of the Schism in Medical Thought. Vol. 1, The Paterns Emerge: Hippocrates to Paracelsus.* Wehawken Book Company, Washington, D.C., 1975.

Coulter, Katherine R., *Portraits of Homoeopathic Medicines: Psychophysical Analyses of Selected Constitutional Types*, North Atlantic Books, Berkeley, 1986.

—*Portraits of Homoeopathic Medicines: Psychophysical Analyses of Selected Constitutional Types*, Vol. 2, North Atlantic Books, Berkeley, 1988.

Cummings, Stephen, and Ullman, Dana, *Everybody's Guide to Homeopathic Medicines*, Jeremy P. Tarcher, Los Angeles, 1984.

Dalichow, Irene, and Booth, Mike, *Aura-Soma. Healing Through Color, Plant, and Crystal Energy*, Hay House, Carlsbad, California, 1996.

Danciger, Elizabeth, *Homeopathy: From Alchemy to Medicine*, Inner Traditions, Rochester, 1989.

Davenas, E., et al., "Human Basophil Degranulation Triggered by Very Dilute Antiserum Against IgE," *Nature*, Vol. 333, June 30, 1988.

Dinshah, Darius, *Let There Be Light*, Second Edition, Dinshah Health Society, Malaga, New Jersey, 1995.

Don, Frank, *Color Magic: Learn to Use Your Personal Color Power*, Destiny Books, New York, 1983.

Eizayaga, Francisco Xavier, M.D., *Treatise on Homoeopathic Medicine*, Ediciones Marecel, Buenos Aires, 1991.

Ghadiali, Colonel Dinshah P., *Spectro-Crome Metry Encyclopedia*, Dinshah Health Society, Malaga, New Jersey, 1992.

Gimbel, Theo, *The Colour Therapy Workbook: A Guide to the Use of Color for Health and Healing*, Element Books, Shaftesbury, Dorset, 1993.

Godwin, Joscelyn, *Harmonies of Heaven and Earth: The Spiritual Dimension of Music from Antiquity to the Avant-Garde*, Inner Traditions, Rochester, Vermont, 1987.

Gorman, James, "Take a Little Deadly Nightshade and You'll Feel Better," *The New York Times Magazine*, (August 30, 1992).

Graham, Lamar B., "Homeopathy: Same As It Ever Was," *The Boston Phoenix*, (July 21, 1989).

Grossinger, Richard, *Planet Medicine: From Stone-Age Shamanism to Post-Industrial Healing*, North Atlantic Books, Berkeley, 1980.

Hahnemann, Samuel, *Organon of Medicine*, Künzu Jost, M.D., Naudé, Alain, and Pendleton, Peter, translators, J.P. Tarcher Inc., Los Angeles, 1982.

Hunt, Roland, *The Seven Keys to Colour Healing*, The C.W. Daniel Company, Saffron Walden, 1963.

Irlen, Helen, *Reading by the Colors: Overcoming Dyslexia and Other Reading Disabilities Through the Irlen Method*, Avery Publishing Group, Garden City Park, 1991.

Junge, Werner, "The Homeopathic Principle," *Mercury: Journal of the Anthroposophical Therapy and Hygiene Association*, No. 11, (June 1991).

Kayser, Hans, *Akroasis. The Theory of World Harmonics*, Plowshare Press, Boston, 1970.

Kent, James Tyler, M.D., *Lectures on Homoeopathic Philosophy*, North Atlantic Books, Richmond, Virginia, 1979.

Kilner, Walter J. *The Human Aura*, The Citadel Press, Secaucus, New Jersey, 1965.

Kleijnen, Jos, Knipschild, Paul, and ter Riet, Gerben, "Clinical Trials of Homeopathy," *British Medical Journal*, (February 9, 1991).

Koenig, Karl, M.D., "Samuel Hahnemann," *Mercury: Journal of the Anthroposophical Therapy and Hygiene Association*, No. 7, (September 1985).

Lawren, Bill, "The Case of the Ghost Molecules," *OMNI*, (June 1992).

Leviton, Richard, "The Healing Energies of Color," *Yoga Journal*, (January/February 1992).

    —"Healing Vibrations," *Yoga Journal*, (January/February 1994).

    —"Homeopathy—How It Works, Why It's So Controversial, and How You Can Benefit," *Yoga Journal*, (March/April 1989).

    —*The Imagination of Pentecost. Rudolf Steiner and Contemporary Spirituality*, Anthroposophic Press, Hudson, 1994.

Liberman, Jacob, *Light: Medicine of the Future,* Bear and Company, Santa Fe, 1991.

Lindenau, Christof, "Life Organization and Thought Organization: Concerning the Dual Nature of the Human Etheric Body," in *Toward a Phenomenology of the Etheric World: Investigations into the Life of Nature and Man,* Jochen Bockemühl, editor, Anthroposophic Press, Spring Valley, 1985.

Lüscher, Dr. Max, *The Lüscher Colour Test,* Scott, Ian A., editor, translator, Pan Books, London, 1970.

MacIvor, Virginia, and LaForest, Sandra, *Vibrations: Healing Through Color, Homoeopathy and Radionics,* Samuel Weiser, York Beach, 1979.

Marti, Ernst, M.D., "Potentizing," *Mercury: Journal of the Anthroposophical Therapy and Hygiene Association,* No. 11, (June 1991).

Mayer, Gladys, *Colour and Healing,* New Knowledge Books, East Grinstead, 1960.

McAuliffe, Kathleen, "Homeopathy, Medicine or Mysticism?" *Self,* (August 1992).

McClellan, Randall, Ph.D., *The Healing Forces of Music, History, Theory and Practice,* Element Books, Shaftesbury, Dorset, 1991.

Nelson, M.V., Bailie, G.R., and Areny, H., "Pharmacists' Perceptions of Alternative Health Apporaches—A Comparison Between U.S. and British Pharmacists," *Journal of Clinical Pharmacy and Therapeutics,* Vol. 15, (1990).

Page, Jake, "Dilutions of Grandeur," *American Health,* (November 1988).

Panos, Maesimund B., M.D., and Heimlich, Jane, *Homeopathic Medicine at Home,* Jeremy P. Tarcher, Los Angeles, 1980.

Pelikan, Wilhelm, "Disease Process and Medicinal Plant," *Journal of Anthroposophic Medicine,* Vol. 5, No. 1, (Spring 1988).

—"The Members of Being in Man and Nature," *Journal of Anthroposophic Medicine,* Vol. 5, No. 1, (Spring 1988).

Pfeiffer, E.E., "Physical and Etheric Energies," *Mercury: Journal of the Anthroposophical Therapy and Hygiene Association,* Spring Valley, No. 2, (April 1976).

Poppelbaum, Hermann, "The Concept and Action of the Etheric Body," in *Toward a Phenomenology of the Etheric World: Investigations into the Life of Nature and Man,* Jochen Bockemühl, editor, Anthroposophic Press, Spring Valley, 1985.

Rawson, D.S., "A Scientific Approach to Homoeopathy, With Special Reference to Potentization," *British Homeopathic Journal,* Vol. 61, No. 2, (1972).

Reilly, David Taylor, et al., "Is Homoeopathy a Placebo Response?" *Lancet,* (October 18, 1986).

Robinson, Karl, M.D., "Why Do We Fall Sick? Is It to Dream?" *Journal of the American Institute of Homeopathy,* Vol. 81, No. 2, (June 1988).

Rodarmor, William, "Modern Homeopathy's Bitter Medicine," *East West,* (November 1984).

Schneider, Vimala, "The Healing Power of Color," *Yoga Journal,* (January/February 1987).

Steiger, Brad, "Taking on the Medical Establishment," *East West,* (May 1987).

Steiner, Rudolf, *Man's Life on Earth and in the Spiritual Worlds,* Anthroposophical Society, London, 1922.

—*Art in the Light of Mystery Wisdom,* Rudolf Steiner Press, London, 1984.

—"The Cosmic Word and Individual Man," single lecture, Rudolf Steiner Nachlassverwaltung, Dornach, Switzerland, May 2, 1923.

—*The Gospel of St. Luke,* Rudolf Steiner Press, London, 1964.

—*The Reappearance of of the Christ in the Etheric,* Anthroposophic Press, Spring Valley, New York, 1983.

—*Cosmosophy, Vol. 1.* Anthroposophic Press, Spring Valley, New York, 1985.

—*The True Nature of the Second Coming,* Rudolf Steiner Press, London, 1971.

Stoff, Jesse A., and Stoff, Sheldon P., "Induced Electrical Changes at Acupuncture Points by Homoeopathic Remedies," *Alternative Medicine,* Vol. 2, Nos. 3/4, (1987).

Tansley, David V., D.C., *Dimensions of Radionics: New Techniques of Instrumented Distant-Healing,* C.W. Daniel Company, Saffron Walden, 1977.

—*The Raiment of Light: A Study of the Human Aura,* Arkana, London, 1987.

Tiller, William A., Ph.D., "Towards a Scientific Rationale of Homeopathy," *Journal of Holistic Medicine,* Vol. 6, No. 2, (Fall 1984).

Twentyman, L.R., "Homoeopathy—An Introduction," *Mercury: Journal of the Anthroposophical Therapy and Hygiene Association,* No. 5, (April 1981).

—"The Problem of Life and Potentization," *Mercury: Journal of the Anthroposophical Therapy and Hygiene Association,* No. 6, (July 1982).

—"The Nature of Homeopathy," in *A Compendium III, Research and Conceptual Basis for the Comprehension of High Dilutional Activity,* Mercury Press, Spring Valley, October 1990.

Uhlman, Marian, "Following Old Route to Health," *Philadelphia Inquirer,* (September 12, 1988).

Ullman, Dana, "Beyond Medical Chauvinism," *San Francisco Examiner* and *San Francisco Chronicle, California Living Magazine,* (August 21, 1983).

—"Homeopathy Conference a Stunning Success," *Homeopathy Today,* Vol. 8, No. 8, (July/August 1988).

—"Principles of Homeopathy," *Co-Evolution Quarterly,* (Spring 1981).

—*Homeopathy: Medicine for the 21st Century,* North Atlantic Books, Berkeley, 1988.

—"Homeopathy in America: A Status Report," *Homeopathic Research Reports,* (Winter 1989-90).

—"British Medical Journal Publishes the Most Significant Review of Homeopathic Research to Date," *Homeopathic Research Reports,* (Winter 1991-92).

—"Homeopathic Research: Scientific Verification of Homeopathic Medicine," *Townsend Letter for Doctors,* (June 1988).

Wall, Vicky, *The Miracle of Colour Healing: Aura Soma Therapy as the Mirror of the Soul,* The Aquarian Press/Thorsons Publishing Group, Wellingborough, 1990.

Wilson, Annie, and Bek, Lilla, *What Colour Are You? The Way to Health Through Colour,* The Aquarian Press/Thorsons Publishing Group, Wellingborough, 1981.

Wood, Betty, *The Healing Power of Colour,* Destiny Books, Rochester, 1984.

Wood, Matthew, *The Magical Staff: The Vitalist Tradition in Western Medicine,* North Atlantic Books, Berkeley, 1992.

Vithoulkas, George, *Homeopathy, Medicine of the New Man,* Arco Publishing, New York, 1979.

—*The Science of Homeopathy,* Grove Press, New York, 1980.

Winston, Julian, "Constantine Hering, M.D.," *The Hahnemannian, Journal of the Homeopathic Medical Society of the State of Pennsylvania,* (March 1988).

Yasgur, Jay, "On Homeopathy—A Modern Day Perspective," *American Pharmacy,* Vol. 24, No. 12, (December 1984).

CHAPTER 7

The Pleomorphic Self:
The Meaning of Illness
and the Elemental Revolt

Opening Pandora's Box:
Why Is There Illness?

We have to begin with asking the biggest question possible: Why is there illness and disease at all? What purpose does it serve in the order of the world and in the life of humans?

For a question this large, we need a large perspective, the kind of instruction the realm of myth and metaphysics offers the discerning. The Greek myths give us matter for thought regarding the original purpose of disease and its teleology through the story of Pandora's box, the source of all contagion. Taken literally, the Greek myths declare that illness is a curse of the gods; read esoterically, it is a profound teaching on why there is illness in the world.

As the Greek legends recount it, Prometheus (his name means "fore-thought"), the Titan who stole fire from his godly colleagues on humanity's behalf, had a brother named Epimetheus (his name means "after-thought"). Prometheus was punished for his transgression of Olympian law by being chained to a rock, where during the day an eagle plucked at his liver. Epimetheus was alarmed at his brother's fate and decided to marry Pandora (her name means "all-giving"): she was beautiful, but idle, mischievous, and foolish, qualities bestowed upon her by Zeus, king of the gods.

After Prometheus stole the heavenly fire, Zeus decided to make him pay for it. In effect, humanity was not meant to have this celestial fire, so Zeus came up with a plan to give humanity the reverse of the stolen fire: a different kind of fire that would burn them alive with trouble, anxiety, and pain. This nemesis would be Pandora, the first woman, who would be the Double and opposite of men, at that time (according to the Greek myths) the only humans alive. Zeus ordered Hephaestus, the smith of Olympus, to fashion a clay woman; into this clay form, the Four Winds breathed life; all the goddesses of Olympus, led by Athena (gray-eyed Goddess of Wisdom, who leapt fully formed from Zeus' brow) added their feminine charms to the clay-sculpted female.

To Pandora came the godly gifts of beauty, grace, dexterity, and cogency, but also lying and deceit. This is why her name also means "all gifts," because she was the recipient of manifold dispensations from the gods. The name "Pandora" also signified the first *gune* or woman, suggesting "she who is the gift of them all" (meaning the Olympian gods) and "she who gives all," a reference to the Earth as Gaia.

Yet Pandora was also a virgin who brought about death, according to classical scholars Laurence Kahn-Lyotard and Nicole Loraux. "First and foremost, Pandora, with her body of a *parthenos aidoie,* forbidden and respectable (but *aidoios* as a neuter noun designates shame itself: the pudendum, the sexual organ), Pandora from whom the female race has sprung; the artifice named woman." For Jean-Pierre Vernant, Pandora is the embodiment (thanks to an avenging Zeus) of evil: "She was evil, but a likable evil clothed in stirring beauty, a *kakon kalon,* the kind of evil one can neither do without nor endure." In this archetypal woman, good and evil, divine and bestial, were "merged and confused," says Vernant.

Zeus sent Pandora, the most beautiful woman ever seen on Earth, as a gift to Epimetheus. At first Epimetheus refused, because Prometheus had warned him to not accept any gifts from Zeus, ever the trickster. Prometheus in his forethought (or precognition) had warned Epimetheus to prevent anyone from opening a certain box (or stone jar) in which he had labored hard to imprison the Spites, entities that meant to plague humanity with illness. He also warned Epimetheus not to welcome Pandora into his house because she would surely seduce him, bringing upon him great misfortune.

Here the names of these two Titans who were twins yet opposites bears true: Prometheus ("fore-thought" or foresight) could guess or see in advance, before the events, while Epimetheus ("after-thought" or hindsight) could understand only too late, after the event had transpired.

The Spites were a family of misery, including Old Age, Labor, Sickness, Insanity, Vice, and Passion. Also known as *Keres,* the Spites were malignant spirits, evil bringers of bodily pollution that made humans unclean, causing blindness, diseases, old age, death, spiritual oblivion, misfortunes, and general troubles. Some sources depicted them as birds of prey similar to Harpies or Sirens. In the *Iliad,* the *Keres* often appeared in battle scenes and at acts of violence as a kind of presiding deity, controlling the destiny of each individual. As such, they were depicted as black-winged creatures of horrible mien, with long pointed nails and daggerlike teeth. The *Keres* were said to tear human corpses to pieces and drink the blood of the wounded and dead.

The *Moirae,* or Fates, embodied the same idea of inexorable destiny. Each human being had its own *moira,* or personification of destiny (karma); so strong was this individually mandated destiny that not even the gods could shift its direction without seriously upsetting the fabric of orderly creation. The concept of the individual *moira* and the specificity of biological fate tends to counterbalance the general attitude of blamelessness supported by the Epimethean (or godly) origin of illness. The gods (or Nature, for our deicidal age) may have generated illness as a legacy for all of humanity, but somehow each of us is individually responsible for the activity of that illness-bearing *moira* in our own body and life.

Homer suggested that the *Keres* were an expression of the destiny (or fate) of heroes, such as Achilles; the *Keres* coexisted with them, personifying the quality of their life and the face of their death. The Greek conception of *Keres* and *Moirae,* in fact, is highly similar to Rudolf Steiner's concept of the *Doppelgänger,* or Ahrimanic Double, who carries around a soul's illness predispositions during the period of incarnation, as described earlier in Chapter 2. In one source, the *Keres* are said to be the daughters of Nyx. She is the Goddess of Night, herself the daughter of Chaos; yet Nyx is also the mother of Aether (as in ether, etheric, "the upper sky") and Hemera (his sister, Day) and a family of abstract forces such as Destiny, the *Keres*, Sleep, Dreams, Reproach, Distress, Nemesis, Deceit, Love, Old Age, and Strife.

This is probably why the early Greeks also pictured Eros (passionate Love or Cupid) as a *Ker* or winged Spite, similar to Old Age and Plague. Strife, for example, is in turn the mother of more troubles: Work, Forgetfulness, Hunger, Pain, Battles, Fights, Murders, Killings, Quarrels, Lies, Stories, Disputes, Lawlessness, and Ruin.

Under Zeus' order, Pandora opened this box (which some say was Zeus' wedding present to her), and out flew the Spites in a thick cloud, stinging her and Epimetheus all over their bodies. "All of its evil contents spread over the Earth and mingled with the good, so that they could be neither foreseen nor recognized," writes Vernant. The Spites swarmed on to attack the entire human race. A seventh Spite—Delusive Hope—used her wily arts of persuasion to discourage a now suffering humanity from committing mass suicide; a variant of the legend says that Hope remained in the box when Pandora at last replaced the lid. "Some evils roved about the world, hidden and invisible," Vernant says. "Others, lurking about the home like the 'beautiful evil' that Pandora was, hid under the deceitful guise of seduction."

There is no need to defend or even comment on the strongly misogynist tendencies in our received version of the Greek myths because none was ever meant. The myth of Pandora's box veils a metaphysical (gender free) truth about the occult origin of illness and its incarnation in both men and women.

There was never a primal woman at fault, but there was a virgin soul who corresponded to Pandora. The goal of this chapter is to explain this process, and to link the Greek *Keres* with contemporary discussions and descriptions of illness, the realm of "germs," drug-resistant mutating bacteria, the disaster of antibiotics, the elemental revolt, bacteriological pleomorphism, and the human astral body.

These connections and the individual topics themselves no doubt will strike most readers as exotic, possibly bizarre, and certainly poorly understood. What do they have to do with medicine? However, by the end of this chapter, I will have presented a strong case that the story elements of Pandora's box represent the key to understanding and healing our environment, from body to landscape.

Pandora's Legacy:
Does Illness Belong to Us?

Let's descend from the Olympian abstractions (or fantasies, some might say) of Pandora's box to the more mundane and familiar world of illness. Contemplating the mystery of disease, Randolph Nesse, M.D., and George Williams, Ph.D., in *Why We Get Sick,* ruminate: "Why, in a body of such exquisite design, are there a thousand flaws and frailties that make us vulnerable to disease?"

They apply the principles of Darwinian evolution to make disease both less and more meaningful; they contend that disease arises from past natural selection and that the human is a bundle of compromises, in which heightened capacities were acquired as a trade-off with increased susceptibility. Cancer, for example, is the price we pay for having tissues capable of self-repair. Illness has an inherent impersonal, or public, significance, favoring and resulting from the evolution of the species, Nesse and Williams contend. "After all, nothing in medicine makes sense except in the light of evolution."

Meanwhile, implicit in the empirical model is the contention that illness is a process uniquely relevant to the individual. Disease and the struggle to resolve it and heal are innately meaningful, even necessary, experiences. Meaningful means you regard illness as a life event that is not arbitrary, random, or mysterious, but specific, purposeful, and informative—an event that has something vital to do with *me,* the experiencer, the recipient. Taking this kind of stance is not customary in allopathy's philosophy of medicine. Yet surely anybody who becomes ill demands answers of one's doctor or one's body: why me, why now, why this way, for how long, and with what outcome?

An understanding of the points of coinciding between a disease process and a life can be the basis of an invigorating insight into causality and intention, if one has the nerve to pursue the event to its core. Disease, says empirical medicine, is heuristic—it can teach you something important. It has the potential to inspire you to investigate its origin, timeliness, appropriateness, and requirements.

So in this chapter I pose what may seem an intimidating question: What does *this* illness have to do with *me?* An insightful answer born of long, careful contemplation could give us the means to radically change the way we position environment—in this case, the human body—in our thinking.

Yet this contemplation is not easy, nor is the balm of insight guaranteed; certainly one has it only at the expense of great pain and suffering. Christina Middlebrook, for example, wrote a memoir *(Seeing the Crab)* about her experience with presumed terminal cancer. Judy, her sister-in-law, was simultaneously dealing with the decline of her husband with prostate cancer. Shaking her fists at the sky, Judy screamed: *"Fuck* you, God!" In effect, Judy was cursing what the Greeks called the *Keres* or *Moirae;* God, or Zeus, may ultimately be to blame, but "he" delegated responsibility to these lower-echelon agents. It is a little consolation to curse God if you are a believer, but as a Jungian therapist, Middlebrook says she came from a "godless" family.

Having no frame of etiological reference, the experience of life-denying illness can be an existential nightmare. Her survival odds were not good, admitted Middlebrook. "Jesus God, a can of worms. Pandora's box spilling like night crawlers from a Styrofoam cup." When Middlebrook's mother criticized her for "not thinking right" about the possibility of a remission, Middlebrook felt enraged. "The mere assumption that good thoughts will affect the outcome of my life or death-revealing bone scans turns me ugly as Medusa." Even so, Middlebrook learned deeply from her cancer initiation: "Cancer has changed me. I take more risks . . . Hideous as it is, cancer has bathed me in love."

Kat Duff similarly regarded her protracted engagement with chronic fatigue syndrome as having alchemical, initiatory elements. The more she probed her illness, the more she suspected it held "deeper mysteries and hidden designs," as she writes in her sickness narrative, *The Alchemy of Illness.* Probably to a greater degree than most other such autobiographical chronicles, Duff's ruminations willingly run with the idea that illness may have a personal purpose. "I suspect it is actually an attempt to embody the whole truth, to remember all of ourselves."

One of the prime labors of illness is to gradually remember various "isolated, frozen fragments of memory" and the "scattered parts of my self and history" and reincorporate them into the present stream of life, identity, and awareness, says Duff. Illness reminds you of what you have forgotten—in her case, a painful experience of infantile incest and sexual abuse—and healing is the act of recollecting your wounds.

The actual physiology of the illness process is therefore a kind of expedient means set in motion by "that deep knowing which operates through the agency of our dreams and flesh, I would call it soul."

As our illness contemplation yields fruit, we begin to see the ways in which longstanding habits of mind might contribute creatively to the design and dynamics of our bodily environment. With this insight comes liberation: if we help shape environment through our (mostly passive, unconscious, or un-self-reflexive) thoughts, then we may use this environment-making power to our advantage and reconfigure our bodily environment according to a pattern of comparative health and vitality.

The tacit requirement of empirical medicine is that we get involved in our environment, that we become active, aware participants in the creation and maintenance of our bodily and psychological environment. At the least, life and its periodic nodes of illness will enlarge itself into a field of meaning.

That illness has meaning and purpose is implicit in the empirical view of medicine. Symptoms exist in the context of unique individuals and their way of living; symptoms are not random, aberrant acts of a mechanistic biology, as allopathy instructs us, but are purposeful agents of a larger intention expressing itself through biology. The disease process is inherently meaningful, empirical physicians contend, provided we're willing to expand our vision of the field of contributing factors.

Here of course we confront one of the archetypal questions of philosophy—cause and effect—from perhaps an unusual perspective. It's a vantage point from which we gain an *insider's* view of the origin of illness; in effect, this is where we learn how to create and change an organic environment with our mind. Let's turn to an actual illness narration to see how some of these elements become conscious in the experience of a person struggling to overcome a serious disease.

Lupus Novice: A Wolf Bite's Aftermath

When Donna Hamil Talman was thirty-four, a wolf bit her. The wolf kept its teeth dug into her for over ten years and didn't ease up until Talman, a successful psychotherapist and educator, a working mother and wife, radically transformed all aspects of her life—her history, thoughts, emotions, expectations, body. The wolf was identified as *lupus erythematosus,* an excruciating autoimmune disease often intractable to conventional medicine and sometimes fatal.

Lupus is a multiple-symptom major illness whose characteristic bodily signature is skin lesions that resemble wolf bites. The wolf lesions indicate that the body's immune system is mistakenly, dangerously, producing antibodies against its own connective tissue. What Talman wanted to know, as does nearly everyone who contracts a life-threatening disease, was *why* did the wolf bite her?

Lupus profoundly shook up Talman's accustomed order of life, but as she eventually realized, it was this very order that precipitated the autoimmune dysfunction as a corrective in the first place. The lupus experience catalyzed her awareness of an unbalanced, unresolved, incomplete part of herself—unfinished psychological business played out in her biology. It was the first lesson in a life course of illness as biography.

"Instead of a rap to beat, lupus slowly came to be a spiritual lesson, a koan," confides Talman. "Whatever else lupus did, it catapulted me beyond my realm of understanding. I was forced to find a new way to make sense of my existence and to explore myself in greater depth than I had ever imagined was possible." Getting well, Talman learned, requires a fundamental, active reorientation to life, a prolonged self-examination in depth. Healing necessitates "a far greater degree of commitment than we have ever before been called upon to make."

The first several years of Talman's lupus experience involved intermittent hospitalizations, a slew of capricious incapacitating symptoms, and regular prednisone medication to enhance adrenal function. She understood that lupus represented a constellation of symptoms. "I needed to move beyond symptom-chasing because lupus is a *systemic* illness." She had to stop thinking allopathically, always seeking after yet another specific, isolated etiology. Talman struggled to gain a broader perspective on the intense body-mind issue that was at play in her—that her life had become.

As buried feelings began to surface, she realized that her emotional bottom line was a tirade against herself: she was never good enough, she was always at fault. "Self-blame ran swift and deep. Day after day self-blaming feelings tugged at me so powerfully that I felt compelled to keep trying to unravel them." The equation became unassailable: it was self attacking self, as self-blame transformed into self-digestion, as psychology became immunology. Talman was playing out this drama of self-destruction equally in the twin theaters of psyche and immune system.

With this initial understanding she sought out Gestalt, psychodrama, and bioenergetics as "active expressive modes that offered the fastest way to work through locked emotions." And the fastest way to unlock those knotted-up emotions, Talman found, was a couple of powerful sessions with the founder of bioenergetics, Alexander Lowen, M.D.

You're a nice hysterical personality and a good girl, Lowen told an astounded Talman in her first session. "But your feelings are all blocked. You hold on for dear life in your jaw. That's where the lupus comes from—a longing. You have been fighting off deep, sad feelings for a long time. Lupus is the holding back of that sadness." Talman was shocked by Lowen's direct recognition of her inner pattern.

Talman converts unconscious, unrecognized emotions into physical symptoms, Lowen later told members of a private clinical seminar in which Talman was the guest patient. "Her outer structure—emphasis on rationality and reality—has to collapse. Then her body won't have to do all the reacting. She has to give up the delusion that her father will rescue her. Despair will manifest itself in deep crying, which is her way out. She has to feel it, to go to the very bottom of it, then she will stop struggling, and healing can begin."

Lowen was essentially right, but he had one more punch reserved for Talman's psyche. Talman had gone to him thinking she was exaggerating her dark side. "He seemed to be saying that not only was I not exaggerating, I was underestimating its size and scope." It's big and it will fight you to the death. But the crucial turning point in many severe illnesses, said Lowen, is the moment the patient accepts the possibility of death from his or her condition. "In the face of death, one unconsciously gives up the neurotic struggle to maintain a facade, which makes more energy available for combating the disease," he wrote Talman.

Talman dropped the facade, accepted the chance of a mortal outcome, healed, and wrote an amazingly candid, edifying account. Today, sixteen years after lupus first bit her, she's symptomless and very insightful about herself. As to the equation lupus equals self-blame played out in biology, Talman entertains this with reservation. "It's too simplistic to try to find a single meaning for illness, a single psychoemotional equation. This would be allopathic thinking disguised as holism. There are more mysteries to the body than we can account for. The personality characteristics of an illness add pieces to our understanding, but it's too reductionist to see this as a single etiology. We don't begin to grasp the power of the mind. From what I've tasted I know I don't even begin to see how powerful our thoughts can be."

The search to impart a meaning to illness may be tantamount to struggling to understand the meaning of life itself, of one's individuality. What do *I* mean? That's what the wolf, clamping into our flesh, compels us to ask. By way of answer, maybe all you get is a haiku, not an expository essay, says Donna Talman. "Lupus compelled me to search the *unknowing* of what my life is about. The inquiry itself is the result, just as they say in meditation the path is the goal. The creative use of metaphor as a tool for understanding intrigues me as a therapist. There is nothing hard and fast, no universal etiology. I don't know if in the end there is a single meaning to lupus or any other illness, and if there is, that meaning is individually variable."

Today everything seems grayer, more paradoxical, after her ten-year lupus initiation, reflects Talman. "I cannot say I am cured, yet in most ways I have never been healthier. The illness has no inherent meaning, but I can make it meaningful. I ask significantly fewer questions these days about cause and effect. Symptoms and emotions interconnect, but I am less clear about the extent to which my emotions stimulate symptoms or are in response to symptoms. The illness has been as much a journey into unknowing as into knowing. We are terribly complex beings."

The Mistake of Turning Disease into Metaphor

I've noted throughout this book, that for allopathy major illness is anomalous, random, invasive, inimical, impersonal, nondiscriminatory—and inherently meaningless. It's an inconvenient incident, "a flat tire on the road of life." Disease is meaningful only in that it debilitates, maims, or kills, and generates astounding medical bills and social dislocation, but besides that cancer, AIDS, and lupus have no more intelligent purpose in a person's life than a stray bullet in wartime. They kill, and that's the meaning, says allopathy.

A philosophy of illness and a wide-ranging discussion of the possibility that it could hold personal meaning and relevance aren't topics mainstream American culture encourages. M.D.s are not Socratically probing the mystery of disease. But as the incidence of major illness accelerates, both degenerative and immune dysfunctional, personal chronicles of the agonizing process of medicalization—survival, "negotiated settlement," victory, or defeat—are becoming popular. Medical patients ("disease victims" or illness novices), such as Talman, are gradually becoming philosophers.

Each disease has a characteristic mark, a signature, that distinguishes it from every other, and patients "can actually feel, experience, and sense" this pathogenic identity, suggests James Buchanan in *Patient Encounters—The Experience of Disease*. We have an uncanny intelligence to somehow know the identity of the disease that may be consuming us; pathologies seem to "reveal themselves in shocking exhibitionism" in all their "texture, tone, and composition" to us while often hiding from the inquiring eyes of the physician. After a while, each patient comes to sense, deep within, the pathological presence of "some dark, primal source" and its ambivalent metabolic fires.

Through a brilliantly executed series of "phenomenological descriptions of disease processes," Buchanan brings us intimately within the lives of patients, all of whom suffer terribly and many of whom die from their pathologies. Buchanan writes with poetic force, although his attitudes are colored by the standard allopathic mechanistic view of disease; yet even from within this limiting perspective his revelations of the "feelings, experiences, and inner dynamics" of each illness are profoundly moving.

The onset of Alzheimer's, acromegaly, porphyria, progeria, carcinoma, and Parkinson's may seem meaningless, suggests Buchanan, but not, if you're the patient, their lived experience. Here is meaning indeed. "To understand a disease, it is not enough to study it; you must also endure it, suffer it, survive it, perhaps even die of it as well."

Buchanan should know: he almost died at age eight when he contracted subacute bacterial endocarditis. The interior experience of endocarditis suggested it was like "clotted bacterial vegetation" burrowing through his heart, suffocating him from within, "as if the greasy, glossy green of the bacterial plant had rooted itself into his very soul and was now sending long shoots of tangled ivy twine throughout the rest of his body." Buchanan felt he was "dying from the inside out as this hungry, greedy plant blossomed forth to replace the child wherein it fed. The very thought of the monster filled him with a nauseous claustrophobia, and yet he had no choice but to submit passively to its will and therein to suffer."

But pay close attention to the life of your suffering, because there may be an important lesson here, says Arthur Frank. Frank, a Ph.D. medical sociologist, offers his reflections on the experience of being ill (heart attack compounded by cancer at age forty) in *At the Will of the Body*. Critical illness leaves no aspect of one's life untouched, says Frank. Illness takes one to the threshold of life and death and recovery is worth "only as much as you learn about the life you are recovering."

Even so there is no exemplary way to be ill, comments Frank. "To seize the opportunities offered by illness, we must live illness actively: we must think about it and talk about it. Only then can we learn it is nothing special. Being ill is just another way of living."

Frank thinks and writes well about illness, but his bittersweet reflections are entirely within the conceptual framework of allopathy. He's a passionate apologist for a Newtonian mechanical view of human life and health. His heart attack taught him "how little control" he has over his body, that he is a vulnerable creature. "Illness is not any kind of enlightenment. Illness is nothing more than the body moving on. I happened to get cancer. That's the strangeness of contingency: neither my body nor my mind knows why these things happened as they did."

Patients may be contingent victims of disease, argues Frank, but their active choice comes in how they experience illness, whether this total engulfment by the "great fish of illness" is in the end meaningful or a nightmare. With too much thinking about illness, however, we confront the danger of "romanticizing" disease, says Frank, turning this willful act of the body into "something it is not."

But as sociologist David Karp points out, illness can become a kind of career and an awareness that one suffers from clinical depression (a comfortable diagnostic parameter) can arise in an "extraordinarily patterned" way. In fact, it's possible to "analyze the depression experience as a 'career' sequence characterized by distinctive identity transformations."

We might make the equivalent mistake of turning disease into a metaphor. That was the position Susan Sontag took in her allopathically inspired essay *Illness as Metaphor*. Sontag's book, while criticizing the metaphorical appendages to illness, helped precipitate a new dialog about the meanings of illness. Sontag lucidly analyzed the degree to which tuberculosis and cancer had wrongly become "spectacularly encumbered by the trappings of metaphor." Illness is not a metaphor and must be demythicized, Sontag insisted. "The most truthful way of regarding illness—and the healthiest way of being ill—is one most purified of, most resistant to, metaphoric thinking."

Cancer carries the most radically negative disease metaphors, argued Sontag. Feelings about evil are easily projected onto a disease, making it adjectival. The popular mythology of cancer sees it as something "unqualifiedly and unredeemably wicked": it's the barbarian within, a shameful, demonic pregnancy, the destructive, putrefying result of emotional withdrawal, inhibition, and sexual repression. The meaning of cancer, said Sontag, is a moral judgment. "Nothing is more punitive than to give a disease a meaning—that meaning being invariably a moralistic one. Any disease whose causality is murky, and for which treatment is ineffectual, tends to be awash in significance."

Sontag's description matches *lupus erythematosus* perfectly. The biochemical causality isn't understood and prednisone, the standard treatment drug, doesn't always work, is addictive, and produces harmful side effects. But for a practicing psychotherapist like Donna Talman, who counseled clients every day in the need for inner examination and who was familiar with Sontag's antimetaphor strictures, disease without meaning was a far more punitive prospect than any mistakes in attributing significance she might make on the road to recovery.

For Talman, lupus compelled her to inquire within. "Knowing myself seemed important in understanding my illness. I read anything I could find that addressed the questions which had begun to obsess me. Was disease random and devoid of meaning? What was the relationship between my body and mind?" More to the point, had she chosen or caused lupus, had she somehow unconsciously incited the wolf to bite—and was the wolf part of herself? Was her illness a biography written in the biology of her body?

For Jungian analyst and psychosomatic consultant Alfred Ziegler, M.D., the answer is *yes,* as he explains in *Archetypal Medicine.* According to Ziegler, disease is the end result of a somatization process whereby psychic contents, images, and archetypes metamorphose into physical, pathological expression, employing biology as agents for their existential, heuristic purposes of mirroring the individual's idea of the self. "We can regard illness as the transformation of recessive [unconscious or suppressed] traits and tendencies into physical suffering," Ziegler comments.

These traits may be inconsistent or capricious, yet they have a tendency to take bodily form (to "somatize") "and to appear as identifiable diseases, as *morbus.*" Especially because we are normally unaware of these deeply submerged personality contents, they tend to take up residence in the body "where they stubbornly clamor for our attention as disease syndromes."

Illness is a fundamental aspect of human nature and highly adaptable to the specific needs or predispositions of the individual, says Ziegler. "Man is extremely resourceful in his search for the necessary disease; the causes he simply conjures up out of thin air." Every human environment is contaminated from the very beginning of existence, because it needs to be this way: "Our dispositions are capable of converting anything into disease noxae.

"Our dispositions lend the 'somatogenic' or 'psychogenic' factors their effectiveness." In other words, if we are predisposed—by fate, karma, destiny, genes, shadow contents, the *Moirae, Keres,* or our Ahrimanic Double—to express a soul content through the flesh, we will find the means (the probable cause) to make it happen in the body ("somatogenic") or mind ("psychogenic"). There is no real end to illness: it is cyclic, recurrent, continual: "We are all chronic patients who from time to time get better."

The role of the physician, says Ziegler, in developing a diagnosis is not a "seeing through, but a living through," a participation in the patient's "cult" of somaticizing recessive traits (shadow contents), transforming archetypes into bodily illnesses. More often than not, our understanding of illness is Epimethean: "Our psychosomatic understanding is oftentimes from hindsight," says Ziegler. To understand it as it happens, or, even better, before the "recessive trait" has transformed the body, to catch the edge of somaticization, is an initiation experience. Should the physician be sufficiently astute and intuitive, one can assist the illness novice in becoming a *physis* initiate.

Paradoxically, very few people seem to want complete health. "In its purest form, health is unbearable in the long run, for it carries too great a responsibility and too much freedom for us to take it upon ourselves unscathed for any length of time," observes Ziegler.

The Intimidation of Becoming Whole

The prospect of being whole and healthy is difficult, even frightening, to most people, contends Carolyn Myss, medical intuitive, counselor, and author of *The Creation of Health* (with C. Norman Shealy, M.D.). "I sometimes think people would rather be semi-healthy, which means with no pain, mobile, functioning, in a close relationship, that this is more important to them than complete health which is enormously intimidating." That's because for many illness is actually a socially validated way to be emotionally expressive, says Myss.

"We cover our emotional life with shame, then we cover our shame with dysfunction or disease that comes out as a language of wounds. We now have a language of intimacy which is a language of wounds. It's how two people know each other. The bridge between people is wound-sharing in a bond of trust, and the science of wounds is called psychology. People get more mileage out of being wounded. I can't do that because I was a battered child, people often say, then give up their power. We're so ashamed to be vulnerable and needy. Illness gives us the first stages of how to structure being emotional men and women without shame. It's the first stage of a new model of being human. Full health is the courage to honor our emotionality."

Full health is a state of emotional maturity we have to work our way up to, often through the intermediate state of illness, says Myss. In Myss' view, the onset of illness can be a positive indication that this process of personal evolution through emotional honesty is under way. But it's facile to categorically say all illness is self-generated. "The widespread principle that we create our illness doesn't equally apply to each person. It depends on the strength and structure of the psyche. We have the option today to make illness a teacher or a destructor. One person is aware he creates his reality and lives by these internal mechanisms. He sees illness as the inside world coming out. But another person less in communication with his inner being sees illness as the outside world coming towards him." Relatively speaking, both perceptions are correct depending on one's level of consciousness awareness.

Often it's the torturous schism between what we intellectually uphold and what we emotionally believe that precipitates an illness. Myss calls this gap our inconsistency. "Illness for some is an experience of recognizing their inconsistencies. The mind usually gets there a long time ahead of the emotions and maybe one's emotional interior doesn't match what her mind says. The juice through which you create your reality comes from the distance between what your head says and what your heart believes. The inconsistencies may be the fears a person won't look at, what they need to change but haven't the courage to face. For others it's a test of faith, a challenge to trust, to not come from negativity."

The starting point for Myss is the fact that illness is psychologically meaningful. But often the meaning can be skewed to the negative according to an outmoded belief in just retribution. Myss calls this belief "Earth justice," by which she means the old moralistic polarity of good and evil, reward and punishment. In this moralistically simplistic equation, health is a reward, illness is a punishment. These are archetypal constructs in our emotional life and hard to shake loose, especially when we think about illness, says Myss. It's the same condition Susan Sontag meant when she said we project evil onto disease to generate negative metaphors.

Many people, Myss claims, are addicted to basically harmful ideas, such as the attitude that there is a just cause for every action. You're ill *because* you ate apples as a child. If you know you're creating your reality, you *should* be immune, and if you're not, you're at fault. "Without finding this cause, they won't move forward. People paralyze their healing process this way. They want everything black and white, straightforward. They need some level of validation. People won't release their hurts, their victim mentality, their self-pity, until the guilty party validates their hurt. But if it's child incest, in which the guilty father is already dead, the woman-daughter can't get that validation and she can't move forward. Her emotional body clings to that experience and she can't rally her healing power."

This simplistic morality that we bring into our thinking about illness prevents us from understanding all the causes for illness, especially the deeper ones, comments Myss. The search for meaning and validation is justified, but we're looking for it in the wrong way, using the wrong model. While we seek meaning in the sense of retribution, payment, or redress, what may be at play instead in our lupus or cancer or childhood trauma is a profound educational opportunity, a spiritual opening created by the tension of the disease. The value of the questioning is that it brings us to the threshold of a new perception. "It's an introduction to Karma 101, but through the door of feeling that you're unjustly punished through an illness," explains Myss.

The quest for personal meaning in illness may introduce us to the rigors and complexities of karma, the theory of long-range effects. "The idea of looking for just validation behind illness is a crude way in which karma is making itself known to us, that a system of justice is working in all life systems and individual illness. The trouble is our awareness isn't wide enough to take in all the facts yet. We're not mature enough yet to see the karmic truth about our interpersonal relations, such as incest, and still be compassionate, and not react according to tribal vengeance, without thinking of reward and punishment."

People who seek meaning in their illness are really asking for a karmic profile, comments Myss—and what if the daughter did the same to her incestuous father in an earlier life? Could she live with that revelation? "The more you pursue it, the more the origins of an illness will reveal themselves. Illness comes to us through our personal mysteries, through our unique karmic history."

We mustn't overlook the fact that our unique karmic history is played out in the social environment, too. That outer world throughout the 1990s was staggeringly unstable. "There's absolutely nothing that signals stability anymore, that makes us feel safe and secure," says Myss. Families, marriages, relationships, careers, economies, national boundaries, even governments, break up and reconfigure as rapidly as clouds. Nature has grown more unpredictably destructive, even indifferent, to human life. Everything in our personal and business life seems to pose a chronic threat.

"We've never been this vulnerable," says Myss. "Our immune system naturally doesn't feel safe either. Immune diseases reflect a feeling nothing is safe or stable anymore. The etiology is human evolution itself. We're not maturing fast enough in awareness to handle the massive physical power we've unlocked in the nuclear age. We've catapulted ourselves into a fast forward to grow into the maturity we need to handle the powers of destruction. We have to get stable inside because we can no longer count on it outside."

Searching for Illness' Final Destiny

Our society has largely turned its back on any philosophy of illness and the teleology of disease is still a foreign idea, says Peter V. Madill, a philosophical M.D. specializing in complex chronic illness in Sebastopol, California. Teleology is an important word for understanding the meaning of illness. It's about final causes, the view that developments are due to a long-range purpose and design and that symptoms and illnesses arise to fulfill that innately spiritual design. Whose design is it? Our greater being, says Madill.

"Illness animates our entire life. Our greater being uses illness to animate these great tensions in our life. It's one of the most potent ways, and often a very destructive way, to break down a person's rigid belief system, to get someone to question their core beliefs of self, their role in life, their religious choices, the impact of the choices of their early conditioning. Identity gets chewed up in illness. It shatters people's security. Illness is a powerful demand for major karmic change. Our society has turned its back on an embracing view of life that gives illness meaning but without blame and guilt. Illness isn't really healed until people discover its meaning and life purpose, until they see its role in their soul journey."

The Swiss *depth* psychologist Carl Jung once expressed the protocols of this delicate communication from inner self to outer persona succinctly. Jung said, "That which we do not bring to consciousness appears in our lives as fate." Madill agrees, and points to the disease process as the most cogent, fateful example. "The greater Self kicks a man with an accident, an illness, even death. These are tools the Self uses if the person isn't responding to the symbols, messages, and symptoms coming from within."

The ancient Western mystery tradition used illness as a tool of initiation, part of what was called "temple medicine"; the old initiates knew that illness is not only a teacher but an individual student's specific teacher. Paracelsus, the great Swiss alchemist, philosopher, and occultist (1493-1541), contended that illness is potentially creative for the patient, as contemporary British homeopath Ralph Twentyman explains: "If healing really comes about, then the patient will have taken a step forward in his psychospiritual development. He will not merely have recovered his static balance, but will have experienced a dynamic metamorphosis of his whole being. His healing will be at least to some extent a new birth, not just a being rid of a discomfort and inconvenience or avoiding of death."

The processes of disease and healing inherently belong to us, says Twentyman. "By constantly falling ill and constantly unfolding a healing activity within ourselves we can take definite steps forward in our development." When we do this we can truly say, as astonishing as it may seem, that we are "blessed" by our illness, adds Dutch physician L.F.C. Mees. "Illness, in spite of the paradox, blesses humanity by making possible his evolution. Even by doing away with the symptoms, we should develop the 'attitude' not of fighting but of taking over the task of the illness."

As participants in the disease process, we facilitate our healing by *taking up the task*—engaging actively in the process—of the illness, by transforming a presumed passive victimization role into a dynamic tool for self-understanding and psychospiritual unfolding, Mees suggests. "Illness is not senseless any longer but becomes a link in man's evolution. Man creates predispositions; illness blesses him by continually taking away the predispositions." Thus illnesses can teach us what needs to be done in consciousness. It is both a consequence of deviations of the "soul-spiritual" life and a forceful aid in personal development.

Illness can never be understood in isolation from the totality of the human, contends Otto Wolff, M.D., one of Europe's leading exponents of anthroposophically extended medicine and the editor of the encyclopedic multivolume *Anthroposophical Approach to Medicine: An Outline of a Spiritual Scientifically Oriented Medicine.* "In a higher sense, every illness is a stage of development for the human being. He must be able to become sick to realize his being. It has the purpose of leading man to himself, enabling him to attain his true manhood."

Healing, says Wolff, is the restitution of the "divine archetype of man"; illness is the path leading to this. "Healing is bringing oneself into harmony with the divine creative force, and one who does not nurture spiritual life is bound eventually to become ill." The transformative process of healing is possible only with the conscious participation of the patient, Wolff stresses.

So when Peter Madill talks about illness in terms of "tools of the Self," he's implying the deep tradition of temple medicine. "In our lifetime I predict it will be conclusively shown that psychological factors will be the most important factors in how we live with illness. With complex immune system illnesses like chronic fatigue syndrome and environmental illness, I've not seen anyone get well without a profound psychological change and without a major revisiting of early life experiences."

That early-life revisiting can be psychologically harrowing, says Madill. He worked with a woman who had an intractable, virtually immedicable condition of environmental illness. She was so acutely sensitive that the minutest trace amounts of volatile chemicals produced bizarre symptoms, even made her unconscious. She had tried all the therapies, had refitted her house, restricted her lifestyle, but she was still unrelievedly reactive. Then she developed uterine bleeding and went into the hospital for surgery. When she received the preanesthesia medication for surgery, the whole EI complex finally unraveled before her.

She went into seizures, but for the first time she gained access to herself as a fourteen-year-old girl, says Madill. She suddenly remembered that her early adolescence was marked by incessant incest. "The incest was such an insult to her body that it locked up all memory of it. Somehow the light preanesthesia worked as a truth serum. When she accessed her repressed memory of this trauma, her sensitivities to the chemicals decreased and she gained a new range of freedom in her lifestyle." The meaning here is that severe trauma persisted physiologically as EI.

With all of his EI patients Madill finds that when they remember their childhood, invariably it was a difficult time of abuse, abandonment, or sexual damage. "As children they never developed a healthy sense of boundaries, a basic trust and knowing that ordinary chemicals might be safe. As a person's boundaries are insulted on the emotional level, the body's physical ability to establish boundaries is depleted." The rest is predictable, says Madill.

The stress leads to hyperventilation, carbon dioxide depletion, a reduction in immunological first-line defense, blood pH imbalance, and a dangerous depletion of minerals and metals necessary for detoxification. With this biochemical systemic collapse and the failure to maintain immunological boundaries, the environment becomes inimical, and EI moves in.

On the Processing Edge with the Dreambody

Maybe immunological failure isn't a disaster of life. Maybe it means we need to be more open, less defended, less bounded. Immunity may be an existential mistake. That's the highly unconventional but provocative view of neo-Jungian therapist Arnold Mindell, Ph.D. Mindell is the innovator of process-oriented therapy, whose principles and case studies he's explained in numerous well-received books.

"Western culture has trouble with the immune system because people have tried to be immune from one another, have tried to stay as individuals," says Mindell. "People aren't open to picking up from other people, to acknowledging that we are not separate. Now we're learning we're not immune, that we're strongly influenced by the world around us. Our immune systems wouldn't have had to do this for us if we could have been more open in the first place."

In Mindell's radical process-oriented model, the increasing prevalence of illness is a revelation of the unconscious through biology. Mindell interprets this unreservedly as a positive sign in the evolution of human consciousness. "Our process orientation understands symptoms; we don't pathologize them. All body experiences in our view are a sign of health, including illness. Body experiences and dreaming are closely related. Symptoms are a statement of dreaming trying to become conscious. Symptoms are dreams happening in the body. Illness is connected with our dreaming process and represents a growing in consciousness, which is health.

There's always some kind of unconscious growth process trying to happen. The more powerful the symptoms, like AIDS or cancer, the more powerful the dreaming process. The fact that Western culture has so many different illnesses today means more people are waking up. The whole culture is waking up during this time of transition and rapid growth in the psyche. There's more dreaming, more potential trying to become available to us. So there's more illness."

According to Mindell, our larger potential communicates to us through dreams. When we continually ignore these vivifying messages, they come back through the body as symptoms and illness. There is a direct continuum from psychological dreaming to physical symptomatology, says Mindell, whose therapy encourages the physical symptoms to speak their symbolic meaning. He calls this holistic context for health and disease the dreambody.

It's the dreambody that holds the revelation of the meaning of illness, Mindell notes. "The meaning of illness is discoverable on an individual basis. It's very possible, as we've seen in thousands of cases. It's a core part, but part of the core process is experiencing the significance of the *energy* behind the symptoms. This energy can be used for other things besides creating symptoms. So we get people in touch with meaning and the energy of their dreambody symptoms."

Mindell cites a recent case in point. A woman had been a minority social activist all her life. Whenever she had to speak in public, her asthma came up so strongly as to almost choke out her voice. Mindell asked her how she would create the asthma symptoms in him. She squeezed his wrists, giving him that same cramping feeling she had in her chest. Mindell realized this was the creative energy behind her asthma. Can you use this same squeezing energy in movement, he next asked her. She stamped her feet, then sang, then suddenly spoke spontaneously in a different, passionate voice. Her asthmatic symptoms disappeared.

"The energy behind her asthma is *passion*," Mindell announced. "You need to connect the meaning with the energy behind the body symptoms. It's an energy that's trying to do many things."

Why does dreaming typically come out as symptoms and not as insight? It's because of our edge, explains Amy Mindell, copractitioner of process-oriented therapy. "Edges are boundaries between our identity, our primary process of consciousness, what's close to our normal awareness, and what's secondary, or unconscious, but trying to come into awareness. The unconscious is anything in any moment that's trying to come into our awareness. It's a body signal arising in that moment wanting integration. New information challenges this in an intense moment of confrontation at the edge. It becomes a question of how much our identity can incorporate that challenging information."

Confrontations at the edge can be exciting or scary, says Mindell. The edge is our rules, our limits, our belief systems, the restrictions of our primary process. "Our creative potential comes up against this edge, this barrier, which deflects it. The edge keeps it out, like a pariah. So it comes up again in different form in dreams, body signals, spontaneous movements, symptoms, illness." The edge is the limit of our identity, the edge of the cliff of our being.

Mindell worked with a woman who felt she had a witch inside her. Mindell asked her to dramatize this witch through her body. She made claws with her hands and a frightful face. Then Mindell asked her what those claw-like hands wanted to do. "This brought her right to her own edge. She moved her hands, grabbed with them, then danced, played, and giggled. She just wanted to feel like a playful child, a side of her she'd never given enough attention to. This information transformed her and she went right past her edge. There was no witch anymore. Her cliff edge disappeared."

In other words, when the dreambody's symbolic communication is comprehended, symptoms and illness assume their inherent meaning.

"The germ is nothing, the terrain is everything"

The illness process needs agents, biological factotums to transform dreambody messages, or what Ziegler called "recessive traits," into bodily diseases. "Man is extremely resourceful in his search for the necessary disease; the causes he simply conjures up out of thin air," said Ziegler, as quoted earlier. Our dispositions—call them genes, shadow contents, dreambody reality, the Self—"lend the 'somatogenic' or 'psychogenic' factors their effectiveness."

What are these factors? By way of answering this, I'd like to return to our discussion of the "myth" of Pandora's box and the issuing Spites (*Keres, Moirae,* or Steiner's Ahrimanic Double) who spread disease, contagion, and bodily misfortune throughout the world. Surely it is not a stretch to regard the *Keres* as a pre-scientific description for what modern science has identified as the multifaceted microbiological kingdom, the presumed agents of myriad diseases—the world of "germs." In the age of AIDS, Ebola hemorrhagic fever, resurgent tuberculosis, and other communicable, infectious diseases, it is small wonder, comments Wayne Biddle in *A Field Guide to Germs,* "that a certain edginess about contagion has crept into daily encounters of all kinds."

In Western allopathic medicine, the germ theory reigns supreme: every infectious illness is mediated by a germ, whether it be bacteria *(Salmonella, Myobacterium tuberculosis, Bordetella pertussis),* fungi *(Candida albicans, Pneumocystis carinii),* protozoa *(Cryptosporidium, Plasmodium),* or the mysterious virus (Coxsackie, Epstein-Barr, swine flu, rhinovirus). We are all exposed, all the time, Biddle says, and it's only the strength of our immune defenses that wards off infection.

The mutability of germs, says Biddle, is astonishing as new, even mutated, generations can mature in minutes. The overuse of antibiotics since 1945 by allopathic physicians has been a "terrible blunder," Biddle adds, because it has compelled the microbial world to adapt in response to killer drugs, thereby creating "microbial freaks that assume unnatural dominance."

Associating germs with illness may be our sole and customary way of regarding microbes, the myriad invisible creatures that co-inhabit our body and planet, but producing disease is only a small aspect of their life activity. They live in the soil, our intestines, the air, on our skin, in our hair and mouths; in fact, microbes make up about 90% of all living material on Earth, where they are responsible for nearly all the chemical changes that occur within all living environments, including all the processes of food digestion and nutrient assimilation.

"In this sense they are of transcendental importance in the terrestrial economy," explains microbiologist John Postgate, "because without them higher organisms would rapidly cease to exist."

Current research indicates that microbes inhabited the planet as early as 3,465 million years ago; like it or not, our physical world, and body, are possible because of the activities of myriad microbes. A bacterium may weigh only 0.000000000001 gram, yet it can kill a blue whale weighing 100 million grams. "In sum, their manifold influences in shaping our history and that of the planet, and in sustaining the world and promoting the quality of life can scarcely be overestimated," comments Bernard Dixon in *Power Unseen*. They colonize and alter the face of the planet and possess an adaptability far superior to anything human beings have—microbes "rule the world," Dixon concludes.

Microbes are not inherently good or bad, prohuman or antihuman, says Postgate; they can be either, depending on circumstances. "Microbes seem to have a faintly alarming or disgusting aura, and the fact that by far the majority are nugatory or even beneficial is rarely understood." When it comes to the human body, there are an estimated thousand billion bacteria spread over 400 species resident, all necessary for our physical well-being. These bacteria all perform functions necessary for the continuance of human life in the body, for which reason, bacteriologists and a growing number of physicians who understand alternative medicine, call them probiotics, or "friendly" bacteria.

The excessive use of antibiotics, understandably, spells their slow destruction. In the human gastrointestinal tract alone there are an estimated 3.5 pounds of probiotics. The colonization of the body by friendly bacteria begins at birth, through consumed foods, such that the probiotic *Bifidobacterium infantis* is present in about 60% of babies born vaginally (by normal means), but in only 9% of babies born by Caesarean section. In other words, not only can antibiotics impede the useful floriation of probiotics, but so can modern birthing practices (plus faulty diet and chronic stress).

In earlier chapters, we reviewed examples of placebo response, PNI, spontaneous remission, and multiple personality disorder, and saw how these indicate a significant, underexploited mutability of the mind-body orchestrated most frequently by unconscious intention. The inevitable inference of this unilateral plasticity of biology, even identity, is that perhaps it represents blooms of a fundamental molecular mutability, a polymorphous and form-changing natural potential.

The question itself instantly highlights a longstanding dialectic in bacteriology and immunology between advocates of monomorphism and pleomorphism over whether bacteria remain always the same or can change shape and nature. An even more intriguing question is this: what is the force or influence that makes microbes change, or be pleomorphic? I'll address this later in the chapter.

The monomorphic school, founded principally on the work of Louis Pasteur (1822-1895), contends that bacterial genera and species are few in number, fixed and unchanging in form and identity—hence *mono* ("one") *morph* ("form"). The pleomorphic school—as in *pleo* ("multiple") *morph* ("forms")—based on the work of Pasteur's contemporary, Antoine Béchamp (1816-1908), argues that bacterial species are numerous, unstable, change form, and have in fact many forms. It's a debate waged at the heart of medicine: do germs cause disease (Pasteur) or does disease cause germs (Béchamp)?

The answer is crucial to the philosophy and practice of therapeutics. In fact, it is one of the most important questions in medicine because how you answer this question directly determines whether consciousness is accorded any efficacy in the human organism.

Contemporary allopathy would have us believe the dialectic was settled long ago with the ascendancy of Pasteur's germ theory of infection and the overthrow of Béchamp's naive pleomorphism, but that's not so. The debate, despite intense, unilateral allopathic suppression, is far from concluded, and the pleomorphic view is once again resurging. As medical historian Harris Coulter positions the dialectic, the monomorphists are the rationalists, "the left-brain bureaucrats who subordinate the data of sense perception to *a priori* theories and *a priori* categories." Monomorphism simplifies the bacteriological realities, thereby making treatment simple and uniform, benefiting the physicians.

The pleomorphists are the empirics, the right-brained thinkers, "always aware of the inherent heterogeneity and diversity of the observed phenomena" and disinterested in rigid, reductionist, classificatory schemes. The empiric pleomorphists usefully complicate bacteriological realities to benefit the patient, making therapeutics more responsive to the particularities of the individual case, says Coulter. "Hence the medical profession as an organized body manifests an instinctive preference for monomorphism, even though individual members may recognize it as nonsense."

The story of Béchamp's pleomorphism represents what Ethyl Douglas Hume, author of *Béchamp or Pasteur?*, calls "a lost chapter in the history of biology." Beginning in 1866, Béchamp, a medical doctor, chemist, pharmacist, university professor, and textbook author, proposed that the smallest units of living matter were microorganisms he called "microzymas," from the Greek, meaning "small ferments." He wasn't the first to propose minute cytological antecedents as "the fundamental unit of the corporate organism"; earlier ad hoc pleomorphists had variously termed them "cell granules," "granulations of the protoplasm," "molecular granulations," and "scintillating corpuscles," but they lacked the improvements in microscopy available to Béchamp.

According to Béchamp, the blood is actually a flowing tissue, not a liquid. The blood cells are mingled with a huge mass of invisible microzymas, which are each surrounded by a membrane of albumin. These are the "molecular microzymian granulations," a basic element of blood. The microzyma is the fundamental element of bodily life; it sustains health, but it can also precipitate illness. What we take to be "disease germs" from the outer environment are in fact, Béchamp argued, microzymas at a later stage in their bacterial evolution but originating from sick human bodies. In effect, Béchamp suggests that all illness is human generated.

All living organisms arise from and are reducible to microzymas, Béchamp contended—including bacteria, which represent fully grown, evolved microzymas. These "molecular granulations" of cells are the formative agents of all cells composing animal and vegetable forms, said Béchamp. Virulent, pathogenic bacteria arise from decaying matter, whose decomposition they aid; then they revert to the microzyma stage again. What pathologists identify as disease germs are in fact diseased microzymas or their evolutionary bacterial forms, said Béchamp.

Depending on the conditions of the body, the microzymas either continue on in "the even tenor of their way," which sustains the health of the organism, or, when the internal environment changes, they "develop morbidly, producing bad fermentative effects and other bodily calamities," as Ethyl Hume explains it. Further, he says, "In a diseased body a change of function in the microzymas may lead to a morbid bacterial evolution."

The microzymas "build up [a person's] bodily frame, preserve it in health, disrupt it in disease," Hume explains, and at death, which marks the end of this "corporate association," the microzymas demolish their former residence, "themselves being set free to continue an independent existence in the earth, the air, or water." To Henry Lindlahr, M.D., one of the founders of twentieth-century naturopathy, Béchamp's theory of the "infinitesimal, minute living organisms" that are as small with respect to cells as electrons are to atoms, gave much rational and scientific validity to what advocates of nature cure had been claiming.

When the internal "soil" is healthy, then microzymas develop into "normal, permanent, specialized cells of the human organism," Lindlahr wrote in 1918 in his *Philosophy of Natural Therapeutics*. "The same microzymas, feeding on morbid materials and systemic poisons in these living bodies develop into bacteria and parasites." In contrast, Pasteur had maintained that healthy tissue is bacteriologically sterile (or ought to be).

However, the function of microzymas is to either build or disintegrate tissue, depending on conditions; if the tissue is healthy, the microzymas support the integrity of life, aiding the anabolic processes; but if the tissue is unhealthy or damaged, the microzymas may evolve into pathogenic, catabolic bacteria and begin decomposing it. By extension, Béchamp argued that microzymas, resident in an individual, could develop into pathogenic organisms—change form, assume more forms, become pleomorphic—in a manner similar to the transformation of tadpole to frog or chrysalis to butterfly, given suitable environmental conditions, namely, the character of the cellular fluids, the vitality of the "soil" of the host organism.

According to Béchamp, the catalyst for the evolutionary shift from microzymas to pathogenic bacteria is the presence of dead, damaged, or unhealthy cells. In other words, bacteria are not form-fixed, or monomorphic, but pleomorphic, and "*reflect* the conditions in which they find themselves rather than create those conditions," explains Walene James in *Immunization: The Reality behind the Myth,* who cogently summarizes Béchamp's views.

In effect, through his numerous experiments, Béchamp showed that the individual pathogenic germ associated as a causal agent in disease is not that but rather its product. He further indicated that what microbiologists had been assuming to be distinctly differentiated species of bacteria were in fact different stages of a microzymian evolution as it assumed bacterial form. Implicit in Béchamp's proposal was the assertion that most disease originates within the human body and is not the result of a pathogenic invasion from the external environment. Microzymas can create illness (by, in effect, transforming into pathogenic bacteria) only in unhealthy terrain, a degenerated internal cellular environment marked by acidity and low oxygenation.

As French physiologist and Béchamp's contemporary Claude Bernard remarked, "The germ is nothing, the terrain is everything."

In this view it is more correct to say there are specific disease conditions rather than specific diseases. Pleomorphism received another endorsement from an iconoclastic European scientist around the same time—Rudolf Steiner. The presence of parasites and bacterial accumulation in a patient indicates that deeper causes are at work, permitting them to remain in place, Steiner explained in 1921.

"Bacilli are never really the cause of illness; they only indicate that the patient has the causes of illness within him." Bacteriological research is important, but only as a foundation for research, Steiner added, because the "actual organic causes lie in the human being himself."

A Manifesto for a New Bacteriology

The history of pleomorphism and its historical dialectic with monomorphism is a long, complex narrative already capably handled by Harris Coulter, so we'll only touch on a few key figures and their observations. Günther Enderlein (1872-1968), a German zoologist and bacteriologist, elaborated his discoveries and pleomorphic principles for more than sixty years of his professional life, devising a program of biological treatments still in use in Europe and, in limited fashion, the United States. In 1925, he set forth his views on pleomorphism in *Bakterien Cyclogenie* ("The Life Cycle of Bacteria").

According to Enderlein, the blood of the healthy human body is filled with "protits" or "centrosomes." These are archaic, nonharmful, nonmoving, plantlike protein life forms that reside in the red and white blood cells, plasma, and other bodily fluids. Seen through a dark-field microscope (which views living blood), protits appear as a pinhead-sized globe or tiny shining point. They live in cooperative harmony, symbiosis, and communication with their host organism as *endobionts.* According to Enderlein, the endobiont, meaning "internal life" (from *endon,* "internal"; *bios,* "life"), is born with the human being, incorporated during the placental stage of life; it comprises two parasitic microbes: the tubercle bacillus and a fungus called *Mucor Racemosus Fresen.*

The fungal parasite unfolds all developmental stages of its life within the human organism, Enderlein postulated; its lower stages (called protitit, protit, and chondrit) are apathogenic, but the higher forms can produce tuberculosis (tubercle bacillus) and carcinomas *(M. R. Fresen).* As the endobionts begin shape shifting and differentiating, "they appear in unimaginable numbers of diverse forms," says Dr. Maria M. Bleker, an Enderlein scholar and curator. "Here we have the progenitors of the masses of bacteria and bacilli which we develop in ourselves, according to Enderlein."

This cycle of development from simple protein lumps to the fungal stage "with its enormous productivity of primitive forms" Enderlein called the cyclogeny. As Dr. Bleker explains, it is our modern civilization—its artificial fertilizers, pollution, preservatives, chemicals, and "false nutrition" of high protein and sugar—that provokes the pleomorphism of the endobionts. Long-term "antibiological nutrition" and its acidification of the blood produces this "endless proliferation" of the endobiont, says Dr. Bleker. "Basically, there is not a multitude of diseases, but only one constitutional disease, namely the constant overacidification of the blood, which disturbs the central regulation of the body, disorienting it," Enderlein wrote.

Disease develops when the pH, or cellular terrain, becomes imbalanced and the indwelling parasites start growing into their more advanced forms. Thus, when the symbiotic equilibrium is disrupted or destroyed—specifically when the pH of the cells gets either too acidic or alkaline due to "counter-biological" diet and lifestyle—they lose their symbiotic nature and start evolving into disease-producing *endobionts*. Factors that can precipitate this move into imbalance include environmental influences, contact with carcinogenic substances, and dietary excesses, Enderlein explained.

When the cellular milieu—the overall biochemical condition of the individual cells—shifts into imbalance, the protits follow suit, said Enderlein. The protits change shape and nature, and become "blood-symbionts," capable of aggressive, hostile behavior toward their host. In effect, reclassified as harmful parasites, these blood-symbionts start producing internal disturbances, which we experience as the symptoms of illness.

Enderlein used the term "endobiont" to indicate the protits' entire sequence of developmental changes—the pleomorphic repertory. An endobiont could have, literally, thousands of different forms. In fact, the endobiont's protean shape-shifting ability led Enderlein to describe them as "a multi-headed hydra."

Like Béchamp, Enderlein proposed a model of bacterial evolution—he called it an "endobiosis complex"—in which, given the suitable conditions (e.g., overconsumption of animal proteins and fats, exposure to carcinogenic materials, excessive substance abuse, environmental toxins), the friendly symbiont evolves precipitously through a virus-bacillus-fungus cycle to become pathogenic, generating a variety of chronic diseases.

According to Enderlein, an "endobiont-induced disease complex," which contributes to the slow degeneration of body cells and tissues, underlies nearly all chronic illnesses, including arthritis, heart disease, diabetes, multiple sclerosis, leukemia, and many more. "That all these numerous diseases are attributable to a single parasite is due solely to the fact that its unusually varied number of different developmental stages are capable of affecting a large number of tissues and organs of the human body," Enderlein said.

For this reason, Enderlein argued that there is only one constitutional illness, namely, the overacidity of the blood; this disturbs the functional balance of all bodily systems and eventually assumes any of a multiplicity of symptoms or disease states.

Examining a Global Bacterial Entity

Technological improvements in fine-resolution microscopy took pleomorphism a step further with the work of Dr. Royal Raymond Rife (1888-1971), an American scientist working in San Diego, California, in the early decades of the twentieth century. Rife developed a superb high-resolution microscope that enabled him to study living specimens rather than dried artifacts in blood, which had been the convention up until his instrumentation breakthrough.

During the 1920s, working at his Rife Research Laboratory in Point Loma, California, Rife produced five different microscopes (comprising fourteen lenses and prisms, a quartz crystal illumination unit—5,682 working parts in all) with magnification capability ranging from 5,000 to 60,000 diameters and a resolution of 31,000 diameters; we must bear in mind that in Rife's time, the best resolution available through any other microscopic system was only 2,000 diameters, so his "Rife Universal Microscope" was an outstanding achievement. Even today's electron microscopes, which have resolutions of about 25,000 diameters and magnifications up to 200,000, cannot work with live specimens. Working with resolutions of 17,000 diameters, Rife was able to study a submicroscopic layer of biology that had never before been visible, including 20,000 lab cultures of living cancer cells obtained from a nearby hospital.

Rife's meticulous observations (preserved in thousands of microphotographs) indicated that bacteria could change into completely different forms through only slight alterations in environment (about two parts per million in cellular composition). Rife's microscopy yielded a highly practical result, too. He discovered that pathogenic bacteria could be devitalized through beaming specific light frequencies at them, which Rife called the "Mortal Oscillatory Rate." First in theory, then in practice, Rife had identified a foolproof cure for cancer, "the cancer cure that worked," says Rife's biographer, Barry Lynes. The Rife Universal Microscope is a "sensational new instrument," declared *Science* in December 1931. "Is a new field about to be opened in the science of bacteriology?" queried the editors of *California and Western Medicine*.

Rife's life specimen microscopy furnished him with copious clinical data arguing for the pleomorphic view of bacteriology. It seemed obvious to him that pathogenic germs are aspects of the disease *process* but not their sole instigators. Health and illness, Rife postulated, depend on the evolutionary status of the "oval, motile, turquoise blue bodies"—probably Béchamp's microzymas and Enderlein's protits—revealed through high-resolution life specimen viewing.

"In reality it is not the bacteria themselves that produce the disease, but we believe it is the chemical constituents of these microorganisms enacting upon the unbalanced cell metabolism of the human body that in actuality produce the disease," said Rife. "We also believe if the metabolism of the human body is perfectly balanced or poised, it is susceptible to no disease."

In 1931, Rife used his Prismatic Microscope to study 20,000 cancerous tissue samples. He claimed that in every instance he observed a "violet-red motile form," which he labeled the BX virus. Subsequent research indicated that this BX virus normally lay dormant and incubatory in a healthy human, but upon a weakening of the physiological state, it would become active and virile. Where there is a cancer tumor in the body, you will also find an active BX viral colony, Rife said.

During the 1930s, Rife perfected his mortal oscillatory rates for cancer and apparently was successful in obtaining remissions in tumors. He focused direct current, short-term electrical spikes through a gas-filled discharge tube (similar to an x-ray cathode) at the infected site on the body. He could adjust the frequency of the discharge to the type of pathogen he was seeking to devitalize. Rife found that his "armament of light"—electric rays, in effect—was capable of completely destroying the BX virus within seconds.

Unfortunately the Rife story had a rotten ending. As Barry Lynes recounts it, the AMA tried to buy into the developmental and distribution rights to Rife's microscope and was refused; then, with hardly a pause, the AMA mounted a nasty suppressive campaign that eventually brought Rife to court with charges of illegal practice of medicine. Rife's prodigious files of microphotographs disappeared, his microscopes were broken, lost, dismantled, or hidden, and he died in obscurity, and if it hadn't been for two key articles (one in 1944, then another in 1976), *nobody* today would have heard of Rife—as opposed to only a few.

Rife's work unequivocally demonstrated the reality of pleomorphism, says Lynes, an advance in medical knowledge that should have won him professional accolades. "This demonstration did more to bring down upon him the wrath of the worst kind of politics of science than any other facet of his work. It violated the strongest of established biological dogmas, that of the germ theory of disease."

It was probably because they were academic scientists and not practicing physicians that University of Montreal bacteriologists Sorin Sonea and Maurice Panisset were not given Rife-style allopathic pillorying when in 1980 they published "a kind of manifesto for a new bacteriology." Their brief book, *A New Bacteriology*, was, in their own estimation, a "radical restructuring" of important aspects of biology, and it garnered some professional favor, being hailed by Boston University bacteriologist Lynn Margulis (an important colleague of James Lovelock) as "an original and profound statement about nature and us."

Sonea and Panisset reject the classificatory convention of separate, isolated bacterial genera and propose that there is a single, dispersed, intracommunicating planetary bacterial superorganism that shares genes; further, they argue that "all bacteria on Earth constitute an essential, actively constructive factor in the biosphere" fundamentally friendly to human life.

Though bacteria, as prokaryotes (cells whose nucleus is unbounded by a membrane, in contrast with eukaryotes whose nucleus is bounded), tend to be genetically incomplete, through a planetary system of gene exchange, they are always able to respond quickly and efficiently to new environmental pressures, even develop resistance to new antibiotics like penicillin, if required. Through this network of genetic transmission and "biological communications network," the "innumerable bacterial strains in nature" are continuously linked.

The global bacterial entity represents an enormous database of bacterial genes, explain Sonea and Panisset, comprising a global genome from which all individual strains may borrow genetically as needed. "The binding force among bacteria is one of constant exchange and permanent choice of information bits, principally genes." It's the possibility of constant gene exchange and a shared total genome, not only at times of reproduction, that actually keeps the bacterial superorganism united; in fact, its stability in large measure is tantamount to planetary biospheric homeostasis. "In this planet-wide association of all living entities, bacteria provide most of the facilities for association, cooperation, and stability, and we should no longer underestimate their role."

The key to a rational estimation of their role depends on how we frame the problem in the first place. Consider the public discussion of the possible (predicted) resurgence of an influenza-flu pandemic as reported by Robin Marantz Henig in the *New York Times Magazine*. The author's tacit medical assumptions themselves, on behalf of allopathic consensual understanding, are the subtext of the article. The influenza virus is "fickle," characterized by fast, random mutations, such that a mere twelve to fifteen weeks are required by the virus to significantly alter its genetic composition.

This is the virus' "terrific trick"—"influenza, long thought to be the most dramatic example of random mutation in all of virology"—enabling it to outstep the scientist's attempts to develop successful vaccines and to "rage through a human population."

As if to seek reassurance through a repetition of common assumptions and possibly to denature the influenza virus, Henig uses the word *random*—qualifying it on occasion with *bizarre* and *unpredictably*—repeatedly. But are its rapid mutations *random*? Surely not if the hypotheses and laboratory demonstrations of 150 years of pleomorphic thinking are valid or if Sonea and Panisset are correct in postulating a global bacterial entity. If anything, the seemingly bizarre, unpredictable, fickle, and swift mutations of the influenza virus will emerge as purposeful, directed, and highly rational, once we reframe the dynamics of bacteriology according to pleomorphic indications.

Aware of the tortuous dialectic between the empiric advocates of pleomorphism and the rationalist proponents of "fixism," or monomorphism—"the intransigence and verbal violence displayed by the various factions in this conflict"—Sonea and Panisset note that it took the notable late-twentieth-century advances in bacterial genetics to make a more convincing case in favor of "more form" (pleomorphic) bacteriology. The proliferation of Linnean categories of bacterial species has been erroneous, the result of "an overly exclusive reductionism" and the "long reign of fixism" that has dominated molecular biology. "Conclusive new facts were required in order to question and overcome the scientific anathema surrounding any theory that even indirectly evoked pleomorphism."

Not only may microbial entities change shape and evolve upward from apathogenic to pathogenic forms, they may do this *very* quickly. The theory is called punctuated equilibrium and was first proposed in 1972 by two paleontologists, and ignored. However, scientists studying 3,000 generations of *Escherichia coli,* a simple bacteria that produces six generations in twenty-four hours, found that it undergoes rapid bursts of change, growth in cell size, and species evolution followed by long periods of stasis, something like 1,000 to 1,700 generations. In response to changes in their environment, the bacteria make all the survival-required genetic mutations as fast as possible, then settle back into a static existence.

This new model of bacteriology may help explain the comparative uproar of change and seeming pathogenicity now under way around us in the microbial kingdom in the form of resurgent old infections and multiple-drug-resistant bacteria.

Somatids—Form-Changing Energy Condensers at the Heart of Life

Scientific anathema can come down hard on pleomorphic heretics, as the recent experience of Quebec scientist Gaston Naessens indicates. The Quebec Medical Corporation took Naessens to court three times from 1985 to 1990 over what turned out to be spurious charges of improper, illegal medical practice and unsubstantiated therapies. The Quebec Medical Corporation dished out the standard AMA-style tactics of discreditation, suppression, name-calling (charlatan, fraud, and quack), and distortion, compounded by glaring ignorance of Naessen's scientific protocols, disregard for the testimony of his patients, and a general paradigmatic arrogance in the face of original work.

"Gaston Naessens' trip to hell was a direct consequence of his having dared to wander into scientific terra incognita," says Christopher Bird, who observed the trials as a journalist. Naessens was acquitted and if anything emerged from the prolonged ordeal with an enhanced international reputation; it also helped matters that the intellectually peripatetic Christopher Bird published a usefully inflammatory account of Naessens' "persecution and trial" in 1991 and that the American Association of Naturopathic Physicians presented him as a featured speaker at their 1992 convention.

In many respects it's the story of Béchamp, Enderlein, and Rife all over again, the self-educated scientist making brilliant, heretical discoveries in relative isolation, then getting ambushed by the medical heavies. Like his predecessors in pleomorphism, Naessens invented a microscope, created an anticancer medicine, and generated a theoretical model to explain it all. As Rife did, Naessens (who was born in 1924) invented a live specimen supermicroscope, which he calls the somatoscope, with magnifications from 4,000 to 30,000 and resolution of 150 angstroms, far in advance of conventional microscopes, excepting the electron microscope (which cannot work with live specimens).

Naessens' somatoscope enables him to witness the activities and transformations of the *somatid* ("tiny body"), the minuscule, precellular basis of biological life, probably the same as Béchamp's microzymas and Enderlein's protits. Somatids are indestructible, fundamentally electrical in nature—tiny, living energy condensers. Using his somatoscope, Naessens observed this "extremely tenuous, elementary particle endowed with a movement of electronegative repulsion" in all biological liquids, but particularly the blood.

"The somatids, one can say, are *precursors* of DNA," Naessens theorizes. He means by this that the somatids act as a "missing link" between the nonliving and the living; the somatid, unlike the virus, which requires a living host to survive, can live autonomously, either in a living body or in a glass test tube.

As Naessens explains, this is possible because whereas the virus is a *particle* of DNA, the somatid is a *precursor* to DNA, "something that leads to its creation"—what might be called a "concretization of energy." The somatids exhibit definite electrical properties, such that the nuclei are positively charged and the membranes are negatively charged. "Somatids are actually tiny living condensers of energy, the smallest ever found." Further, Naessens contends that each of our internal organs possesses somatids specifically adapted to the functional needs of that organ; yet at the same time, the entire "family," or physiological ensemble, of somatids collectively circulates throughout the body.

Somatids exhibit a sixteen-stage pleomorphic life cycle, all of which Naessens has documented with microphotographs and live-action video. The first three forms (somatids, spores, double spores) are noninjurious within the host, but as they enter the fourth (bacterial form) and proceed through the remaining twelve transformations, their pleomorphic activity is coincident with the onset and progression of disease. Stages 4 to 16 are the pathological phases of the somatid cycle, precipitated by trauma, which weakens and destabilizes the immune system.

Knowledge of this fundamental form-changing cycle enables Naessens to prediagnose by as much as eighteen months the onset of pathologies in a host organism. "In the blood of healthy persons, we observe somatids, spores, and double spores," explains Naessens. In healthy individuals the otherwise natural, inevitable progression of the complete sixteen-phase pleomorphic cycle of the somatid is blocked by the presence of an inhibitor in the blood called trephone "a proliferative hormone indispensable to cellular division."

If, owing to stress, trauma, or other biological disturbance, the concentration of trephone inhibitors in the blood diminishes, and the somatid cycle continues past stage three, "one sees the appearance of diverse forms of bacteria." According to Naessens, initiation of "cancerization" happens daily, in the form of "an acceleration and anarchic multiplication of one or several cells" generating a precancerous entity, but this is regularly deactivated by a healthy immune system. "In this fashion, we develop a small cancer daily, but our immune system rids us of it."

But if the immune system is already weakened and deficient, then this new, precancerous entity of anarchic cells reaches a critical mass and emits a substance (Naessens calls it cocancerogenic K Factor, or CKF) that paralyzes the immune system and enables it to draw off nitrogen from the organism for its own sustenance.

Naessens' remedy is brilliant for its simplicity. He uses a camphor-based, nontoxic herbal product called 714-X injected intralymphatically that suppresses CKF and feeds the cancer with nitrogen, in effect distracting it long enough for the immune system to regain competence sufficient to destroy the cancerous entity. As of 1991, Naessens' 714-X treatment had arrested and reversed the progress of more than 1,000 cancer cases, plus a couple of dozen AIDS cases. In light of this, cancer should not be considered "a cellular disease isolated from general biological disorders," says Naessens, but a progressive disease "linked to conditions of the organism." In fact, according to Otto Wolff, M.D., Ph.D., anthroposophical physician and educator, bacteria and viruses are innate conditions of the human organism, too.

"Fundamentally speaking, bacteria and viruses are 'merely' special cases of human cells; bacteria are really cytoplasm and viruses are DNA or RNA; that is, bacteria belong to cytoplasm and viruses to the cell nucleus." Infectious diseases (in which bacteria and viruses become inimical), allergies, and cancer, says Wolff, are immunological problems centered on the need for self-protection, which means that "one is always dealing with a spiritual problem, for the self is the spiritual core of the essential human being." Corroborating Naessens, Wolff adds that the best medicine is that which encourages the organism, coping with disease, to develop its own restorative, curative powers, a useful struggle that will result in "better health, a true sign that healing has occurred."

Pleomorphic Terrain: Mutability in the Microbiological Kingdom

Developments in the medical world are rapidly vindicating the controversial presumptions of such bacteriological radicals as Béchamp, Enderlein, Sonea, Panisset, and Naessens. Numerous signs indicate that the bacteriological world is virtually in revolt against allopathic medicine. Our world is suddenly rife with old plagues resurging and new ones emerging, says Laurie Garrett in her best-selling alarmist book, *The Coming Plague*. She warns us of the resurgence of old and newly mutated microbial infectious diseases. The apparent successes of modern medicine and immunology have lulled us into a complacency in which we find ourselves suddenly vulnerable to a quickly evolving, possibly unpredictable, microbiological kingdom.

It's as if our immune system is being attacked on all fronts, by eruptions of newly discovered diseases (Hantavirus in New Mexico); epidemics of old diseases in new places (cholera in Latin America); and disease spawned by technology (toxic shock syndrome from tampons); diseases spread by animals (Lyme disease). Meningitis is rampant in Brazil, hemorrhagic fever sweeps through Bolivia, tuberculosis returns in America. To an allopathic frame of mind, it's the revenge of the germs.

"The mutability of bacteria, coupled with their ability to pass around and share genetic trumps in a microscopic game of cards, seemed to increasingly leave *Homo sapiens* holding losing hands," writes Garrett. Our standard antibiotics are no longer effective against infectious diseases because they are now multiple-drug resistant.

The most dramatic example of this is tuberculosis, once nearly eradicated from the Western world, now back with considerable potency. Tuberculosis in its pathological heyday took 100,000 American lives yearly until doctors brought it under control with antibiotics in the 1940s—or so they thought. New York City hospitals in 1992 estimated that 25% of their TB patients failed to respond to most or all of the standard antibiotics commonly used against TB infections. TB, which generally has a 50% mortality rate, is coming back, fast, often as a corollary to AIDS, as an opportunistic infection; worse, it's coming back resistant to most standard drugs developed to treat it.

Incidence of TB had been declining steadily in the past forty years—in 1953, there were 84,000 new cases; in 1985, about 22,000—but by 1990 the number had started climbing again, to nearly 26,000 throughout the U.S. from the inner cities to the countryside. That's a 9.4% increase in one year's time, the largest percentage increase since TB epidemiological data was first collected in 1953; since 1985, incidence of TB cases in the U.S. has increased a total of 18%. As of mid 1996, health experts estimated that one-third of the world's population has a latent TB infection, and of the 8 million people who develop active cases each year, 3 million die.

As medical writer Frank Ryan, M.D., notes, the "forgotten plague" has returned. "The entire world was facing a new and very frightening tuberculosis threat," he discovered in 1992, and it was strangely linked to the AIDS epidemic. "How utterly incredible to discover that the new virus of AIDS was coming together with this equally dangerous if more ancient enemy, in the most sinister alliance imaginable."

What's far more troublesome about the TB resurgence is that it is increasingly multiple-drug-resistant (MDR), a new and far more virulent strain than the original TB. In a mid-1992 study, 34% of TB patients in New York City were unresponsive to one first-choice drug, while 19% failed to respond to two standard anti-TB drugs; in some cases, patients exhibit TB strains that are resistant to nine of the eleven most commonly used antibiotics in TB treatment. Meanwhile, an estimated 25% to 50% of TB patients in New York City are also infected with AIDS. Further, the case fatality rate of MDR-TB patients is now estimated at 40% to 60%, and in HIV-positive patients, it can be higher than 80%. As Barry Bloom and Christopher Murray note in *Science,* "The resurgence of TB is severely complicated by emerging drug resistance."

Tuberculosis isn't the only old infectious scourge to suddenly, anachronistically, reappear in our midst, just after our medical establishment has congratulated itself on its epidemiological conquests. The incidence of syphilis has doubled in the last decade, from 70 cases per 100,000 individuals in 1981 to 140/100,000 in 1990. The outbreak of measles increased in New York City alone from 135 confirmed cases in 1989 to 1,108 in 1991. Infection with hepatitis B virus increased an estimated 77% among young adults in the 1980s, becoming the first infectious disease to become more widespread in America after the introduction of a vaccine.

In August 1993, scientists became alarmed with a new strain of cholera spreading through India and Bangladesh that might pose a worldwide danger of epidemic. In fact, since 1817, cholera has circumnavigated the globe almost seven times, leaving, on its latest resurgence as a "tireless traveler," 10,000 dead since 1991, when it made landfall again in Peru.

In October 1995, Pasteur Institute spokesman Bernard Le Guenno warned readers of *Scientific American* that new emerging forms of hemorrhagic fever viruses, such as Ebola, Hantavirus, and Dengue fever, are being discovered every year, and that human-induced environmental changes may be favoring their spread. These pathogenic viruses—arenavirus, filovirus, flavivirus, bunyavirus—may not be new, only changed, because "what appear to be novel viruses are generally viruses that have existed for millions of years and merely come to light when environmental conditions change."

Among those changes is the accelerating destruction of the world's rainforests.

It's not just TB, syphilis, measles, hepatitis, and cholera infections that are resurging with a strong resistance to standard antibiotics; the microbes that cause pneumonia, surgical wound infections, meningitis, otitis media, gonorrhea, malaria, urinary tract infections, and severe diarrhea are joining the list of what *Science* recently called the "top ten drug-resistant microbes." As Mitchell Cohen of CDC's Division of Bacterial and Mycotic Diseases wrote in *Science*, "Such issues have raised the concern that we may be approaching the postantimicrobial area . . . in which infectious disease wards housing untreatable conditions will be seen again."

The situation has grown so grave that allopathic physicians themselves are forced to admit that the proliferation of multiple-drug-resistant microbial strains of infectious diseases believed to

have been eradicated or brought under control may have been produced by an excessive use of allopathic antibiotics. "Long-term use
of antibiotics may pose a greater risk of antimicrobial resistance
than short-term therapeutic or prophylactic use," comments
Cohen. "In this respect, efforts should be made to decrease inappropriate antimicrobial use in humans. Curative medicine is, in a
sense, a failure of preventive medicine," Cohen adds, by which he
means antibiotics used inordinately to "cure" infections may have
failed in the long term to prevent disease. That's not good news to
the antibiotics merchants.

Antibiotics are *big* business, with worldwide sales (1995) of $2.3
billion, or about 10% of the total drug industry annual income of
$23 billion. In the U.S., some 160 antibiotics are routinely sold and
used; researchers race to develop, patent, and release new antibiotics, lured by the market prospect of reaping somewhere between
$200 million yearly (for a "niche" antibiotic) to $1 billion (for a
broad-ranging drug). The anomalous mutations of the microbial
world, producing multiple-drug-resistant strains of germs, is interfering with the steady flow of cash for antibiotics.

But biotechnology firms are staging a "counterattack on resistant bacteria," riposting the microbiological mutability with a new
generation of even more virulent killer drugs. Disease-producing
bacteria can be "diabolical" in their ability to foil the action of
antibiotics, writes *New York Times* columnist Lawrence Fisher. All
160 of the existing antibiotics have at least one strain of bacteria
that is partially or fully resistant to it. "The time is right and the
need is great," commented one biotech executive. New research
into molecular biology reveals areas of bacterial vulnerability—
such as the identification of essential enzymes within bacteria—
targets against which newly crafted antibiotics will attack.

In fact, the language used by both scientists and medical journalists in reporting these developments is militaristic and strategic. A
new TB drug called isoniazid is engineered to attack the regulatory
mechanism of the TB bacterium by deactivating key enzymes and
cell wall building process. Isoniazid, researchers hope, is sufficiently
cleverly designed to preempt the bacteria's ability to shape-shift into
a nonresponsive form. These same scientists, according to *Science
News*, have begun to *"entice* the disease and its chemical *assailants*
into *yielding* some of their elusive *secrets"* and to find out what molecular mechanisms enable TB "to *resist* them [italics added]."

The language is strikingly similar to the way American intelligence officers might discuss the obscure but probably unfriendly intentions of North Korea or Iraq. The TB bacterium—nearly all disease bacteria, in fact—is the enemy; while its annihilation is a given; it's just a matter of time and manipulation until the appropriate antibiotic "proportional response" is fitted to the microbe.

One reasonably wonders—but it is unreasonable to common sense—if microbes have a mind (and agenda) of their own, at this point in the estranged relationship between humans and microbes. In mid 1996, a "baffling" new intestinal ailment called cyclospora suddenly appeared in eight states. It was believed to be produced from a protozoan parasite called *Cyclospora cayetanensis,* and it could set up weeks of debilitating fatigue, appetite and weight loss, intestinal cramps, diarrhea, and nausea.

Again, the reportorial language (*The New York Times,* in this case) illustrates the mainstream attitude about "illness-producing" microbes and their seemingly inimical intent. Public health officials were *"mystified* by the outbreak of an intestinal infection caused by an *exotic* microbe" whose *"sudden* appearance" and unknown transmission vector *"baffled"* health experts"; moreover, experts were taking the cases "very *seriously"* acknowledging the presence of "a *newly recognized* illness" the size of whose "public health *threat"* remained to be seen (italics added).

We have become mortally afraid of microbes in a world in which, paradoxically, we cannot survive without them. We have broken our covenant with them and, worse still, forgotten there ever was one.

"The cells began to function as autonomous units"

As a species, we are at war with the microbiological world. Antibiotics are our weapons, death of infectious microbes is our goal. But where is it all headed?

The popular film *Outbreak* and best-selling book, *The Hot Zone,* both attest to the growing uneasiness and fear that the microbial kingdom may be in the early stages of a lethal revolt against humanity. Patrick Lynch's novel, *Carriers* (1995), depicts the war of humanity against nature; a plague in the form of an airborne virus from the rainforest attacks Indonesia. A kind of hemorrhagic fever, it rapidly and gruesomely deconstructs the human organism within hours, as blood seeps out of all body orifices.

Once again, science fiction roams far ahead of Western science in contemplating the likely extrapolations of current developments. Greg Bear's *Blood Music* is highly instructive in this regard, extrapolating a possible future scenario from today's reality of multiple-drug-resistant microbes. In Bear's future, the microbes take over the planet and colonize, even transform, human beings, according to their agenda. *Blood Music* explores the results of merging recombinant DNA engineering and psychoneuroimmunology (PNI) to train white blood cells *in vitro* for higher-intelligence activities.

In the book, Vergil Ulam is a renegade scientist working in a fictional La Jolla, California, lab with the assignment to develop biochips (called MABs, medically applicable biochips). These are autonomous organic computers, "the incorporation of protein molecular circuitry with silicon electronics." Ulam has an even more exciting idea of his own: biologics. It is dangerous, bold, and far ahead of what his company is willing to explore.

Ulam begins working with genetically altered human B cell lymphocytes—his own—because he is intrigued with the possibility of cells developing intellects, becoming "intellectual cells." Surely this is feasible, Ulam reasoned, because, referring to immunological memory, "in almost every living cell there was already a functioning computer with a huge memory."

Ulam wants to create "billions of capable cellular computers." He inserts a biologic string of codons generated by computer into *Escherichia coli,* a standard laboratory template. *E. coli* in turn elaborated and enhanced them, such that "the computing capacity of even bacterial DNA was enormous." Contemplating his *E. coli* mutations, he felt himself to be more their servant than creator, as the "cells began to function as autonomous units"; they began thinking for themselves and developing their "complex brains."

Next, Ulam took the best biologic sequences of *E. coli* and incorporated them with extracts of his own B cell lymphocytes and trained them to interact with one another and their environment; soon they were "busily engaged in an orgy of genetic exchange," he found. Every lymphocyte has the potential intellectual capacity of a rhesus monkey. "They were his children, drawn from his own blood, carefully nurtured, operated upon."

Not long after, Ulam is fired from the lab, but before leaving, he injects a vial of trained lymphocytes into his arm. With this, he begins an astounding process of physical transformation.

Ulam becomes much healthier in appearance; he changes his diet, eliminating all junk food as the lymphocytes spread their intelligent biologic to other cells in his body. As his spine and ribs begin to fuse, he realizes: "I'm being rebuilt from the inside out." Ulam begins to suspect he has been seduced by the selfish genes in the bacterial world. "So they won't have to rely on us anymore. The ultimate selfish gene . . . Emergence. Coming-out party. Tempting somebody, anybody, into giving it what it wanted." Their intelligent chatter, exchange of information—this is the blood music he hears. Ulam is their creator, deity, and ultimate frontier; to him, they are noöcytes, mind cells equivalent to "a thousand civilizations."

From within their interior universe, they begin speaking to him across the cellular-human threshold, seeking more information. In the eyes of his peers, Ulam has created "a disease that thinks, an intelligent plague." He deliberately spreads this "infection" to a only few people, but within a month the entire United States is infected and all its people "killed": that is, transformed, absorbed into the noöcytic civilization. The talking disease spreads through every infection vector known to epidemiologists, seemingly directing its own growth.

In a few days, their numbers have grown to a billion trillion: "That is the number of intelligent beings on the face of the Earth at this moment—neglecting, of course, the entirely negligible human population." The noöcytes completely transform the physical landscape of America, overgrowing it like a mold, digesting, eventually dissolving it all. As the noöcytes communicate with another host, named Bernard, they explain that the concept and experience of individuality is distributed throughout their totality as an interchangeable identity.

With this comes a sobering possibility: "Perhaps his humanity was coming to an end." The noöcytes tell Bernard his soul is already encoded as one of them, and that parts of him have been encoded and distributed; what remains uncoded are his "mental fragments." "You already are one of us," they tell him.

A physicist named Gogarty outlines the noöcytes' intention. Through concentrated information processing, or observation, they want to change the nature of space-time. With billions of trillions of individual cogitators, far more mental power than humans ever mustered, the noöcytes can alter the nature and timber of the universe.

This is due to the reality-fixing power of the observer effect. We don't discover physical laws, but collaborate with the universe on them. The theory becomes a template and the universe conforms with this description of reality for a while if the theory doesn't contradict the known facts from the past. The universe is information, so observers and theorizers can fix the shape of events if their mental powers are intense enough.

Gogarty says there is no absolute reality, only temporarily appropriate hypotheses; reality has no underpinnings other than momentarily expedient accommodations to theories and models. "A theory that works can determine reality for only so long, and then the universe must ring a few changes." This the noöcytes achieve. Mathematics prevent them from expanding any further than the North American continent, however. If their numbers kept growing, they would create a singularity, a black hole of thought, "a portion of space-time much too closely observed" and their evolution would be frozen.

This would distort time and destroy the Earth and them as well. "They've learned how to create isolated pockets of observation, very powerful. They *delude* trillions of observers into establishing a small, temporary pocket of altered space time." But they have to take their focus away from the world long enough so it can reshape itself; otherwise it remains frozen under their observation. Reality can't be observed to change, but has to change outside the eye of observation.

It turns out none of the humans is actually killed, at least, not their consciousness. "They don't destroy anything. They can keep everything inside them, in memory" and these memories can be revisited holographically in a kind of virtual reality. The human memories become part of the communal intelligence of the noöcytes. Bernard travels through the noöcytes' thought universe—the blood music—in which there are many equivalent duplicates of his mental contents. Individual identity is holographically multiple, and a kind of shared illusion. In the thought universe, or noösphere, Bernard meets Ulam, or about one-third of him in terms of his mental contents; there everything they experience is generated by thinking as simulation, or memory reconstruction.

The memories, or human information, are stored across millennia in the introns of the genes, the empty junk spaces: "highly condensed memory storage." Bernard eventually loses his human form and dissolves and physically disappears, though he can still communicate through the computer. "I am a theme in their art, their wonderful living fictions. They have duplicated me a million times over . . . There is no longer an original. I can go off in a million directions, lead a million lives (and not just in the blood music—in a universe of Thought, Imagination, Fantasy!), and then gather my selves together, hold a conference, and start all over again. Narcissism beyond pride, propinquitous, far grander than simply living forever."

The noöcytes next master information storage in subatomic spaces, to the submicroscale, where it's more efficient to store memory compactly than in molecular domains; it's stored in the structure of space-time itself. Gogarty says: "What is matter, after all, but a standing wave of information in the vacuum?" First, the noöcytes made Southern California disappear, then the entire planet and all the moons of the solar system were reabsorbed into the planets. "When its time came, the cities, towns, and villages— the homes and huts and tents—were as empty as shed cocoons.

"The Noösphere shook loose its wings. Where the wings touched, the stars themselves danced, celebrated, became burning flakes of snow." Intelligence is freed from matter and humanity from the Earth through the directed agency of the bacteriological kingdom that only needed a genetic boost from humanity to complete its long-intended evolutionary agenda to create a nonmaterial, superintelligent thought organism capable of creating reality, says Bear.

The Astral Body—The Great Fomenter of Trouble

The daily headlines, the scientific studies and books, and even science fiction imagination all suggest that the microbiological kingdom is in some kind of elemental revolt against humanity as its master environment. In a previous chapter, we examined how the etheric domain, of the body and outer environment, acts as the interface for subtle energies seeking to influence our environment.

In effect, the etheric emerged as a necessary agent in this exchange by which different dimensions of our environment— again, physical body and physical world—interact. Similarly, we need an agent that handles the interface between the pleomorphic microbiological domain and the panoply of human illness.

To address this need for an interfacing agent, we turn to another aspect of the metaphysical model of the human being, as described in many esoteric schools. The etheric body or energy field deals with thoughts and our thinking process, with the dynamic weaving of pictures. What about emotions? Do they have a body or site of activity all their own in the human organization? Imagine if you could see the totality of all the emotions you have felt in your life, even the ones you were barely aware of, such as emotions experienced during dreaming and other states of relative unconsciousness.

Imagine if you could see them all at once, expressed as a human body or perhaps a human wearing a cloak made of these strong feelings. This is more than an imagination; it is actually an occult reality. Most commonly, this is called the astral (or emotional) body.

Although the astral body has been known to occult schools for millennia, in the late nineteenth century, theosophical writers began tentatively introducing the term into Western consciousness. The astral body, more than anything else, is the vehicle for experiencing *sensation* based on the fulfillment of "all varieties" of desires and emotions "to the fullest possible extent, the highest as well as the lowest," explained British theosophist A. E. Powell in the 1920s.

Not only does the astral body make sensation possible, it serves as an independent (though interconnected with the whole human being) body for consciousness and action. Presently, only the clairvoyantly gifted ordinarily perceive the astral body. According to Powell, the astral body of the undeveloped person will appear as a "cloudy, loosely organized, vaguely outlined mass of astral matter . . . gross, dark in color, and dense."

In such a person, the astral body mostly permeates the physical form, up to 99% in ordinary humans; that part of the astral body that enclouds the physical body is called the aura and consists of various colors. In highly developed beings, the aura may extend a considerable distance beyond the body; according to legend, the astral aura of Gautama Buddha was three miles in radius. The specific hue of color correlates with specific emotions and the general state of emotional development of the individual, Powell said. The aura's colors constantly play through it, "corresponding to and being the expression in astral matter of feelings, passions, and emotions." In ordinary humans, the auric field may have nine different, somewhat conflicting, vibratory rates; this number can even reach 100, indicating emotional chaos, says Powell.

Here "the whole surface [is] broken up into a multiplicity of little whirlpools and crosscurrents, all battling one against another in mad confusion." An astral body that vibrates in fifty contradictory ways is both ugly and seriously annoying, said Powell. "It may be compared to a physical body suffering from an aggravated form of palsy, with all its muscles jerking simultaneously in different directions." In the aura of a young child, a clairvoyant may potentially read out the soul's life agenda. "In it may also be seen lying latent the germs and tendencies brought over from his last life, some of them evil, some good," said Powell.

A similar relationship exists with the planet itself, according to theosophical thought. The Earth, too, has a subtle enveloping sphere filled with astral light. This light passively reflects back whatever it receives. As such, it is "the great terrestrial crucible, in which the vile emanations of the earth (moral and physical) upon which the Astral Light is fed, are all converted into their subtlest essence, and radiated back intensified, thus becoming epidemics—moral, psychic, and physical," commented theosophical luminary and occultist, H. P. Blavatsky in 1892.

Powell offers an additional observation of keen interest to our exploration. Although couched in the now mostly outmoded vocabulary of theosophical occult chemistry, Powell states that every physical atom floats in a sea of astral matter that surrounds and fills every gap ("interstice") in physical matter, that is, the gaps between atoms. The astral world is a condition of nature, not a locality, Powell states. A single physical atom is made of the whirling force of an estimated 14 billion "bubbles in koilon," which is a theosophical term for astral atoms.

An astral atom consists of 495 bubbles; a chemical atom of hydrogen contains 882 astral atoms; and in essence, electrons are astral atoms. Astral atoms, in turn, are comprised of mental atoms, representing a higher order of rarified energy. Whether the specificities of Powell's description are accurate or not, the concept of an astral antecedent for the atoms underlying physical matter is worth keeping in mind as we proceed.

There is more to this astral body than our emotions; here is the origin of the category of emotions itself. The astral body is the "starry" connection with cosmic influences—*aster*, meaning "star" as in the luminous, even phosphoric, appearance of astral matter—and represents the animal kingdom and the element of air living within the human constitution, according to Rudolf Steiner. The astral body, said Steiner, is the realm of emotions and effect and the dialectic of sympathy and antipathy (feeling and thinking); it consumes etheric life forces to make consciousness possible. As Hermann Poppelbaum notes, astral forces "transform mere vitality into sentience."

As our affective life, the astral body is what other traditions call the human soul, the seat of affective sentience, that is, consciousness and the sense of self based on how we feel. The life of feeling itself becomes the locus of identity in the experience of the astral body by a human. But as everyone knows, the nature and structure of human emotions are deeply generic, similar across the species. Although each person incorporates individual contents and emphases into this generic emotional matrix, the parameters of joy, grief, anger, despair, hope, and dismay remain uniform across the species.

British neuropsychologist Manfred Clynes coined the term *sentics* as a way of modeling the "biological basis of emotion communication." By *sentic,* which derives from the Latin *sentire,* which is the root of sentiment and sensation, Clynes wanted to identify a specific brain state (program or mathematical formula called an algorithm) called an "essentic form" and a corresponding mode of expression, uniform across the species and both measurable and mappable by electronic means. Such maps Clynes called sentograms, and these represent what he called the "essentic forms of emotions."

Using a device he invented called a Computer of Average Transients, Clynes was able to prepare graphs based on actual physiological readings recorded by computer from individuals experiencing emotions that illustrated the expressive nature of different emotions, such as love, hate, grief, joy, reverence, anger, and passion. Essentic forms (which resemble the dips and curves produced in a galvanic skin response lie-detector test) are a general (and generic) frame for the spectrum of human emotions. "The production and recognition of essentic forms are governed by inherent data-processing programs of the central nervous system, biologically coordinated so that a precisely produced form is correspondingly recognized," Clynes explained.

The purpose of this complex arrangement is to enable communication of emotional states between humans. "This ingenious biologic design allows individuals to recognize the expression of essentic form in other individuals and makes it possible for emotions to be communicated as qualities of experience." No doubt, but as our discussion proceeds, Clynes' essentic forms may also help to facilitate communication between human emotional states and pleomorphic bacteriological forms.

Clynes' sentic research helps us model how human emotional states are uniform across the species, even electronically or geometrically bounded. But where do they come from, ultimately? Once again, we must be prepared to take a much larger view of life than one would expect in a discussion of medicine in order to encompass profound realities such as the origin of human emotions. According to the occult research of Rudolf Steiner, the astral body comes from (and still is) the great spiritual life of the stars in us.

As the human etheric body is the residency of the plant kingdom within the human organism, the animal kingdom finds its legitimate place in the astral body and its protégé, the human organs. In the astral body, we find the influences of the constellations; in the human organs, we find the zoomorphic presence of the zodiacal constellations. The astral body emerges from the *Tierkreis*, the "animal circle" of the zodiac of bull, fish, lion, crab, ram, scorpion, and goat, said Steiner. "Our animal nature is above all what gives us our organs, which even in number are very similar to the organs of the higher animals. Man forms his own organism—his inner organs—out of the sum total of the animal group-souls."

By *animal group-souls*, Steiner refers to the collective seat of self-identity in the animal kingdom; whereas individual humans can establish an authentic sense of self within their unique individuality, with animals the "I consciousness" isn't lodged in individual members of, say, the lion species, but in a kind of single, archetypal lion soul that embodies the essence of "lion-ness."

For example, there is the lion's anger, the rabbit's fear, the wolf's greed, the lamb's patience, the sloth's mental apathy—these are "features of the human soul, but they are inseparably bound up with the bodily forms that go with them," notes the Dutch anthroposophist Wilhelm Pelikan, M.D. "Animal bodies are the symbols of psychic qualities become flesh," Pelikan notes. The lion group soul lives as the human heart with the emotional quality of courage; the bull group soul lives as the human throat and neck with the quality of obduracy.

In other words, human emotions are based in or have reference to our various internal organs and their antecedents represent certain expressive qualities of individual animals. The astral body's emotional anatomy is thus bounded by the twelve signs of the zodiac; conversely, the twelvefold zodiacal qualities are metaphorical glyphs (Clynes' essentic forms) for the fundamental emotional structure and tone of the human. Astrology, when correctly understood, can be an instructive guide because we are dealing with intelligences and processes of significance, as Steiner reminds us. "It is important to realize that when we refer to the zodiac we are speaking of spiritual beings."

Astonishingly, Steiner further declared that all the forces of the cosmos—to him, they are sentient, volitional agencies, "great spiritual beings," what other traditions might call angels—contributed to the creation of the archetypal human. The animal kingdom represents cast-off aspects of the human, remnants from the process of formation. Once man, during the period of cosmic evolution, contained all the animals within; later, the man, as the evolving human, cast out the fish, birds, reptiles, mammals, and apes—"and then he himself continued to advance," said Steiner.

This of course turns Darwinian evolution upside down. Unlike Darwin, who asserted that humanity evolved from the ape kingdom, the animal species most apparently similar to the human, Steiner reported, on the strength of his clairvoyant spiritual-scientific investigations, that the animals are in fact "prematurely congealed" aspects of the emotionality of the human as it was evolving into its completed form. Reversing Darwinism, Steiner argued that the animals evolved out of the human and are differentiated parts of humanity. If anything, the higher apes evolved out of the human during its process of phylogenetic consolidation.

Here's how Steiner explained it in his *At the Gates of Spiritual Science:* "Man has therefore always been man and not ape; he separated off the whole animal kingdom from himself so that he might become more truly human. It was as though you gradually strained all the dye-stuffs out of a colored liquid and left only clear water behind." In other words, when we survey the full range of the animal kingdom, here we see the emotional, affective differentiation of the astral and inner organological nature of the human. The animals *live in us* as the generic core of the astral, emotional body; the animal kingdom as we encounter it in the outside world represents our emotionality in living projection. When as a human we look at the animal world, we might say, as Steiner suggests: "I carried all that within myself and cast it out from my own being."

Putting it in the Aboriginal framework, we might say: Opossum Dreaming, Raccoon Dreaming, Dolphin Dreaming—these are all elements of our Human Dreaming. Human consciousness, when fully commissioned, dreams the entire multispecies natural environment. The entire animal kingdom is part of my humanness, affective core components of my astral body and its organological extensions. Thus totemism, as the Aborigines understand it, is inherently linked to both environment and human consciousness; even better, it's correct. All of this of course is opposite to how we normally see the world, but Steiner was the master of metaphysical reversals.

The natural elemental world lives in and as us, as humans. In the mineral world, then, we behold the constituents of our skeletal, material composition; in the plant kingdom, we behold the dynamic thought processes of our etheric body; in the animal kingdom, we behold the assertive emotionality of our astral body. As humans we are the embodiment of the living environment around us, as paradoxical as it sounds. Wilhelm Pelikan put it this way: "The world *is* in the mineral; it *lives* in the plant; it *experiences* in the animal; in man it comprehends itself, and in this sense man is the 'core of nature.'"

Human consciousness establishes the vital self-reflexive presence in this threefold world environment, the human voice declaring on behalf of all Creation, as the mystical traditions have always taught us, "I am!" During the course of phylogenetic human evolution, we spun the whole world out of ourselves, Steiner observes; we can find traces in everything we perceive around us in the environment, the traces of our own being. "Evolution had to take its course in this way, through a process of splitting off, because Man was to become an inward being; he had to put all this out of himself in order that he might be able to see his own self."

Within the fourfold human, the astral body is the great fomenter of troubles, which manifest as illness. As quoted earlier, "The heart makes no mistakes, but the astral body makes many," notes Steiner. "The passions and desires of the astral body surge against the physical body and overpower it." The astral body impresses its passions onto the etheric body and in effect works to influence, even redirect, its thought processes and blueprint for the physical organism.

Put more simply, in this relationship, our emotions (astral body) can put pressure on our thoughts (etheric body) and thereby influence, often negatively, our physical body. This shouldn't surprise us too much, for the PNI studies of conventional science, visited in an earlier chapter, have demonstrated precisely this interaction, just in more materialistic terms.

The Pure and Chaste Pandora in the Garden of Eden

Let's return to the myth of Pandora and her box of diseases. Now that the subject of the human astral body has been introduced, this might give us a vantage point for opening up the metaphysical truth veiled by the myth of Pandora.

Pandora's name meant, in effect, "all the gods' gifts." Pandora was divinely gifted, her constitution was an endowment of the gods, or shall we say, of the myriad stars of the heavens. In Steiner's cosmology, stars are the cast-off physical remains of great spiritual beings whose field of influence is the vast expanse of the cosmos itself. In effect, stars *are* spiritual beings, according to Steiner's research.

If we say that Pandora was made of stars, that is, of the contributions of numerous gods and spiritual beings who were the stars of the Olympian firmament, we make it possible to reconstrue Pandora. There are other ancient myths, notably from the Gnostic tradition, that explain how numerous spiritual beings—some texts give their number as 365—contributed elements to comprise the total human being, under construction. A Gnostic fragment called *The Apocryphon of John* states that 365 angels "all worked on it [the human form—'the first, perfect Man'] until, limb for limb, the natural and the material body was completed by them . . . And all the angels and demons worked until they had constructed the natural body." Pandora is thus an image of the pure and chaste human astral form—the body of stars—before the onset of sickness, illnesses, disease, and physical death.

The Western mystery tradition and its most recent expression, anthroposophy, has a term for this pure and chaste astral body. Ancient initiates and later Christian esotericists called it the *Virgin Sophia*. In essence, this refers to pure, unfettered, unhindered cognition of cosmic reality and the intelligence of the stars. It is the quality of consciousness available to human souls before they enter material embodiment, and afterward, as well, provided some effort is made. That's why *Sophia* means "divine wisdom."

When Christian esotericists spoke of an initiation experience called the purification (or catharsis) of Sophia, they meant the purging, clarification, and reshaping of the astral body, the removal of all the taints and errors that have blemished it, rendering it unable to comprehend the realities of existence. The use of the Gnostic term *Sophia* links this idea with the emotions. In the Gnostic saga, Sophia, wanting a direct glimpse of God, or perfect Creation, left the realm of complete unity to wander in the lower worlds.

There she experienced her anguished isolation from God as four basic emotions, including grief, fear, bewilderment, and ignorance. These emotions were so strong they became the basis of substance in its fourfold expression of earth, fire, air, and water. Sophia's fifth emotion, conversion, was a turning back, a return to the unity she had left; this emotion corresponds to ether, what we have described as the etheric realm. As such, Sophia became the Soul of the World and the archetype for the human soul (the celestially generated astral body). In this view, Sophia's passions are the basis of matter and the human soul.

Many in the Judeo-Christian West are not familiar with the Gnostic myth of Sophia, but they are quite at home with the Biblical story of Adam, Eve, and the Serpent in the Garden of Eden. This is probably the most abused and willfully misinterpreted initiate truth ever, thanks to institutionalized Christianity. Exoterically seen, the Garden of Eden was a paradise of virginity; there were no taints upon humanity, no disease or illness, no evil nor death. I maintain that esoterically in the figures of Adam and Eve we are dealing with another equivalent expression of Pandora. But before proceeding further, we must deconstruct the gender bias of these stories.

Esoteric tradition maintains that in this paradisiacal state, there was no biological gender; Adam and Eve were a single unified human soul without distinguishing sexual characteristics. Adam was not a "man," nor was Eve a "woman." Similarly, Pandora was not a female; Pandora is an ancient image of the composite unified human soul richly endowed by the gods, angels, stars, or cosmic spiritual beings. At this point, there was no planet Earth, no material physical world, no biological human bodies.

The paradise of virginity that was Eden is the pure and chaste astral body before its experience (or fall) in the realm of physical substance. It is Sophia before she experienced her five matter-forming emotions. In the standard Biblical rendition, the Serpent tempts Eve with an apple from the Tree of the Knowledge of Good and Evil; she succumbs, eats of it, and God throws her and Adam out of Eden. This subject is exceedingly complex and worthy of its own lengthy book; therefore, I will compress the interpretation to its barest essentials.

The Serpent offered Adam/Eve the power to manifest their desires in substance, in effect, to create the world of matter according to their passions, and to experience the delights of this manifestation in similar bodies of substance. The Serpent opened an astonishing and intoxicating vista of the possibilities of free will (cocreative potency) wielded in a realm of virginal substance. Only in physical matter could this field of dreams be realized. The much-lamented Fall from grace is nothing other than a negativistic way of describing the voluntary incarnation of the pure and chaste human soul (Pandora) into the world of substance formed of the primordial passions of Sophia.

The incarnation of the "polymorphous perversity" of desire was the consequential opening of Pandora's box. Of course it wasn't literally a box. If it has to correspond to anything, it must be to the apple the Serpent offered. The apple wasn't packed with disease-generating Spites, but it did generate a new level of cognition, a troubling *knowledge*. Just as the material world would now be peopled by humans (Pandora's progeny), so would it need its microbial factotums to run all of its physical processes. The Spites *(Keres)* of illness that flew pell-mell out of Pandora's box were the whole of the entire microbiological kingdom, entirely necessary to the newly created physical world.

More precisely put, according to pleomorphic theory, it was the undifferentiated microzymas, protits, or somatids that flew out of the box. Pandora needed agents to effect her desires in this world of substance. She made a covenant with them. Here we have the first surprising vista of a link between the astral body and the pleomorphic terrain, between feelings and microbes. Human emotion, or the configuration and dynamics of the astral body—Clynes' essentic forms—is the force that directs the pleomorphically perverse microbial kingdom, which are now the agents of human desire.

Let us say that to call Pandora's box the apple of the Garden of Eden is but a metaphorical window. The apple, when consumed, conveys perilous knowledge and awareness. However, let's work the factotums of pleomorphism—Béchamp's microzymas, Enderlein's protits, and Naessen's somatids—into this picture. As Béchamp explained, "the microzyma is at the beginning of all organization." Every organism "may be reduced to the microzyma."

The human physical organism comprises a "united multiplicity" of little bodies, "each possessed of its own independent being," Béchamp's biographer, E. Douglas Hume, explained. Hume says that insofar as every organism is reducible to its core constituency of microzymas, "life exists in the germ before it develops organs." Further, "It is because the microzymas are endowed with an individual independent life that there are in the different centers of the body differing microzymas, with varying functions."

We may draw two intriguing inferences from these remarks. First, Pandora's box indicates a new *context* for human life, namely, the living physical cell. This is the "box" or container filled with an inestimable number of microzymas, protits, or somatids, the basic constituents of biological life. This is the primal germ plasm that precedes organ development, as described by Hume. Second, some type of working, contractual arrangement between Pandora, as the incarnating human astral soul and consciousness, and the *Keres,* as the formative, pleomorphic agents was required. Béchamp's concept of microzymian "independence" clearly suggests this, however strange it may seem.

The origin of disease would follow from a serious contractual breech in this human-elemental partnership. It would be the result of a sundering of the covenant. As humans violated the contract, the apathogenic microzymas, protits, or somatids started shape-shifting and form-changing into the pathogenic Spites.

To put the matter concisely, all the trouble began (and still continues) when the force of emotions hits the cells. This opened the "box" and made the material world very much an interactive place, a field of desires enacted by the *Keres* on humanity's behalf. Pleomorphic theory implies that, historically speaking, humanity has generated every describable illness known to medicine; it has cocreated, in concert with the *Keres,* the metamorphosis of microzymas into the myriad bacteria, viruses, fungi, and molds believed to be associated with pathology. However, the reverse must also be true.

Humanity should be able to convert all pathologies back into their apathogenic state by renegotiating the incarnational contract with the elemental *Keres*.

Let us presume that, at the outset, the arrangement between Pandora, as the human soul now in matter, and the Spites, the pleomorphic elementals, was collegial, cooperative, efficient, and reciprocal. There was no illness or disease *yet*. In fact, the probable scenario is reminiscent of Enderlein's protits that remain nonharmful and apathogenic as long as the cellular milieu (pH) remains stable. The *Keres* would not turn spiteful and pathogenic until full human consciousness began to wane and parts of human awareness began to live in the shadows—that is, until part of the human became unconscious and the organismic milieu became unstable.

In a remarkable sense, modern pleomorphic theory seems to recapitulate the "fable" of Pandora and the boxful of Spites.

The Human I—Holder of the Knowledge of Good and Evil

The incarnation of Edenic Pandora into the world of substance could only happen with a profound transmutation in its own organization. Edenic Pandora may have been richly endowed with emotions, desires, passions, and dreams, all of which were a reflection of the great life of cosmic spiritual beings, but she needed a dynamic center, a point of identity and mediation. Steiner called this the Ego.

The Ego or "I" (not to be confused with Freudian conceptions of the ego as the restricted personality at war with its instincts) is the individual spark of spiritual creative energy and self-consciousness, corresponding to the Promethean element of fire. The Ego is actively expressed in the blood and immune system. The I seizes the "warmth organism" of the human, through the blood, and seizes the sense of biological self, through the immune system; the I enables the human to stand erect and speak intelligible words.

The Ego—what Steiner meant by the "clear water" left behind after straining out the colored liquids, as cited above—holds and introduces the master blueprint for the physically incarnate human. The Ego is what makes a man or woman humanly unique and more than merely a sentient but not self-aware culmination of mineral, plant, and animal energies. Pandora lacked self-awareness; she was copiously endowed by the gods from the Tree of Life, but lacked the reflexive self-awareness to partake of the Tree of the Knowledge of Good and Evil.

The Ego is needed to master the *knowledge* of the fundamental duality of existence, the good and evil of life. The Ego's knowledge enables it to exercise free will to produce either good or evil. Pandora, the pure and chaste virgin Sophia, had to be good because she knew of nothing else. Ego-endowed humans living in material bodies are morally ambivalent: we can go either way. In effect, it is the free-willing Ego that enables us to get sick and aberrate our contract with the *Keres*.

In his pleomorphic theory of protits, Enderlein said that these microflora remain harmless and neutral until the pH of the cell changes, shifting out of balance (7.0) into a more acid (6.9-0.1) or alkaline (7.1-14) state. When this happens, the protits become pathogenic endobionts. We could restate this principle of pleomorphism mythologically: When Pandora opens (expresses strong emotions) the box (shifts the cellular pH), the *Keres* (harmless protits) become Spites (pathogenic endobionts), producing "endobiont-induced disease complexes" (contagion). According to Steiner, the human I is similarly subject to "acidic" and "alkalinic" tendencies of a spiritual nature.

In Steiner's model, the human I is constantly pulled and buffeted and tempted by two opposing forces. The *Luciferic* force influences the human I to expand, inflate, glorify, to desert the physical world for a rarefied nonmaterial realm of imagination, fancy, passion, and illusion. The *Ahrimanic* force influences the human I to contract, condense, materialize, concretize, to deny the spiritual underpinnings and to take material reality as the totality of existence. The Luciferic *inflates,* the Ahrimanic *contracts;* for Steiner, both represent states of imbalance for the human.

In terms of disease processes, the Luciferic works through inflammation, the fever process, typical of childhood illnesses, while the Ahrimanic acts through the sclerotic, hardening process, typified by mid-life cancer. Steiner's dialectical model of Lucifer and Ahriman is central to his cosmology, in fact, to all aspects of anthroposophy; as such, it is far too complex to explain even cursorily here, other than to state that in his view, it represents a fundamental fact of life at all levels of creation.

Creating the Ahrimanic Double, a Great Stalking Shadow Body of Illness

Ideally, the human I remains poised and balanced between these two powerfully opposing spiritual forces. More realistically, most of the time, we are swayed in one or the other direction. It is regrettably simplistic to put it this way, given the complexity of Steiner's theories, but let's say as we depart from the mediating center, where the I ought to dwell, and drift toward either the Ahrimanic or Luciferic pole of expression, then the *Keres* in Pandora's box (the pleomorphic cellular denizens in association with the astral body) become activated and *act accordingly,* generating illness and disease.

What most acutely causes us to drift to either the Ahrimanic or Luciferic pole is a diminution of consciousness. Unconsciousness is the precipitator of the pleomorphic generation of illness; put differently, an inability to be aware of the contents and activities of our own astral body, or field of dreams and desires—Arnold Mindell's *dreambody.* When we are unaware of what our astral body is doing, feeling, conspiring, or desiring, then we are similarly unaware of the *reciprocal* activities of its pleomorphic agents, the *Keres* microbes.

It is an inimical sleight of hand for which we are the sleepwalking magicians casting noxious spells against ourselves.

In other words, Luciferic or Ahrimanic deviations enable, even direct, the *Keres* to change shape and nature, and to manifest illnesses. They don't produce illness willfully out of spite against humanity; rather, it is the unavoidable consequence of our transgression of biochemical, spiritual balance that makes them undergo their pleomorphic permutations. The *Keres* are agents of *unconscious* human astral desire; in practical terms, they have no consciousness other than what humans endow them with. They are at our service in this world of substance; when we live like the Prodigal Son, the *Keres* automatically proliferate disease as a consequence of our imbalance.

This unawareness of the contents and activities of the astral body is nearly universal among humans. It is the sorry state of consciousness indicated by the negativistic Biblical expression, the Fall; put more positively, it is the strenuous challenge of our physical embodiment to surmount this extreme tendency to fall asleep to our spiritual processes and to wake up and actually direct them from an I residing in the mediating center.

In theory—that is, in the original scheme of things—the I is supposed to act as a calm spiritual center of moral gravity amidst the passionate tumult of the astral body. The I is supposed to impart the knowledge and ramifications of good and evil to the astral body, which would otherwise recognize neither, only the continuous amoral fulfillment of its protean desires.

The knowledge of good and evil informs us that in terms of cosmic law, certain acts are proscribed and others permitted; certain acts favor spiritual awakening and others impede; some actions, seen broadly, are correct and others incorrect. Incorrect actions change the spiritual pH of the individual and activate the Spites, inducing their endobiontic transformations into pathogens. It should be clear by now that the theory of pleomorphism opens a window into how the astral body affects the physical world, how desires engage microbes to act accordingly, how desire metamorphoses substance.

"After all, nothing in medicine makes sense except in the light of evolution," state Randolph Nesse, M.D., and George Williams, Ph.D., in *Why We Get Sick*. It's worth quoting again because in a way they perhaps did not intend, their idea of Darwinian evolution as applied to medicine aids us in this exploration of how the astral body works with the microbial domain. Seen over time, such as multiple lives, the cumulative effect of the astral-directed actions of the *Keres* is what Steiner earlier called the Ahrimanic Double—a great stalking shadow body of illness and disease.

Few people have seen their own Ahrimanic Double. Who would want to, for it is a truly frightening perception. Earlier, I asked the reader to imagine a body made of all our known and unknown emotions. Imagine now a body comprising all the emotions, desires, passions, rages, hatreds ever experienced by the Ego over its entire career of incarnation, most likely thousands of lifetimes. Imagine further, that this body is a roiling tumult of unexpiated amoral astral desires, of murderous, bestial impulses, libidinous excesses, and every essentic emotion that the human is capable of experiencing. Remember, too, that these are all seeds of diseases, visages of the *Keres*.

It would not be unreasonable to label this apparition monstrous; indeed, in magical and occult circles, the unexpiated astral body is regarded as quite the monster. On the other hand, the process of occult initiation—encountering the Minotaur at the center of the labyrinth, slaying the dragon, taming the lion—involves not so much the ritual "slaying" of the beast within but the purging and expiation of the emotionally feral contents of the astral body, the cumulative residue of astral desires impacting the world of substance. We might call this the inventory of our likely disease states.

In Christian esotericism and in anthroposophy, this tortuous process is called Encountering the Lesser Guardian of the Threshold. It says that our own astral body—our unique historical accumulation of emotions and their effects—stands before us as a feral, chthonic monster (potentially) barring us from entry into the sublime supersensible realm. Should we sneak past this rightful guardian, we are subject to unending illusion and misperception, because the very guardian we thought we had eluded becomes a dirty filter through which we perceive the spiritual world.

If the guardian is transparent, as a result of our hard, initiatory purging of our unconscious emotionality, then we have a chance to see true and clear in this spiritual domain; but if the guardian is still a "monster," we will see nothing other than monster-generated illusions and nightmares.

The emotional residues in the astral body are the poisonous seeds (or catalysts) that turn the *Keres* spiteful (pathogenic). Encountering the guardian can be "a revelation of the incompletion, the imperfection, the fundamental immaturity of our inner being," as I wrote in *The Imagination of Pentecost,* which explores this theme in far greater detail. "The density of unfulfilled emotionality and unredeemed karma within the inner self can 'seem horrifying,' especially when its energies seem at every moment to be trying to entangle or capture us with tentacles." This guardian is our own self-created Angel of Death, "a spectral form made of 'the hitherto invisible results' of our actions, feelings, and thoughts."

This is why in the mystery initiation, one gains knowledge about one's astral propensities *and* disease tendencies—because they are two sides of one hand. They are part of the same package of self-knowledge. But it works both ways. When we voluntarily, consciously engage ourselves in finding the meaning and appropriateness of an illness and see through the pathogenicity to the precipitating astral emotion, then we are simultaneously purging the flawed Sophia and encountering the Lesser Guardian of the Threshold.

When understood as a rational expression of the dreambody from the reservoir of the Ahrimanic double, illness can be a means for spiritual awakening.

The New Plagues: Spectral Legacy of the Mexican Mysteries?

To return to a vocabulary used earlier, the *physis* is the interface for the dialectic between karma—the contents of our Ahrimanic Double—and the pleomorphism of the *Keres*—their shape-shifting from harmless to pathogenic—in the living context of a human body. The search for the meaning of illness promises a potential revelation of the contents of the Ahrimanic Double and of the way the astral body cocreates disease states.

This search opens a vista upon the pleomorphic terrain and the primal symbiosis between humans and microbes. As such, it affords a glimpse of how consciousness shapes the bodily environment, in this case, how astral consciousness negatively affects the physical body and its prime constituents, the microzymas. How does this exchange work beyond the vale of illness? In the next chapter, we'll explore how consciousness interacts with substance to create and sustain an overall environment.

With each of our karmically destined illnesses, we have the opportunity to remove yet one more taint from our astral body and to come one step closer to restoring a harmonious relationship with the *Keres*. An individual human illness, correctly engaged, can actually contribute positively toward a restitution of the intended relationship between the embodied human and the cellularly encased *Keres*. This is an elemental redemption brought about by a human I on behalf of the ancient contractual relationship with the *Keres*. We begin to see how environment, inner and outer, comprises a series of exchanges between human consciousness and the fundamental form-builders of nature, the microzymas.

As Douglas Hume, Béchamp's biographer, put it: "Thus, while our own shortcomings are first reflected on them [the microzymas], so their ensuing corruption afterwards revenges itself upon us." To exclude consciousness from the dynamics of environment, as allopathic thinking uniformly intends, is to kill nature, humanity, and the *Keres,* and to replace it with a dead world of automatons. Within the old Mexican Mysteries, nobody was admitted to the higher grades without committing ritual murder, said Rudolf Steiner.

Specifically, the murder had to do with the ritual excision of a victim's stomach. "Certain experiences arose from the act of having cut into the living organism with such consummate [surgical?] skill, and under such special conditions," Steiner said. On the basis of this experience, the initiate could build up one's knowledge of the mechanization of the Earth—"mastery of the mechanistic element in everything living . . . a purely mechanistic realm, a great dead realm in which no Ego could have a place"—which was the goal of these mysteries.

This tends to place the "emerging viruses" and the "coming plague" in a different, if spectral, light. AIDS, Ebola, Hanta, Dengue, Gulf War disease, Lyme disease, MDR tuberculosis, cholera, meningitis—is this evidence of the global microzymian entity in revolt? If so, who is the astral magician casting the word spells that set these aberrations in motion, turning peaceful *Keres* into malignant Spites? Whose Ahrimanic Double is carrying these toxic seeds of disease, capable of infecting the planet? Might it be the secret bearers of the corrupt Mexican Mysteries still working on American physical and etheric soil? It may be unconscious to us, but is it unconscious to those at the source?

Recent evidence regarding the anomaly of Gulf War Syndrome (GWS) forces us to ask the same hard question we posed for AIDS: is it an accident of nature or is it a deliberate laboratory-generated malady? GWS may be the result of genetically engineered germ warfare, according to Garth Nicolson, Ph.D., professor of pathology and internal medicine and chairman of the tumor biology department at the M.D. Anderson Cancer Center in Houston, Texas. Dr. Nicolson contends that researchers developed the GWS microbe by combining a gene from the HIV virus with a mycoplasma (a minute cellular component, probably identical to the microzyma) to produce a new superpathogenic microbe new to nature.

According to Nicolson, this disease agent was generated in a secret U.S. lab then sold to the Iraqi government to use as germ warfare against the Iranians during their protracted conflict in the 1980s. With 6,000 dead, 15,000 infected, and symptoms similar to chronic fatigue syndrome, the U.S. government still adamantly denies even the existence of GWS as a specific disease. "This is a huge cover-up of immense proportions," states Nicolson. "A lot of people are not happy about this getting out."

Reading the Occult Language
of the Pleomorphic *Keres*

Might there be a rational, coherent system or language here? Might the *Keres*, even in their spiritually distorted, pleomorphically altered pathogenic states have some lawful order to them? Might the *Keres* as disease agents have corresponding essentic forms, as Manfred Clynes describes for human emotions? Might there be an essentic language of disease states?

Let's assume that each emotion, passion, or desire has a describable sentic shape, as Clynes demonstrated; his essentic forms were demonstrable in the physical world of computerized printouts. Let's assume that each astral feeling has a similar essentic form, a "thought form," to use the term from theosophy and magic.

Earlier, I described Hans Jenny's work with cymatics, the ability of sounds to shape physical matter. In a similar fashion, strong thoughts or emotions can shape astral substance, generating distinct morphologies called thought forms. Annie Besant and Charles Leadbeater, both occultists, psychics, and leaders in the Theosophical Society at the close of the nineteenth century, discussed the nature and generation of thought forms. The "elemental essence" that surrounds us responds readily to the influence of human thought, such that "every impulse sent out, either from the mental body or from the astral body of man, immediately clothes itself in a temporary vehicle of this vitalized matter," wrote Besant and Leadbeater in 1901.

"Such a thought or impulse becomes for the time a kind of living creature, the thought-force being the soul, and the vivified matter the body." This thought-form may also be called an "elemental," added Besant and Leadbeater. Where cymatics describes sound-shapes, theosophical occultism describes *thought-shapes*. Every distinct thought produces both a radiating vibration and a floating form, said A. E. Powell. He described thought-forms as "elementals formed unconsciously," as usually short-lived "entities of intense activity."

According to Powell, "The desire and thought of a man seize upon the plastic elemental essence and mould it instantly into a living being of appropriate form." These forms may last for a few minutes to several days, depending on how much focused energy and emotional charge were spent in their creation. Here's how it works. If you have a strong thought with respect to yourself (as distinct from ill-will directed toward another person), this thought hovers about you as if in a heavy cloud, always ready to react with your consciousness when you enter a moment of mental passivity, Leadbeater and Besant explained.

When you are disengaged from the normal outer-directed activities of the day, this self-generated thought-form, which lives in your astral body, can now impress itself upon your awareness. If it was a sexual desire, the impression of this astral thought-form upon your waking awareness may seem as if you are being tempted by the devil, as many used to think. "Yet the truth is that the temptation is from without only in appearance, since it is nothing but the natural reaction upon him of his own thought-forms. Each man travels through space enclosed within a case of his own building, surrounded by a mass of forms created by his habitual thoughts."

Leadbeater, who was clairvoyant, describes many thought-forms he had observed. Watchful and angry jealousy in the aura of a man he observed appeared to him as a brownish-green snake with raised head, "its curious shape shows the eagerness with which the man is watching its object." There are three principles with respect to generating thought-forms, state Besant and Leadbeater: the quality of the thought determines its color; the type of thought determines its form; and the clarity and definiteness of thought determines its clearness. For the purposes of understanding, we might substitute Leadbeater and Besant's "case" of thought-forms with Pandora's "box" of *Kerean* contagion.

Here is a fourth principle, not described by Besant and Leadbeater. If you take a thought-form and mount it on a microbe, you get an illness word. The Ebola virus, for example, is a simple, almost elegant, looped shape; a thought-form can range from an amorphous color blob to a geometrical shape. When a thought-form rides a microbe, a disease word is activated. Put differently, if you want to generate a *Keres*, which means a pleomorphically activated pathogen, affix a thought-form to a specific microbial form, and off it goes, spreading a specific disease state.

Let's penetrate even deeper into this mystery, by juxtaposing two thoughts presented above. First, A. E. Powell's statement that a single physical atom is made of the whirling force of an estimated 14 billion "bubbles in koilon," or astral atoms. Here we see a possible mechanism by which astral content—our feelings, sensations, passions, desires—can affect physical matter. Second, Gaston

Naessens states that somatids are tiny concretizations of energy, precursors to DNA, the electrically charged, autonomous link between the living and inorganic; somatids lead to the generation of the genetic code. "Somatids are actually tiny living condensers of energy, the smallest ever found," Naessens said.

Here is the link: *connect astral atoms with somatids*. Do this and you have a possible mechanism by which the astral body directs the pleomorphic expression of cellular and corporate identity. You have the key to the pleomorphic self. Astral atoms directly affect the configuration of physical atoms; the quality of atomic spin— metaphorically, the emotional "baggage" on board—in turn affects the somatid DNA precursors. DNA becomes the cellular facto-tum—in magical parlance, the "familiar"—for the astral atoms.

Let's shift vocabularies to get another illuminating angle. In this connection, we behold how the Ahrimanic Double talks to the *Keres* and has them do its bidding.

This is what we might call the sequence of magical communica-tion between the astral body (Pandora as generator of thought-forms) and the microbiological kingdom (the box of *Keres*). The thought-form clicks onto the *Keres* and in effect produces a new form; this merging of the two precipitates the change in cellular pH (or internal milieu) necessary to activate the protit, empower-ing it to become endobiontically active. In effect, you have a mag-ical spell for producing states of physical deformity and degeneration. Here the Ahrimanic Double is the black magician, casting disease spells upon the *Keres*.

Seen from this viewpoint, Pandora's box is filled with an illness language, the letters of contagion. It is a catabolic language; it tears down the physical organism; it deconstructs its lawful processes; it generates sickness. It is, paramountly, an *unconscious* magical spell, cast by an astral body of which we are unaware, upon a microbio-logical kingdom of which we are also unaware, to produce deleteri-ous results upon our physical organisms, of which we are, at long last, painfully aware. Such is the protean life of our pleomorphic self.

The *Keres* are in revolt against millennia of human abrogation of the original contract. I speak metaphorically, of course. But the proliferation of multiple-drug-resistant (MDR) bacteria is the expression of elemental revolt. The *Keres* will no longer tolerate the regime of antibiotics. Both Béchamp and Sonea and Panisset sug-gested that the microzymas or global bacterial entity are capable of independent action. MDR microbes are a token of that *Kerean*/microzymian independence; Greg Bear's *Blood Music* is a full-scale "science fiction" orchestration of what could happen.

References

Altman, Lawrence K. "Outbreak of Intestinal Ailment is Baffling," *The New York Times,* (June 20, 1996).

Bailey, Alice, *Esoteric Healing,* Lucis Publishing Co., New York, 1953.

Bear, Greg, *Blood Music,* Arbor House, New York, 1985.

Begley, Sharon, "Desperation Drugs," *Newsweek,* (August 7, 1989).

Besant, Annie, and Leadbeater, C.W. *Thought-Forms,* Theosophical Publishing House, Adyar, (India), 1925 (Quest Books reprint, 1969).

Biddle, Wayne, *A Field Guide to Germs,* Henry Holt and Company, New York, 1995.

Bird, Christopher, *The Persecution and Trial of Gaston Naessens,* H.J. Kramer, Tiburon, 1991.

Blavatsky, H. P., *The Theosophical Glossary,* The Theosophy Company, Los Angeles, 1990.

Bleker, Maria-M., Dr., med. *Blood Examination in Darkfield,* Semmelweis-Verlag, Hoya, Germany, 1993.

Bos, Arie, M.D., *AIDS,* Hawthorn Press, Stroud (England), 1989.

Buchanan, James H., *Patient Encounters: The Experience of Disease,* Henry Holt and Company, New York, 1989.

Chaitow, Leon, N.D., D.O., and Trenev, Natasha, *Probiotics: The Revolutionary "Friendly Bacteria" Way to Vital Health and Well-Being,* Thorsons Publishing Group, Wellingborough, (UK), 1990.

Chopra, Deepak, M.D., *Unconditional Life: Mastering the Forces that Shape Personal Reality,* Bantam, New York, 1991.

Clynes, Manfred, *Sentics, The Touch of the Emotions.* Prism Press, Bridport (England), 1989.

Cowley, Geoffrey, "AIDS, The Next Ten Years," *Newsweek,* (June 25, 1990).

Dienstfrey, Harris, *Where the Mind Meets the Body*, HarperCollins, New York, 1991.

Dixon, Bernard, *Power Unseen. How Microbes Rule the World*, W. H. Freeman, New York, 1994.

Dossey, Larry, M.D., *Meaning and Medicine: A Doctor's Tales of Breakthrough and Healing*, Bantam, New York, 1991.

Duff, Kat, *The Alchemy of Illness*, Bell Tower/Harmony Books, New York, 1993.

Enby, Eric, with Peter Gosch and Michael Sheehan, *Hidden Killers: The Revolutionary Medical Discoveries of Professor Guenther Enderlein*, S and G. Communications, Saratoga, CA, 1990.

Fisher, Lawrence M., "Biotech Counterattack on Resistant Bacteria," *The New York Times*, (April 26, 1996).

Frank, Arthur, *At the Will of the Body: Reflections on Illness*, Houghton Mifflin, Boston, 1991.

Flaskamp, Herbert, Dr., Med. "Enderlein's Endobiosis in its Holistic Aspect," *Explore!* Vol. 7, No. 2, (1996).

Garrett, Laurie, *The Coming Plague: Newly Emerging Diseases in a World Out of Balance*, Farrar, Straus and Giroux, New York, 1994.

Gelman, David, "AIDS," *Newsweek*, (August 12, 1985).

Graves, Robert, *The Greek Myths, Vol. I*, Penguin Books, Baltimore, 1955.

Grimal, Pierre, *The Concise Dictionary of Classical Mythology*, Basil Blackwell, Oxford, 1990.

Henig, Robin Marantz, "Flu Pandemic," *The New York Times Magazine*, (November 29, 1992).

Hume, E. Douglas, *Béchamp or Pasteur? A Lost Chapter in the History of Biology*, C.W. Daniel Company, London, 1923.

James, Walene, *Immunization: The Reality Behind the Myth*, Bergin and Garvey, South Hadley, 1988.

Kahn-Lyotard, Laurence and Loraux, Nicole, "Death in Greek Myths," in *Greek and Egyptian Mythologies*, compiled by Yves Bonnefoy, The University of Chicago Press, Chicago, 1992.

Karp, David A., *Speaking of Sadness. Depression, Disconnection, and the Meanings of Illness*, Oxford University Press, New York, 1996.

Le Guenno, Bernard, "Emerging Viruses," *Scientific American,* (October 1995).

Leviton, Richard, "What Does Illness Mean?" *Yoga Journal,* (November/December 1991).

—"Beating the Odds," *East West,* (July 1990).

—*The Imagination of Pentecost: Rudolf Steiner and Contemporary Spirituality,* Anthroposophic Press, Hudson, New York, 1994.

—"Gulf War Syndrome, Thanks to Biological Germ Warfare," *Alternative Medicine Digest,* No. 11, (March 1996).

Lynes, Barry, with Crane, John, *The Cancer Cure That Worked!,* Marcus Books, Toronto, 1987.

Mees, L.F.C., M.D., *Blessed By Illness,* Anthroposophic Press, Hudson, 1983.

Middlebrook, Christina, *Seeing the Crab: A Memoir of Dying,* Basic Books, New York, 1996.

Mindell, Arnold, *The Leader as Martial Artist—An Introduction to Deep Democracy,* HarperSanFrancisco, 1992.

Nesse, Randolph M., M.D., and Williams, George C., Ph.D., *Why We Get Sick, The New Science of Darwinian Medicine,* Vintage Books, New York, 1996.

Poppelbaum, Hermann, "The Concept and Action of the Etheric Body," in *Toward a Phenomenology of the Etheric World: Investigations into the Life of Nature and Man,* Jochen Bockemühl, editor, Anthroposophic Press, Spring Valley, 1985.

Postgate, John, *Microbes and Man, Third Edition,* Cambridge University Press, New York, 1992.

Powell, A.E., *The Astral Body, and Other Astral Phenomena,* Quest/Theosophical Publishing House, London, 1965.

"Probiotics: The Friendly Bacteria," in *Alternative Medicine: The Definitive Guide,* The Burton Goldberg Group, Fife, WA, 1994.

Rennie, John, "Trends in Parasitology—Living Together," *Scientific American,* (January 1992).

Rietschel, Ernst Theodor, and Brade, Helmut, "Bacterial Endotoxins," *Scientific American,* (August 1992).

Robinson, James M., General Editor, *The Nag Hammadi Library in English.* Harper and Row, San Francisco, 1988.

Sheehan, Michael, "The Enderlein Alternative," *Body Mind and Spirit,* (May/June 1992).

—"Was Pasteur Wrong?" *Natural Health,* (January/February 1992).

Silverstein, Arthur M., *A History of Immunology,* Academic Press, San Diego, 1989.

Sonea, Sorin, and Panisset, Maurice, *A New Bacteriology,* Jones and Bartlett Publishers, Boston, 1983.

Sontag, Susan, *Illness as Metaphor,* Farrar, Straus, and Giroux, New York, 1978.

Steiner, Rudolf, *Anthroposophical Spiritual Science and Medical Therapy,* Mercury Press, Spring Valley, New York.

—*The Reappearance of the Christ in the Etheric,* Anthroposophic Press, Spring Valley, NY, 1983.

Sternberg, S. "Penetrating the Secrets of Tuberculosis," *Science News,* Vol. 149, (June 15, 1996).

—"Cholera Hides a Sinister Stowaway," *Science News,* (June 29, 1996).

Talman, Donna Hamil, *Heartsearch—Toward Healing Lupus,* North Atlantic Books, Berkeley, 1991.

Tate, David, *Health, Hope and Healing,* M. Evans and Company, New York, 1989.

Twentyman, L.R., "Homoeopathy—An Introduction," *Mercury, Journal of the Anthroposophical Therapy and Hygiene Association,* No. 5, (April 1981).

—"The Nature of Homeopathy," in *The Science and Art of Healing,* Floris Books, Edinburgh, 1989.

Vassilatos, Gerry, "Ultra Microscopes and Cure Rays, Dr. Royal R. Rife," *Borderlands: Journal of Borderland Science,* Vol. LII, No. 1, (First Quarter 1996).

Vernant, Jean-Pierre, "Sacrifice in Greek Myths," in *Greek and Egyptian Mythologies,* compiled by Yves Bonnefoy, The University of Chicago Press, Chicago, 1992.

Wolff, Otto, M.D., Ph.D., "Bacteria, Viruses, and Immunological Problems: An Anthroposophical Approach," *The Journal of Anthroposophic Medicine,* Vol. 4, No. 2, (Autumn 1987).

Yoon, Carol Kaesuk, "Bacteria Seen to Evolve in Spurts," *The New York Times,* (June 25, 1996).

Ziegler, Alfred J., *Archetypal Medicine,* trans. by Gary V. Hartman, Spring Publications, Dallas, 1983.

CHAPTER 8

Incarnation Redeemed: The Battle for the Control of Substance

The Spinning Eyes of the Astral Body

At this point in our exploration of the mysteries of the human environment—the complete and extended *human* form—we need to probe deeper into the origin of the astral body. In the previous chapter, we learned that, in theosophical occult chemical terms, astral atoms, as agents of the astral light, combine to form physical atoms in the building up of material substance. Every physical object has its astral counterpart, explained theosophist A. E. Powell; the human physical form has its astral counterpart.

Now we need to ask, from what does the human astral body derive? The answer takes us seemingly out of the domain of human embodiment into the cosmos and the planets. The link is another subject long known to esoteric studies and now tentatively and somewhat superficially discussed in public forums: *chakras.* It is by understanding the nature of the chakras that we can comprehend the terrestrial-cosmic relationships implicit in the astral body.

Throughout the ages, the secrets of the chakra system have been depicted in Eastern images and veiled in Western metaphors. In the Indian Tantra, the cosmos is an interwoven vibratory web of sound created by the tinkling anklets of a dancing Shakti, the divine female and mother of Kundalini. Her rhythms spin the fabric of the universe into seven primary layers or force centers, which become the human chakras. Gautama Buddha, addressing his students, tied a silk handkerchief into six knots to indicate how the human ego binds up the essential unity of mind through the knots of the chakras. The interior channels for subtle energy in the human body are named after India's three great rivers—Ganges, Yamuna, Sarasvati—that flow upward (in the spine) to Mount Meru, the sacred mountain in the Himalayas (head).

In the West, esoteric Christianity called the chakras (meaning, literally, "spinning wheels") the Seven Churches in Asia or the Seven Seals of the Apocalypse. The medieval alchemists knew them variously as the Seven Interior Stars, the secret vessels of the art of transmutation, the "many fine instruments made in the house," the islands in the sea of the inner life, the seven planets, the seven metals, or the seven burning lamps. The Rosicrucians saw them as the seven roses. For the twentieth-century Bulgarian teacher Omraam Mikaîl Aôvanhov, the chakras are the fruits of the Tree (spine) of the Knowledge of Good and Evil.

But in recent decades those fruits have been openly acknowledged and described in Western texts. Chakras are the psychic, generic matrix from which the unique form of the human mind-body is created. They are superphysical centers, rapidly spinning vortices, flower wheels or color whirlpools through which energies pulsate rhythmically "in constant harmonic motion," says medical clairvoyant Dora Kunz. The chakras, or *padmas,* are differing centers of consciousness, vitality, and "subtle centers of operation" for *Tattvik* energy, meaning, the energetic quality of one of the four elements (from *Tattwas:* earth, water, fire, air), explained Tantric scholar Arthur Avalon.

For Rudolf Steiner, the lotus blossoms are the sense organs of the soul, the eyes of the astral body. Chakras, for scientist-yogi Christopher Hills, are "vortices of psychic electricity" and "psychic electricity stations," biological prisms through which kundalini is differentiated into the human organism. For theosophist C. W. Leadbeater, chakras are saucer-like depressions or small circles in the surface of the etheric body that glow dully in the ordinary human but "when awakened and vivified they are seen as blazing, coruscating whirlpools, resembling miniature suns." For Tibetan scholar Lama Anagarika Govinda, chakras represent the elementary structure, form-potentialities, and dimensionality of the universe, "from the organs of dark, subconscious, but cosmically powerful primordial forces to those of a radiant, enlightened consciousness."

The anatomical models of the chakra system vary somewhat among the traditional Tantric, Tibetan, and Western sources. Whether it is the ancient Hindu rishis or twentieth-century clairvoyants, perception of the chakras has always been a matter of heightened awareness. The classic Tantric texts describe six principal centers as belonging to Shakti, and a seventh, the crown chakra, as the seat of Shiva. In Tibetan teachings, there are five centers, but it's understood that two chakras are complexes—the brow and crown centers—making seven. Some Hindu savants say each of the seven major chakras has seven microchakras, making an additional forty-nine minor centers.

In *Esoteric Healing,* Alice Bailey accounts for twenty-one minor etheric centers (in places like the palms, the soles of the feet, behind the knees and eyes) and forty-nine smaller etheric centers. The energy lines or subtle nerve channels, called *nadis,* which are the conduits for vital energy (prana), are copious; the ancient texts claim there are between 72,000 and 350,000 nadis in the etheric body. Malvin Artley, a researcher in the Alice Bailey tradition, suggests that the principal fourteen *nadis* are equivalent to the fourteen meridians of acupuncture and are "vessels for consciousness." Their intersections form an estimated 176 pairs of lesser chakras, or 352 individual points, as acupuncture meridians are bilateral, running along both sides of the body. If the etheric body comprises a complex web of force lines, some commentators suggest that the chakras are like sparkling jewels set into the fishnet fabric.

Chakras have several correspondences with the physical body, including the autonomic nerve plexuses, the endocrine glands, the major physiological systems, and the five senses. Disease, whether psychological or pathological, can be seen diagnostically as a manifestation of chakra dysfunction. In *The Chakras and the Human Energy Fields,* clairvoyant Dora Kunz and medical doctor Shafica Karagulla documented more than 200 cases in which the correlation between chakra and disease through the endocrine system was apparent.

Rudolf Steiner noted that in undeveloped people the lotus flowers are "dark in color, motionless, and inert," but when a student begins spiritual exercises, the chakras become more luminous and begin revolving. C. W. Leadbeater said that in the "more evolved" individual, the chakras may be "glowing and pulsating with living light, so that an enormously greater amount of energy passes through them."

In a sense, the pulsating living light of the spinning chakras is the pure astral form of the five subtle elements that comprise the material world, as filtered and modified by individual human experience and conscious development. The chakras represent a *nexus* between the seemingly interior world of human-embodied consciousness and the seemingly exterior world of nature-embodied process and energy—or might we feel sufficiently emboldened to suggest that this exterior environment—literally, the physical world around us, the stars and planets—is similarly a residence for consciousness?

If we are willing to grant this (or even tentatively entertain its possibility), then we have opened a doorway into environment (of any kind—human body or world body) as the lawful residence for consciousness.

Body Cosmology:
The Planets within the Human

Consistent throughout these varying models of the chakras is the understanding that they mediate, transform, and transmit spiritual energies into the materialized dimensions of life, even into cellular physiology. Mention energy, and you open the door to the vast subject of *kundalini*.

The Hindu scriptures provide a convenient model for approaching the subject of energy. Invariably it is given a cosmic origin. The source of all energy, gross or subtle, is Shakti, the divine mother, say the Tantric texts. Shakti as cosmic energy is the primal life force underlying all creation—electricity, magnetism, supreme consciousness, or pure bliss. The whole world—matter, life, mind—is Shakti's body; our environment is the manifest expression of "her" energy. Shakti's consort and polar opposite is Shiva, pure consciousness without form or movement, absolute blissful contemplation. Ultimately, their relationship is one of union, and the human theater for this cosmic union is the chakra system.

Within the human, kundalini and *prana* are aspects of cosmic Shakti. Kundalini is fiery, creative energy coiled in a state of resting potential and dormancy in the human root chakra. Prana is Shakti as active, life-supporting energy constantly in circulation through the *nadis*. Here we may accurately substitute *physis, dynamis,* or *Qi* for *prana* to get a more familiar foothold on the concept. Energy and consciousness are stepped-down in progressive stages in the human astral body. Another way of putting this is to say that the chakras represent the archetypal formative forces of the five elements underlying matter: earth (solidity), water (fluidity), fire, air, and ether (*akasha* or space).

These primordial forces—manifestations of Shakti that the Tantric texts call *Tattwas*—are the basis for our thoughts, feelings, desires, sensations, perceptions, personal identity, and life as embodied humans. They represent the conditioned energies that create the primary elements of the human body and, ultimately, our wakeful awareness as individuals.

Again a substitution of names awards us with clarity: substitute the Gnostic Sophia for the Hindu Shakti and her "passions" for *Tattwas* and the concept comes clear. Sophia (Shakti) is the source of energy that flows through the cosmos, enlivening individual beings through her transduced essence called *physis (prana). Physis* is Sophia in the human embodied context (through the portal of the astral chakras), invigorating the human organization with pure cosmic intelligence. From this link alone, you can sense how the energy that heals is also the energy that informs: *physis* is the healing stream of Sophianic intelligence.

Esotericists who discuss the chakras explain that they exist in relationship to what were once called the seven sacred planets: Saturn, Jupiter, Mars, Venus, Mercury, Moon, and Sun. Each chakra is energetically linked to a planet; more precisely, the seven planets form and energize the chakras within the human astral organism. That's why anciently the chakras were known as the Seven Planets. Picture it this way: ribbony bands of light connect each of the human's seven chakras with its host planet. According to this theory, kundalini (Shakti) flows through this planetary network and is sequentially stepped down (transduced) until it reaches the root reservoir.

Remember, these are energy transfigurations occurring in a plane that *precedes* physical matter as we know it. Any discussion of chakras, correctly put, deals with activities *prior* to the manifestation of material substance, whether it be the human body or the physical planet.

For example, let's consider the correlation of the planet Saturn and the root chakra, located at the perineum-anus and known as *Muladhara*. This chakra expresses the energetic quality and formative force of the element of earth: solidity, containment, firmness, substantiality, fixity, gravity, density, mass—crystallized energy. As such, the earth element is the root support for consciousness and the existence and activity of the other four elements (water, fire, air, ether) in the human psyche and constitution. Saturn, according to exoteric astrology, is the planet of obstacles, responsible for the laws of karma, the limitations of form, and the contractions of matter.

But the root chakra bears an astonishing secret: it is the reservoir of Kundalini, World Mother, the divine creative force whose name literally means "coiled." Expressed alternatively, the *Muladhara* chakra is Sophia's abode in the lower worlds. Through kundalini, "the creative divine fire has entered the region of fixed earth," explains Werner Bohm in *Chakras—Roots of Power.* The earth element is the final emanation of kundalini as mother of the *Tattwas.* "When she had produced all types of form, and all the *Tattwas* also, there was nothing more for her to do but to coil herself up and go to sleep."

In other words, the five elements are differentiated expressions of one energy: they are the life of Shakti. The Tantric texts say: "It is she who maintains all the beings of the world by means of inspiration and expiration, and shines in the cavity of the Root Lotus like a chain of brilliant lights."

Remembering to substitute *Sophia* for *Shakti,* we begin to see what is at stake in the matter of chakras. The planets and chakras are equivalent knots and contractions tied in the flow of cosmic energy, whether it be known as Shakti or Sophia. These "knots" are both the planets (as macrocosmic energy transducers) and the chakras (as microcosmic energy transducers); they differentiate pure energy into seven conditions and five elements.

The ramification of this model is important. It instructs us that physical substance is created from the energy of the seven planets; more precisely, physical substance is the differentiation of the energies and qualities of the seven planets. There are planets within the human body and in every atom of physical matter. The energy and qualities of the planets inform substance.

For this reason, Rudolf Steiner spoke of the human's "inner cosmic system." Here the principal organs (liver, spleen, kidneys, stomach, lungs, heart, gall bladder) correspond to the seven planets. For reasons that were not in any way arbitrary but based on occult perception, Steiner attributed the kidneys to Venus, the liver to Jupiter, the stomach to the Moon, the gall bladder to Mars, the spleen to Saturn.

Steiner established these correlations as a correspondence of *activity:* the liver is a "Jupiter-activity" in the body. "On the same basis on which these names were chosen for the activities here referred to, occult knowledge sees in the heart and the blood-system belonging to it something in the human organism which merits the name Sun," Steiner explained. An organ is a deposition of physical matter within a system of supersensible forces not physically visible, Steiner explained. These supersensible forces include astral energy streaming from the planets, impacting the fishnet webbing of the etheric body. "Through the inclusion of physical matter in the supersensible system of forces, the organ becomes a physical thing."

Lest this seem confusing, Steiner was not saying that the chakras, with their planetary antecedents, are the same as the material organs, with their planetary streams. Let's simply say that the energies of the seven planets have multiple hierarchical roles in the elaboration of the human organization.

What we have provisionally established at this point is that at a more subtle level of our being and, potentially, of our awareness, too, there live the great planets of the solar system. To comprehend subtle energies, of course, we must school ourselves in thinking subtly. When I say "planets," I refer to what we might designate as the energy essence or quality of that great solar body, perhaps even its astral nimbus as a constituency in the human organism.

Soon we will learn that the planets are not "dumb" constituents either, but highly vocal and articulate.

The Voice of the Planets Echoing along the Human Spine

In the Tantric iconography for the chakras, they are consistently depicted as multipetaled lotus flowers, and on each petal there is a Sanskrit letter, expressed phonetically. Ascending from the root chakra to the throat, each chakra has a greater number of petals:

four in the root, six in the sacral, ten in the solar plexus, twelve in the heart, sixteen at the throat, then only two at the brow. It turns out that this, too, is not arbitrary, but linguistically precise.

As the Sanskrit alphabet—universally considered a sacred, even God-bestowed language—has fifty letters, the chakra system is a cymatic tableau of a sacred alphabet. The fifty letters/sounds of the Sanskrit alphabet essentially create, form, and activate the fifty petals of the first six chakras, from root to brow. That's why, as a kind of open secret, the vowels and consonants of Sanskrit are displayed on the individual petals of the six chakras in the Tantric icons. In the vibratory alphabet that is Sanskrit, their sounds *are* the petals and chakras themselves.

So it makes sense, for somebody wishing to stimulate the chakras, to chant their sounds as given by Sanskrit, says Sanskrit scholar Vyas Houston and director of the American Sanskrit Institute in Warwick, New York. "The Sanskrit alphabet is a coherent selection of the most pure, distinct and focused sounds that can be made by the human vocal instrument." The remarkable fact is that as a body of coherent sounds it "reconverts the mind into pure energy," which makes Sanskrit "the ultimate tool for approaching the study of the Self."

Consider the *Visuddha,* or throat chakra: its sixteen petals *are* the fourteen Sanskrit vowel sounds and two variations—simple, basic sounds like *um, am, om, aim, em, rm.* This means the alphabet, as a spoken energy body, begins at the throat; by extension, it implies that cosmic creation was spoken forth from the larynx as well—Shiva's, presumably.

The fifty individual sounds—of the petals, of Sanskrit—represent pure energy, or seed sounds, that expand into language. All the mantras of the Vedas and Tantra are implicit in these seed sounds because "sound is the primary vehicle in the yogic tradition to expand individual consciousness into cosmic awareness." Sanskrit is sometimes called the "garland of letters," notes Houston, but this garland is a necklace of sound beads around the neck of Shiva whose speech is called *Devavani,* the speech of the Gods.

Coming into manifestation and incarnation, moving from the crown to the root, the fifty petal sounds create the five elements and the stages (chakras) of consciousness (as thoughts, feelings, and sensations) they represent in human experience. But the primary seed mantras, which are single syllables assigned to the core of each of the first five chakras—*Lam, Vam, Ram, Yam, Ham*—represent stages through which kundalini converts matter (expressed as the particular formative force of the element in each chakra) to energy through sound. At the Ajna, or brow chakra, the primary bija is *AUM*, which represents all the sounds (and chakras) in one—"the whole alphabet in one single sound."

Again, jumping vocabularies to clarify the point, this is Sophia's language, the creative sounds of her element and world-forming speech, sounding along the virtual solar system along the human spine.

The Word-Mist of the Etheric Body

There are letters and words in the human etheric body, too. Rudolf Steiner explained its mechanism by way of introducing a new art-dance form called eurythmy, or "beautiful movement."

The impetus to develop the beautiful gesture speech of eurythmy came to Steiner in 1911. All artistic creation has a supersensible origin, he declared, representing a spiritual revelation of the secrets of cosmos through the human being. Formerly such things were revealed only through the mysteries, the mother of art; now Rudolf Steiner perceived the implicit gestures of speech and gave them visible form as choreographed arm and hand movements. Eurythmy is the language of the etheric body made visible.

If you pronounce the alphabet out loud from *a* to *z*, you produce a complicated air-form made of letters—a complex word, explained Steiner in 1924. This word form is the human etheric body; the etheric body is woven of spoken letters, and these are the origins of the eurythmy gestures. The physical body in effect is made of the shape-forming energies of the alphabet. The human form is a *spoken* sculptural shape; the etheric body's life is a perpetual speaking—a kind of ontological filibuster—of the human physical form, a speaking that maintains the life, structure, dynamism, and intelligence of the physical body.

When the etheric body "speaks," it doesn't use the tongue but the limbs; when the larynx makes words, the etheric body dances them. "This etheric man is the Word which contains within it the entire alphabet, born from out of the creative human larynx. So if we were to go through the whole alphabet, we should in the consecutive sounds, unfold the mystery of man. In speech the human being himself is fashioned." After all, *In the beginning was the Word,* our Western traditions continually remind us; Eastern traditions have always emphasized the creative force of mantras, or sacred spoken syllables.

All words lead back to the Word. But with Steiner's observation, these old formulations spring into new meaning. "God eurythmetizes, and as the result of His eurythmy there arises the form of man." The human is the Word made flesh—eurythmy gives us a fresh angle of comprehension for the truth and mechanics of this ancient statement.

According to this view, the human being is a spoken word. The speaking is the activity of the etheric body, but the voice that speaks comes from on high. Through the larynx, the human can recapitulate this etheric word formation by creating a mirror image of its own etheric letter-filled form. In single words we encounter fragments of the human being, but when the entire alphabet is uttered from beginning to end, the entire universe is thereby expressed through the larynx—"that most wonderful organ which is present in the etheric body and which is the womb of the Word," said Steiner.

The alphabet—Steiner did not believe it mattered which Western language was used, such as German or English, as the effect would be the same—is an expression of the mystery of the human and of our roots in the universe. The individual letters of the alphabet are images of cosmic energies, of the great spiritual lives of the stars, Steiner said. "When the alphabet was spoken out of the original, instinctive, human wisdom, it was astronomy that was expressed." Through studying the letters of the alphabet, the mysteries of astronomy and the fixed stars were relayed to students. The conclave of stars is a "wonderful cosmic instrument" upon which the planets play music.

The human etheric body is in effect a cosmic musical experience arising out of the cosmic mists, said Steiner. This is more than metaphorical.

Clairvoyants who have observed the human etheric body leaving and reentering the physical form have described it as a mist. "A coffin-shaped drift of grey mist . . . spreading itself [to] take form . . . a silvery strand of mist connected the grey wraith with the body on the bed . . . the grey drifting mist drew nearer and was gradually absorbed into the physical form"—such is the way British occultist

Dion Fortune described the etheric body. It is a marvel: this malleable grey drifting mist is filled with words, the musical alphabet of stellar consonants, the sound shapes from stars for the human form.

This grey mist is also alive with ceaselessly weaving picture-activities and living thoughts. As with the astral body and its chakras originating in the planets, the etheric form also precedes the physical body and the appearance of all material substance. From this we appreciate that substance, whether it be that forming the human body or the outer environment, is made of the stars and planets. With our environment, either inbody or worldy, we are dealing with the galaxy on Earth. "We are faced by the great mystery of the extent to which Man is an actual pictured microcosm of the reality of the macrocosm," Steiner said.

Astronomy is the textbook for understanding physiology, physiology is a doorway opening into a mystical astronomy, and astrology is the interpretive language of meaning for this matrix.

Could we hear it, we would behold in our own etheric body a kind of cosmic music, Steiner said. It is a resounding music made of the "consonants" of the fixed stars of the zodiac, just as the astral body comprises the "vowels" of the seven planets. In the planets we behold vowels comprising the astral body; in the stars of the zodiac, we behold consonants comprising the etheric body. The grammar of their interaction informs the physical organism. In other words, at the core of the human organism are the energies of the planets and stars. In fact, the dynamics of this grammar explain both the relationship of the astral and etheric bodies and the stars with the planets.

If you understand one, you comprehend both. Implicit in the body is the cosmos; were we to apprehend the reality of our inner molecular life, we would behold the galaxy.

This possibility offers a vista of a new approach to healing, or perhaps merely illuminates the archetypal dimensions of true spiritual healing. In *Leah,* Stuart Perrin writes engagingly about his efforts to heal a woman with cancer using the spiritual energy principles he had learned from his guru. Above the head of Leah, the woman with cancer, he perceived a golden aura that, upon his watching, transformed into a burning disc. Perrin saw that Leah's chakras were connected to the acupuncture meridians crisscrossing her body and that their particular configuration was similar to the array of stars and planets.

"Leah's body reflected the design of the universe," Perrin says. He saw the chakras move around a light as if at the center of the universe, in the same manner that the planets move about the Sun, and believed that if he could move the energy from the Sun down to the chakras and through the meridians to Leah's cells, it would realign her system and drive out the cancer. "The tumor couldn't thrive in a body that had realigned itself with the flow of energy in the universe."

It all makes sense when you adopt a different view of the world. "Self-knowledge is knowledge of the world, and world knowledge is knowledge of the self," Rudolf Steiner explained. The great life of the macrocosm pulses within each of us as our own inner being, he said, because all that is within us was once outside as the world. The human being is woven out of all the materials of the cosmos; each of us is a shrunken, contracted universe, "intergrown with the entire cosmic structure" despite the fact that each of us feels independent and physically defined. Human organology is a mirror of the cosmos, Steiner explained, and a doorway into that vast realm.

The cosmos "outside" us is a seed of our own physical organism as we "bear the whole cosmos within us when we incarnate"; conversely, when we leave the physical form, we cognize the cosmos as our own physical body and its organs "spread out boundlessly, expanded to a universe." Were we able to see our etheric body objectively, we would behold the zodiac and its multitude of constellations, said Steiner, for whom this perception was not theoretical but an experiential reality.

Nor was it merely an intriguing theory for the hero of Michael Murphy's classic tale of inner exploration, *Jacob Atabet*. Atabet, though ostensibly a fictional character, was an intrepid explorer of the inner stars, planets, "molecular samadhi," and "internal music" of his own organism. Through Atabet, Murphy pursued the goal of "making the unconscious conscious right down to the original Quantum." If we could remember how our bodies were originally made, "we would win a new freedom and mastery in this form of spirit we call matter." Jacob Atabet sought the transfiguration of the body, "the appropriation by the flesh of the glories."

His extended meditation practice, recounted in journal form in Murphy's text, was the progressive extension of wakeful awareness and control to his organs, cells, molecules, and fundamental forces comprising his body. In his unrelenting descent into matter, Atabet sought to dismember his organism through all its layers of tissues, cells, molecules, elements, atoms, and beyond, to be able to remember its origins, knowing that, ultimately, "our deepest self made it in the first place."

Atabet penetrated the matter of his own being—his body is "all time remembered"—seeking the "first day" of creation and "the place where matter is rising from mind."

Why bother? Because when you reach that awesome moment at the secret of matter in which material bursts forth from mind, this might conceivably change the human relationship with the physical forces of the world, says Atabet. "A new control might be won over gravity, entropy, aging and death, over the formation of atomic particles." This is nothing less than a new basis—more likely, the actual basis—for a reordering of environment.

The Great Etheric Organism of Man and Earth

But where does the Earth fit into this remarkable scheme of shared identity between the human and cosmos? By now, we have encountered numerous clues suggesting a profound intimacy, if not equivalence, between the human and the planet. It's central to the argument of this book—and particularly this section, which sees self *as* environment—that this relationship be made perfectly clear. We'll discover that in essence this similarity is found by way of the etheric and astral organizations of each.

In an earlier section, we considered the Gaia Hypothesis, which informed us that the Earth is a self-regulating, homeostatic planetary organism; James Lovelock, the model's promulgator, was not willing to extend sentience and reflexive self-awareness to the planet. Certainly he (and all of conventional science) would balk at the proposition that the Earth might have a similar subtle anatomy as the human, namely, that it possesses both an etheric and an astral body, and that through these, it is connected—"wired," if you like—to the solar system and stars.

However, anthroposophists such as scientist Guenther Wachsmuth, a contemporary of Steiner, felt sufficiently emboldened (backed by decades of his own rigorous research and unhindered thinking) to state in 1923 that the Earth indeed does have an etheric body comprising etheric formative forces. The Earth is not an inert cosmic corpse, as maintained by modern scientific conceptions, but a great living world organism. "We have seen that the living earth organism shows an etheric system of forces in which processes of breathing and circulation take place corresponding to similar life-processes in the human organism, and in a reciprocal relationship with these."

Great reciprocal relationships exist between the rhythms of the "etheric environing world" and the human inner world, said Wachsmuth; in effect, both the human organism and the planetary organism are actually a copy of that "great world organism, the macrocosm" of stars of the zodiac and the planets.

Etheric forces—anthroposophy describes four different kinds— are polarized north-south (with a rhythmical process involving the other two, in the middle section) in exactly the same way around the planet and the human body, Wachsmuth explained. All levels of being—cosmos, Earth, and the human—are built up "according to the same will, through the same etheric forces, and of the same substances." The human being "living within the general laws of the macrocosm, is shaped in his organism by the same etheric formative forces which are also active in the organic structure of the cosmos." The etheric body of a single person is an individual modification and unique adaptation of the "etheric life current of the earth."

We must remember, from what we have established to this point, that when we mention etheric forces and bodies we are implying the presence and activities of all the fixed stars of the zodiac. Another anthroposophical scientist named Rudolf Hauschka, D.Sc., wanted to find out to what degree it was provable that stellar and planetary influences affected the material world. It was part of his inquiry into the nature of substance. He found that "the surrounding universe plays a part in the processes that bring matter into being and again dematerialize it," including the mineral kingdom.

Dr. Hauschka studied the mineral content of cress seeds prior to germinating and afterward, particularly with respect to phosphorus and potassium. Two weeks after germination, he burned the seedlings and analyzed the ash; no fertilizer or nutrients of any kind had been applied to the cress while they were growing. He repeated this monthly with new batches from June to December. Dr. Hauschka found that the phosphorus and potassium content of the seeds rose and fell in rhythmical intervals according to the phases of the Moon. The results showed "a characteristic rhythm of even alternation, with the full Moon favoring the emerging of substance and the new Moon favoring its disappearance."

Our physical world, and all its elements and molecular configurations, is the congealed incarnation of cosmic processes and energies. The elements that comprise our physical organism are no different from those comprising the material world, and we have established that at the preatomic level of these elements reside the stars and planets. It is not stretching matters to declare that at the heart of things, the galaxy lives on Earth. Rudolf Steiner taught (and meticulously explained) that the mineral kingdom comprises the human skeleton, the plant kingdom makes up the human etheric body, and the animal kingdom constitutes the human astral body.

Seen in mirror image, the physical world is planetary expression of the human organization. In the realm of minerals and stones, we behold the building blocks of our own skeletal system; in the plant kingdom, we see the dynamism of our etheric body made manifest; and in the realm of animals, we witness the zoological differentiation of our emotional-soul nature.

The Earth and the human organism were congealed out of the same atmosphere, explains Paul Scharff, M.D., an anthroposophical physician and philosopher. "Out of the living albuminous substance of the atmosphere, man's inner organs are brought about," he explains. "The inner organs are constituted at the same time the Earth formation comes about. This is an immense process of the unfolding of Man and Earth simultaneously."

The entire spiritual world of stars, planets, and cosmic intelligences had to work to produce the evolution of materiality we take for granted as our world and body today, says Scharff. "The substances of the Earth, as we know them today, are the expression and by-products of the actual evolution of this process which makes singular, individual Ego birth possible."

As Scharff depicts it, "the evolution of substance, the transformation of the atmosphere, the bringing about of the Earth itself, is then seen as an act of Man."

The Mystery of the Logos of the Stars Is Revealed at Golgotha

In effect, our material world was created *for* and *from* us out of cosmic energies. Both human and planet began their incarnations comprising *pure* forces of all the cosmos; we might say, with some regret, that the history of our subsequent incarnation has been the chronicle of the deposition of toxins and the degradation of our environment. From this point forward, with any mention of the word "environment," let us now understand this to mean any habitation for consciousness, whether it be the human or planetary form or any of the intervening hierarchies of nature.

As to "whose" consciousness, it would be tautological to say "human" consciousness, for this is a modification of something archetypal, and we have seen how all the stars, planets, and spiritual agencies of the cosmos have collectively contributed to the generation of the complete human being on all levels of being. The logic of this model itself requires us to grant consciousness of some kind to this constituency. Perhaps we can arrive at a conception of "whose" consciousness inhabits environment by examining the word *astrology*.

Earlier, I suggested that astrology is the interpretive language of meaning for the matrix of physiology and astronomy, inner body and outer world. Literally, astrology means the logos *(logy)* of the stars *(aster)*, the meaning, relationships, purpose, rationale, matrix, invisible connecting link, and articulate totality of all that comprises the cosmos.

Divining the nature of the *Logos* was at the heart of the classical philosophical and initiation streams of Greece and, later, the pure impulse behind earliest Christianity. "The first, primal beginning was the Logos becoming aware of itself," explains Hungarian anthroposophist educator, Georg Kühlewind. The Logos emerges out of nothing, at the very beginning of creation, as the first sight that penetrates back to its beginning, says Kühlewind. The Logos is the first-born of creation, the very first cognition, the point of coherence, the act of cognition itself, the primal beginning: "the Creator himself *becomes* through the first creation, the Logos."

The Logos is the *knowing* of all the subsequent activities of all the spiritual hierarchies, stars, planets, and other rarified spiritual beings of the cosmos, who they are, what they're doing, and *why*. It is full consciousness; it is the total illumination of the unconscious—the human etheric and astral organizations—by Christ, the quintessential "I" consciousness of creation permeating the divinely granted Ego in Man. It is Sophia waking up in matter and substance, expiating her emotions, and remembering *why* and seeing *what*.

This, after all, was the whole purpose, mythologically speaking, of her leaving the plenitude in the first place. The Christ completes her vision, and with this, substance is redeemed and all environments born anew. The flow of cosmic intelligence throughout the world of substance goes on unimpeded; Sophia, as cosmic intelligence infusing substance, wakes up in this context and provides total knowing (gnosis) to all willing humans. Or, if you prefer the Hindu vocabulary, Shakti unites with Shiva and all of creation is completed as an oroboric whole.

Certainly, this is an abstract expression and an even more abstract experience, yet Kühlewind argues otherwise. "To become aware of the Logos is to become aware of the Logos in oneself . . . the Logos in him [individual humans] allows him to look back to the origin of the Logos." The active being of the Logos dwells in every human being and is at the basis of all communication; the Logos is "God's voice." Later, men and women with a more anthropomorphic state of mind gave the Logos another name: *Christ*.

We must be exceedingly careful from here on in to abandon all our preconceived ideas about the nature of this Christ. It may be obvious to some, but perhaps not to all, that the Christ is not a property of the Christian Church, that the Christ's ontological reality may be entirely opposite its appropriation and reification by an institution that has become increasingly, over the course of its 2,000-year history, the perfect embodiment of the Antichrist.

The Christ was known and sought for millennia before the advent of heretical and then orthodox Christianity; in the earliest days of the Western mystery initiation tradition, the Christ was a name for the great spiritual being of the Sun. Candidates for initiation and illumination sought an experience—in effect, an irradiation and permeation—with this exalted spiritual being, or as Steiner says, this cosmic "fact."

For the Christ as Logos is indeed a *fact* of the cosmos; as the first-born point of cognition and of absolute *self*-knowledge, and as the Voice and Word behind all speaking and the proliferation of tongues across humanity. Insofar as the planets inform the human astral body (as vowels) and the zodiacal stars comprise the human etheric body (as consonants), the Christ-Logos inhabits the human organization as the archetypal I, or Ego—that point of reflexive, knowing self-awareness at the core of consciousness that says, continually and with every act of cognition or speaking: *I AM!*

As such, the Christ-Logos is antecedent to both astral and etheric levels of human (or planetary) expression; this means that this cosmic fact is the *perfect model* for the central organizing principle of consciousness and substance in any expression of material environment, whether it be human or world. The Christ is the Logos of the stars—the pivotal point of first cognition—and the stars are the energy essence at the heart of all atoms, elements, substances, molecules, cells, tissues, organs, bodies, and creatures of the environment.

This tells us that consciousness is the core of all substance—the "first day" of creation, "the place where matter is rising from mind," as Michael Murphy's hero, Jacob Atabet, says.

Remember, whatever is "outside" is also "inside." The Logos in the cosmos is also the Logos in the human being who is the miniaturization of this same cosmos. The human form is "the vesture of the Logos," said Steiner. "Everything is an incarnation of the Logos," all things in the world—mineral, plant, animal kingdoms, the stars and planets, and human intelligence that encompasses the world—"first come forth into existence from the Logos."

Therefore, if you want to *know*, the Logos is the place and the means to do it. This knowing was made a lot easier 2,000 years ago in the culmination of a public initiation drama called the Mystery of Golgotha.

Exoterically, the Romans executed Rabbi Jesus; esoterically, they enabled the Christ to permanently infuse the Earth's etheric plane for the future benefit of all. Prior to Golgotha, initiates had to "travel" (by clairvoyant perception) to the Logos; now the Logos had come to where even the uninitiated dwelled, appearing in human form in the world of substance.

The Christ bore the *perfect* astral and etheric bodies, which, since the "Fall" from Eden into the world of substance and desire-fulfillment, had become rather sullied and vitiated, respectively. The Christ redeemed the generic archetype of both human bodies and left the energy of all future redemptions for individual humans in the etheric body of the Earth itself. All we had to do was reach into the etheric world with our eyes wide open and our attention calm and focused and the clarification and enlivening of our etheric body was at hand. Even better, the event at Golgotha ensured that this reaching into the etheric for redemption would be a hundred-fold easier for every woman and man willing to try.

Before the Mystery of Golgotha, the Logos was only an appearance. With the physical incarnation of the Christ on Earth and the completion of the Mystery of Golgotha, Christ united with this cosmic appearance and made it tangible through its own being. Through Golgotha, "the apparent Logos [was] born upon Earth as real Logos," said Rudolf Steiner. Golgotha, of course, is the notorious hill of skulls in Jerusalem, site of the crucifixion of Jesus Christ. But to esotericists, this was only the fourth act (preceded by birth, baptism, and transfiguration) in a five-part mystery play; the fifth was the ascension, the glories made visible.

Part of that glory involved the potential transmutation of human blood, the carrier of "I" consciousness and the molecular context for individuality in the body and the interface between the world of substance and the etheric and astral worlds. Through Christ's blood shed on the cross, Christ became one with Earth and humanity. Master Jesus' blood, sanctified by its Christ permeation, literally entered the substance of this planet. The Sun Being imparted this cosmic essence—the living Ego or "I" consciousness—to the Earth and was forevermore present.

As a result of the Christ Event, men and women could comprehend the Christ-Logos, virtually any time, any place—and on their own, without priests or apostles, and today, without gurus. The Logos, expressed as the Ego or "I," is the basis for human freedom. The cognitive basis is more important than the bodily sense of freedom because as you construe the world, based on the activities of the "I," so you act in the world. If your "I" is fast asleep, so are your cognitive abilities, and the concept of freedom and thus the need to have its reality are moot points.

As the Christ awakens within each individual human, so does one's blood literally become a transmuting medium carrying the force of the awakening Christ to the trillions of cells in their pleomorphic domain that comprise our organism. The Ego finds its highest expression in the Christ, who is called the Son of Man; the tangible blood of the consummate I-being is a priceless elixir for both planet and humanity. This elixir can both heal and illumine; in fact, every healing *is* an illumination of the astral body and an enlivening of the etheric.

Consciousness heals, and the Christ-Logos is the consummate healer because it carries the perfect model of the resurrected human, resanctified, redeemed, and reconstituted after the confusing, traumatic history of human incarnation since Eden.

There is no purer or more efficacious medicine: it is pristine *physis*. That is why the Mystery of Golgotha has profound implications for the practice of medicine and the destiny of human freedom in our times.

Why Everybody Is Out to Get Alternative Medicine

So what on Earth does the Mystery of Golgotha have to do with the political struggles of alternative medicine in America? A very great deal. Ever since this momentous occulted event—occulted in the sense that few at the time appreciated its planet-changing and humanity-altering significance—a dialectical struggle has been waged over its legacy.

One set of forces has striven to bring it forward into human evolution as a quickening influence; the other set of forces has worked strenuously to suppress it and to kill the Christ forevermore on this planet. One side in this dialectic seeks to redeem the physician as the master of soul-enlivening *physis;* the other side seeks to degrade the physician into an agent of soul death. Shall the physician be the wielder of *physis* or the dispenser of *rigor mortis?* These are large topics, and approaching them with understanding is a bit like climbing a stepped pyramid, which is how we'll address them, in a logical, stepwise fashion.

Why is everybody out to get alternative medicine? This of course is a question that cuts both ways. As I documented in Chapter 1, increasing numbers of Americans are moving toward the acceptance and regular use of various modalities within the portmanteau category called alternative medicine. For the most part, these modalities honor and support the *physis* as the source of healing; this pro-*physis* camp is known as the empirics.

Concurrently, vested medical economic powers are waging an intensive campaign involving propaganda and regulatory fascism against alternative medicine. By and large, these powers—the medical establishment of big drug companies, insurance corporations, government agencies (FDA, NIH, NCI), trade groups (AMA), and their attack dogs (various "quack buster" groups)—do not acknowledge the therapeutic efficacy of the *physis* and wish to impose upon the body various artificial and mechanical agents.

This *anti-physis* camp is known as the rationalists whose philosophy is allopathy. The dialectical struggle of the empirics versus the rationalists has played out over the last several thousand years in Western culture, building in political intensity since 1850, but it has come to its final urgent crisis in America. At stake is *human* consciousness, the "I" in the body.

But why such a pitched battle? As a foundation, let's not overlook the obvious: money. Almost $1 trillion a year is at stake, every year, and the medical honeypot grows by about 6% every year. In 1994, national health care spending in the U.S. was $949.4 billion, or 13.7% of this country's Gross National Product (GNP); that's about $3,510 per citizen, up 30.6% since 1990. Of the nearly one trillion dollars, hospitals got $338.5 billion in revenue and doctors took in $189.4 billion. To put this in perspective, when U.S. health care expenditures were announced for 1992 (about $838.5 billion), *Fortune* called this "the world's seventh-largest economy." This $838 billion represented 14% of our GNP compared to 12.2% in 1990, 5% in 1950, and only 4% of GNP in 1940.

In terms of 1989 Gross Domestic Product (GDP, the value of products made in the U.S.) health care was 11.8%, more than any of the other twenty-three member nations of the Organization for Economic Cooperation and Development, including Canada, which spent 8.7% of GDP and sixteen other countries that spent less than 8%. During the 1980s, U.S. health care per capita spending increases (46%) exceeded those of Canada (43%), Japan (38%), France (35%), England (27%), and Germany (22%). In 1990, U.S. health care climbed to 12% of GNP, while defense, which had never been higher (since 1965) than 8% (in 1970) dipped to 6% and education dipped to about 5.8%.

The American health care industry, says Janice Castro in *Time*, is a "gridlock of powerful constituencies" consisting of giant pharmaceutical corporations, hospitals, doctors, the AMA and its affiliate professional organizations, insurance companies, and a powerful senior citizens lobby. "We got what we wished for, a medical miracle system—but all its perilous side effects, too," says Castro. Chief among these side effects are the facts that it is practically unaffordable and it does not heal anybody. When it comes to reversing chronic illness, the empirics today have the winning therapeutic track record, while the allopaths have a résumé of dismal failures.

When it comes to market control, dominance, and regulatory preeminence, the allopaths win hands down and the bolder, innovative empirics practice virtually on the lam in the United States.

The allopathic establishment is out to "get" alternative medicine because it wants to protect its trillion-dollar market turf in the U.S. There is a fantastic amount of money in pills. "As they say in Hollywood, I'm talking structure here—a health-care system that each day is devoted less to the art of medicine and more to the delivery of pills," wrote Greg Critser in *Harper's.* To get their message across, the U.S. pharmaceutical industry spends more than $10 billion a year on drug promotion. "Our media and medical establishment are drunk on it," Critser notes, because $10 billion "buys a lot of understanding." But understanding is not the same as therapeutic efficacy. Allopathic drugs may sell, but they don't work as well as the competition.

In the nineteenth century, the homeopaths and herbalists had a greater financial market share than the allopaths because they were more successful at reversing the leading contagious diseases of that century. The allopaths eventually changed that, not from superior medical practice, but through superior political control. Today, the allopaths again are feckless in the face of pervasive immune system failures, cancers, and multiple chronic-illness syndromes; in contrast, the empirics practicing alternative medicine in the U.S. (and Europe) are registering impressive therapeutic successes against *all* disease categories, at far less cost, without toxic drugs, and with no "side effects."

There are no surprise "side effects" when the physician works with the *physis;* there is only rational, purposeful healing and illumination. Even better, it's healing at a cost we can afford.

Thus, an estimated 33% to 40% of Americans want to "get" alternative medicine because they see the proof that it works without bankrupting anyone; and they're willing to spend about $11 billion of their own money—not insurers'—to get it. That was in 1990. Extrapolate these figures ten years forward and you begin to see that the allopaths will no longer be able to lay claim to the trillion-dollar bounty for "treating" the American *physis.*

Why the Conspirators Want to Control the *Physis* of Americans

The first level in the multileveled conspiracy against the *physis* in the guise of alternative medicine is crude financial gain. For the sake of $1 trillion, the allopathic medical establishment will do whatever is necessary to quash the therapeutic competition. Outwardly, it's in the name of science and efficacy; inwardly, it's simply for the money.

Thus at varying degrees of conscious, deliberate, and willful participation, individuals within the U.S. government, physician trade groups, pharmaceutical corporations, meretriciously labeled "consumer watchdog" groups, and the insurance companies are actively working together to suppress alternative medicine.

No doubt most of the individuals involved believe they are simply supporting the scientific status quo against pseudomedical mavericks; most probably have no inkling of the degree to which they themselves are unconscious pawns of more deeply entrenched interests that manipulate events, regulatory agencies, and medical practice unseen. Their agenda entails a more sophisticated goal than mere money: they want total social control.

The signs are everywhere that people are beginning to suspect that social and political events happen the way they do on account of somebody's careful planning, in fact, as the result of a group of somebody's strategizing. Anyone who watches *The X-Files* even a few times quickly picks up the threads and lexicon of a deeply hidden multifaceted conspiracy operating somewhere within our government.

It's not just *The X-Files;* other popular television shows such as *The Lazarus Man* and *Nowhere Man* similarly have supported the claims of conspiracy theorists. To many mainstream social critics, these shows are among the "quirkiest" on television; whether it's the government or a powerful shadow organization, forces are out to ruthlessly suppress the truth. "Either way, the most provocative trend is the conspiracy series, in which spunky heroes fight a mysterious Big Brother," comments *New York Times* critic Caryn James.

Conspiracy theory is now rampant and no doubt accurate evidence is so intermingled with paranoid, sometimes hysterical, exaggeration and projection that it becomes exceedingly difficult to negotiate one's way through the thicket of allegations. However, the chief value of this category of observation is the way it instills reasonable doubt in the validity of presumed social and political reality. It's the reasonable suspicion that events of a different order are going on behind the veil of perception that is of *keen* value and may be the chief contribution of the many conspiracy-theory explicators.

The more we can learn to think flexibly, discerningly, and acutely, the freer we become of the intricately conceived and masterfully executed mass brainwashing that political culture represents.

As Kevin Costner said in *JFK*, "We're through the looking glass. We have to think like the CIA now. White is black and black is white."

The theorists span a peculiar spectrum, from espousals of suppressed UFO technology to insidious plots by the Federal Reserve to steal all our money. A. Ralph Epperson presents what used to be called in the 1960s the John Bircher ultraconservative right-wing view in *The Unseen Hand: An Introduction to the Conspiratorial View of History*. At the other end of the spectrum, former U.S. Navy intelligence officer Milton William Cooper presents the ultra leftist's alien infiltration model in *Behold a Pale Horse*.

Despite the seeming disparity in overt political stances, both Epperson and Cooper meet in agreement when it comes to the presumed existence of secret societies, hidden government agencies, and collusion at high levels to deny Americans their rights. The goal is control over the citizenry and the conversion of a democracy into a dictatorship, says Epperson. "The Conspiracy uses government to get control of the government, and total government control is their goal," he asserts. According to Epperson, a major reason for the increasing presence of synthetic substances in the American food supply since 1945 and the overall shift from natural to chemicalized foods is a cartel agreement between Germany's giant chemical concern, I.G. Farben and at least six major U.S. food companies. I.G. Farben "either owns outright or has had a substantial financial interest in or has had other cartel agreements" with at least six major U.S. pharmaceutical companies.

This collusion of corporate interests also helps explain why laetrile was outlawed in the early 1980s despite sufficient evidence proving its efficacy and legal status in twenty-two other nations. Also known as amygdalin or vitamin B17, laetrile is a potent anticancer remedy found in apricot pits and at least a dozen other nuts and berries. G. Edward Griffin, writing in his now classic account of the laetrile debacle, *World Without Cancer*, said that the U.S. medical establishment wanted all tests seeking to validate laetrile to fail. "There are far more people making a living from cancer than are dying from it. If the riddle were to be solved by a simple vitamin, this gigantic commercial and political industry could be wiped out overnight." When it comes to medicines, the U.S. citizen does not have the legal right over his own body or to put what he chooses into it, concludes Epperson. I.G. Farben, incidentally, was the principal supplier to the German Nazi government of poisonous gases used in the extermination camps.

A Worldwide Cartel to Suppress Competition against Drug-Based Medicine

If any single name can stand for this level of the conspiracy against alternative medicine, it is I.G. Farben, with headquarters in Frankfurt, Germany. The business interests and manipulations of this multinational corporation, first formally organized in 1926 to control nearly the entire German drug and chemicals industry, are central to the opposition to alternative medicine at the end of the twentieth century.

I.G. Farben was not a single company but an interlocking web of dozens of companies around the world; in fact, by 1940, not only did I.G. Farben's operations straddle ninety-three countries, but it was Europe's largest industrial corporation and the world's largest chemical manufacturer. In the U.S., I.G. Farben had commercial interests or outright ownership in dozens of major companies, many of them in pharmaceuticals. Its name itself—I.G.—indicates the "cartel" nature of its business operations: *Interessen Gemeinschaft,* meaning "community of interests." Nearly all manufactured chemicals, including drugs, require coal tar or crude oil as a component, and in this simple fact you can begin to see the desirability of Rockefeller's oil interests becoming linked with I.G. Farben's chemicals.

The goal of a cartel is to eliminate all competition and to restrict free enterprise in the marketplace so that prices may be fixed at a level assuring maximum profits to cartel members. The best conceivable arrangement is to control both drugs and oil. In 1927, John D. Rockefeller's Standard Oil of New Jersey—a giant among American corporations—signed a cartel agreement with I.G. Farben; Rockefeller would sell oil but not drugs, while I.G. Farben would stay out of oil and only sell chemicals. Over the decades, the line between these two categories would blur, and the Rockefeller/Farben cartel would reap profits from both.

From this concept alone, you can begin to see why a global cartel would work to discourage—squash—all small-scale, enterprising, non-drug-oriented (non-petrochemical-based) approaches to medicine. They wouldn't be able to control the money flow otherwise and success in an alternative medicinal product—laetrile, Hoxsey herbs, antineoplastons—could eventually undercut their monopoly.

As G. Edward Griffin concludes, after poring through reports of U.S. government hearings on these topics conducted between 1928 and 1946, "The reality, therefore, is that government becomes the tool of the very forces that, supposedly, it is regulating." For "government," substitute NCI, FDA (and all twenty-one branches of the National Institutes of Health), and you can see why it is axiomatic for these organizations supposedly working *for* the American public to take all possible steps to suppress any innovations that might threaten the global drug (and oil) edifice they represent.

It is also highly revealing to note that during the 1930s, when Nazi Germany was preparing for war, I.G. Farben used its cartel interests in the U.S. to suppress or censure (through canceling advertisements) the publication of any information critical of or unfavorable to Nazi Germany. There is no reason to suppose that such media manipulation ever stopped with the end of that war. The fact that most mainstream American media consistently and routinely deride, make fun of, or seriously criticize alternative medicine, despite the facts of its success and efficacy, suggests that the next generation of I.G. Farben interests are pulling the strings in editorial offices across the country. The use of alternative medicine runs against the financial interests of the cartel.

There is still another factor that illustrates how a global cartel can strangle alternative medicine. According to Griffin's research, as of 1974, the Rockefeller interests included "vast" stock holdings in the first and third largest insurance companies in the U.S., namely, Metropolitan and Equitable; they also maintained a strong presence (through board of directors membership) in the Traveler's and several other insurers. Rockefeller/Farben control in the insurance sector, which no doubt continues, camouflaged, to this day, enables the cartel to complete the squeeze on alternative medicine by preventing its practice from being reimbursed by insurance policies across the country.

Open competition among different brands of vitamins, for example, was to be discouraged, as was over-the-counter sales of medicines. Making drugs available only by doctor's prescriptions, Griffins explains, suited the cartel as a long-range strategy because by this set-up, they could continually raise the prices and tightly control the market. Griffin states: "In the specialized field of drugs and pharmaceuticals, the Rockefeller influence is substantial, if not dominant."

The recent FDA push to reclassify all nutritional and herbal supplements as drugs requiring massively expensive clinical research and, if they passed this stage, prescriptions, is a perfect example of a regulatory change that would materially benefit the Rockefeller/Farben cartel and help put alternative medicine out of business. Cartels do exist today, as they did during the time of Nazi Germany, Griffins states; the names and ownership lists may have changed, but the interests remain the same. "The pharmaceutical industry, far from being exempt from this influence, has been at the center of it from the very beginning."

Griffin adds that by the time the Nazis began preparations for war, I.G. Farben had gained control over a major portion of America's pharmaceutical industry. Decades earlier, John D. Rockefeller had learned from his I.G. Farben colleagues that pharmaceutical drugs could become a source of fantastic profits especially if the competition factor were eliminated from the picture.

Rockefeller money, incidentally, was instrumental in eliminating homeopathy and naturopathy and their medical institutions from America for fifty years via the infamous Flexner Report in 1910. Abraham Flexner, M.D., prepared this report, highly damaging to all forms of alternative medicine, while employed by Andrew Carnegie and John D. Rockefeller. This report unfairly criticized homeopathic and naturopathic medical colleges for not meeting criteria specific to conventional medical training, thereby enabling new licensing and accreditation laws to squeeze hundreds of alternative medical colleges out of business.

The end result of this study was that U.S. medical schools became intensively drug-oriented and all research became focused on developing new drugs. In this way, major investors such as Rockefeller would start seeing a return on their investments in chemicalized medicine.

The Invisible World Government and Their "Created Crises"

William Cooper's message in *Behold a Pale Horse* is not that different from the scenarios of Griffin or Epperson, although he uses different evidence and presumptions to formulate it. "I must warn you, however, that I have found evidence that the secret societies were planning as far back as 1917 to invent an artificial threat from outer space in order to bring humanity together in a one-world government which they call the New World Order," Cooper cautions. He adds that we are being manipulated by a cabal of government agencies and extraterrestrial aliens for the purposes of creating this one-world government "and the partial enslavement of the human race."

Somewhat supporting the views of both Epperson and Cooper is the report of another self-described former U.S. intelligence officer, Dr. John Coleman, in *The Conspirators' Hierarchy*. According to his research, which he says involved short-term access to highly classified documents, the governments of both the U.S. and Britain (and probably others) are run by "an upper level parallel government" that he calls the Committee of 300.

Numerous business corporations, prominent individuals, and quasipublic international organizations, such as the Club of Rome, the Council on Foreign Relations, the Trilateral Commission, and the Bilderbergs, comprise the Committee's secret membership. It is an invisible government with a major bureaucracy made of numerous think tanks and front organizations that "run" businesses and government leaders. They have been at this for at least 150 years, although they were formally organized around 1897, Coleman adds.

The Committee's goal is the creation of a world government, which they seek to achieve through the "pending conquest and control of the world" through manipulated economic recessions, depressions, conflicts, and wars that create "masses of people all over the world who will become its 'welfare' recipients of the future," claims Coleman. Among its strategies is a ploy to render individuals apathetic and maladapted, full of inner conflict with respect to public events, and thereby incapable of responding willfully. The Committee orchestrates crises, conflicts, distractions, even disasters so that they may then demonstrate their competence in managing these created crises, Coleman explains. "This will confuse and demoralize the population to the extent where faced with too many choices, apathy on a massive scale will result." Our maladaptive responses then enable the Committee to "govern our reaction to created events."

Even better, the cumulative effective of constant manipulation is to make Americans "dazed, apathetic, and eventually fall asleep in the thick of battle." This in turn plays into a more recessed but potent goal, says Coleman: "Control of each and every person through means of mind control and what [former U.S. National Security Adviser Zbigniew] Brzezinski calls 'technotronics,' which would create human-like robots and a system of terror."

Let's pursue Coleman's model of "created crises" that enable government agencies to demonstrate their competence at crisis management into the field of current medical research, specifically, AIDS. In a lengthy front-page article that is blushingly propagandistic in its lush hyperbole for allopathic medicine, the *Wall Street Journal* recently reported on a new "drug cocktail" that may be effective against the HIV virus. The drug cocktail is a combined dose of a new protease inhibitor (that blocks the activity of an enzyme involved in the reproduction of HIV cells) with two other drugs based on the notorious AZT. As of mid-1996, about 60,000 Americans had already received the treatment and drug companies were lathering at the prospects of getting the estimated 650,000 to 900,000 other Americans infected with HIV enrolled in the miracle program as well.

Yearly costs for the new drug (made by three companies: Invirase, by Hoffman-La Roche; Norvir, by Abbott Laboratories; and Crixivan, by Merck and Co.) run up to $16,000, and patients must stay on them for years, possibly for their remaining lifetime. The *Journal's* descriptive language was beyond the hyperbolic: remarkable, potential for rescuing people, astonished and inspired, current wellspring of hope, incredibly effective, emboldened, historic undertaking, enthusiasm, encouraging, exciting, jubilant experiences, recent abundance of good news, difficult to restrain their optimism.

Prior to this development, absolutely nothing had been effective against HIV, the *Journal* said, dutifully oblivious of the documented successes of alternative medicine against AIDS. "It is the first time any medical therapy has shown the potential for rescuing people on the verge of succumbing to the disease." A research physician at New York University's medical school was quoted as saying, "It now appears at the very least, we may finally have the tools to turn [AIDS] into a long-term manageable and treatable disease."

Frankly, one's mouth hangs open at this display of verbal excess lavished on a new set of allopathic drugs. It is inconceivable that the *Journal* would deploy such fulsome praise for an herb that had been clinically proven to augment the immune system. The primary point here is this: if AIDS in fact is a laboratory-concocted disease, one of Coleman's "created crises," then the advent of some form of successful allopathic therapy is the Committee's "crisis management" for their secretly contrived "global disaster."

The scheme is so venal it is impressive. It satisfies the first two levels of the conspiracy against alternative medicine. The drug companies stand to make $16 billion on the AIDS market, while the Committee is one step closer toward total social control.

With minor exceptions, Epperson, Cooper, and Coleman do not focus their Hydra-headed conspiracy theories upon the practice of medicine. Their concern is the steady usurpation by government and business cartels of our political rights. The evidence and assertions they lay before the reader are highly suggestive and may support a discussion of yet more veiled strategies that use medicine as a tool. The overt goal of the conspirators, of course, is control of the populace.

As the chain-smoking "cancer man" and field agent for the unnamed secret society told FBI agent Fox Mulder on *The X-Files,* "We give them their pleasures and they give us their authority." But then as indefatigable conspiracy researcher agent Mulder says, "The truth is out there."

The key question unaddressed by both Epperson and Cooper is this: What interest, besides financial gain, does it serve the "conspiracy" to invisibly support the enforcement of monopolistic allopathic medicine? Cooper's seemingly paranoid remark about "partial enslavement" is oddly appropriate. Let us see how allopathic medicine makes "partial enslavement" possible.

The essence of allopathic medicine is to ignore, sidestep, or suppress the *physis* by introducing alien or contrary substances into the body to counter the disease process. Allopathy reifies the physician into a role of total body authority; the patient's proper role is as passive recipient of allopathic interventions, be they surgery, drugs, radiation, transplants, or implants. The quintessential allopathic intervention is the antibiotic: it literally kills life.

Allopathic medicine opposes consciousness in the body; it denies the "I" a place of biological residence and physiological efficacy. It's more than a matter of medical philosophy; the debate was over long ago. The war has been on for some time; allopathic medicines are molecular assassins seeking to eradicate the *physis* wherever possible. Allopathic drugs wage a campaign of cellular terrorism in the human organism, sowing fear and distrust of the corporate body and its chief officer, consciousness.

Allopathy schools its patients in the anonymous, invasive, soulless etiology of illness: illness is disconnected from the individual's life, meaning, and direction. It is an inconvenient interruption, an irrational assault, a fixable flaw in the machinery. It has nothing to do with *you;* in fact, you, as a point of consciousness and Logos embodiment, have nothing to do with anything in your body, especially any diseases that might latch onto it. After all, consciousness is a mere by-product of the physiological processes in the organic brain; it has no therapeutic efficacy, nor is it a reliable, "objective" indicator of symptoms.

As for healing, consciousness is impotent. You hear this every day, either overtly or slyly through the allopathic propaganda campaign; most Americans come to believe it after perpetual subliminal reinforcement. When sickness or disease arise in the human being, one's will to respond is already disarmed; the *physis* has already been kneecapped.

Add to this the antiwill milieu of multiple vaccinations of infants in their first two to six months. Infants are inoculated with virulent disease strains before their immune systems have fully developed; parental failure to make sure this happens actually results in arrest or at least harassment in many states. You have here a picture of state-enforced unilateral assault against the human being; a program of government-endorsed molecular war against the *physis* in literally the first few days of incarnation.

Not only is the adult human dissuaded from assuming responsibility or participation for the illness process, but the infant human is prevented at the molecular level even from formulating the basis of a true individuality that could undertake this responsibility and participation later in life. Infant vaccinations commandeer the immune system so that the human "I" can never find a home in the body and so that biologically based consciousness will always be attenuated and unfree.

The immune system, after all, is the physiological theater whereby the body negotiates on a biochemical level what is self and not self. Metaphorically speaking, these antigens are okay, these are "outta here," and the net balance is *me.* That's essentially how immunology works, according to modern science. In other words, immune response involves a determination of identity. The *physis* reacts flexibly to a constant barrage of possibly inimical influences yet always in accordance with a reference point: an integral biological interpretation of self. This interpretation is founded in consciousness and its focal point, the human "I."

Contributions are made by the human astral body, too, which we have already identified as the great troublemaker. Even so, it's still *my* troublemaker, not the soulless factotum of allopathic assault medicines.

Allopathy has a destructive effect on the immune system, leaving the body weaker and less capable of dealing with disease and of differentiating against friendly and inimical microorganisms based on a self-interpretation. The long-term effect of allopathic drugs is to undermine individualized immune response, substituting for it a generic, drug-modulated reaction. The drugs get rid of the symptoms in the given moment, but down the road, they progressively weaken the patient and the *physis* staggers. All of this affects your sense of self, your innate "I-ness"; you could end up with a perverted, fragmented, confused, or manipulated and generic identity.

People become incapable of thinking for themselves, of developing and entertaining independent thoughts; it takes far less to control them in this state, and a prescription for Prozac will be much appreciated.

Who's going to oppose Big Brother when you can't even fend off unfriendly germs on your own, when your immune system belongs to Big Brother and its doctors and you've been undermined from within? This is control over humans at the cellular level, administered by "physicians" and enforced by the state. Seen this way, Cooper's "partial enslavement" and Coleman's semirobotic apathy no longer seem so outrageous a proposition.

Perverting the Disease Process— The Occult Offense

At the first level of presumed conspiracy against alternative medicine, there is money, and at the second level, there is social control. However, as we will see, agents acting on each successive level are still the unconscious pawns of manipulators at yet more recessed levels. Conventional doctors and their trade groups and government regulatory affiliates are the unconscious agents of more recessed power wielders, which we could expediently label

Big Brother. Yet Big Brother, whose focus is absolute social control, is again the puppet of superior, even more occulted, powers.

This time I use the term "occult" in the more traditional esoteric sense, as in occult lodges and brotherhoods of White and Black magicians. Here we enter problematic territory. Any "occult lodge" that people have heard of is of no magical importance, or else it is a front for something quite different. Strictly speaking, you will never hear of a real occult lodge unless you are one of its members. That's why they are *occult:* the average person never even suspects their existence, yet you see the fruits of their actions almost every day.

As British occultist Dion Fortune once observed in the 1930s, "There are those who are concerned with the inner governance of the world; not its politics and wire-pullings, but with the secret spiritual influences that rule the minds of men."

The idea that behind politics you find magic (both White and Black) may surprise many and of course it is, as always, impossible to prove in the conventional sense of secret documents and smoking guns. That is, unless you accept the testimony of someone who could have belonged to such a lodge, could in fact have been in charge of one, but chose instead to reveal some of their machinations to the public. I am referring to the Austrian initiate, Rudolf Steiner.

According to Steiner's clairvoyant research, the Spiritualism effusion that burst into the materialistic nineteenth century in 1848, and ran to the end of the century, was entirely a sleight of hand staged, manipulated, then abandoned by the occult brotherhoods of America and Europe. After long discussions, these occult lodges purposefully introduced Spiritualism, with its mediumship and presumed conversation with the dead; their goal was to leaven the materialism of Western culture with a sensing of the invisible, supersensible realm and the elemental semisentient forces of nature normally beyond the ken of perception.

According to Steiner, the lodges secretly trained mediums in the mechanisms of seances; they arranged with "dead" spirits on the astral plane to participate in materializations; and they even sent their own astral Doubles to "miraculously" appear before the credulous as the risen dead. The gullible quickly believed they were in fact conversing with the authentic vocal dead, and missed the lodges' point altogether. Instead of forming more dynamic pictures of the supersensible, people began construing life after death as mere extensions of life in bodies.

Eventually, when the White brotherhoods abandoned the project, the Black brotherhoods took it over and perverted it for their own ends. At the risk of being simplistic, it is somewhat accurate to distinguish the White from the Black along these lines: White lodges work on behalf of the enlightenment and spiritual welfare of an evolving humanity, using the light for uplifting, healing, humanitarian purposes; Black lodges work to undermine human freedom and conscious evolution, using the light to deaden, pervert, and manipulate purposes. The Brothers of the Left schemed to block the introduction of the idea of reincarnation into Western culture and to keep intellectual life at the dense level of materialistic concepts.

Ultimately, the Black lodges plotted to interfere with the lawful progression of humanity by obstructing the etheric cognition of the Christ in every woman and man, Steiner explained. They used various means, including many that are gruesome and abhorrent such as the generation of astral vampires and demonic spirits that possessed human bodies. Ever they strove to prevent people from becoming aware of the presence of the Christ in the Earth's etheric realm and to thereby block the Mystery of Golgotha from being assimilated into Western culture.

Why bother doing this? Because once you perceive the etheric Christ through the development of your own etheric clairvoyance, you become an *independent* thinker, free from the deadening materialism, erroneous thoughts, and insipid atheism of mainstream culture. You begin to be able to construe the world afresh, free from all the priesthoods of organized consensus social reality. You become a threat to the establishment, as was Jesus Christ to both the Roman authorities and Judaic patriarchs. Even better, you become master of yourself, of *all* your bodies—physical, etheric, astral, Ego, and beyond, a universe on two legs.

Vaccinating the Christ out of the Human Body

We must remember the secret equation operative here: thinking *is* the legitimate life of the etheric body. Truly liberated thinking is the same as etheric clairvoyance and its picture-consciousness; this in turn is profoundly healing for the physical organism: it is pure medicine, the *physis* unfettered, the thinking cure.

The resurrection of Christ in human form at Golgotha entailed the reenlivening of the human *physis*. Etheric clairvoyance elevates humans to the threshold of conscious participation in the cosmos, as a recapitulation of the resurrection. Here we rightfully assume our birthright as individualized Logos, the "I" consciousness in me, another Christ in human form. Alternative medicine, as we know it, is transcended because we have unlocked the source of all healing: the *wholeness* of the Christ-Logos within.

We may sensibly assume the Black brotherhoods, then and now, strenuously oppose humans taking up the implications of the Mystery of Golgotha. Through allopathy and its anti-*physis* medicines, the Black brotherhoods can effectively block the flowering of etheric clairvoyance and the incarnation of the Christ-Logos and its all-healing "I" in individual humans. Suppress the *physis* and block the Christ's entry into human biology and you stifle the chance of human freedom, game, set, and match.

In effect, allopathy is able to vaccinate the Christ out of the human blood and to inoculate humans with the Antichrist in their nanotechnological form as Ahrimanic elementals. These are unredeemably foreign to the human organization; they are outside of nature, abominations spawned by human beings, something new and strange in the cosmos, and forever outcasts.

These elementals take the form of the myriad toxins, pollutants, environmental estrogens, carcinogens, silicone, synthetic chemicals, and nuclear and x-ray radiation—all the human-made poisons that are now rampant in our environment, both bodily and terrestrial. Everybody knows (though many professionally deny it) that environmental pollutants are toxic and thus terribly bad for human, animal, and plant health. Clinical studies increasingly implicate them as causal agents in cancer and numerous chronic immune system dysfunctional illnesses. But they pose an even more serious, but unacknowledged, threat to human well-being.

Ahrimanic elementals are perverting the lawfulness of the disease process and the communication channels between the human astral body and the pleomorphic microbial terrain. Through this, they also block the lawful, natural commerce between the human astral body and the human physical self; as the etheric and astral organizations are the unconscious, any interference in the flow of information between these two realms keeps the so-called waking human in the dark and unaware of (immune from) the unconscious and its contents.

An unexamined unconscious is the perfect context for black-magic manipulations, on an individual or global scale. If you're unaware of where it's happening, there's no way you can ever see anybody doing anything to you there, because you are unconscious of your unconscious.

Negative Entities in Your Aura Are Making You Sick

There is another dimension to the activities of the Ahrimanic elementals and a perfectly veiled place for us to be oblivious of life-compromising events. This is the role of negative energies or entities in the human energy field. The Ahrimanic elementals are the interface for demonic influences operating inimically in the human aura. At the end of the 1990s, attention within the progressive reaches of psychology and alternative medicine gradually became focused on the possible role of negative energies or so-called demonic entities in the human etheric and astral fields as sources of disease and dysfunction. The corresponding therapy became known as spirit releasement.

Shakuntala Modi, M.D., a board-certified psychiatrist, shocked the alternative medicine world in 1997 when she published *Remarkable Healings: A Psychiatrist Discovers Unsuspected Roots of Mental and Physical Illness*. Dr. Modi presented the results of her interviews with hundreds of patients while they were under clinical hypnosis. These patients reported a phantasmagoria of weird presences and distortions of their energy field, or aura, including the presence of what has classically been referred to—and dismissed—as demonic entities.

However, according to Dr. Modi's empirical research and tabulation, such entities, whatever their ultimate ontological origin might be, seem to be potent agents in illness. "Demons in my patients seems to be the single most common cause for most psychiatric problems," says Dr. Modi. They can suck out a patient's life force, making them feel chronically sick and tired. "They use energy absorbers, a type of black, sticky, liquid type of substance, which can absorb the patients' vital energy, causing chronic fatigue," Dr. Modi reports. Other effects can include elevation or depression of blood pressure, certain forms of cancer, (stomach and intestinal are cited), digestive problems, inflammation, ulcers, circulatory problems, breathing disorders, and pain anywhere in the body.

In the course of her hypnosis, Dr. Modi claims she was able to interview the demons themselves, to ask them their purpose in harassing the patients. Their typical answer, though incredible, is also instructive: "It is my job to make him miserable and to make sure he does not achieve his true potential." Another said: "My job is to work deep within the organs and cause hidden pain and discomfort that are not detected easily." Yet another boasted: "They all are simply like puppets in our hands and we have fun in manipulating them . . . We do not want people to learn about us and how they can free themselves from us through prayers and other means."

With this demonic interface in mind, let's return to the activities of the Ahrimanic elementals. You find an even grimmer scenario of the Ahrimanic deconstruction of the living human being in the ravages of Ebola hemorrhagic fever, as described by Richard Preston in *The Hot Zone*. Once the virus enters the human bloodstream, it undergoes extreme amplification, such that a single eyedropper of the person's blood may likely contain 100 million particles of the virus. "During this process, the body is partly transformed into virus particles," writes Preston. "In other words, the host is possessed by a life form that is attempting to convert the host into *itself*. Brain damage wipes away the victim's personality and all details of individual character vanish. He is becoming an automaton."

The Ahrimanic elementals have adulterated, even blocked, the initiation process inherent in any disease event; as such, they are interfering with the natural egress of the astral level of consciousness into the material body. Insofar as the astral body is the seat of the emotions and the life of Sophia, the soul of the world, these foreign agents are *killing the soul* in the human being.

The purpose of killing the soul is to transform humans into biological automatons incapable of self-reflection or conscience. You need a soul to have an activated conscience; without a conscience, you have no empathy for other humans and life is no longer precious but eminently expendable. Soulless humans have no moral qualms, about anything.

The medical murder of the soul was predicted in 1917 when Rudolf Steiner made an unsettling forecast about the future of Western medicine. He offered this six years after the development of the typhoid vaccine. "The soul will be abolished by means of a medicament in the form of a vaccine which will be injected into the human organism in earliest infancy, if possible, immediately after birth, to ensure that this human body never has the idea that a soul and a spirit exist. Materialistic doctors will be entrusted with the task of driving souls out of human beings."

In the future (Steiner's future, but our present), doctors will vaccinate bodies "so that these bodies will not allow the inclination toward spiritual ideas to develop" and so that the humans inhabiting these soulless bodies will only perceive the physical surfaces of the world.

The soul will be made nonexistent with the aid of a drug, Steiner added, as scientists invent a vaccine "to influence the organism as early as possible, preferably as soon as it is born, so that this human body never gets the idea that there is a soul and a spirit." Then as the human soul begins to progressively withdraw from the human body, the body becomes vulnerable to being filled with something else. Since humans will no longer be able to take up spiritual impulses, through the soul, "the body will be filled with demonic powers" because the degree of spiritual emptiness that now possesses their bodies makes it possible that "a powerful Ahrimanic spirit can live in them."

Scientists are rapidly closing in on one of the longstanding goals of vaccine research: a single-dose inoculation given to children shortly after birth to provide a lifetime of immunity against all major illnesses (at least ten). The supervaccine represents childhood immunology's "Holy Grail," according to leaders in this field. Advances in developing biodegradable microcapsules may allow for the sequential time-release of antigens, proteins, and disease toxins within the human body. This way scientists can kill the soul before it even enters the infant's body, all in one injection.

Driving Souls out of the Body through Medicine

The process of driving souls out of bodies through medicine is happening all around us (and to us), yet it is so pervasive it is easy to miss it. Foreign proteins enter, souls leave, and the body is bereft and increasingly unhuman. Signs of the protracted assault are everywhere. You can sense the veiled activity of the Ahrimanic elementals all around you in Western culture today. If you step back and look at current events from a slightly different angle, you begin to see the tracks of their movements. Something quite nasty is trying to infiltrate our culture, consciousness, and body from every possible point of entry.

Consider the recent products of pop culture: on television, there are shows such as *Sliders, The Legacy: Poltergeist,* and *The Outer Limits.* The normal parameters of consensus reality dissolve into a bizarre fourth dimension of time-travel, shape-shifting, dimensional jumps, occult rituals, and ET visitations. At the movies, UFO movies are resurgent, but this time, the ETs are hostile and have no interest in phoning home.

In *The Arrival* and *Independence Day,* completely hostile ETs invade and attack the Earth. In *The Frighteners,* a congeries of ghouls, phantoms, and demons thoroughly haunt a house, threatening to completely defile the domestic order. In *The Terminator 2: Judgment Day,* future humans have been supplanted by self-aware, utterly soulless robots made of liquid steel; these "terminators" are merciless killers, capable of instantly assuming the shape of any human. In mass-market literature, Ann Rice's *Vampire Chronicles* are wildly popular; a vampire named Lestat spins his autobiography of the damned and ghostly, enthralling millions, with his spectral, subhuman memoirs. Charm aside, he is still an astral parasite.

Meanwhile, newspapers and television almost obsessively give us reports of ruthless, unrelenting terrorism, random killings, instantaneous madness, sustained mayhem, a world unrelievedly gone to hell. Signs of the new disorder of the day around the world, indeed. Add to this the accelerating procession of presumed "natural" disasters such as forest fires, earthquakes, tornadoes, hurricanes, droughts, and floods. Surely it is clear that something entirely foreign and inimical is assaulting us on every front: it is the energy of the Ahrimanic elementals deconstructing the *physis* in humans and nature, hell-bent to drive the soul out of the body and the life out of nature.

As Dr. Modi's revelations of demonic activities in the human aura suggest, the negative entities veiled but active in the human sphere help the Ahrimanic elementals in their nasty work.

Their strategy is quite effective. Use the anti-*physis* medicines of allopathy and the anti-*physis* synthetic chemicals of technology to drive a wedge between the physical and astral expressions of the human. By this means they can *mechanize* the disease process and leave the soul no place of efficacy or access. Nobody likes being sick, yet disease has its lawful place in the scheme of human life as a catalyst for initiation leading toward illumination.

One could compile an inventory of diseases and make correlations with states of spiritual imbalance and corresponding styles and contents of initiation. Remember, illness is one way of making contact with the astral body and its legacy of unfulfilled desires and unexpiated wishes.

Illness can be a doorway into the presence of Sophia, the great Soul and Wisdom of the World, the mother of the elements, whose body is made of stars and planets and is the repository of all cosmic intelligence—what everything is, what's going on, and why. The purification of the Virgin Sophia is a rigorous cleansing of the once chaste, epistemologically clean astral body; it redeems the tragicomedy of the "Fall" from Eden into incarnation.

The product of this catharsis is a soulful incarnation of the elements of matter and the entry of Sophia into the world of substance. Imagine: Sophia present in every cell, molecule, atom, quark—Creation is so precious that the Soul of the World should incarnate into its minutest areas.

Even better, this Sophianic purification is the preliminary step in the *redemption* of all substance. The purified Sophia becomes able to cognize and identify with the Christ-Logos, which, in the Gnostic philosophy of Sophia, was her heavenly consort; their celestial union was called a syzygy, and it was meant to be consummated within human consciousness. The marriage of Sophia and Christ-Logos is to take place in *human* consciousness: this is the redemption of substance and the validation of incarnation. But much has to go right before this grand event can happen.

The purgation of illness must be preserved as a human right. Illness as initiation on behalf of the syzygy of the Soul of the World and the Christ-Logos—certainly this is a different way of viewing matters.

Now into this rational and, shall we say, "divinely mandated" scheme, the Ahrimanic elements insert a wedge that severely interferes with the Christed initiation of Sophia, the astral soul in humans. The Ahrimanic elementals have no rightful place in the exchange between astral and microbial in the context of the human organism. Metaphorically, it's like postatomic explosion nuclear radiation in the landscape; its half-life runs into the hundreds of thousands of years. It remains there, entirely toxic, incapable of decomposition, irredeemably noxious to human life, virtually permanently.

The disease-initiation process has been commandeered from human beings and our collegial pleomorphic microbes by the Ahrimanic elementals and perverted into mechanized soul-killing. It comes down to this: shall the Christ-Logos permeate substance or the Ahrimanic elementals? This is how the line is drawn in the battle for the control of substance with the environment, bodily and terrestrial, as the spoils of war. Will consciousness incarnate in the multileveled environment or will it be blocked?

Here is a grim scenario of what happens when an Ahrimanic elemental in the guise of a synthetic drug begins to commandeer a human being. An illicit street drug, known as "crank" or "ice" (methamphetamine) and completely synthetic, is being called "the most malignant, addictive drug known to mankind" by public health officials. Crank is a fast-acting brain stimulant that can persist for eight to twenty-four hours in brain cells; the trouble is it can cause psychotic and violent reactions in users, rendering them, in action and appearance, exactly like a paranoid schizophrenic. In 1994 alone, over 400 deaths were attributed to suicide or overdose under the influence of this drug; it can also produce a form of fatal meningitis. In 1995, about 35% of people sent to Iowa jails were users, as were 90% of those committed to the mental health facility in a single Iowa county, very much become the field of bad dreams. Similar statistics are showing up in San Diego.

As a result, "good people go bad in Iowa and a drug is being blamed," writes *New York Times* journalist Dirk Johnson, and "the drug is now making its way across America, ruining lives and families." In other words, people are initially attracted to the fast brain high the drug offers; soon they are addicted and before they know it, the drug has commandeered their physiology and has begun destroying their brain. Fundamentally, this story is not different from the theme of *The Arrival* and *Independence Day*: inimical intruders seek to capture and destroy the human environment.

Whether the Ahrimanic elementals wear the nonhuman face of synthetic drugs or ETs does not matter very much in this imperialist scenario. The elementals have their own ruthless agenda, and human freedom has no place in it.

The Ahrimanic elementals do not correspond to naturally arising astral desires of an evolving humanity; they are aberrant implants deliberately inserted where they do not belong. They force the disease process to run along unintended channels; the salutary shock of initiation is perverted into the horror of soul death. Synthetic chemicals have become so pervasive in the world environment and human bodies since 1945, states Theo Colborn in *Our Stolen Future,* that "it is no longer possible to define a normal, unaltered human physiology."

Further, Colborn notes that "there is no clean, uncontaminated place, nor any human being who hasn't acquired a considerable load of persistent hormone-disrupting chemicals." Synthetic chemicals alter the chemistry of human bodies and meteorological and geophysical processes of the environment. The average human being today has an estimated 250 chemical contaminants in his body fat. These chemicals not only act as carcinogens, but they are transgenerational, passed from mother to fetus, disrupting hormone-regulated processes.

Physiological incursions at this level of penetration are perilously close to the source of planetary energy and influence within the human organization, as we recall the close correlation between the planets, chakras, and the human endocrine system.

Load enough endocrine-disrupting chemicals into the body and you begin to eclipse the beneficial influence of the planets at a molecular level, thereby shutting another door to a rightful cosmic source of nourishment. Add to this situation the anti-*physis* medicines that render the etheric body impotent and ravaged. Here allopathy succeeds in shutting out the starlight that forms the etheric web and illuminates our thinking. The result is etherically dead, astrally impotent human bodies imprisoned on an Earth effectively isolated from the solar system and cosmos.

The whole enterprise of generating synthetic chemicals is a global blind experiment, Colborn argues, in which every human is a guinea pig. Even worse, there are no experimental controls—subjects or terrestrial landscapes left unaltered—"to help us understand what these chemicals are doing." There may be no controls (anymore, or in the hands of the public health authorities, as opposed to the black magicians), but it is quite possible that some people know exactly what these chemicals are doing.

An Invidious New Factor in Pandora's Box

Something unnatural has been added to Pandora's box and even the *Keres* have been derailed. Such an insertion can only be the result of black magic practiced on a global level with the intent of deconstructing the human being, killing the soul in the body, and mechanizing, roboticizing the human. Traditionally, such an invidious project was called evil. Conspiracy theories always come perilously close to what might be called the paranoid. This is unavoidable and somewhat regrettable.

However, we may take counsel in the rational observation that if the world is orderly, purposeful, and logical—that is, permeated with the Logos—it must be 100% so; anything less, and the world is sundered, with one half being rational, and other, random. This means if we propose to make the case for the world being deliberately planned and executed, it must be 100% so at *all* levels of manifestation.

We must grant that there are ever deeper, more recessed, levels of purposeful operation, of which we normally see only the final consequences, the Punch and Judy show of consensus reality.

Can doctors and scientists knowingly be evil? Yes, in some cases. Consider the Nazi doctors. According to Trevor Ravenscroft in *The Spear of Destiny*, Nazi physicians homeopathically potentized the ashes of the testicles, spleens, and skin of virile young Jews then spread them on the landscape to drive the Jewish population out of Germany. It was Hitler's idea, based on his (distorted) studies in homeopathy blended with black magic. Nazi physicians made an infernal vaccine of the potentized ashes of male Jews and inoculated the inmates of Buchenwald concentration camp in an attempt to develop a human-based pest control system.

German physicians had a role of "extraordinary importance in general for the Nazi killing project," observes Robert Jay Lifton, who documented their unpardonable transgressions of the Hippocratic Oath in *The Nazi Doctors*. These doctors occupied a central role in Nazi genocidal projects, "based on biological visions that justified genocide as a means of national and racial healing." Lifton chronicles the "Nazification of the German medical profession," in which fairly ordinary doctors willingly cooperated in a state-mandated program of demonic medicalized killing. They may have been ordinary, but they were also soul-dead, because, of the several dozen surviving Nazi doctors Lifton interviewed, "not a single former Nazi doctor . . . arrived at a clear ethical evaluation of what he had done . . . [Each] morally speaking, was not quite present."

Let us not forget, too, the allegations of Leonard Horowitz in *Emerging Viruses* that AIDS and Ebola might be designer diseases, generated in taxpayer-funded government laboratories for ruthless population control. If Dr. Horowitz is correct, then allopathic physicians in this century knowingly participated in an unarguably evil enterprise of medicalized killing that is not much different from the corrupt heart-rendering Mexican Mysteries of an older, equally sinister America.

As a coda to this observation, let me introduce another element from the practice of magic. Magicians, especially those of the Left, or Black, side, work with "familiars." These are more or less servile factotums either trained or forced to do the bidding of the opera-tor. These familiars may be various elemental beings, either natur-al or generated, or the restless, unexpiated dead. But how about recruiting familiars from the living world of microbes?

Here's a new way to wage biological warfare against drug-resis-tant bacteria. According to Carl R. Merril of the National Institute of Mental Health Neuroscience Research Center in Washington, D.C. (part of the NIH-Public Health Service within the Depart-ment of Health and Human Services), you can use viruses to kill bacteria. It's called phage therapy and was first proposed in 1915 by a French bacteriologist.

A virus is injected into a living organism (clinical studies were performed on mice); it multiplies exponentially, making more than a million copies of itself in twenty-four hours; soon the bacteria are dead, their cell walls burst. The downside is that phages (the virus agents used in this manner) carry genes that produce disease and the bacterial debris from the bursT-cell walls can be toxic to the host. Merril and colleagues contend they've found ways to circum-vent these problems.

"It's a biological warfare that's probably been going on since life evolved on Earth," he says. He can see no reason why scientists shouldn't (italics added) *use it* to our benefit" or invest the neces-sary time and money "to build up the armament of phages *to do what we need to do.*" After all, allopathic scientists have already declared total war on the microbial kingdom; analogically speak-ing, why not use the equivalent of Iran (virus phage) to fight the drug-resistant Iraq (bacteria) to our benefit, as the U.S. did during the 1980s? If they destroy each other, so much the better.

Or how about using the molecular equivalent of a mad suicide bomber to deliver something lethal to the cells? U.S. scientists are experimenting with how *Shigella flexneri,* a prime infectious agent in food poisoning, might deliver a DNA vaccine to theoretically stimulate human immunity for diseases, from tuberculosis to AIDS. The genes, carried by disabled *Shigella* (their replication gene is deactivated), once inside the body, code human cells to produce antigens by way of building immune defense. Ideally, the host will swallow the genetically engineered DNA delivery system.

As an alternative to the *Shigella,* whose presence might disrupt a human cell's genome, scientists are also looking into encapsulating plasmid DNA (which means, prebent into a hula-hoop shape) in microscopic spheres of a biopolymer called PLG. This is more of a Trojan horse approach. The PLG carries the DNA vaccine, protecting it from digestion by intestinal acids and enzymes, until the right moment. Then the biopolymer degrades and the genetically engineered vaccine goes to work; yet another Ahrimanic elemental is injected into the human organism.

To give the scenario its final surrealist gloss, one scientist notes: "It's a very safe and innocuous material [PLG] that has been used in medicine for a long time." As ever, the prime site of experimentation and the ultimate destination of all allopathic "innovations" is the human organism.

The Dark Benefits of Failure
at a Planetary Level

At this point we need to probe deeper and come up with reasons for *why* this effort is being made at this time. The world, however complex, baffling, and mysterious, is still rational and purposeful, even if the rationality surpasses conventional understanding and belief systems. A compelling reason for the opponents of human development into free-willing Christed individuals to adulterate and mechanize the disease/healing process would be to block the awareness of and fulfillment of individual karma. The issue of karma, or destiny, is a vexed, confused subject in the West, and possibly in the East as well.

It is, of course, inherently transpersonal or multipersonal in scope; it presupposes a continuity of incident, memory, intention, debt, and momentum through time and bodies. Illness may be seen to have a karmic, or multiple-lifetimes, component; the experience of diabetes, for example, may be both a necessity (as a kind of debt compensation or unavoidable result of erroneous ways of living) and an opportunity for soul reform. Even though most of the major events in our lives seem like meaningless ambushes or unlooked-for moments of grace from an invisible, ambivalent "fate," from the viewpoint of the soul, they are scheduled items on the life agenda for our edification as embodied personalities.

Thus, karmic fulfillment and soul redemption through the illness process can be an initiatory event necessary for the unfolding of one's full humanness. The astral body being the vehicle for the karmic agenda, when you block the communication between one's astral and etheric/physical organism, you are blocking the working out of that person's karma through biology, the *only* place where it may be resolved. It would serve the Black brotherhoods to block karmic fulfillment and, even better, to completely confuse the subject among supposedly educated people, because it would be another way to murder the soul, keep the soul out of the biological human, and defeat the freeing of the human will. It served the brotherhoods of the Left well in the nineteenth century when, according to Rudolf Steiner, the American Spiritualists and lodges "wanted to let the teaching of reincarnation disappear [and] mediumship was a means to this end and so that method was adopted."

Follow the logic through and you'll find the connection. Block the spiritual teachings on reincarnation, with its general principles of karma, by creating materialistic psychic distractions and you block individuals from discovering their karma and its specific agenda for them. Or in our day, since you can't block the teachings, you can completely confuse them, fostering misconceptions, glamour, illusion, falsehood, and psychic disinformation.

The result is that people form occultly mistaken views on reincarnation and remain snared in illusion, even worse off than if they had remained ignorant altogether of the subject. If a person remains unaware of, confused about, or misdirected regarding one's karma, there is no possibility of becoming truly free while living as a biologically embodied human. You remain subject to the veiled agenda, ambushes, appointments, and upsetting events of your own karma. You are in effect hostage to your astral body. As nearly everyone else is as well, the psychic living conditions are a morass of astral affects.

Then prevent the disease process from revealing its soul/astral qualities; keep it mechanized, materialistic, and interventionary, and you prevent it from revealing its initiatory quality. Keep the superintendents of illness, medicine, and "healing" equally ignorant and materialistic, and you effectively keep everyone in the dark, living like automatons, like golems, humanlike figures of clay animated only with the uttering of a magical spell.

Who shall be the human-awakening astral magician: the soul/Sophia within every human or the Black brotherhoods using humans as familiars to keep the world a dead and darkened place?

If the Black brotherhoods win, you become unable to fully incarnate, to fully enter your body, to permeate every cell and molecule with your awakened soul qualities. You remain, practically speaking, the walking unborn; you are never a complete human; you are easily manipulated and influenced; you are not likely to progress with open, discriminating eyes across the Threshold into the supersensible worlds. You are most unlikely to be able to speak *as* the Logos to and re-create worlds with your Christed voice. Because you—and all of us—are the voice for the living Earth, the planet, too, remains dumb, mute, and hostage to its cosmic astral body.

It becomes unable to fulfill its purpose in the solar system, which is to be the generative larynx of bright new worlds spoken into existence by freely willing individualized humans. This planetary failure serves the interests of the Black brotherhoods.

The HAARP That Hurts the Angels' Ears

The black magic assault on the human environment also seeks to deconstruct the terrestrial expression of environment. The outer environment is as polluted with Ahrimanic elementals as is the human body. Might there be a lawful process of nature that is being blocked as the result, similar to the way the Ahrimanic elementals interpose themselves between the astral body and the microbial kingdom? The answer is yes.

The process in question is the interchange between celestial intelligences and the spirits of nature, more colloquially known as gnomes, undines, sylphs, and salamanders. These elemental nature spirits are the sentient agents of Sophia in the world of the four elements at the level of etheric substance. Their affiliations with the elements are as follows: gnomes/earth; undines/water; sylphs/air; salamanders/fire.

Probe the facade of nature and you will encounter these etheric denizens. World folklore, especially Celtic, Teutonic, and Scandinavian, has amply chronicled human interactions with these spirits. The lovely flowering of Scotland's new age Findhorn in the early 1970s focused the attention of a generation on these old archetypes of an intelligent nature; even the great god Pan made a cameo appearance in the Findhorn epiphanies.

In recent years, the presence of the elemental nature spirits is gradually insinuating itself into mainstream cultural awareness. In the film, *Labyrinth* (1986), a teenage girl must negotiate a devilish labyrinth to rescue her abducted infant brother, aided only by an ambivalent dwarf (i.e., gnome). *Splash* (1984) portrays a winsome mermaid (i.e., undine) whose charms win over a man. In *The Secret Garden* (1994), a lush but neglected flower garden proves wonderfully healing for several children; the nature spirits are practically seeable through the sparkling greenery that is their domain.

The elemental beings help to create the plant kingdom. "They are involved with the Earth and the Heavens coming into relation with the plant . . . [to serve] the nourishment of animal and man," explains Paul Scharff, M.D. In effect, the elemental spirits are the pantheistic "faces" behind what atheistic science later called the "forces" of nature. "It is the elemental beings who bring about the states of matter," Scharff says. "It is their working as forces in relation to substance that brings about the four states of matter."

These elemental beings toil within the etheric realm to create the four states of matter that comprise the world of substance—both our bodies and our terrestrial habitat—on behalf of humanity. But in doing this, they make a voluntary sacrifice that only humans can redeem for them. "Through the incarnation of Man, elemental beings come to be chained into the existence and workings of Earth and Earth kingdoms," says Scharff. "In turn, they need to be liberated to be returned to the higher spiritual world where they can continue their evolution."

As humans, we are responsible for freeing these "fallen beings" whose task is to build up substance for the incarnation and illumination of humankind. They create and sustain a world for us, but we must help them eventually pass on to a greater world.

The degree to which this idea strikes us as preposterous indicates how far we have deviated from this ancient pact between the subtle kingdoms of nature and our own humanness. But it's worse than oblivious neglect. We have interposed the Ahrimanic elementals between the nature Spirits and our physical environment.

Environmental pollution acts to seal out the gnomes, undines, sylphs, and salamanders from their rightful access into the world of substance; where it doesn't seal off their access, it distorts their energies and activities.

There is no longer any safe, uncontaminated place anywhere on the planet, says Theo Colborn. The once pristine Arctic is as polluted as steel industry-ravaged Gary, Indiana. PCBs—invented in 1929 as a family of 209 chemicals known collectively as polychlorinated biphenyls—are "world travelers," notes Colborn; they can travel through ecosystems and migrate over long distances. Thus we have laid a chemicalized blight on the landscape, interfering with the natural transduction of celestial energies through the kingdoms of the nature spirits and into the plant kingdom.

Modern technological civilization has further intruded upon the etheric domain of the elemental spirits through the deployment of various forms of extremely low frequency (ELF) electromagnetic wave technologies, microwave radar towers, and military adaptations of futuristic technology conceived by Nikola Tesla earlier in the century. The most flagrant example of this is called HAARP, for High-frequency Active Auroral Research Program, installed in Alaska by the U.S. Defense Department and scheduled for activation in 1998. Officials say the giant radio telescope is a benign academic project designed to change the ionosphere to improve global electronic communications by deploying a focused and steerable electromagnetic beam to heat the ionosphere.

Alaskan residents such as Nick Begich and Jeane Manning think the consequences will not be benign. HAARP's "super-powerful radio-wave beam may irreparably damage the planet's atmosphere and severely disrupt our mental and physical health," as they explain in *Angels Don't Play This HAARP.* The device will beam a billion watts of radiated power into the ionosphere, the protective "soap-bubble" membrane extending from 30 to 300 miles above the planet; these beams will then bounce back onto the Earth as long waves and penetrate our bodies, the oceans, everything. HAARP's real target is the electrojet, a "river of electricity" that flows through the atmosphere into the polar icecap. This electrojet will become a "vibrating artificial antenna for sending electromagnetic radiation raining down" on the Earth, say Begich and Manning.

The project may be "the most dramatic geophysical manipulation since atmospheric explosions of nuclear bombs." The HAARP "skybuster" could represent an unprecedented act of global vandalism; it also holds the potential for geophysical warfare by creating localized environmental instabilities and selective weather modification at the molecular level. Between 1945 and 1960, nuclear and hydrogen explosions sundered the fabric of matter and deposited in the environment a great deal of utterly toxic materials that are glacially slow to decompose.

Now HAARP—itself preceded no doubt by fifty years of undisclosed experimentation with similar neo-Teslan scalar wave technologies—will begin deconstructing the electromagnetic basis of the planetary environment. Soon the planet will be entirely unfit for true humans; only the downgraded mutants will survive. Developments such as these make the task of the nature spirits close to insuperable; these developments may also interpose severe obstacles between the natural commerce of humans and elemental beings in the *cocreation* of the environment, also part of the original pact.

It is worth our attention to re-examine the increasing incidence of "natural" disasters, such as floods, tornadoes, hurricanes, droughts, fires, and earthquakes, that have beset the U.S. and many other areas of the world in the last fifteen years. If we subscribe to the proposition that the universe is orderly, rational, and purposeful, then we must grant, however outlandish it seems, a degree of deliberateness to acts that insurance companies euphemistically call "acts of God."

For example, in Raymond Buckland's occult novel, *Cardinal's Sin,* a Vatican cardinal seeks revenge against the U.S. by using black magic to unleash terrific storms, earthquakes, floods, and fires. The elemental forces are natural, but their intensity is forced by the magic. "It was the storm, but a hundred times more powerful than it should have been," says a character. "It's almost as though nature itself was crying out to me. I picked up agony, confusion, and anger." In the film *Under Siege II: Dark Territory* (1995), a U.S. satellite is commandeered by terrorists who use it to create an earthquake.

Rumors abound that the intelligence and military communities of the U.S., the former Soviet Union, and other countries, have the means to generate earthquakes in targeted regions as a form of invisible terrorism. One must be particularly suspicious of any such events occurring on January 17 (such as the Northridge, California, earthquake of 1994 or the Kobe, Japan, earthquake of

1995) as this date represents a kind of black magic *Mardi Gras,* as it has for centuries. At least seventy years ago, Nikola Tesla demonstrated that scalar waves and other "technotronic" energies could produce localized geological imbalances. Nor may we discount the possibility of Black lodges manipulating the weather by commanding elementals to stir up fires (salamanders) or winds (sylphs) as a "favor" to their proteges, the Committee of 300 or whatever umbrella term we prefer to use to indicate the invisible government.

Terrorism in the form of "natural" disasters, though expensive in terms of relief management, pay fabulous dividends in terms of demonstrating the government's crisis management expertise.

We must also credit the possibility that if the Earth has an etheric field, might it not also have an astral layer, and if the planet's astral "body" is anything like that of the average human's—a roiling tumult of conflicting passions—might not this powerful energy configuration have serious effects on the weather? It is not necessarily unfounded to propose that there is a feedback loop between the human and planetary astral fields such that, to an extent, what the planetary astral body serves back to us in the form of meteorological disturbances may reflect what we, as a collectivity of men and women in a region, have roiling, oblivious to us, in our own astral-emotional bodies.

The result is weather by astral resonance, generated partly by a global (or regional) collective unconscious. And what's to say it's not manipulated and modulated along the way by those who have the technological or magical means?

Waging Star Wars in the Body— Conspiracy at High Levels

Something of importance to the cosmos has to be done through humans living on Earth, and at this juncture, medicine will either effectively block it or facilitate it. Nothing is more crucial in our time than the outcome.

As I touched on earlier, what's at stake is the incarnation of the Christ-Logos in human beings and the redemption of Sophia in the world of substance—the Mystery of Golgotha completed, globally. Success in this project will mean the emergence of truly *free* human beings, awake and knowledgeable within the world of substance, capable of willing freely as the living embodiments of complete cosmic intelligence. It will be the Word made Flesh becoming capable of the Flesh made Word again. The human will become a free-willing creator who creates by speaking.

Stars and planets and the Logos of it all will speak through each man and woman, and these Logos-speaking men and women will be in a position to re-create the environment along new lines. When the environment is re-created in this way, the Earth itself is reborn. We will know neither ourselves nor our home at the end of this epiphanous day.

Globally, every day there will be perpetual acts of White magic as the Flesh becomes Word again, illuminating all the hierarchies of creation, words returning mellifluously to the Word. In this scenario of liberation, empiric medicine is the midwife. As a result of its intelligent ministrations, like scarlet ink, the Christ permeates all the parchment layers of our being, Sophia, *physis*, and physical organism, quickening consciousness in this ultimate environment.

Alternatively, if the forces opposing this project prevail and permanently lock out the Logos on this planet and kill the Christ forevermore on Earth, then this shuts out the rest of creation. Blocked will be the "voices" of the planets and stars and their subsidiary elemental beings, the vowels and consonants of cosmic intelligence. Blocked will be the entirety of the etheric and astral levels of existence and with these, the soul of Sophia, the inner voice and wisdom of all substance, the conscience in humans. The inner life of humans will wither and die out; allopathic medicine will have triumphed in killing the soul in the human body.

This will imprison human beings in a deadening, opaque materialistic environment in which the ingress of spiritual light is blocked at all apertures. Humans will become organic automatons, easily programmed, decisively manipulated. Sophia will die within her body of substance and her four states of matter will grow dark. Humans will have no access to cosmic intelligence and will languish in a wasteland of ignorance and fear out of having no inkling of their origin, identity, or destiny—prodigal sons who never come home again on account of having utterly forgotten there is a royal home to return to.

It will probably be even worse than this because we must figure in the consequences of an unimpeded medicine-assisted organic *mutation* of the human through allopathic experimentation, toxic drug therapies, and the cumulative effect of a myriad Ahrimanic elementals given free reign. It will be a unilateral deconstruction of the spiritual aspects of the human being. Could we now see ourselves in this possible future, we wouldn't know ourselves. In this scenario of enslavement, rational medicine and its allopathic black magic "familiar" will be the executioner, killing the *physis* to starve Sophia and deny the Christ.

It is hard to conceive how this second scenario will benefit any human being living on Earth, for who could escape this? This outcome might be a bit more than the Black lodges bargained for, for these masters of the dark forces would also have to live within this spiritually denuded environment. We must always ask: Whom does the arrangement benefit? Surely this grim scenario could only benefit those who would *not* have to live within its confines or who would not be affected by its biological parameters. Logically, this points to something nonhuman or transhuman, in either case, not "people" are we know them.

We can answer this question by way of posing yet another one: If there are stars and planets in our body and planetary environment, and if there is this great dialectical struggle under way for the human soul, might there be certain stars that are against the emergence of human freedom? Might the human mind-body organism be a theater of war for a strange form of star wars waged within the human flesh?

There are by now many theories and assertions regarding extraterrestrial (ET) involvement in the history and current affairs of the Earth. Numerous books, television series, movies, and other expressions of popular culture attest to the suspected and, increasingly, presumed ET presence. The almond-eyed "greys" are the most familiar aliens—emotionless abductors or celestial savants, depending on your orientation. The government officially denies all such allegations but frankly, it's unlikely that anyone believes them. After all, *The X-Files* has hammered home the idea of a grand alien-government conspiracy for seven seasons and a full-length movie. In the 1980s, the general tone of the presumption of ET influence was favorable, benign, optimistic, even expectant, but in the 1990s, the cultural attitude has shifted toward a darker, sinister, manipulative scenario.

First they came to instruct, now they come to abduct; where formerly humans emerged transformed from the epiphanous close encounter of the third kind, now they struggle to fill in missing time and remove the implants. What is true versus what is delusional in these matters becomes harder to discern; occupying a mind-deranging middle ground is the considerable amount of disinformation purposefully generated by what many presume to be a collusion of ETs and governmental agencies.

Any allegations as to extraterrestrial agency are inherently shocking, if not fantastic, when it comes to naming names and indicating origins. One explanation put forward is that the prime ET agitators against human evolution are called Anunnaki who come from the planet Nibiru; this planet used to be an outer planet associated with Sirius (in Canis Major), and now is the unknown thirteenth planet in our own solar system, with a 3,600-year solar orbit.

According to Barbara Hand Clow, astrological counselor, psychic, and author, and proponent of this theory, the Anunnaki first began investigating Earth some 450,000 years ago; their activity as the "World Management Team" consists of manipulating humans within the already vexing materiality of three dimensions, says Clow. "The Anunnaki thought you [human beings on Earth] would become robots they could control with their thought, but instead you are dying."

The Anunnaki manipulate the uranium deposits on the planet and the radioactive residuals of an atomic war that was once waged on this planet, Clow writes. Their intention is to make Earth a radioactive planet and to use radiation as an "emotional frequency retardant" to block the articulation and resolution of human emotional bodies, which is to say, human astral bodies.

The Anunnaki use radiation to set up belief systems of limitation within the human emotional field; this in turn becomes the suitable precondition for illness, disease, and degeneration. "Uranium sticks emotions in your bodies, and then they run amok and become cancerous. But these tumors transmute radiation, they process it by means of cancer in your bodies, and the frequency of tumors indicates how polluted your environment really is."

The Anunnaki's goal is quotidian: world control. Their means are insidious: to block and distort memory. The true history of the planet and its human inhabitants—Clow calls these the myths of "Gaia's consciousness"—is registered in the Earth's etheric body, but the Anunnaki work to adulterate this information. "Instead, hoping to distract you from the real truth in these stories, the Anunnaki distort these original records by laying down one layer after another of distorted information in the pathways." According to Clow, the Anunnaki use allopathic medicine to keep humans in the dark. "It is more subtle to heal in the glands, and glandular healing techniques will end up being the way to bypass the more gross mechanisms of Anunnaki allopathic medicine."

Clow further suggests that the Anunnaki direct humans through the control allopathic doctors exert over human blood. This encompasses blood transfusions and the spilling of blood (both real, as in war, and simulated, as in movies). All of the Anunnaki manipulations of human beings in matter transpire in fourth-dimensional reality, conveniently beyond our ordinary perception. They also quite successfully interfere with what should be the natural relationship between three-dimensional (3D) humans and two-dimensional (2D) elementals, what we called earlier the *Keres*. "The 4D intelligences have crafted a great big smokescreen . . . just to keep you from seeing the brilliant 2D elementals!"

Clow's scenario of Anunnaki interference with human life and destiny helps us to conceive of the possibility of a conspiracy waged against humans at high levels, in this case, from a multidimensional platform beyond our common awareness. Clow outlines the involvement of other ET intelligences, such as the Pleiadians (our benefactors) and the Vegans from the constellation Lyra (of ambivalent intent). There are other scenarios for ET involvement and manipulation put forward by other writers, but all we need to take away from these allegations is the sense of probable manipulation of our reality from a dimension beyond our experience.

The fruit of such manipulation, whether it be benign or malign, is the total human being inhabiting and vivifying an organism whose substance is ultimately drawn from the stars and planets. In effect, our inner life consists of majestic and fearsome star wars roiling within our human body.

As Above, So Below, and in the Middle, Too

Leaving aside the specificity of which ETs from which location are the prime players, let's focus for the moment on discerning what their agenda might be and how allopathic medicine might be a principal tool in its achievement. As a starting point, let's presume that the ETs represent the fourth layer of the conspiracy against the whole human being, that behind the money-grabbers, social controllers, and black magicians, there is this even more occulted, inimical influence—the puppet masters themselves.

To understand the motives of this fourth conspiratorial layer, we must conceptualize globally. We must think in terms of how the totality of human beings on this planet affects the dynamics of the solar system and cosmos. Surely, if reality is orderly and rational, the Earth and the entirety of its residential human collectivity has a *purpose* to fulfill in the cosmos. Above, I suggested that one way to describe the presumed purpose of humanity is to be the living context for the incarnation of the Logos in the world of substance.

Something similar might be intended for the living planet as well; after all, the blood of Jesus Christ flowed at Golgotha to fructify the materialized Earth. From this confluence of interest and Christed initiation we might reasonably suppose that humanity and planet have a synchronous, possibly synergistic, purpose, namely, the redemption of substance and the illumination of environment. True to the Hermetic principle *As Above, So Below,* which is to say, the human is the microcosmic expression of the macrocosm, our fate as humans and the Earth's fate as a planet are exquisitely codependent.

To help make this clear, we must amend the Hermetic axiom just quoted to read: *As Above, So Below, and in the Middle, Too.* The middle is our planet where we find the galaxy on Earth.

Earlier, we touched on the concept of there being an equivalent etheric and astral topography for the planet, mirroring that in the human, which in turn mirrors that which exists as the cosmic foundation for life and existence. This view was supported by Rudolf Steiner and other anthroposophical researchers. Let's return to Clow's model for clarification on this point. The true history of the planet and its human inhabitants—Clow calls these the myths of "Gaia's consciousness"—is registered in the Earth's etheric body, but the Anunnaki work to adulterate this information. Clow adds that the precise places in Earth's etheric body where these myths and true memories of ancient times on the planet are deposited are called "vortexes," or what popular culture now scantily knows as sacred power points in the landscape.

The vortexes, which contain "records of stellar intelligence, the Galactic Mind," connect the Earth's "telluric fields with all dimensions." Long ago, individual plant and animal species were generated out of these vortexes at the places where pathways originating in the vortexes crisscrossed in the landscape. These generative line crossings are known by various names, such as *song lines* by the Australian Aborigines and the *lung mei* (dragon lines) in Chinese geomancy. In essence, the total planetary configuration of vortexes and energy pathways was once known as the Web of Life, says Clow.

Among proponents of geomancy, the Web is also referred to as the planetary grid. "Now the Web has become the Net that blocks travel by stellar intelligences in the pathways," Clow writes. In our time, the Web has tightened and almost closed up due to so many layers of Anunnaki lies. "Now the Earth vortexes are clogged and very inaccessible to higher dimensions, and that is why they need clearing."

Let's consider the implications of what Clow suggests. Behind the physical landscape there is another etheric or astral terrain with a purposeful configuration of energy lines and vortexes. Analogically, we might usefully compare this topography to that which is described in acupuncture: throughout the human body run numerous energy lines (meridians) carrying vital life force *(Qi)*, accessible at some 1,000 treatment nodes (acupoints). What Clow calls "energy pathways" the European geomantic tradition calls "ley lines," and what she terms "vortexes" we might, analogically, call acupoints in the landscape—*geopoints,* if you will.

Clow further suggests that at least part of the function of this Web of Life topography of ley lines and geopoints is to convey "stellar intelligence"—information, energy, codings, revelations from the stars vitally necessary for both human and planetary life.

As seemingly fantastic to everyday common sense as Clow's notion of a planetary Web of Life containing ley lines, geopoints, and insertion points for stellar intelligence, we find precedence and confirmation for the allegation in what British geomancers call a "landscape zodiac" or "template of the stars." There are many kinds of vortexes in the planetary grid, and one of them is the landscape zodiac.

In Britain, a fair amount of attention has been accorded one particular landscape zodiac. It is in the form of a huge, elliptical *zodiakos kyklos* or twelvefold circle of tumbling zodiacal animals and effigies, located in and around Glastonbury, Somerset, in the southwest of England. It's been called various names: Star-Spangled Avalon, Somerset's Star Fields, King Arthur's Round Table, the Glastonbury Zodiac, or as one commentator has it, drawing on Hebrew scholarship, *Shamarsheth,* meaning, "The Watch of the Heavens Established."

Earth mystery advocates claim that this is the anomalous presence of a terrestrial starwheel made of twelve earthen effigies accurately patterned and sequenced with their celestial counterparts (e.g., Taurus, Gemini, Cancer, Leo, etc.). All of this is laid out like a cookie-cutter template upon a circle thirty miles in diameter with Glastonbury in the middle. Within these massive landscape effigies (each several miles wide) are hundreds of numinous geopoints that receive "starlight" from many dozens of stars above. Among those who have heard of it, Glastonbury's Temple of the Stars has attracted equal measures of enthusiasm and skepticism.

The knowledge of the extent and operation of Glastonbury's zodiac was for long a guarded Druid secret. Aside from the isolated studies of the sixteenth-century Elizabethan astrologer, scholar, and occultist, Dr. John Dee, little awareness of landscape zodiacs was publicly expressed until the twentieth century, when the outlines of the Somerset starry domain first began to be sketched.

The indefatigably curious Dee immersed himself in matters of occult history and Druidic esotericism and allegedly made sufficient visits to the Somerset zodiac to prepare charts and a commentary, circa 1580, regarding this strange phenomenon. Dee noted the unusual arrangements of prehistoric earthworks in the Glastonbury area and the way they apparently represented the standard images of the constellations of the zodiac. "The starres which agree with their reproductions," Dee wrote, "on the ground do lye onlie on the celestial path of the Sonne, moon and planets . . . thus is astrologie and astronomie carefullie and exactley married and measured in a scientific reconstruction of the heavens which shews that the ancients understode all which today the lerned know to be factes."

The Glastonbury landscape zodiac wouldn't be publicly rediscovered until 1929, when a Canadian artist named Katherine Maltwood perceived a Somerset landscape replete with mythological giants. Maltwood had been preparing illustrations for a medieval French Grail text reportedly composed at Glastonbury Abbey and, as she discovered, it was apparently meticulously referenced to the local landscape, as if it were a handbook to an esoteric topology written in mythic code. She remembered reading the thirteenth-century antiquarian William of Malmesbury's gnomic comment that Glastonbury was "a heavenly sanctuary on Earth."

Maltwood had aerial photographs prepared of the Somerset terrain, then in what must have been a grand moment of inspiration, Maltwood *saw,* imaginatively, overlaid on the photos like a delicate patterned doily, the complete zodiacal circle of images. She saw the standard "skeletal" morphologies for the signs of the zodiacal twelve, Aquarius, Pisces, Aries, and the rest; their outlines were etched in streams, earthworks, drainage ditches, hedges, tracks, pastures, hills, mounds, and stone walls. Somehow, when seen from above, the ordinary domesticated features of the local British landscape outlined the images of the signs of the zodiac.

More remarkably, in some unconscious way, local farmers, road-makers, and grazers had maintained this landscape tapestry intact over the centuries. For Maltwood, mystically giddy and spiritually appalled by her discovery, this landscape feature impressed her as "a laboratory of thought and mystery."

It wouldn't be until the late 1970s that Maltwood's ideas were taken up again in earnest. Then landscape zodiac research was renewed, sparked in part by a more comprehensive, sympathetic treatment by another intrepid English woman, Mary Caine, in her *The Glastonbury Zodiac—Key to the Mysteries of Britain.* Caine extended Maltwood's bold claims by stating that the Somerset temple was not only the original, presumably mythic, Round Table of King Arthur, but also the template origin of Egyptian, Greek, Chaldean, and Celtic mythologies. Further, said Caine, this Somerset landscape Round Table had archeoastronomical significance: it was "a table of measurements charting the movements of the earth and heavens" such that "myths and maths were united in a splendid space-time scheme." The Somerset zodiac would be the first of *many* to be rediscovered; others have been identified elsewhere in England and France such as Rennes le Chateau near the Pyrenees.

The purpose of the zodiac is to display in a majestic tableau "the star-lore of all the ages, the source of all religious teachings," plainly depicting "the Fatherhood of God, the Brotherhood of Man," the process of creation, evolution, and resurrection, exemplified by a variety of mythic heroes, said Caine. "By such parables were the initiates in the Mysteries instructed. Well might our Zodiac have been prepared by God himself for the salvation of men." For Glastonbury mystical exegete Robert Coon, the Somerset star temple is "a Grand Ideal latent in the Somerset landscape," keyed to the spiritual-magical unfoldment of human consciousness and based on the Hebrew behind Qabala, the occult side of ancient Judaism.

"Each star temple within the Somerset zodiac represents a progressive stage of initiation," proposes Coon, who suggests that formerly men and women purposefully transited the starry landscape as part of a cycle of initiations and perhaps akin to what native Americans call the vision quest.

Geomantic information, such as indicated by Clow, Dee, Maltwood, Caine, and Coon, has been more of an open secret than anything innately elitist. Initiation in the mystery tradition or occult lodges in the West has necessarily involved the development and use of psychic or clairvoyant capacities, and if one wants to proceed very far in penetrating the mysteries of the bodily or planetary environment, the flowering of some degree of clairvoyant cognition is necessary. That's what makes it a mystery tradition: its content is not immediately apparent but only gradually revealed in accordance with the candidate's degree of preparation and cognitive flexibility.

This can't be helped: just as the human aura is only perceivable by the sensitive, intuitive, or psychic, so, too, are the subtle energetic aspects of our planet only "visible" to the clairvoyant.

Geomancy necessitates heightened perception and enhanced cognition. This of course is a major epistemological obstacle for Western science and its affiliate, allopathic medical thinking. Those familiar with the books of Carlos Castaneda recounting his initiation at the hands of Don Juan Matus, may have surmised that his training was serially referenced to specific landscape sites in the Sonoran district of Mexico. Even though he never overtly discussed the matter, Don Juan seemed to be intimately aware of their psychic potency and used them to facilitate the necessary shifts in Castaneda's consciousness.

In its simplest sense, the concept of a landscape zodiac refers to the presence upon a circular portion of the landscape of a subtle template of the twelve standard constellations (or houses) of the zodiac plus many dozen others. These form a miniature galaxy in the landscape, a living if subtle spiritual presence and an essential component in the planetary body of Gaia. They appear to be designed and intentioned that human interaction with this star map matrix is not only possible but necessary, essential for the well-being of Gaia as a planetary being.

This implies that not only was Castaneda's interaction with landscape sites in the Sonoran desert of benefit to his own initiation, but that they somehow contributed usefully to the tenor of being for all living organisms in that environment.

Just as the human totality is not complete without the indwelling of the Logos, so the zodiacal matrix is complete only with the insertion of a similar level of Logos consciousness. This can only come from human beings acting on behalf of the Logos, *as* the Logos. Here you have the galactic milieu of stars and planets present within a numinous terrain, awaiting fulfillment. The Logos gives it all coherency.

In a sense, the Earth, with its landscape zodiacs, is a big round version of the human being, with the same occult anatomy and physiology, the same fundamental configuration of etheric and astral energy fields. If so, then the Earth similarly needs an Ego, "I" consciousness, or Logos presence just as the human physical, etheric, and astral organizations require to complete the total human being.

Grid Wars in the Human Galaxy on Earth

The landscape zodiac is a miniaturized, holographic, experiential mirror image of Cosmic Man. By *Cosmic Man* I refer to the archetypal original ideal (pregenderized) human whose body is the cosmos, the stars, planets, and all the spiritual intelligences and hierarchies. You might think of this in terms of Adam and Eve as a composite being, along the lines suggested in an earlier chapter.

Alternately, Cosmic Man is Steiner's "gigantic being" whose body first appeared as the cosmos; from our perspective it's the original template from which each of the billions of humans who have ever walked Gaia have been fashioned. Cosmic Man comprises the three worlds of mineral, plants, and animals, or physical, etheric, and astral spheres; in other words, the formative expressions of the entire natural world, the planetary environment.

The zodiac is *miniaturized* for an obvious reason: the galaxy is vast, Earth is comparatively small, and miniaturization takes up minimal space while affording maximum content. Miniaturization also enables multiple sites; there are several hundred landscape zodiacs distributed around the planet.

The zodiac is *holographic* in that information about the entire system (the galaxy above) is distributed uniformly throughout the miniaturized system (the landscape zodiac below). Technically, one has simultaneous access to many expressions (i.e., different zodiacs) of this same system and to the original as well.

It's *experiential* because as commentators like Caine, Roberts, and Coon suggest, the zodiacal domain involves a high degree of interaction and participation, and in some cases, initiation. It's the epitome of environmental empiricism, inviting direct engagement.

Finally, the landscape zodiac is a *mirror image* because its key intention is to reveal an image of Cosmic Man through its stellar-terrestrial body. It's a bit like a hall of mirrors, potentially vertiginous but ultimately enlightening. As an individual man or woman, you look into the mirror of the landscape zodiac and behold Cosmic Man of which *you* are the living expression. All the stars in the galaxy add up to you—and me, and each other individual human who has ever breathed air on the planet. All the spiritual hierarchies of angels have their mandated residency and function within your human organism. That is what "microcosm" means, however shocking.

We can behold this in the zodiacal mirrors upon the surface of Earth. Our looking in fact completes the circuit, providing the essential missing ingredient: the presence of consciousness, of the human "I" that makes the whole system aware of itself and self-knowing.

The analogy of the hologram is useful here. One feature of the hologram is that it packs enormous information into a small space and codes it in an unfamiliar form, in this case, as wavy, squiggly contour lines that represent wave diffraction patterns but don't seem to resemble anything else. According to holographic technology, when light is projected onto the holographic plate, it reveals its original image. If we make a hologram of an apple, the holographic plate wouldn't look like an apple; it would be meaningless contour lines. But when we shine light on the plate, a virtual (or astral) image of the apple appears in space. So the hologram is an intermediate, coded information state veiling its original form.

According to this analogy, the landscape zodiac and its prototype, the galaxy, are holographically encoded. Coherent light reveals their original content: the image of Cosmic Man. The coherent light is human consciousness or the Ego. When the myriad stars of the galaxy are cognized by the application of the light of consciousness, you behold the image of Man. The mystical tradition calls this the experience of cosmic consciousness; Buddhism calls it awakening to Buddha Mind. Awakening can happen in any dimensional expression of the hologram; when it's in the geomantic, it especially benefits Earth.

The zodiac is the lock, consciousness is the key, and geomancy is the hand that turns the key to open the door. The landscape zodiac, when perceived clairvoyantly, is a mirror image of everything that constitutes the human being, from mineralized anatomy to the "I" consciousness of the Ego. As such, it is the prime theater in which the battle for the control of substance in all expressions of environment is waged. Star wars for the simultaneous control of human and planet are played out in the same grid theater—the galaxy on Earth and as the human.

We must learn to think on multiple channels through holographic analogies, to construe the human and planet as isomorphic, same in essence, different in shape.

The human has an unconscious, so does the planet. The human has an astral body, so does the planet. The human has a complex interconnected web of meridians and acupoints, so does the planet. The human has chakras and planet-points in its aura, so does the planet. The human is a microcosmic expression of the galaxy, so is the planet. The human is the target of black magic manipulations, so is the planet. The human may be the recipient of an Ahrimanizing influence, so is the planet. The human needs to awaken, so does the planet. The human's efforts to awaken may be opposed by a consortium of interests, and so may the planet's.

The theater for opposition to planetary awakening is the landscape zodiac. Star maps in the landscape have a spiritual purpose, yet they can be used to accomplish political ends, either for good or bad, depending on whether they favor the unfoldment of human free will. The purposeful use of such etheric fixtures is necessarily occult; when it's directed toward promoting the good, it is white magic; when it's focused toward suppressing human free will, it is black magic. Both have happened, continually, over the course of the planet, and this dialectic continues through the present time.

Rumors circulate that Hitler's geopolitical goal, during the period 1933 through 1945, was to gain control over the pivotal grid locations (landscape zodiacs and related features) in Europe as a base for controlling even larger areas of the planet. As it is fairly well known today that Hitler had many Black occultists on his staff, the outcome, had he won World War II, would have been grim. Similarly, but this time on the white magic side of the picture, the Knights Templar also were aware of the etheric geography of Europe and the Mideast and sought to keep the routes and sites free for human spiritual development. The construction of numerous Gothic cathedrals—precisely situated and designed according to the canons of "sacred" geometry—throughout Europe was part of their plan of maximizing the grid's potential for human spiritual upliftment.

In our own time, conflicts in Jerusalem, Lhasa, Baghdad, Sarajevo, and elsewhere, are attributable to planetary grid issues. It is not an exaggeration to suggest that the world's history might be usefully reconstructed based on a knowledge of etheric geography and geopolitical goals occultly pursued. Under any circumstances, this is not an easy subject to broach; for the purposes of this book, we can limit the discussion to a focus on how this feature of etheric geography can be used either to support or suppress the inhabitation by consciousness of its rightful environment.

How can an etheric landscape zodiac be used to suppress consciousness? By resonance. I have established that the essence of such a terrestrial star map is a copy of a cosmic image of Man; this same image is livingly embodied by every human being that has lived and is living today. Numerous stars and the planets inhabit and, literally, inform both the human and the planetary body. A precise and fluid and perpetual feedback loop exists between the three domains involved: above (cosmos), below (human), and middle (planet), as based on the same basic morphology. Astrology, properly, maturely, and occultly understood, is an appropriate descriptive language for this feedback system.

The matter of appropriate and ineluctable *timing* operates in the human and planetary realms, whether it's a health crisis in an individual or a spate of terrorist bombings in a country.

Referring to the layout of Mayan temple sites, Frank Waters wrote: "The alignment of sites and buildings thus helped to align the lives of the people with the structure and nature of Creation, and the source of man's own consciousness." The landscape zodiac can broker influences to humans living within its environs in two ways. First, there is the natural, perpetual transmission of astrologically described energies and influences from star point in the landscape to star point within the human mind-body organization. Second, there is the willful *addition* of forces and pressures through this matrix through the agency of other humans or other intelligences.

Sundering the Web
of Reciprocal Maintenance

Let's take Lhasa, for example, the political and spiritual capital of Tibet. There is a landscape zodiac in its midst; the city is expertly designed in accordance with its geomantic endowment.

From the Potala, the Dalai Lama's residence and seat of government, spiritual influences of a beneficent kind can be transmitted through the Lhasa zodiac out into a significant portion of Tibet. According to ancient legend, most of Tibet's landscape was taken up with a "Supine Demoness" *(srinmo yaksi)* whose head faces east and whose feet face west; her heart lay in Lhasa. Since the usurpation of Tibet by Communist China in the 1950s, great efforts were made to deconstruct much of Tibet's templic structure and to secularize Lhasa. The Chinese may have been venal, but they weren't occultly stupid. The best way to defeat a spiritually based country is to adulterate or deactivate their templic transmission points, in this case, Lhasa, chiefly, then the many other subsidiary sites around the "Demoness'" landscape body. Not only does this block the transmission and flow of beneficent spiritual influences through Tibet, but it blocks the contribution of this zodiac to the global etheric condition.

We must conceive of each of the planet's numerous landscape zodiacs as vital organs in the global organism. The more of these that are blocked, adulterated, deactivated, or destroyed, the less consciousness (cosmic intelligence) can flow through the system, and the planet remains stagnantly asleep. But as the planet goes, so go we; as more planetary grid points become coopted by black occultists, it becomes increasingly difficult for humans to remember *who* they are, as cosmically originated beings, *why* they are here on the planet, and *how* to wake up and reclaim total health.

From the viewpoint of the Black brotherhoods, this is precisely the point: they would prefer we stay asleep and submit with minimal awareness to the mechanization of life and automatization of consciousness. This is, after all, the Ahrimanic goal. The plan works best when nobody, or very few, are aware of it; the fastest way to keep things secret is either to suppress it outright or, even better, to distort it by way of disinformation, sending the gullible on end-less diversions and digressions. This makes it practically impossible for humans to fulfill their properly mandated responsibility: to par-ticipate in the web of *reciprocal maintenance.*

The concept of reciprocal maintenance has been elaborated in different wisdom traditions, including that of Russian metaphysi-cian G. I. Gurdjieff. Animals, humans, nature spirits, the planetary spirit, and celestial beings mutually support one another in an inter-dependent web, said Gurdjieff. As J. G. Bennett, a Gurdjieffian explicator, explained, "Full renewal requires full mutuality. It is by Universal giving and receiving of energies that Cosmic Harmony is maintained. The commandment becomes: 'Fill your place in the Cosmic Harmony or perish.'"

On a global level, the way we as humans can fulfill our role in the web of reciprocal maintenance is through infusing the body and planet with consciousness, awareness, self-reflexivity—by inhabiting our material environment with that which is rightfully, inalterably *human.* First, we must stop bifurcating the world into body and planet. Both are identical, except for shape, and both comprise the galaxy of cosmic intelligence with the Christ Ego at the core. Sec-ond, we must extend awareness into the physical body and plane-tary landscape. Western science and medicine have hoodwinked us into believing both are inert, unresponsive environments, subject to anomalous perturbations (illness or storms) and best suited for mechanical manipulation by experts, be they priests, scientists, or doctors. We believe this at our peril. Third, we must work to heal both domains simultaneously and equally; in essence, they are one and the same environment—our human environment.

Probably the most vivid example indicating how out of touch we have become with this web of reciprocal maintenance is the near-ly global fear that has arisen in the face of rampant, drug-resistant or newly mutated infectious microbes. Microbes may be the unseen power that runs the biological world, but they should be ruled by humans, the seen power that embodies the spiritual world. As I indicated earlier, in the best of circumstances, things running this way are the fruit of initiation and inner development. In our time, our oblivion of this initiatory necessity is compounded by willful distortions and adulterations of the web by black occultists to make it doubly hard for humans to struggle into awareness and competency.

Unfortunately, the World—humanity, the planet, the solar system—urgently needs us to surmount these considerable obstacles, wake up, and infuse our bodily and planetary environment with consciousness. Again, Frank Waters expressed it well. Given the fact that consciousness informs every cell in the human body and the Earth, "it is not too difficult to believe that all our planets contribute to the higher consciousness of the solar system, and it, in turn, to the consciousness of the living body of the galaxy which embraces it."

Put simply, we must all get mystical fast to catch up with what's been done to our environment while we were sleeping. It may seem a long way from the freedom to practice and receive alternative medicine, but, truly, it is only an injection away. Medicine is the gatekeeper of our future.

The Unpurified Astral Body Is Like a Golem

In the ninth century A.D., when reports of the American continent reached the spiritual leaders of Europe and their occult advisers from the secret societies, it was decided that the occult energy of the American landscape was too formidable for Europeans as they were at the time.

The American landscape would have prematurely introduced Europeans to the Ahrimanic influence of the Double—their karmic body—and produced damage to their souls. Presumably, this influence was successfully accommodated, if not mastered, by the native Americans already living on the American continent. Now evidently it was necessary to expose the European soul to Ahrimanic America, and for this exposure to proceed, it was necessary for the previous landscape masters to fade away.

Some centuries later, beginning in 1492, the date of the official European discovery of America, this Ahrimanizing influence was evidently judged more manageable, and immigrants began spreading across the large continent. Up until the twentieth century, it was primarily Europeans who arrived; in the last 100 years, representatives from nearly everywhere else have come.

Now in the 1990s, the U.S. is preeminently the country of immigrants, a global nation comprising citizens from quite possibly every known nationality. In effect, people whose country of origin might be Germany to Borneo, Mongolia to Chile, Norway to Gabon, are now each American citizens, subject to the powerful influence of the landscape. Politically, few will argue that one goal of the American polyglot population is to construct a global democratic commonwealth, with citizens of every nationality enjoying equal rights and opportunities under the law.

Yet it's not America, the McDonaldized melting pot of world cultures; the nation of immigrants is also a land of the New Regionalism, according to *The New York Times*. The Northeast maintains its ties to Europe, Miami is the conduit to Latin America, Texas is the Mexico link, and the West Coast stays cozy with the Pacific Rim. America is fast becoming a world country.

Lest this sound like a recitation of civic boosterism, we must remember the roots of democracy are biochemical and immunological. To live, act, move, and speak as individuals, one must be able to elaborate one's individuality at the molecular level. There must be democracy in the immune system—here negotiations between self and not-self are continuously made, resulting in idiosyncratic individuality—for there to be freedom at the political.

Evidence has been presented in this book suggesting that there is considerable opposition to this unfoldment and that one of the prime vectors of this organized opposition to human soul growth is state-mandated allopathic medicine.

The Double, as we learned in Chapter 2, is a spiritualized copy of an individual human, bearing its endowment of illness, desire, and karma. It is a shadow copy of ourselves—in fact, it is a lot more than we take ourselves to be—lurking in the unconscious. The Double is akin to the concepts of alter ego, phantom, shadow, mirror image of the self, the darker, unacknowledged aspects of the self, or the deceptive image of one's own shape—another you, if somewhat distorted. The Double accompanies humans under the threshold of consciousness, subliminally; though we encounter it every night during sleep, during our waking daytime consciousness, we are oblivious of the Double.

Basically, the Double is the human astral body, that troublesome repository of desires, wishes, rages, passions, sympathies, antipathies, memories, intentions—our total being, past karma, and personal destiny. The Double is the bearer of our karmic liabilities, long-held intentions, aspirations, and vows as well as injuries and unfulfilled desires. The Double, as astral body, is chiefly the body of sympathies and antipathies, likes and dislikes, the inchoate emotional vortex of Sophia, *humanized*. Mythologically speaking, it is the "body of shame" Adam and Eve assumed in Eden after consuming the golden apple.

More precisely, it is the body that is capable of knowing evil and goodness, and of choosing between the two. It is the ambivalent fruit of the Tree of the *Knowledge* of Good and Evil.

Were we able to behold a person in whom the astral body was well developed, stated theosophical occultist Annie Besant, "the astral body is clearly outlined and definitely organized, bearing the likeness of the man, and the man is able to use it as a vehicle." The astral body of the undeveloped human, says Besant, is more of a "shapeless mass," unable to travel far from the physical body and not too active as a vehicle of consciousness. Besant explains that after death, when the physical and etheric bodies have dissolved away, the astral body rearranges itself according to a sevenfold stratification of concentric shells, of which the densest lies on the outside.

The common conception of Hell—summarized vividly in Dante's *Divine Comedy*—is based on this occult reality. Depending on a human's spiritual development and refinement of the astral body while alive, so is his "confinement" with an astral shell of postbiological existence. "Until this shell [belonging to a man of "very low and animal tendencies" and hence of "the grossest and densest kind of astral matter"] is disintegrated to a great extent the man must remain imprisoned in that section of the astral world, and suffer the annoyances of that most undesirable locality," says Besant.

Whatever content of the astral body remains unexpiated at death, continues as a latent germ or tendency that *must* be incorporated in the next astral body that individual forms in preparation for a new human birth, Besant explains. "We never begin a new life with a clean sheet on which to write an entirely new story; we do but begin a new chapter which must develop the old plot." This old plot is the basic script for the astral body doing business as the Double.

Known to occultists throughout time, the Double has gradually been brought to limited public awareness in the past thirty years. The inveterate inner explorer Robert Monroe described the "Second Body" vividly in his now classic *Journeys Out of the Body*, which recounts astral incursions he experienced during the approximate period 1958 to 1970. At first, Monroe thought he was being followed by an inimical spirit; it took a number of encounters before he figured out that this "someone, a body, warm and alive, pressed against my back the moment I left the physical body" was his own Double.

The Double, or Second Body, Monroe learned empirically, resembles "a filmy piece of grey chiffon" and has a "strange rubbery elasticity" and may assume any shape its owner desires. He also learned that his Second Body was capable of moving and acting independently of his physical body, that to an extent, his conscious mind was able to direct it, and that some sensory inputs registered in the Second Body were incapable of translation into the physical. "There are unfolding areas of knowledge and concepts completely beyond the comprehension of the conscious mind of this experimenter," Monroe concluded.

In his next book, *Far Journeys*, Monroe recounted his astral anthropology among the "rings" beyond the physical plane. These are multiple layers of sentient human life, quite reminiscent of Dante's hierarchy of Hell, Purgatory, and Heaven in *The Divine Comedy* or for that matter, the Buddhist Wheel of Life and its six realms (blissful gods to despondent hungry ghosts).

Monroe describes his out-of-the-body experiences of "cruising the rings," sampling the quality of "life" and awareness at different layers of the astral world. He encountered the Dreamers (still physically embodied, but dreaming), the Locked-Ins (dead, but they don't know it). Out beyond this, Monroe found a layer of "stunned" souls, who know they're deceased but short of options for the next step. In the outermost ring Monroe found the Last-Timers, souls preparing for a final incarnation. The analogy is not stretched to compare Monroe's multiple rings with a sixty-channel cable television hookup. Cruising the rings, surfing the channels—in either case, one is able to view astral life from a position of relative detachment.

The Double, or human astral body, is the Lesser Guardian of the Threshold, as Rudolf Steiner explained. It stands with its "old plot" like Cerberus at the liminal gates of initiation and the supersensible worlds, be our experience of them heavenly or hellish. According to Steiner's concept of "geographic medicine" and etheric geography, the American landscape gives a resident's apprehension of the Double a distinctly Ahrimanic quality.

There are two effects at play here. First, a heightened activity of the human astral body, an enhanced potential to become aware of it, and a nearly guaranteed propensity to be strongly influenced by it. The trouble is, to be influenced unknowingly by the astral body is quite dangerous, both spiritually and socially. Consider the fact that with America as a *world* country, there are present on American soil humans with astral bodies representing every nuance of human culture, folklore, history, and human darkness that exist on the planet.

Formerly these variations observed national borders and were in effect chaperoned by the national tutelary folk soul, or presiding archangelic influence that maintained subtle sociological and spiritual gates between conflicting astralities. But today, the borders are soft, fluid, permeable—melting. So America is also a country of world astrality, probably a unique condition in the history of the Earth. Further, as the norm for human behavior, regrettably, is not to expiate, purify, cleanse, and render conscious the astral body but to be buffeted and directed by it, we have the occult makings of a highly turbulent, chaotic psychic atmosphere.

Set this into a landscape whose geographic energy heightens the astral body and you have a collective unconscious of activated but unexpiated astral bodies. It is a bit like a nation of *golems*. A *golem*, according to Jewish mystical tradition, is a fake human being, a simulacrum made of clay, made as a factotum by a rabbi or black magician who animates the human clod with a magical word. In the famous folklore tale, *The Golem of Prague*, one such golem cuts loose of its rabbinical control and starts creating major trouble in the medieval city.

During the late-1500s, Rabbi Judah Loew of Prague wanted to find a way to stop the harassment of the Jews. One night in 1580 Rabbi Loew dreamed of a Hebrew text that advised him to make a "golem of clay to destroy those tearing Israel's heart." One night, after a week of fasting and prayer, Rabbi Loew and two assistants went to the banks of the River Moldau. Using river clay, they fashioned a full-grown man lying on his back; on his forehead they wrote *Emet*, which is Hebrew for "truth," and on his tongue they slipped a piece of paper bearing the unspeakable Name of God. Then the good rabbi circumambulated the clay figure seven times, reciting mystical combinations of Hebrew letters. Soon the body glowed like burning goals and mist rose off its form; then it breathed and opened its eyes.

Thus the golem was born, this shapeless mass conjured and animated by magic to resemble a man. Mind you, he may have been a "fake" human, but he was as strong as ten, invulnerable to fire or flood, capable of being invisible, and basically indestructible. Rabbi Loew employed him as his servant and factotum, especially when Jews were in physical danger or being plotted against. Nobody knew the golem was not a real man, but once the Rabbi's wife mistakenly bade him fetch water. He emptied so many buckets of river water in their house he nearly drowned them all. Eventually "Joseph," for so they named the golem, had done everything Rabbi Loew envisioned to protect the life of Jews in Prague.

During a special ceremony, Rabbi Loew erased the letter "E" from his forehead (because *met* means "dead") and removed the slip of paper from his tongue, and the golem collapsed into a lifeless lump of clay, which they buried in the attic.

Everything ran smoothly for Rabbi Loew, but not for Rabbi Jaffe in Poland. His golem, trained to light Sabbath fires, got out of hand and nearly burned the village down. It was the same with Elijah Baal Shem of Chelm; he had to deftly remove the magical *shem* from his golem's tongue because he had run amok and was trying to destroy the world. Normally the rabbi removed the *shem* every Sabbath eve, turning his golem back to inanimate clay, but one Friday night he forgot and the golem started running about town, shaking the houses, breaking the windows. Eventually, they were able to stop it and decommission the golem for good.

Perhaps this is why the golem figure slips so easily into the image of Frankenstein, the artificial human run amok, the monster offspring. We see it as well in the Sorcerer's Apprentice, in alchemy's homunculus in the retort, and in the macabre story by Jorge Luis Borges in which a man laboriously dreams up a man and gives him life only to find that he, too, is not singed when he walks through fire—meaning he, too, is a golem.

Likening the golem to the unpurifed astral body has more than analogical merit. Consider how things normally work. A person believes that his attention—available consciousness—is situated in his personality as it inhabits the physical body. The true seat for and identity of consciousness is the Ego, or "I," and the intermediary state, which interacts with both, is the astral body. However, if a person in his normal waking state is functionally unaware of his astral body and if the Ego remains remote and aloof from the astral organization, in effect, the astral body is somewhat independent although it is largely programmed according to the necessities of fulfilling its "old plot" and karmic liabilities.

As such, the astral body runs on automatic pilot, spiritually unsuperintended, a lot like the golem named Joseph who nearly drowned everybody by repetitively—unconsciously—filling buckets of water. He lacked an Ego, the self-aware equilibrating center of consciousness.

The second effect is that the heightening of the activity of the astral body assumes an *Ahrimanic* cast. American astrality is Ahrimanic. This means a tendency to materialize everything, to lock out the spirit, to squeeze it into material parameters, to exalt physicalized or mechanized intelligence at the expense of cosmic intelligence. Ahriman seeks to densify everything, to bury it under the gravity of unconscious matter, heredity, separatist, racial, tribal, "blood," and conflicting, parochial victim identities—a Balkanization of the soul. This state of mind fosters an intelligence riveted on only tangible things, materialistic science founded on measure, number, and weight, and anti-*physis* allopathic medicine based on false, illusory data about the human being.

Ahrimanic means a contraction into time and single lifetime, body-based identity—the self that is skin deep. It is also about the apotheosis of personality the American specializes in: celebrity. In Ahrimanic America, everyone desires their narcissistic fifteen minutes of fame, and increasingly, many achieve this televised ephemerality. American culture has become a franchise of the celebrity cult—planet Hollywood—and the Ahrimanic geography supports it. Ahriman is the contraction into unmystical preening selfhood, a world made of oneself—the prima donna lifestyle.

Freedom in Ahrimanic America means "the proud feeling of manifesting [oneself] in the action," Steiner explained; it's like walking around with a video camera perpetually filming oneself throughout the day. Ahrimanic geography seeks to hold humans spellbound and permanently fastened in a sense-bound way to the materialized Earth, having turned all spiritual truths into boringly visible stone. The soul under an Ahrimanic enchantment requires not edification but entertainment.

As Steiner wrote, "The Ahrimanic powers succeed in ensuring that the Ego is only very loosely connected with the human being." All the better to keep us golems.

Ahrimanic America:
Watching the Double on TV

Coincident with the influx of individuals from every part of the world onto American Ahrimanic soil was the development of first movies, then television. Other than allopathic medicine, there is probably no other perfect vehicle for imparting an Ahrimanic influence upon the human soul than these two mediums. As Marshall McLuhan rightly declared, the medium *is* the message; in this case, the message of the medium of movies and television is the astral plane, that roiling cinematic tableau of human life, past, present, and future.

Consider the technology itself and its buried revelation: dramatic, flowing images—stories—are projected through light onto a screen or through a specific bandwidth in the electromagnetic spectrum and decoded electronically for projection onto a screen. The revelation of the medium of movies and television is that the astral plane—the human astral body—is an interactive tableau in light set in motion by human feelings.

On the astral plane, life *is* a movie, because you can see personal events and dramas in their fourth dimension—as a flowing time tableau. Here life events make sense because they can be viewed in a time context: you can see the beginning and end, the causes and motivations; in ordinary three-dimensional life, these crucial factors of the story are usually veiled, making it hard to see the sense in a great deal that happens. Thus movies by their medium impart the message of the reality of the postdeath astral review.

Occultists such as Rudolf Steiner assure us that following death, one is obligated to review all the events of life, both in the daytime and dreamtime: this is the actual contents, in full, of the astral body. During this review, motives and causes are revealed and the outcomes of karmic liabilities fulfilled, or not, become painfully evident. This process is condensed and materialized in making a movie; when we see the movie for what it is, it becomes a vehicle for initiation, at least once. Remembering his experience of watching movies in a large theater as a youth, William Irwin Thompson observes that "the movie theater became for me a ritual of initiation, the Paleolithic cave of Lascaux and the ancient Greek mysteries of Eleusis in one."

Robert Monroe could cruise the spectacle of the astral rings in the same way that we can flip channels on our cable-equipped television and watch soap operas to nightmares. In a sense, but not literally, the astral plane is the same intangible place as television programs in transit from network to set. Both, from our perspective, are located somewhere in the vast electromagnetic field spectrum of frequencies; as soon as we have the means—clairvoyance or a television set, respectively—to tune in, we can watch the action.

Film, but more intensively, television, present the reality of the astral plane through its technological medium. More importantly—but troublingly so—they serve up the manifold treacheries and violences of our uncleansed collectively unconscious astral body. All it requires is a moment's self-reflexivity while watching television to get the message from the Ahrimanic Double. If we can switch from following the entertaining drama to realizing that this drama carries an educational content, namely, a portion of our Ahrimanic cultural Double that desperately requires purgation and redemption. The trouble is, if you don't become aware of it, it runs your life.

Coast to coast, it's a televisionized—and televised—country. As cultural critic William Irwin Thompson notes, Americans have replaced culture with Disneyworld, historical reality with CNN, and incarnation with Gnostic technologies such as virtual reality and artificial intelligence. Europe lacks it but America has it in spades: "an electronic *Umwelt* in which history is replaced with movies, education is replaced with entertainment, and nature is replaced with technology," says Thompson. American Disneyland culture has become "a commercial from which there is no escape."

Our shadow is served up nonstop twenty-four hours a day on television, expressing repetitive content as if stuck on a single low-life astral "ring" that specializes in violence, murder, mayhem, deceit, greed, horror, rape, torture, mutilation, revenge, brutality, cruelty, depravity, and the like. Sexual interests of all kinds find their expression in movies, available as videos for television viewing. Disasters, both contrived and real—from *The Towering Inferno* to the Oklahoma City bombing, from *Fearless* to TWA Flight 800—are available for our titillation or shock.

At this point, practically *anything* conceivable is watchable on television, and Hollywood will spend fabulous sums to make it happen, such as $60 million for *Independence Day* and $100 million for *Waterworld,* and still greater amounts for *Titanic* and *Star Wars: The Phantom Menace*. Action movies—Sylvester Stallone's *Judge Dredd,*

Arnold Schwartzenegger's *Eraser*—have surpassed the state of being visually stupendous and unrelentingly stimulating, and have become almost numbing. Ghosts, ghouls, phantoms, vampires, goblins, extraterrestrials, fairies, gnomes, angels—all have been given virtual reality as moving images on television. Similarly, anomalies of space-time, serial lifetimes, lucid dreaming. multiple identities, and shape-shifting have been simulated for movies.

Even allopathic medicine has its astral "ring" devoted to perpetual self-glorification, as indicated by the runaway popularity of *E.R., Chicago Hope,* and *Rescue 911.* These shows portray—erroneously, as we noted in Chapter 1—the heroic, emergency side of modern medicine, with its chest thumpings and last-minute cardiac resuscitations of dying patients by skilled doctors and nurses.

The opportunity of having our collective astral shadow portrayed daily on television is that we can see it, acknowledge, accept, redeem, and transmute it for the benefit of all. The liability is that few consider watching television to be a vehicle for occult initiation and take the stimuli into their own being without conscious discrimination; once inside, it roils, revs, stirs, shakes, disrupts, and incites the soul like poisoned candy or toxic fruit. Random shootings and unpremeditated violence may be results of this subliminal churning of unprepared souls. Completing the feedback loop, this unexamined astral content churns up, filters, distorts, and seriously influences our waking consciousness, deepening the Ahrimanic spell.

There is another occult drawback to this medium. The phenomenon of television itself is highly Ahrimanic: it reduces the Sophia of the soul, which is the positive, exultant, celestial side of the astral body, to an electronic, mechanized intelligence. TV gives us the astral plane in a plastic box. Meanwhile, the spiritual realities and dangers of the astral plane are purposefully obfuscated because such images and statements do not please the commercial sponsors. For the world's population converged upon Ahrimanic America, the medium of television is an ambivalent initiator, the Lesser Guardian of the Threshold with an attitude, the psychopomp of the uncritical unconscious masses.

The trouble is, this is a virtual initiation; television is only a simulacrum of the astral plane; a movie star or TV celebrity is no more a psychopomp than a *golem* is a rabbi—or a human being.

Television and film give you a preimagined world; they preempt the internal imaginal process of finding images to render supersensible realities. This medium has the tendency to sidetrack, distract, or deactivate the faculty of developing imaginative cognition, giving one and all a predetermined content. The trouble is, this is a content regarding an illusory realm. The images fed into one from television and movies circulate through the etheric and astral bodies, leaving vivid impressions.

Were you able to observe the etheric body after watching an action film, you would behold a virtual replay of the film in the etheric configuration about eight inches from the physical body. The film's moving images form a kind of coating over the natural picture-making activities of the etheric body; the film's emotional content acts like seeds in the astral body, sprouting little flowers of distorted emotionality.

As a result, and given enough viewing of this medium, you will never be able to develop authentic imaginal cognition. Hence, you cannot authentically and purely perceive or enter the supersensible worlds because you will always be looking through the human-made picture-emotion fog. The images that lodge in the etheric and astral body make it harder for legitimate messages and content to percolate into waking consciousness. It becomes harder to have dialogue with your soul to understand life purpose, destiny, and perhaps the meaning of illness as it arises.

The karmic dialogue is somewhat obstructed, but so is the healing process that should be transmitted from the etheric body. If it is full of somebody else's imaginal pictures, your own natural healing potential—the therapeutic word force of the etheric form—is no longer available in full strength. Illness could result, and once established, could be harder to shift on account of the weighty influence of the film of Ahrimanic pictures.

Not watching television or the movies does not exempt one from contact with this initiating Ahrimanic Double, for it has already permeated American culture. It *is* American culture and you live within its atmosphere. Welcome to planet Hollywood, what's your dream?

The Cyberspace Cerebral Delusion: Spiritually Dead on Arrival

The 1990s was the decade of Internet, cyberspace, the World Wide Web, and an unprecedented amount of hyperbole, even bombast, about it all. The modem has emerged as the deus ex machina of world brotherhood, the global nexus among PC-wired minds. According to culture critic Mark Slouka, the cyberspace debut represents an assault on human identity, place, community, and reality—it is a road to unreality, "marking our growing separation from reality," Slouka says.

Cyberspace whisks us away, as electronically digitized minds, from our sense of place within a community and our connection to a particular landscape, and it deposits us in a nonlocal synthetic mind realm—"a computer-induced hallucination" set in "electronically generated space." No longer is it the avant-garde science fiction writers such as William Gibson who speak of uploading one's mind to the Net, leaving the body behind. Virtual reality developments increasingly approach this fantasy with the technological means to make it an actuality. "Physical presence would become optional; in time, an affectation," Slouka suggests, extrapolating cyberspace philosophy into the near future.

With human physical presence rendered irrelevant and therefore, ontologically obsolete, so, too, will planet Earth become irksome baggage in the posthuman cyberspace *hegira*. These attitudes, of course, are quintessentially Ahrimanic, and would fulfill Ahriman's intention of reifying, if not apotheosizing, human intelligence through technological means into a separate disembodied machine-generated sphere. Let's not overlook the obvious: strip away the hyperbole and you remember that computers are machines, mechanical contrivances.

Pull the plug out of the socket, and cyberspace dissolves away into the near nothingness it always was. "Near" because cyberspace is not completely unreal; like television, this technological medium has a message. Pierre Teilhard de Chardin called it the Noösphere—the global human mind. The trouble is, you can't get there from here using electronically contrived cyberspace. Spiritually, it is a dead end; it is a cerebral auto-da-fé, electronic suicide for neurotransmitters. It is no more real—or nourishing—than a *picture* of cake. Not surprisingly, Ahrimanic America is leading the world in the pursuit of this Noöspheric chimera.

Technology can imitate, literalize, mechanize, contrive, but it will never be a substitute for the real thing—the sensory-free global web of human intelligence. The reason you can't get to the Noösphere through your Macintosh is that the ticket of admission is an activated etheric body and a purified astral body. The true consort of human minds at a place removed—transcendent to—body-based life is perennial; is the realm of spiritual initiates. The Celtic Grail legend once gave it a name: *Sarras,* the spiritual city where initiates grounded their experiences of the ineffable Holy Grail.

Cyberspace is a simulacrum of Sarras: it may deliver a vague, almost homeopathic, taste of Noöspheric bliss, but it will never be realer than virtual. The other fallacy of cyberspace is that you can come as you are—the unexamined, unexpurgated personality; in Sarras, only those who can maneuver as "I's," spiritually awake Egos, ever get past the front door. The danger is that cyberspace is a fantastic distraction that will deliver its adherents nowhere; being nowhere, it will be double hard to retrace one's steps back onto the true—ontologically real—path, and doubly hard to muster the willpower to rely on one's spiritual exertions rather than some megabyte petard to get with *real* reality.

As with the planet Hollywood seduction, cyberspaced America bears a mixed message. It could represent the spiritual eclipse of humankind, as concentrated in multicultural America, by massive cognitive illusions, dumping us in mental Wasteland. Yet a distraction or seduction always implies a hunger, an unsatisfied yearning, an inarticulate wish. Speaking of addictions, Emily Dickinson once wrote: "Narcotics cannot still the tooth that nibbles at the Soul."

The best technology can give us are Ahrimanic reductions: television for an experience of the astral plane; cyberspace for a taste of the Noösphere. Given the choice, wouldn't we prefer the original?

Finding the Soul of the World: Why the Fate of the Environment Will Be Settled in America

Planet Hollywood, cyberspaced America, this Ahrimanic nation—it could also represent the first steps of a breaking through the veil of materiality into an awareness of the soul of the world. America *could* emerge, not as despoiler, but as redeemer of the environment. It's by no means guaranteed.

The matter of "care of the soul" emerged in the 1990s as a salutary counterbalance to the hyperbole of cyberspace. The word itself—*soul*—came as a welcome return home to our own Western philosophical tradition, after nearly four decades of enchantment with Eastern spiritual traditions. Like everything in America, "soul" is already in danger of trivialization by the lures of commerce. Psychotherapist Robert Sardello, for one, is trying to preserve the purity of soul so it might be of genuine benefit to the spiritually hungry.

Soul is not limited to individuals and their interior life alone, but to the soul of the world, which Sardello describes as "a way of referring to the inseparable conjunction of individual and world." Soul wisdom, Sardello explains, is the capacity by which self-knowledge develops simultaneously, if not identically, "with an objective sense of the inner qualities of the outer world." This conjunction makes it possible—makes it *urgent*—that we learn to see through events, both in our inner life and in the outer world, and appreciate the subtle "circulation" and constant "re-creation" by which both world and self are continually remade. *Soul* is the name for this circulating force that animates self and world for the renewal and regeneration of both, says Sardello.

The emerging science of psychoneuroimmunology has shown a skeptical West how consciousness can effect, illumine, or sicken, the human body. Similarly, the Green philosophy of deep ecology, DharmaGaia, and ecofeminism have pointed the way for a reengagement with the interiority of the outer world. Rudolf Steiner's anthroposophy and the preliminary indications of a spiritualized geomancy (briefly sketched in this book) suggest how consciousness might simultaneously extend itself into both expressions of environment, body, and world.

In any scenario, what is most needed is the active presence of the human "I," that point of self-reflexive consciousness both beyond and within the individual. *Not I, but the Christ in me,* St. Paul declared on the road to Damascus, summarizing his conversion experience. *The Christed I in me and the world,* we might say. Medicine—our relation to the body—needs to be infused with this "Christed I" as does ecology—our relation with the environment. Into the world of stars resident in both the human body and the humanized planet, the Logos—the "Christed I"—must incarnate. It is our will to see to it that this happens, for only we can do it.

In this effort, Ahrimanic America may well make or break the entire project. Will the geographic medicine of the American landscape be too potent to swallow, or have we swallowed it wholesale without ever reading the label? Will the cold priests of the degenerate Mexican Mysteries prevail, metaphorically excising the hearts of Americans, or will the new hierophants of Sophia have the day, regenerating the soul of Man and of the world? Whether our fate is apocalypse or eucatastrophe, breakdown or break-through, we will know in this lifetime.

Finding ways to shift the balance in favor of a eucatastrophic breakthrough—a happy, if transcendent, "ending" which of course is a beginning—is the mission of this book. Once we awaken to the dialectic in which we are enmeshed, then we can take action. Cognition *is* action, let us not forget; perhaps it is three-quarters of the corrective action we need to take. Change the inner first, then reconfigure the outer. Cognitive reform first, then social, legislative reform. Then we may have an environment worthy of human con-sciousness, and one that can help it flourish on this planet.

Transfiguring Our Web of Environmental Relations

What would happen if empiric, holistic medicine became the main-stream form of medicine, instead of the up-and-coming alternative? How would this change our thinking about our body and our envi-ronment? Let's extrapolate the possible—one hopes probable—results from making one political change in our current medical set up: repeal the Medical Practices acts in the different states and restructure medical licensure so that all qualified health practitioners could practice openly and be reimbursed by insurers. How might this single change (which could result, by the way, from concentrated grassroots consumer lobbying) reconfigure the field of our environ-mental relations? If the empiric model became our consensus way of thinking about health and illness, how would things be different?

First, the transformation in attitude from allopathic passivity to empiric activity generates an awareness of self-responsibility in the resolution of illness and the co-creation of healthy environments.

An implicit emphasis in holistic, empiric medicine is that the dis-ability, illness, or disease underway in one's organism is relevant to one's life, one's sense of self, and how one has lived. It's also pre-scriptive of how one ought to live to avoid reproducing the condi-tion in the future.

I don't want to slip into the reductionist oversimplification of saying we *cause* all our illnesses, *make* all our accidents, and *produce* all our bodily woes because many of the effects we experience today were generated by "causes" yesterday. But that "yesterday" may be a multi-factorial complexity far in the past. To rationally account for the etiology of illness we need to understand the dreambody process, physics' model of quantum synchronicity, and a coherent theory of karma, multiple lifetime causality, and what the Buddhists call codependent origination. Provisionally, the safest and possibly most descriptive position to take is to invoke the image of *co-creation*: numerous interdependent factors over time in conjunction with our intention (conscious or unconscious) precipitate events in our body and life.

Empiricism counsels us to develop a fundamentally new attitude about such events, to adopt a philosophical stance that allows the inherent meaning and purpose of illness or any singificant bodily event to be revealed and discharged. Empiricism contends after all that the cosmos is innately rational, that it makes sense, that this rationality is distributed uniformly throughout every system and level of reality, and that this sense can be comprehended by anybody, with a little effort. Empiricism tells us there is a cognitive, teleological component to illness, a dreambody communication pertinent to our spiritual unfoldment waiting to be deciphered.

Here a little bit of the inherent medicine as Mystery revelation returns as a dynamic understanding. Illness or discomfort becomes an invitation for self-inquiry: why is this happening to me at this time? Clearly this requires a new activist attitude in the face of the health, illness, and healing process, a personal commitment to include these factors as legitimate, meaningful elements, even keys, in our growth, insight, development, and life fulfillment. An example here will help flesh out this idea.

I have a friend, a man in his mid-forties, who is otherwise healthy but has had problems with his back for two decades. He's a reasonably strong man though of medium build and height but for years he's had problems keeping his vertebrae in the right place in his spine. Chiropractors call this dislocation of vertebrae a subluxation; since his mid-twenties he's had a lot of subluxations and seen a lot of chiropractors but until recently his vertebral column was decidedly recidivistic and the chiropractic merely palliative. Chiropractic adjustments would fail to hold, his vertebral alignment would slip out again, and his problem remained chronic.

Does this problem have anything to do with him, with who he is, his identity, or issues about his identity? Empiricism says yes, decidedly. He hadn't seen a chiropractor for a couple years when he threw his neck out quite painfully one day. He made an appointment to visit the best chiropractor in his community, a doctor known for his holistic approach to structural problems. The doctor's treatment program called for a major restructuring of my friend's vertebral column from the pelvis up; when the pelvic foundation is set correctly, the rest of the structure will follow and maintain the alignment, the chiropractor told him.

Concurrently my friend became aware that the chronic instability of his spine might mirror something similarly uncertain within him. He saw that in a profound sense he had not been assuming sufficient responsibility for his *standing* in the world, for *supporting* himself, for being *upright* about his beliefs, for assuming an independent financial *posture*, and for truly inhabiting his body, allowing his Ego to *structure* his bearing as a person in the world. Note that these issues all involve structure, the psychological equivalent of vertebral alignment.

His Ego was not holding his body (and self) erect in the world. His dreams, meditations, journal work, and conversations with friends consistently alerted him to the necessity of taking these long unresolved issues in hand and standing upright on his own in his life. His intuition told him that should he bring them to resolution his chiropractic adjustment would finally hold and his spine at last would be set right. He realized that this was the perfect time in his life to resolve a complex problem that was expressing itself in multiple ways in his life, in his spine and his psyche. He knew he was ready to work with a good chiropractor to help with the physical aspect of an inner psychospiritual shift. His lack of vertebral integrity was a reflection of his lack of firm resolve, commitment, and responsibility to fully incarnate and, spiritually, to take the upright posture.

With this understanding as a strategy, he worked on his attitudes as his chiropractor worked on his spinal column. After three months the changes were dramatic. His entire body posture, his bearing, how he held himself, how he walked—all this was new and reformed. Naturally his chiropractor deserved a lot of credit for a competent adjustment program but my friend knew—and his chiropractor concurred—that the chiropractic work was lastingly successful only because he had been willing to do the complementary inner, psychological work at the same time so that his strengthened sense of self could work from within as an etheric force to support the corrected vertebral alignments.

Together, my friend and his chiropractor co-created a new vertebral alignment; the doctor used his skill to make the adjustments, my friend used his introspection to understand how to purge the psychological attitudes that were undermining the structural integrity of his body and life, knowing the ultimate source of good posture is the Ego.

Second, patient participation in the therapeutic processes of holistic medicine generates awareness of the life force—Hahnemann's dynamis *or the* physis— *and its role in environmental healing.*

Through his experience with chiropractic, my friend learned that there is an additional factor at play in the restitution and maintenance of health. His chiropractor's skill, his own rigorous introspection plus the innate healing response of his organism, what Hahnemann called the *dynamis*, the earlier Empiric tradition called the *physis*, and what holistic medicine today generally calls the etheric life force.

Something intangible, invisible, yet powerful nonetheless cooperates with our intentions and the physician's ministrations to restore our health. Inevitably our discovery of the existence and efficacy of the *physis* within the human organism inspires us to seek it in the ecological environment, to develop a sensitivity for the etheric life force in the natural world. Suddenly the old, discredited Nordic fairy tales and Celtic folk legends about industrious nature spirits take on a new face of probability; perhaps we remember stories we first heard back in the 1970s from the Findhorn Community in northern Scotland and their fabulous gardening success in cooperation with nature spirits and landscape devas; or more recently, we encounter information coming from the Perelandra Gardens in Virginia where Michaelle Small-Wright mapped out the modes of cooperative interaction between human gardeners and intelligences within Nature.

We appreciate how we might be able to communicate with the formative forces behind the physical aspects of nature and together co-create new environmental configurations in the flower garden or the landscape. We can take instruction from two prominent Western empiric scientists, Paracelsus and Goethe, whose appreciation of the *dynamis* in nature prompted a lifetime of research.

Paracelsus (1493-1541), the 16th century Swiss alchemist, physician, and esotericist, spoke of the *essentia* behind plant phenomena, the irreducible fundamental quality. He wrote also of the "Archaeus, the inner firmament," by which he meant the human etheric body enlivened by forces out of the cosmos, and thereby securing the link between endarkened matter and enlightened spirit. "He tried passionately throughout his life to come to know this directly through his senses, through studying phenomena themselves in their living activity," explains Alice Barton Wulsin, M.D.

With his "doctrine of signatures," Paracelsus explained how the plant's outer form is a physical signature of its inner etheric essence; the practical significance here is that correspondences between plant morphology and human form could reveal clues for untapped healing properties. Paracelsus' doctrine of signatures, says Richard Katz of the Flower Essence Society, implies "a cosmology that says plant forms reflect celestial forces which are also reflected in human organs. It's a matter of seeing cosmic principles written in the script of nature."

Extracting ideas about nature from the living botanical script similarly occupied Germany's great 19th century poet, dramatist, and natural scientist, Johann Wolfgang Goethe (1749-1832). Goethe adopted a living, meditative approach to science, particularly to the study of plants. Through an intense contemplation of the essence of the plant as a metamorphic process and activity over time, Goethe arrived at the perception of the "archetypal plant:" that all plants, regardless of shape, size, and climatological variation, equally express a fundamental quality, an archetypal plantness—the *Urpflanze*. "He sought the ideas which live in the things. When he observed nature, it then brought ideas to meet him," wrote Steiner, who spent seven years editing Goethe's scientific papers and wrote several books about Goethe's epistemology.

"He therefore could only think it to be filled with ideas. He tries to find his bearings within the manifoldness of the plant's being and arrives at his sensible-supersensible archetypal plant," wrote Steiner in *Goethe's World View*. Understanding the archetypal or symbolic plant as a time sequence brings one closer to its true being, explains Richard Katz, who applies the Goethean approach in his flower essence research. "When you watch a plant unfold during the growing season, then you begin to live in the time fabric of the plant, which is its etheric domain, and this reveals its essence."

Third, patients and physicians appreciate the source of their remedies in a revitalized Nature.

Let's say for example that our awakened interest in empiric medicine and the etheric life force it mediates takes us into herbalism, the use of prepared plant extracts for medicinal purposes. Herbalism has environmental, even planetary ramifications because as the planet's original pharmacopoeia, herbalism depends on the world's plant kingdom as its source of medicines.

When they contemplate the planet's vast botanical germplasm economic botanists like James Duke, formerly of the U.S. Department of Agriculture, speak of "promising phytomedicinals." These are undiscovered and unexploited plant extracts that could hold stunning remedial, even curative, properties for many of humanity's medical problems. For example, only about 10% (or 27,000) of world plant species have been used in traditional medicines so far, so it's vital for the future of pharmacognosy (drug development from plants), botanists like Duke contend, to keep studying the world's plant genetic resources for new herbal medicines. There is one obstacle in this approach giving the project urgency: traditional human cultures (indigenous tribal people) and their medicinal folkways are rapidly vanishing, along with their homes, the tropical rainforests with their prodigious plant and animal resources.

Understandably, ethnobotanists have been calling for the preservation of the rainforests as a valuable phytomedicinal resource for years. "Somewhere in the tropics there are probably compounds that will alleviate or correct every ailment known to mankind," says Duke. "Once we have investigated and analysed the tropical species as intensively as temperate species, I predict we'll find many more important medicinal species in the tropics. Already there are hundreds of well-known biologically active compounds from the thousands of tropical species that are used as folk or proven medicines." If Duke has a slogan, it's "Save the rainforest, it might save us," because the more plant species still extant and unexploited, the greater the chance of finding new medicines.

As viewers of the film *Medicine Man* well know, the search for promising phytomedicinals in the biotically rich rainforests is literally a race against the bulldozers and chainsaws. As a reclusive pharmacognosist in the movie, Sean Connery rushed to identify a remarkable antitumor agent produced through the interaction of ants with a flower found at the top of a rare tree before the living laboratory was slashed and burned before his eyes. Unfortunately, the argument that rainforests must be preserved for exploitation of their undiscovered medicinal plants is often more abstract than economically persuasive, whether it's the local farmers or the big bosses of development. However, recent good news from a demonstration study in Belize indicates it is demonstrably more profitable to farm the rainforest for phytomedicinals than for agriculture or timber.

Researchers from Yale University and the New York Botanical Garden demonstrated that Belize farmers harvesting medicinal plants from one acre as part of a sustainable yearly cycle involving 30 acres, could reap from $294 to $1346 in income, compared to $137/acre in Brazil and $117/acre in Guatemala for agricultural clearing; even the highest paying pine plantation in the tropics only nets $1289/acre. "We wanted to identify what is valuable to the small farmer today because he decides whether to cut his piece of the forest to feed his family or to use it in another way to derive income," noted Dr. Michael Balick, one of the project's directors. "If it is a good business," comments Hugh Iltis, botanist at the University of Wisconsin, "people will eventually try to plant pure populations of what they are selling, and you would end up with a drug garden."

Here we see a direct connection between our choice of medical paradigm and practical steps towards the resolution of grievous world environmental problems, in this case rainforest destruction. This is the way the world market works: if as Americans we wish to save the rainforests for their phytomedicinal treasures one of the most powerful things we can do is to support American herbalism on all fronts—research, development, legalization, licensing, therapeutic applications, popularization—because this demand for herbs will become a major driving force that ultimately persuades the individual Costa Rican farmer that it's worthwhile to keep his acreage in plants instead of a cattle feedlot.

This of course is what the UN's World Health Organization (WHO) has been advocating in international resolutions for almost two decades—"Save plants that save lives," which means saving their environments, too. WHO encourages Third World governments to inventory, study, and preserve their indigenous phytomedicinals and herbal medical folkways as well. "Making full and proper use of their traditional systems of medicine represents an important step for countries that are attempting to improve the health of their peoples," noted Olayiwola Akerle, M.D., WHO's traditional medicine program manager.

Fourth, as we work closely with the plant kingdom and its etheric forces, this translates into a search for more environment-friendly methods of agriculture such as biodynamics.

In developing his principles of anthroposophical medicine Rudolf Steiner emphasized the importance of M.D.s working directly with the forces and plants of nature that formed the pharmacopoeia. He also outlined the necessity of instituting a profounder approach to food production and agriculture, a system he called biodynamics.

Anthroposophic medicine is a multileveled science of holism encompassing clinic and garden, observes Gerald Karnow, M.D., practicing physician at the Fellowship Community, an innovative, Steiner-based, elderly-care facility in Spring Valley, New York. "We work towards recognizing a lawful relationship between processes in the human and nature." The anthroposophic physician must *know* one's remedies inside out—literally, how they grow in the garden as a basis for understanding how they might work in the human organism. It sounds strange at first, but anthroposophic doctors learn that the garden is in the human.

This means in order to prescribe, for example, *Equisetum* (horsetail) for a kidney dysfunction, you must understand the living process of horsetail and its dynamic relation with the human kidney and its life and illness process. A materialist understanding of pharmaceuticals simply doesn't work here. "You're seeing an aspect of the person as a dynamic plant activity. The etheric body is the plant world in us as a process. So as physicians we need to know the life dynamics of nature."

That's why Karnow spends a lot of time in Fellowship's extensive gardens. It's a little like living in a large drugstore to get familiar with the medicines; in this case the botanical kingdom is the pharmacy. So if the plant world is your environmental pharmacy, then as a prudent physician-gardener, you take measures to maximize the etheric vitality of the botanicals you grow. Life forces in the "outer" environment are potentiated to effect healing in the life force body in the "inner" environment of the human. This is the basis of yet another Steiner innovation called biodynamic agriculture.

Many people in fact first hear about Anthroposophy through biodynamics, Steiner's brilliant contribution to gardening and farming, which he first formulated in 1924. Steiner emphasized many of the points now commonly associated with organic gardening: the crucial importance of living, healthy soil, the use of natural compost and humus, crop diversity and rotation, companion planting of herbs and flowers with vegetables, the abstention from chemical fertilizers and sprays. Biodynamics recognizes the farm as a living organism, as a complete individuality of crops, land, animals, and farmers. But Steiner went still further, illuminating the scope of agriculture from a "supersensible" viewpoint just as he sought to leaven the practice of medicine.

"You are seeking the spirit in nature," he told his agricultural audience in Koberwitz, Germany, in 1924. The biodynamic approach seeks to harmonize cosmic, telluric, and spiritual influences—Steiner called them all "formative forces"—on the activities of soil and plant. Biodynamics enhances the well-being of the planet, through working appropriately with the energies of Nature, and the human, through the production of foods rich in life-force. In this way biodynamics is a fundamental support for spiritual unfolding. "So long as one feeds on food from unhealthy soil," Steiner observed, "the spirit will lack the stamina to free itself from the prison of the body."

Inversely, working with the spirit in nature will yield a sustainable, ecological agriculture, capable of supporting the earth, its farmers, and consumers. It's a message gradually catching on where between Germany and Holland alone there are 1090 commercial biodynamic farms comprising 43,511 acres (1989 figures); considerable interest in biodynamic practices also has been shown in Australia. As Herbert Koepf, head of the School of Biodynamics and Earth Sciences at Emerson College in England, puts it: "Its general application creates a form of agriculture that truly serves earth and humanity."

Fifth, the inextricable interdependency of bodily and ecological environments irresistibly impels us to protect, preserve, and nurture both.

As we understand, directly in our bodies and lives, the living relationships between personal health and global environment, we are irresistibly moved to protect both. Our empiric tutorial has forged a dynamic new body politic, a co-creative response to environment at all levels of expression because we know that wherever we look, what we see is part of us. Through direct experience and heightened cognition we have become environmentally politicized.

Our political attitudes have been changed *from within*, based the hallmarks of the empiric tradition, experience and insight—from "enlivened thinking" and "etheric cognition," if you will—which now form the basis of an unshakeable conviction of the wholeness of life. We know that we can co-create a healthy, supportive environment at any level. As with our first point above, this idea is best presented as an anecdote.

A few years ago I visited Mt. Shasta in northern California during the first week of January. I went to this snowbound logging town, dominated by a 14,000 foot twin-peaked old volcano and New Age millennialist prophecy, for the purposes of tuning into the Epiphany celebration through this renowned planetary nodal point. Traditionally, Epiphany, a spiritual festival older than Christmas, marks the time when the Christ manifested before the Three Magi; esoterically, it marks the moment when the Christ incarnated into Master Jesus at age 30, thus being truly born on earth. So I thought if I tramped around Shasta's snowfields in a meditative frame of mind, I might have a vision of how to relate to the question mark of the new decade and its demands. I vividly remember my first impressions . . . .

It's predawn as I arrive at Bunny Flat Meadows at 6900 feet and 9 miles up the mountain access road. I park my car, strap on the snowshoes, and set off slowly more or less on top of the thick snow. I feel the raw sheer spiritual presence of Mt. Shasta: it's not just a big mountain, it's a big, alarming presence. The mountain is absolutely veiled in mist and I can't see more than fifty feet ahead of me. Apparently there's nobody else up here this morning, so I have Shasta's invisibility—and the blowing wind and drizzle—to myself. I find a ledge and sit down on my snowshoes for meditation. I visualize a single pinpoint of blazing light at my midpoint, visualize Mt. Shasta as a radiant node on the bluewhite globe of Gaia, and "put" both inside my star for incubation.

Here my environmental relations get turned inside out. I am on the outside and the world is on the inside. Momentarily I assume the position of spiritual mother to planet Gaia. I breathe as Love from Above to this image of Mt. Shasta as an aperture on Gaia with both enwombed within the star inside me. You're safe and loved, I tell Her, as we await the coming of the Light. With this gesture my relationship to the mountain and its awesome numinosity is reversed. It's not Mt. Shasta's sheer presence that is intimidating; it is my presence—the Buddha Nature in me that is terrifying.

Time passes, dawn arrives, then I'm treated to a morning glory. In a single moment the clouds blow away from the topmost snowpeaks and a magnificently pristine Shasta is revealed, lit by the morning sun and towering over the weaving mists. How astonishingly beautiful you've become, how celestial your snowy crags appear, how unaccountably newborn you seem, I say to the mountain, as if Shasta were a bride prepared for a June wedding. Now I understand that elegant phrase by Henri Corbin, "spiritual body, celestial earth."

As the wind gradually unwraps all of Mt. Shasta, I catch myself for an instant as I realize I'm talking out loud to a mountain—or am I? "This Tathagata is the Miracle Body, the Dharma Body, and so forth," declared the great Japanese Zen Master Bassui, that 14th century ontological terror of all aspiring Zen students. "The Buddha body fills the Dharma worlds, appearing before all people everywhere. This Buddha body is unchanging truth, clear and wonderful. It is the original mind of everyone. Simply stop thoughts which seek this mind elsewhere, return to yourself and look directly, and you will see the Tathagata. Look! Look! Who is this master that is seeing and hearing right now?"

References

Aïvanhov, Omraam Mikhaël, *Man's Subtle Bodies and Centres*, Editions Prosveta, Frejus Cedex (France), 1987.

Artley, Malvin N., Jr., *Bodies of Fire: A Thousand Points of Light*, University of Seven Rays Publishing House, Jersey City Heights, 1992.

Avalon, Arthur, *The Serpent Power: The Secrets of Tantric and Shaktic Yoga*, Dover Publications, New York, 1974.

Bailey, Alice, *Esoteric Healing, Vol. IV, A Treatise on the Seven Rays*, Lucis Publishing Company, New York, 1953.

Begich, Nick, and Manning, Jeane, *Angels Don't Play This Haarp: Advances in Tesla Technology*, Earthpulse Press, Anchorage, 1995.

Bennett, J.G., *Gurdjieff: Making a New World*, Turnstone Books, London, 1973.

Besant, Annie, *Man and His Bodies*, Theosophical Manual No. VII, Theosophical Publishing House, Adyar, India, 1912.

Bohm, Werner, *Chakras—Roots of Power*, Samuel Weiser, York Beach, 1991.

Breaux, Charles, *Journey into Consciousness, The Chakras, Tantra, and Jungian Psychology,* Nicholas-Hays, York Beach, 1989.

Buckland, Raymond, *Cardinal's Sin,* Llewellyn Publications, St. Paul, 1996.

Caine, Mary, *The Glastonbury Zodiac,* Grael Communications, Torquay, 1978.

Castro, Janice, "Condition: Critical," *Time,* (November 25, 1991).

Coon, Robert, *Elliptical Navigations Through the Multitudinous Aethyrs of Avalon,* Excalibur Press, Street, 1984.

Clow, Barbara Hand, *The Pleiadian Agenda: A New Cosmology for the Age of Light,* Bear and Company, Santa Fe, 1995.

Coleman, Dr. John, *The Conspirators' Hierarchy: The Committee of 300,* Second Edition, Joseph Publishing Company, Carson City, 1992.

Cooper, Milton William, *Behold a Pale Horse,* Light Technology Publishing, Sedona, 1991.

Critser, Greg, "Oh, How Happy We Will Be, Pills, Paradise, and the Profits of the Drug Companies," *Harper's Magazine,* (June 1996).

Deacon, Richard, *John Dee: Scientist, Geographer, Astrologer and Secret Agent to Elizabeth I,* Muller, London, 1968.

Epperson, A. Ralph, *The Unseen Hand: An Introduction to the Conspiratorial View of History,* Publius Press, Tucson, 1985.

Faltermayer, Edmund, "Let's Really Cure the Health System," *Fortune,* (March 23, 1992).

Fortune, Dion, *The Secrets of Doctor Taverner,* The Aquarian Press/Thorsons, Wellingborough (UK), 1989.

—*Moon Magic,* The Aquarian Press/Thorsons, Wellingborough (UK), 1989.

Freudenheim, Milt, "Drugs Cost Less in Canada Than in U.S., Study Finds," *The New York Times,* (October 22, 1992).

—"Canadians See Rise in Drug Costs," *The New York Times,* (November 16, 1992).

—"Two Large Drug Makers in Profit Rise," *The New York Times,* (October 16, 1992).

—"The Unquiet Future of Commercial Health Insurance," *The New York Times,* (July 12, 1992).

—"Health Care a Growing Burden," *The New York Times,* (January 29, 1991).

Griffin, G. Edward, *World Without Cancer: The Story of Vitamin B17.* American Media, Westlake Village, CA, 1974.

Govinda, Lama Anagarika, *Foundations of Tibetan Mysticism,* Samuel Weiser, York Beach, 1969.

Harrison, C.G., *The Transcendental Universe,* Lindisfarne Press, Hudson, 1993.

Hayschka, Rudolf, *The Nature of Substance,* Rudolf Steiner Press, London, 1983.

Hills, Christopher, "Is Kundalini Real?" in *Kundalini. Evolution and Enlightenment,* edited by John White, Paragon House, New York, 1990.

Johnson, Dirk, "Good People Go Bad in Iowa, and a Drug is Being Blamed," *The New York Times,* (February 22, 1996).

Karagulla, Shafica, M.D., and Kunz, Dora van Gelder, *The Chakras and the Human Energy Fields,* Quest/Theosophical Publishing House, Wheaton, 1989.

Kühlewind, Georg, *Becoming Aware of the Logos,* Inner Traditions/ Lindisfarne Press, West Stockbridge, MA, 1985.

James, Caryn, "TV Nourishes the Appetite of Conspiracy Enthusiasts," *The New York Times,* (February 26, 1996).

Leadbeater, C.W., *The Chakras. A Monograph,* The Theosophical Publishing House, Adyar (India), 1969.

Leary, Warren E., "Researchers Closing in on a Single-Dose Vaccine for Children," *The New York Times,* (March 29, 1994).

Leviton, Richard, "The ABCs of Movement," *Yoga Journal,* (July/August, 1993).

—"Landscape Mysteries and Healing Gaia—A Precis of Spiritual Geomancy," *West Coast Astrologer-Geomancer,* No. 3, (April-May 1992).

—"Ley Lines and The Meaning of Adam," in *Anti-Gravity and the World Grid,* edited by David Hatcher Childress, Adventures Unlimited Press, Stelle, 1987.

—"Walking in Albion: Chronicles of Plan-Net Geomancy, Part 1: Child of the Ancient Giant," *The Quest,* (Spring 1992).

—"Walking in Albion: Chronicles of Plan-Net Geomancy, Part II: Child of the Maturing Eagle," *The Quest,* (Summer 1992).

—"Zodiacal Circles of Light," *Timetrack*, No. 4, (June-July 1992).

—*A Primer on Landscape Zodiacs and the Discipline of Spiritual Geomancy*, Blazing Star Enterprises, Goshen, MA, 1991.

—"A Tree of Life Grows at Eden: Celestial Memories in the Landscape in Western New York," *Network of Light*, Vol. 6, Issue 1, (April/May 1991).

Lifton, Robert Jay, *The Nazi Doctors, Medical Killing and the Psychology of Genocide*, Basic Books, New York, 1986.

Maltwood, Katherine, *A Guide to Glastonbury's Temple of the Stars*, James Clarke and Co., Cambridge, 1982.

—*The Enchantments of Britain*, James Clarke and Co., Cambridge, 1982.

Modi, Shauntala, M.D., *Remarkable Healings: A Psychiatrist Discovers Unsuspected Roots of Mental and Physical Illness*, Hampton Roads, Charlottesville, VA, 1997.

Monroe, Robert A., *Journeys Out of the Body*, Anchor Press/Doubleday, Garden City, NY, 1977.

—*Far Journeys*, Doubleday and Company, Garden City, NY, 1985.

Myerson, Allen R., "America's Quiet Rebellion Against McDonaldization," *The New York Times*, (July 28, 1996).

Murphy, Michael, *Jacob Atabet*, Jeremey P. Tarcher, Los Angeles, 1977.

Pear, Robert, "Cost of Health Care is Increasing More Slowly, Report Says," *The New York Times*, (May 28, 1996).

Perrin, Stuart, *Leah. A Story of Meditation and Healing*, Wisdom Publications, Newburyport, 1988.

Preston, Richard, *The Hot Zone*, Random House, New York, 1994.

Ravenscroft, Trevor, *The Spear of Destiny: The Occult Power Behind the Spear Which Pierced the Side of Christ*, Samuel Weiser, York Beach, 1982.

Sardello, Robert, *Facing the World with Soul: The Reimagination of Modern Life*, Lindisfarne Press, Hudson, 1992.

Scharff, Paul, M.D., *Agriculture*, Fellowship Community, Spring Valley, unpublished manuscript, 1992.

—"Elemental Beings in Nature, in the Hierarchies, with Man,

and the Social Domain," unpublished lecture, Spring Valley, September 5, 1995.

Scott, Mary, *Kundalini in the Physical World*, Arkana/Penguin, New York, 1983.

Slouka, Mark, *War of the Worlds, Cyberspace and the High-Tech Assault on Reality*, Basic Books, New York, 1995.

Steiner, Rudolf, *An Introduction to Eurythmy*, Anthroposophic Press, Hudson, 1984.

—*An Occult Physiology*, Rudolf Steiner Press, London, 1951.

—*Cosmosophy, Vol. I*, Anthroposophic Press, Spring Valley, 1985.

—*Eurythmy as Visible Speech*, Rudolf Steiner Press, London, 1984.

—*Knowledge of the Higher Worlds and Its Attainment*, Anthroposophic Press, Spring Valley, 1947.

—*Philosophy, Cosmology, and Religion*, Anthroposophic Press, Spring Valley, 1984.

—*The Alphabet*, Mercury Press, Spring Valley, 1982.

—*The Inner Nature of Music and the Experience of Tone*, Anthroposophic Press, Hudson, 1983.

—*The Occult Movement in the Nineteenth Century*, Rudolf Steiner Press, London, 1973.

—*The Fall of the Spirits of Darkness*, Rudolf Steiner Press, Bristol, 1993.

Tansley, David V., *Subtle Body: Essence and Shadow*, Thames and Hudson, London, 1977.

Thompson, William Irwin, *The American Replacement of Nature: The Outrageous Evolution of Economic Life*, Doubleday, New York, 1991.

Travis, John, "Biological Warfare," *Science News*, Vol. 149, (June 1, 1996).

—"Swallowing Shigella," *Science News*, Vol. 149, (May 11, 1996).

Wachsmuth, Guenther, *The Etheric Formative Forces in Cosmos, Earth and Man*, Anthroposophic Press, New York, 1932.

Waldholz, Michael, "Strong Medicine: New Drug 'Cocktails' Mark Exciting Turn in the War on AIDS," *The Wall Street Journal*, (June 14, 1996).

Waters, Frank, *Mountain Dialogues*, Sage Books, Swallow Press, University of Ohio, Athens, Ohio, 1981.

Index

Index

Index

Hampton Roads Publishing Company

... for the evolving human spirit

Hampton Roads Publishing Company
publishes books on a variety of subjects including
metaphysics, health, complementary medicine,
visionary fiction, and other related topics.

For a copy of our latest catalog,
call toll-free, 800-766-8009,
or send your name and address to:

Hampton Roads Publishing Company, Inc.
1125 Stoney Ridge Road
Charlottesville, VA 22902
e-mail: hrpc@hrpub.com
www.hrpub.com